# NEUROIMAGING FOR CLINICIANS – COMBINING RESEARCH AND PRACTICE

Edited by **Julio F. P. Peres**

**Neuroimaging for Clinicians – Combining Research and Practice**
Edited by Julio F. P. Peres

**Published by InTech**
Janeza Trdine 9, 51000 Rijeka, Croatia



**Publishing Process Manager** Sandra Bakic

**Technical Editor** Teodora Smiljanic

**Cover Designer** InTech Design Team

Additional hard copies can be obtained from orders@intechopen.com

Neuroimaging for Clinicians – Combining Research and Practice, Edited by Julio F. P. Peres
p. cm.
ISBN 978-953-307-450-4

For EU product safety concerns:
IN TECH d.o.o., Prolaz Marije Krucifikse Kozulić 3, 51000 Rijeka, Croatia,
info@intechopen.com or visit our website at intechopen.com.

# Meet the editor

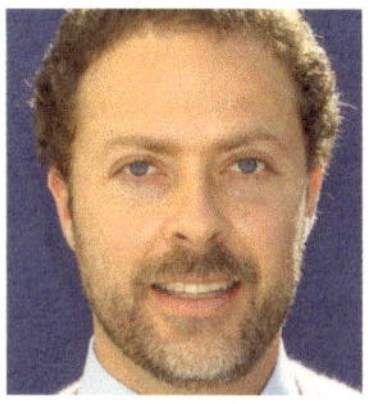

Julio Fernando Prieto Peres is a neuroscientist and a psychologist with twenty years of clinical experience. As a clinician-researcher, he combines psychology with neuroscience and develops his interest in the neurobiological consequences of psychotherapy, having used functional neuroimaging to show the cerebral effects of subjective processing mediated by psychotherapy as part of his doctorate and two postdoctoral programs. Julio earned a PhD in Neuroscience and Behavior from the Institute of Psychology at Universidade de São Paulo, and post-doctorates in Diagnostic Imaging from the University of Pennsylvania and Escola Paulista de Medicina, Universidade Federal de São Paulo (UNIFESP). His published work includes papers on psychotherapy, resilience, coping, and functional neuroimaging. In addition to his research at the Institute of Psychiatry at Universidade de São Paulo, he is the professor in charge of Clinical Psychotraumatology training for doctors and psychologists at Hospital Pérola Byington. Author of the book Trauma e Superação [Trauma and Coping] published in Brazil by Roca.

# Contents

**Preface XI**

**Part 1 Amnestic Disorders 1**

Chapter 1 **Neuroimaging in Dementia and Other Amnestic Disorders 3**
Leonardo Caixeta, Bruno Galafassi Ghini and Julio F. P. Peres, PsyD, PhD.

Chapter 2 **Degeneration of the Human Nervous System and Magnetic Resonance Neuroimaging 15**
Lulé Dorothée and Ludolph Albert Christian

Chapter 3 **Early Detection of Alzheimer's Disease with Cognitive Neuroscience Methods 37**
Jinglong Wu, Chunlin Li and Jiajia Yang

Chapter 4 **Staining of Amyloid Beta (Abeta) Using (Immuno) Histochemical Techniques and Abeta42 Specific Peptides 59**
Thomas van Groen, Inga Kadish, Aileen Funke and Dieter Willbold

**Part 2 Sexual Disorders 71**

Chapter 5 **Magnetic Resonance Techniques in Study of Sexual Stimuli Processing in Paedophilia 73**
Juan Antonio Becerra-García

**Part 3 Systems & Networks 87**

Chapter 6 **Functional Anatomy, Physiology and Clinical Aspects of Basal Ganglia 89**
Edward Jacek Gorzelańczyk

Chapter 7 **Cognitive Integration in the Human Primary Sensory and Motor Areas: An Overview 107**
Jozina B. De Graaf and Mireille Bonnard

Chapter 8 **Ciliopathies: Primary Cilia and Signaling Pathways in Mammalian Development 125**
Carmen Carrascosa Romero, José Luis Guerrero Solano and Carlos De Cabo De La Vega

Chapter 9 **Review of Printed and Electronic Stereotactic Atlases of the Human Brain 145**
Eduardo Joaquim Lopes Alho, Lea Grinberg, Helmut Heinsen and Erich Talamoni Fonoff

**Part 4 Procedures & Neuroscience 173**

Chapter 10 **Intracranial Arterial Collateralization: Relevance in Neuro-Endovascular Procedures 175**
Peng R. Chen, Adnan H. Siddiqui and Peng Roc Chen

Chapter 11 **Haemolytic-Uraemic Syndrome: Neurologic Symptoms, Neuroimaging and Neurocognitive Outcome 203**
Ana Roche Martínez, Pilar Póo Argüelles, Marta Maristany Cucurella, Antonio Jiménez Llort, Juan A Camacho and Jaume Campistol Plana

Chapter 12 **Clinical and Genetic Aspects in Patients with Idiopathic Parkinson Disease 219**
Arben Taravari, Marija Milanovska, Igor Petrov, Vera Petrova, Merita Ismajli-Marku, Besim Memedi, Fadil Cana and Fatmir Mexhiti

Chapter 13 **New Insights for a Better Understanding of the Pusher Behavior: From Clinical to Neuroimaging Features 239**
Taiza E.G. Santos-Pontelli, Octavio M. Pontes-Neto and Joao P. Leite

Chapter 14 **Neurosonological Evaluation of the Acute Stroke Patients 259**
Giovanni Malferrari and Marialuisa Zedde

Chapter 15 **Is There a Place for Clinical Neurophysiology Assessments in Synucleinopathies? 299**
M. Onofrj, L. Bonanni, A. Thomas, L. Ricciardi, F. Ciccocioppo, D. Monaco V. Onofrj and F. Anzellotti

Chapter 16 **How fMRI Technology Contributes to the Advancement of Research in Mental Imagery: A Review 329**
Marta Olivetti Belardinelli, Massimiliano Palmiero and Rosalia Di Matteo

**Part 5 Post Traumatic Stress Disorder 347**

Chapter 17 **Stress Shaping Brains: Higher Order DNA/Chromosome Mechanisms Underlying Epigenetic Programming of the Brain Transcriptome 349**
George S. Gericke

Chapter 18 **Abnormal Brain Density in Victims of Rape with PTSD in Mainland China: A Voxel-Based Analysis of Magnetic Resonance Imaging Study 375**
Shuang Ge Sui, Ling Jiang Li, Yan Zhang, Ming Xiang Wu and Mark E. King

Chapter 19 **PTSD, Neuroimaging and Psychotherapy: A Fruitful Encounter 395**
Julio F.P. Peres, PsyD, PhD.

# Preface

Researchers and practitioners successfully joining forces to integrate science with practice while enhancing patient care and treatment.

What could be more fascinating than exploring the mind and human behavior? Neuroscience is one of the fastest-evolving areas in healthcare, in particular neuroimaging. There has been an exponential surge in the number of neuroimaging publications addressing common health conditions as researchers increasingly report valuable findings that enable new and effective interventions. Alongside this growing literature, the scope and diversity of research is broadening in terms of both scientific focus and methods.

In many cases, clinical practice has been quick to absorb imaging techniques. However, in several countries the prevailing trend among those who support healthcare and science does tend to widen the gap between researchers and clinicians. Practitioners are not usually involved in research, and vice versa, which detracts from the potential for synergy and more efficacious contributions, despite both groups being ultimately complementary and interdependent. Modern neuroimaging offers tremendous opportunities for gaining fresh insights, with key developments that will almost certainly lead directly to clinical applications. Therefore, it was only a matter of time before a new neuroimaging book such as this one would gather the latest clinical and research work for their mutual benefit.

*Neuroimaging for clinicians* sourced 19 chapters from some of the world's top brain-imaging researchers and clinicians to provide a timely review of the state of the art in neuroimaging, covering radiology, neurology, psychiatry, psychology, and geriatrics. Contributors from China, Brazil, France, Germany, Italy, Japan, Macedonia, Poland, Spain, South Africa, and the United States of America have collaborated enthusiastically and efficiently to create this reader-friendly but comprehensive work covering the diagnosis, pathophysiology, and effective treatment of several common health conditions, with many explanatory figures, tables and boxes to enhance legibility and make the book clinically useful.

Countless hours have gone into writing these chapters, and our profound appreciation is in order for their consistent advice on the use of neuroimaging in diagnostic work-ups for conditions such as acute stroke, cell biology, ciliopathies, cognitive integration, dementia and other amnestic disorders, haemolytic-uraemic syndrome, mental imagery, sexual disorders, spondylotic myelopathy, Parkinson's disease, and post traumatic stress disorder. All of the latter have been situated within a conceptual framework that highlights relations between the biological, psychological, and environmental levels of analysis.

I would also like to apologize to readers who may feel that their particular area of interest has been overlooked, perhaps inevitably so, given the wide range of ongoing work.

Finally, *Neuroimaging for clinicians* is highly recommended for both clinicians and researchers and it is a must-read for specialists in neurology, geriatrics, psychiatry, and psychology, who need a means of integrating neuroscience with their everyday practice of managing patients. We hope this will enable researchers and practitioners to work together and integrate science with practice. For the sake of our patients, we hope this book helps detect and treat illness and life-threatening conditions to provide much-needed relief.

**Julio F.P. Peres, PsyD, PhD.**
Radiology Clinic – Universidade Federal de São Paulo, SP,
Psychotraumatology Clinic - Hospital Perola Byington, SP,
Brazil

# Part 1

## Amnestic Disorders

# 1

# Neuroimaging in Dementia and Other Amnestic Disorders

Leonardo Caixeta[1], Bruno Galafassi Ghini[2] and Julio F. P. Peres, PsyD, PhD.[3,4]
[1]*Psychiatric Cognitive Unit of the Hospital das Clínicas of the Federal University of Goiás,*
[2]*Centro de Diagnóstico por Imagem, Goiânia-GO,*
[3]*Radiology Clinic – Universidade Federal de São Paulo, SP,*
[4]*Psychotraumatology Clinic - Hospital Perola Byington, SP,*
*Brazil*

## 1. Introduction

Neuroimaging has revolutionized the field of cognitive neuroscience. Early studies of brain-behavior relationships relied on a precise neurological examination as the basis for hypothesizing the site of brain damage that was responsible for a given behavioral syndrome. Episodic amnesia, for example, clearly implicated the hippocampus as the site of recent memory abilities.

Clinicopathological correlations were the earliest means of obtaining precise data on the site of damage causing a specific neurobehavioral syndrome (D'Esposito & Wills, 2000). In 1861, Paul Broca's observations of nonfluent aphasia in the setting of left inferior frontal gyrus damage cemented the belief that this brain region was critical for speech output (Broca, 1861). The advent of structural brain imaging more than 100 years after Broca's observations, first with computed tomography (CT) and later with magnetic resonance imaging (MRI), paved the way for more precise anatomical localization of the cognitive deficits that are manifest after brain injury.

Anatomical analyses of Broca's aphasia using structural neuroimaging (Naeser et al., 1989, Dronkers, 1996, Alexander et al., 1990) have more precisely determined that damage restricted to the inferior frontal gyrus causes only a transient aphasia, with recovery within weeks to months. Instead, damage to deep white matter and insular cortex causes persistent nonfluency. Noninvasive, structural neuroimaging provides the remarkable power to detail anatomical pathology in every stroke patient without re-lying upon the infrequently obtained autopsy.

Neuroimaging is a powerful tool for creative exploration of the epidemiology, diagnostic sensitivity, progression and therapeutic efficacy in many brain diseases featured by memory impairment (Apostolova & Thompson, 2008). Some consider modern functional neuroimaging methods as useful tools to establish similarities and differences between different forms of amnesias with respect to their brain correlates, while others consider them adequate for constituting groups of patients in a research perspective, but still out of reach for the practitioner (Celsis, 2000).

## 2. Neuroimaging techniques

Functional neuroimaging, broadly defined as techniques that provide measures of brain activity, has further increased our ability to study the neural basis of cognition and behavior. Functional neuroimaging dates back to the use of electrophysiological methods such as electroencephalography (EEG). However, the lack of spatial resolution in these methods (i.e., often limited to hemispheric or anterior-posterior differences) did not allow testing hypotheses regarding the precise anatomical location of a brain region subserving a given cognitive process (D'Esposito & Wills, 2000, Galin & Ornstein, 1972).

The modern era of functional brain imaging, bringing markedly improved spatial resolution, was introduced first in the mid-1970s using the xenon cerebral blood flow technique and later in the mid-1980s using positron emission tomography (Mazziotta & Phelps, 1984, Petersen et al., 1988). In more recent years, functional magnetic resonance imaging (fMRI) has rapidly emerged as an extremely powerful technique with many advantages over positron emission tomography (PET) for studying cognition.

In dementia evaluation, the most commonly used tracers are 99mTc-HMPAO for SPECT brain perfusion and 18F-FDG for PET glucose's metabolism. For practical purposes, the clinical analysis of brain perfusion and glucose metabolism are equivalent, so that hypoperfusion areas in brain SPECT roughly correspond to glucolytic hypometabolism in PET.

The different syndromes and diseases presenting with dementia have different patterns of brain perfusion abnormalities, so we can distinguish them with good specificity.

## 3. Normal aging

Brain aging is characterized by numerous physiological, structural, functional, and neurocognitive changes. The interplay of these various processes is complex and characterized by large interindividual differences. The level of cognitive functioning achieved by a group of elderly is largely determined by the health of individuals within this group (Aine et al., 2011). Individuals with a history of hypertension, for example, are likely to have multiple white matter insults which compromise cognitive functioning, independent of aging processes. The health of the elderly group has not been well-documented in most previous studies and elderly participants are rarely excluded, or placed into a separate group, due to health-related problems (Caserta et al., 2009). In addition, recent results show that white matter tracts within the frontal and temporal lobes, regions critical for higher cognitive functions, continue to mature well into the 4th decade of life (Aine et al., 2011). This suggests that a young age group may not be the best control group for understanding aging effects on the brain since development is ongoing within this age range.

Functional neuroimaging studies of cognitively intact older adults have consistently shown volume loss and loss of white matter structural integrity, particularly in prefrontal cortex, which may be associated with cognitive decline (Caserta et al., 2009). For instance, age-related deficits in working memory (WM) and episodic memory abilities are related to changes in prefrontal cortex (PFC) function. Reviews of these neuroimaging studies have generally concluded that with age there is a reduction in the hemispheric specialization of cognitive function in the frontal lobes that may either be due to dedifferentiation of function, deficits in function and/or functional reorganization and compensation. While data are incomplete, another consistent finding has been a decline in other cognitive domains, such as arithmetic/numerical ability and perceptual speed. Alternatively, other cognitive functions such as verbal ability, word knowledge, and semantic memory remain quite preserved even to old age (Caserta et al., 2009).

Some functional neuroimaging studies on normal aging showed the involvement of different patterns of activation in comparison with control populations, such as increased frontal activity. These differences have been interpreted as reflecting the implementation of compensatory processes (Kalpouzos et al., 2008). Some authors (Rajah & D'Esposito, 2005) argue that in normal ageing distinct PFC regions exhibit different patterns of functional change, suggesting that age-related changes in PFC function are not homogeneous in nature. Specifically, these authors hypothesize that normal ageing is related to the differentiation of cortical function in a bilateral ventral PFC and deficits in function in right dorsal and anterior PFC (Rajah & D'Esposito, 2005). As a result of these changes, functional compensation in left dorsal and anterior PFC may occur.

Factors identified for healthy cognitive (brain) aging are multifactorial, and likely incorporate biological systems as well as cognitive reserve (i.e. the capability of an individual to cope with a task in order to optimize his/her performance by the recruitment of different neural networks and/or by using alternative cognitive strategies).

## 4. Mild cognitive impairment (MCI)

Mild cognitive impairment (MCI), a transitional state between normal aging and dementia, carries a four- to sixfold increased risk of future diagnosis of dementia (Caixeta, 2006). As complete drug-induced reversal of AD symptoms seems unlikely, researchers are now focusing on the earliest stages of AD where a therapeutic intervention is likely to realize the greatest impact. Recently neuroimaging has received significant scientific consideration as a promising in vivo disease-tracking modality that can also provide potential surrogate biomarkers for therapeutic trials (Apostolova & Thompson, 2008).

Evidence to date indicates that functional brain decline precedes structural decline in prodromal dementia, including adults with MCI (Jak et al., 2009). Therefore, functional neuroimaging techniques may offer the unique ability to detect early functional brain changes in at-risk adults and identify the neurophysiological markers that best predict dementia conversion.

While several volumetric techniques laid the foundation of the neuroimaging research in AD and MCI, more precise computational anatomy techniques have recently become available. This new technology detects and visualizes discrete changes in cortical and hippocampal integrity and tracks the spread of AD pathology throughout the living brain. Related methods can visualize regionally specific correlations between brain atrophy and important proxy measures of disease such as neuropsychological tests, age of onset or factors that may influence disease progression (Apostolova & Thompson, 2008).

Given that AD neuropathology preferentially targets the medial temporal lobe (MTL) early in the course of the disease, thereby resulting in the hallmark episodic memory decline, and amnestic MCI is thought to represent prodromal AD, the majority of fMRI studies of MCI involve memory processing (particularly encoding) in amnestic samples (Jak et al., 2009). No known fMRI studies have been published focusing on other clinical subtypes of MCI. While several studies demonstrate increased blood oxygen level dependent (BOLD) response in the MTL (Dickerson et al., 2004, Hamalainen et al., 2007; Kircher et al., 2007; Sperling, 2007), others report decreased MTL activity in MCI (Johnson et al., 2006; Mandzia et al., 2009). These discrepant findings have been interpreted as reflecting bimodal functional activity whereby less impaired MCI subjects show increased BOLD response in the hippocampus corresponding to a slight or moderate neuronal dysfunction, and more impaired MCI subjects demonstrate decreased BOLD response—similar to the levels observed in mild AD patients—as the cortical neuronal networks become more severely impaired with greater disease progression (Dickerson et al., 2004, Hamalainen et al., 2007; Johnson et al., 2006). However, this interpretation is primarily derived from cross-sectional studies and can only adequately be tested with longitudinal designs.

Few longitudinal fMRI studies of MCI have been reported. Although these studies are often limited by small sample sizes, they demonstrate promise for the use of fMRI to detect early AD. Those MCI patients who converted to AD showed a stronger relationship between brain activity in the left superior parietal lobe and the left precuneus during an angle discrimination task in the context of comparable performance (Vannini et al., 2007). Similarly, despite equivalent memory performance, Dickerson et al. (2004) reported that MCI patients who subsequently declined during a 2.5-year follow-up period demonstrated increased right parahippocampal gyrus activity during picture encoding. In a more recent study, the same research group reported increased hippocampal activation predicted greater degree and rate of cognitive decline during a 6-year follow-up period, even after controlling for baseline level of impairment (Miller et al., 2008).

Mandzia et al. (2009) reported that MTL activation during recognition was positively correlated with behavioral performance. However, unlike their healthy peers, MCI adults did not show a strong relationship between MTL activity during picture encoding and subsequent retrieval success, highlighting the complexity of the relationship between BOLD signal and effectiveness of encoding strategies. In contrast, Johnson et al. (2006) found reduced BOLD signal change in the right hippocampus during picture encoding and in the posterior cingulate during recognition of learned items in an amnestic MCI group despite comparable performance to their healthy peers. However, when activation corresponding only to successfully learned words was examined, an increase in hippocampal activity was seen, suggesting that an increase in MTL activity may support successful memory encoding (Kircher et al., 2007). Similarly, a positive correlation between extent of parahippocampal and hippocampal activation and memory performance was found in MCI but, in a paradoxical fashion, greater clinical impairment, was also associated with recruitment of a larger region of the right parahippocampal gyrus during encoding (Dickerson et al., 2004). Data from Johnson et al. (2004) provided further evidence for hippocampal dysfunction in MCI, suggesting that adults with MCI do not habituate to increasingly familiar items in the same manner as healthy older adults who show expected reductions in BOLD response to repeated items over time.

Despite the prevalence of studies examining medial temporal cortex function supporting memory, other cortical areas have also been implicated in MCI. For example, a reduction in functional activity in the posterior cingulate cortex (PCC) during recognition and episodic retrieval of previously learned line drawings (Johnson et al., 2006) and object working memory, but not during self-appraisal, has implicated this region in the memory retrieval difficulty seen in amnestic MCI. The degradation of PCC functioning in MCI is not surprising given that PET metabolic alterations in the temporoparietal cortices and in the posterior cingulate have been reported in MCI and AD as well as in nondemented young and middle-aged adults at genetic risk for AD (Jak et al., 2009). Similarly, dedifferentiation in the retrosplenial cortex during the retrieval of recent versus remote autobiographical memories and during episodic versus semantic memory retrieval has been reported in amnestic MCI, further implicating the medial posterior cortex in MCI (Jak et al., 2009). Additionally, the neural substrates of visual working memory, self-appraisal, and emotional working memory in MCI have also been examined, and generally implicate a greater number of cortical regions (Jak et al., 2009). However, results are varied and highlight the need for greater attention to other cognitive processes in MCI in order to more fully understand changes in cortical functioning that may signal impending cognitive decline.

## 5. Dementias

### 5.1 Alzheimer's disease

AD is the commonest form of dementia worldwide. It manifests with relentlessly progressive cognitive decline presenting initially as memory loss and then spreads to affect all other cognitive faculties and the patients' ability to conduct an independent lifestyle (Caixeta, 2006).
Post-mortem examination reveals abundant cortical and hippocampal neuritic plaques (NP) and neurofibrillary tangles (NFT) as well as pancerebellar atrophy upon gross inspection of the brain. The neuronal degeneration pattern in Alzheimer's disease (AD) spreads from the temporal mesial areas to the posterior regions of the cingulate cortex and then to the parietal lobes and the rest of the temporal lobes, asymmetrically or not. Pre-mortem, AD-associated brain changes can be clinically evaluated with the help of neuroimaging. They consist of global dysfunction with an early predilection for the hippocampal region and the temporo-parietal cortical areas (Caixeta, 2006). In advanced cases, the hypoperfusion pattern may reach the frontal lobes, but even in these cases the perfusion remains normal in thalamus, basal ganglia, motor cortex and occipital lobes.

Among patients presenting with bilateral parietotemporal hypoperfusion, 82% have AD, while the rest are due to Parkinson dementia or cerebrovascular disease. On the other hand, in patients with diagnosed AD, 100% have hypoconcentration of 18F-FDG and 90% have parietal and temporal hypoperfusion with 99mTc-HMPAO. These typical findings are also found among those with early AD, while hippocampal hypoperfusion as only finding has low specificity for AD diagnosis. In individuals with mild cognitive impairment, the posterior cingulate hypometabolism can predict who is going to develop AD. However, not all patients with AD have Bilateral parietotemporal hypoperfusion. In a study conducted by our group in 104 patients fulfilling NINCDS-ADRDA criteria for probable AD, bilateral parietotemporal hypoperfusion was more frequent in patients with severe AD, in those with early onset of the symptoms, and in men (Nitrini et al., 2000).

### 5.2 Lewy body dementia

The metabolic defects described in this disease are very close to those found in AD, but there is also hypoperfusion in the occipital lobes. One must have in mind that a patient with AD and cerebrovascular disease can mimic the LBD pattern, and it's not uncommon to find these pathologies at the same patient (Caixeta, 2006).

### 5.3 Vascular dementia

Arteriosclerotic brain disease presents as multiple focal areas of hypoperfusion randomly distributed in the cortex, also compromising subcortical structures. This particular pattern is never been observed in A.D., but the dual pathology is described as being present in 4 to 10% of patients. The differential diagnosis is AIDS dementia complex. When cerebrovascular disease is predominantly microangiopathic there is significantly more diffuse cortical hypoperfusion and ventricle enlargement (Caixeta, 2006).

### 5.4 Frontotemporal lobar degeneration

Patients with the different diseases in this group present severe bilateral hypoperfusion in the frontal lobes, predominantly in the mesial structures (Caixeta & Nitrini, 2001). There is also perfusion deficit in the anterior regions of the temporal lobes and each subtype has other characteristic findings, like asymmetrical parietal hypoperfusion in primary progressive aphasia.

Also depressive disorders and transient global amnesia can show prefrontal symmetric hypoperfusion, but there is unilateral basal ganglia hypoperfusion in the later, more commonly in the right. Also Huntington's disease can show bilateral frontotemporal hypoperfusion, but it presents later in the progression of the disease, while the first sign is severe bilateral basal ganglia hypoperfusion.

### 5.5 Dementia associated with parkinsonism

As described in Lewy body dementia, idiopathic Parkinson disease with dementia can show hypoperfusion patterns similar to those observed in AD, but basal ganglia hypoperfusion is far more frequent, as is frontal precentral hypoperfusion (Caixeta & Vieira, 2008).

Corticobasal degeneration presents as bilateral asymmetrical frontal, parietal and basal ganglia hypoperfusion. Supranuclear palsy also presents frontal hypoperfusion, predominantly in the mesial regions, but what specifically distinguishes this disease is symmetric severe basal ganglia hypoperfusion.

Multiple system atrophy has a very specific finding, which is cerebelar hypoperfusion, besides symmetric basal ganglia hypoperfusion.

Hippocampal hypoperfusion with bilateral frontal and parietal hypoperfusion is found in normal pressure hydrocephalus.

## 6. Other amnesic syndromes

### 6.1 Transient global amnesia

Almost 60 years after its initial description, transient global amnesia (TGA) remains one of the most enigmatic syndromes in clinical neurology.

Recent diffusion-weighted imaging (DWI) data suggest that a transient perturbation of hippocampal function is the functional correlate of TGA because focal diffusion lesions can be selectively detected in the CA1 field of the hippocampal cornu ammonis. The vulnerability of CA1 neurons to metabolic stress plays, therefore, a pivotal part in the pathophysiological cascade, leading to an impairment of hippocampal function during TGA (Bartsch et al., 2006, Bartsch & Deuschl, 2010). The maximum level of detection of these lesions is 24–72 h after onset of symptoms. Although the diagnosis of TGA is primarily a clinical one, neuroimaging in TGA can positively support the diagnosis.

Although various factors, such as migraine, focal ischemia, venous flow abnormalities, and epileptic phenomena, have been suggested to be involved in the pathophysiology of TGA, the factors triggering the emergence of these lesions are still elusive. (Bartsch & Deuschl, 2010).

To date, data from MRI has not found evidence for structural sequelae of these hippocampal lesions, and recent neuropsychological findings have also not found evidence for clinically relevant chronic neuropsychological deficits.

Quantitative imaging of changes of regional cerebral glucose, oxygen metabolism, or cerebrovascular blood flow in TGA have been studied by use of PET and single photon emission computed tomography (SPECT). In some studies, mesiotemporal flow changes have been described (Guillery et al., 2002, Eustache et al., 2000, Warren et al., 2000). However, most studies have also noted concomitant decreased or increased changes in cerebral blood flow in other anatomical structures, such as unilateral or bilateral thalamic, prefrontal, frontal, amygdalian, striatal, cerebellar, occipital, precentral, and postcentral areas (Nardone et al., 2004, Eustache et al., 2000). In some studies, either no mesiotemporal changes, no cerebral changes, or a global hypoperfusion were detected (Chung et al., 2009, Fujii et al., 1989). In summary, the imaging data derived from PET and SPECT studies are difficult to compare and interpret. Most changes normalised on follow-up examination. The variabilities in PET and SPECT are probably associated with differences in the study designs, such as the imaging protocol and resolution, and the latency of scanning, frequently done days or weeks after the acute TGA and thus not covering the initial pathophysiological event. A correlation between SPECT and MRI in the time window of 24–73 h after onset has been found in a study including only six patients. In five patients, a predominant hypoperfusion in the cerebellar vermis was observed in combination with punctuate DWI lesions in the hippocampus, whereas in another patient a bilateral hypoperfusion in the temporal lobes was detected by use of SPECT (Bartsch & Deuschl, 2010). Functional MRI was used in two patients during an acute TGA to assess memory function and cerebral activation patterns. In both patients, there was reduced or no activation in temporal lobe structures during encoding of visual scenes or recognition of old scenes, thus reflecting the functional impairment of temporal lobe structures (Bartsch & Deuschl, 2010).

Use of structural imaging with MRI has detected abnormalities in memory-relevant structures of the mesiotemporal region. Early results have been inconsistent and controversial about the type and location of signal abnormalities described in some patients (Matsui et al., 2002, Huber et al., 2002). Recent data from studies that used high-resolution MRI have shown that focal hyperintense lesions correlating to restricted diffusion in the lateral hippocampus can now be reliably detected (Bartsch et al., 2006, 2007). The detection rate of these lesions can be improved by up to 85% with optimised MRI parameters and by acknowledging the time course of the lesion.

### 6.2 Psychogenic amnesias

Commonly, memory disturbances are related to organic brain damage. Nevertheless, especially the old psychiatric literature provides numerous examples of patients with selective amnesia due to what at that time was preferentially named hysteria (Markowitsch, 2003) and which implied that both environmental circumstances and personality traits influence bodily and brain states to a considerable degree. Awareness of the existence of relations between cognition, soma, and psyche has increased especially in recent times and has created the research branch named cognitive neuropsychiatry. Within this branch, psychopathologic processes, deviating from normal information processing, are studied with a combination of methods derived from neurology, psychiatry, psychology, neurobiology, and neuroinformatics in order to provide a deeper understanding of psychic disease processes (Halligan & David, 2001).

Modern imaging methods have helped to establish similarities between organic and functional (psychogenic) amnesias with respect to their brain correlates. In fact, it was found that also environmental-related amnesias—caused by stress and trauma situations with which individuals cannot cope appropriately—may alter the brain's metabolism in a predictable way and that even therapy-induced reestablishments of memory may be related to gains in brain metabolism. These results support the view, according to Markowitsch (1996), that organic and functional amnesias are two sides of the same coin Markowitsch, 1996. H.J. Markowitsch, Organic and psychogenic retrograde amnesia: two sides of the same coin?. Neurocase (1996), pp. 357–371. Full Text via CrossRef | View Record in Scopus | Cited By in Scopus (69). According this author, both kinds of phenomena may derive from a common brain mechanism leading to blockade, disruption, or disconnection mechanisms affecting the processes of memory and disintegrating widespread memory networks in the brain. This disintegration may be a consequence of "mechanical alterations" in the brain of organic amnesics and may be a consequence of biochemical alterations in the brain of psychogenic amnesics. For these, such processes may be induced during autobiographical information processing by desynchronization memory patterns, resulting in the reduction of discomfort for the subject.
Functional amnesias and psychogenic amnesias are discussed and their symptomatology is compared to that of organic amnesias. The term "mnestic block syndrome" (Markowitsch, 2003) is introduced and defined as a syndrome of its own. Experimental data, obtained especially with functional imaging methods, are presented to elucidate changes in neural activation during functional amnesic states.
Functional amnesic states, confined to a patient's biography, can be triggered by environmentally induced stress and trauma, leading to lasting inability to retrieve autobiographical events. Such an impairment may be identified at the brain level using functional imaging techniques (Markowitsch, 2003).

### 6.3 Illusory memories

A key point of agreement between cognitive and biological theories is that memories do not preserve a literal representation of the world; memories are constructed from fragments of information that are distributed across different brain regions, and depend on influences operating in the present as well as the past. Memory illusions and distortions have long been of interest to psychology researchers studying memory, but neuropsychologists and neuroscientists have paid relatively little attention to them (Schacter, 1996).
Memory distortions and illusions have long been of interest to psychopathology, dating to the classic 1932 study by Bartlett on the reconstructive nature of memory. Three decades later, Neisser (1967) put forward similar ideas. His monograph stimulated intensive interest on the part of cognitive psychologists in questions concerning memory distortions, resulting in many striking demonstrations of erroneous remembering in laboratory studies. Cognitive studies concerning memory distortion continued through the 1980s and have grown dramatically during the 1990s, inspired in part by controversies over the accuracy of memories retrieved in psychotherapy and effects of suggestive questioning on the reliability of childrens' recollections (Peres et al., 2008, Schacter, 1996).
Neuroimaging studies have highlighted important issues related to structural and functional brain changes found in sufferers of psychological trauma that may influence their ability to synthesize, categorize, and integrate traumatic memories (Peres et al., 2008).
A number of neuropsychologists have noted that damage to the ventromedial aspects of the frontal lobes and basal forebrain are often associated with the memory distortion known as

confabulation, where patients describe detailed recollections of events that never happened (Johnson, 1991, Moscovitch, 1997). Moscovitch (1997) has contended that confabulation arises as a result of impairment to strategic retrieval and monitoring processes that depend on frontal regions.

Illusory memory conjunctions appear to be attributable to inadequate binding of features at the time of encoding, a process that likely depends on the hippocampal formation.

Schacter et al. (1996) conducted a PET study using a specific paradigm: before scanning, subjects listened to a long list of words that were grouped into semantic categories that each included 20 associates of a non-presented critical lure; then was administered yes/no recognition tests in separate 60-sec scans for old words that had appeared on the study list ("true targets"), critical lures that had not appeared but were related to previously presented words ("false targets"), and new words that had not appeared and were not systematically related to previously presented words ("true target controls" and "false target controls," respectively); in a separate passive fixation scan, subjects simply looked at a crosshair for 60 sec. Compared to the passive fixation condition, both accurate recognition of true targets and illusory recognition of false targets were accompanied by significant blood flow increases in many of the same brain regions, including bilateral anterior/dorsolateral frontal cortex, precuneus, bilateral cerebellum, and the left medial temporal lobe, in the vicinity of the parahippocampal gyrus. This latter observation is intriguing in light of previously mentioned findings that amnesic patients with medial temporal damage exhibited little false recognition of critical lures and that medial temporal blood flow increases are associated with successful recollection (23, 51, 52). However, the evidence linking parahippocampal gyrus activation with episodic recognition (as opposed to visual or lexical processing) was equivocal, so this finding must be viewed cautiously pending further research.

Direct comparison between veridical and illusory recognition in this paper yielded virtually no significant findings, suggesting that brain activity during the two forms of recognition is quite similar. Nonetheless, the authors did observe some suggestive differences. Veridical recognition was accompanied by significantly greater blood flow than illusory recognition in the vicinity of the left supramarginal gyrus and superior temporal gyrus. Previous PET studies have implicated these regions in the processing and storage of phonological information (cf., refs. 81, 82, 83). Moreover, studies of brain-damaged patients have linked the supramarginal gyrus with disruptions of phonological analysis and retrieval (84). In light of these observations, authors hypothesized that temporoparietal increases associated with veridical recognition may reflect subjects' recognition of having heard or rehearsed the target words at the time of study; no such auditory/phonological information was available for critical lures. Although alternative interpretations are possible, this idea fits with the previously mentioned finding reported by Norman and Schacter (74) that people report more extensive memories of having heard or thought about presented words than critical lures.

One further suggestive finding from this PET study relates to the previously mentioned observations of a link between frontal lobe impairments and heightened susceptibility to false recognition. The authors found that false recognition was associated with trends for greater blood flow increases in inferior frontal regions (orbitofrontal cortex) bilaterally and right anterior prefrontal cortex than was veridical recognition. One possible interpretation of this finding is that subjects were trying to oppose or inhibit the sense of familiarity or recollection associated with the critical lures. That is, when subjects were deciding whether a critical lure had appeared previously, they likely experienced a strong feeling that it did. At the same time, knowing that many associatively related items were on the list, they may have engaged in effortful retrieval processes as they tried to remember specific information about the test item's appearance in the study list.

## 7. References

Aine CJ, Sanfratello L, Adair JC, Knoefel JE, Caprihan A, Stephen JM. Development and Decline of Memory Functions in Normal, Pathological and Healthy Successful Aging. Brain Topogr. 2011; 24: 135-142.

Alexander MP, Naeser MA, Palumbo C. Broca's area aphasias: aphasia after lesions including the frontal operculum. Neurology 1990;40:353-362.

Apostolova LG, Thompson PM. Mapping progressive brain structural changes in early Alzheimer's disease and mild cognitive impairment. Neuropsychologia. 2008;46(6):1597-612.

Bartlett F C. Remembering. Cambridge, U.K.: Cambridge Univ. Press; 1932.

Bartsch T, Alfke K, Stingele R, et al. Selective affection of hippocampal CA-1 neurons in patients with transient global amnesia without long-term sequelae, Brain 129 (2006), pp. 2874–2884.

Bartsch T, Alfke K, Deuschl G, Jansen O. Evolution of hippocampal CA-1 diffusion lesions in transient global amnesia, Ann Neurol 62 (2007), pp. 475–480.

Bartsch T, Deuschl G. Transient global amnesia: functional anatomy and clinical implications. Lancet Neurol. 2010; 9(2):205-14.

Broca P. Remarques sur le siège de la faculté du langage articulé suivies d'une observation d'amphémie (perte de al parole). Bull Mem Soc Anat Paris 1861;36-45.

Caixeta L, Nitrini R. Subtipos clínicos da demência frontotemporal. Arq Neuropsiquiatr. 2001 Sep;59(3-A):577-81.

Caixeta L. Demência - Abordagem Multidisciplinar. São Paulo, Atheneu, 2006. ISBN 85-7379-864-5.

Caixeta L, Vieira RT. Demência na doença de Parkinson. Rev Bras Psiquiatr. 2008 Dec;30(4):375-83.

Caserta MT, Bannon Y, Fernandez F, Giunta B, Schoenberg MR, Tan J. Normal brain aging clinical, immunological, neuropsychological, and neuroimaging features. Int Rev Neurobiol. 2009;84:1-19.

Celsis P. Age-related cognitive decline, mild cognitive impairment or preclinical Alzheimer's disease? Ann Med. 2000 Feb;32(1):6-14.

Chung YA, Jeong J, Yang DW, et al.. A Tc-99m SPECT study of regional cerebral blood flow in patients with transient global amnesia, Neuroimage 47 (2009), pp. 50–55.

D'Esposito M, Wills H. Functional Imaging of Neurocognition. Semin Neurol 20(4):487-498, 2000.

Dickerson BC, Salat DH, Bates JF, Atiya M, Killiany RJ, Greve DN, Dale AM, Stern CE, Blacker D, Albert MS, Sperling RA. Medial temporal lobe function and structure in mild cognitive impairment. Ann Neurol. 2004;56:27–35.

Dronkers NF. A new brain region for coordinating speech articulation. Nature 1996;384:159-161.

Eustache F, Desgranges B, Aupee AM, Guillery B, Baron JC. Functional neuroanatomy of amnesia: positron emission tomography studies, Microsc Res Tech 51 (2000), pp. 94–100.

Fujii K, Sadoshima S, Ishitsuka T, et al. Regional cerebral blood flow and metabolism in patients with transient global amnesia: a positron emission tomography study, J Neurol Neurosurg Psychiatry 52 (1989), pp. 622–630.

Galin D, Ornstein R. Lateral specialization of cognitive mode: an EEG study. Psychophysiology 1972;9:412-418

Guillery B, Desgranges B, de la Sayette V, Landeau B, Eustache F, Baron JC. Transient global amnesia: concomitant episodic memory and positron emission tomography assessment in two additional patients, Neurosci Lett 325 (2002), pp. 62–66.

Halligan PW, David AS. Cognitive neuropsychiatry: towards a scientific psychopathology. Nat. Rev. Neurosci. 2 (2001), pp. 209–215.

Hamalainen A, Pihlajamaki M, Tanila H, Hanninen T, Niskanen E, Tervo S, Karjalainen PA, Vanninen RL, Soininen H. Increased fMRI responses during encoding in mild cognitive impairment. Neurobiol Aging. 2007;28:1889–1903.

Huber R, Aschoff AJ, Ludolph AC, Riepe MW. Transient global amnesia. Evidence against vascular ischemic etiology from diffusion weighted imaging, J Neurol 249 (2002), pp. 1520–1524.

Ingvar DH, Schwartz MS. Blood flow patterns induced in the dominant hemisphere by speech and reading. Brain 1974;97: 273-278

Jak AJ, Bangen KJ, Wierenga CE, Delano-Wood L, Corey-Bloom J, Bondi MW. Contributions of neuropsychology and neuroimaging to understanding clinical subtypes of mild cognitive impairment. Int Rev Neurobiol. 2009;84:81-103.

Johnson M K. In: Awareness of Deficit After Brain Injury: Clinical and Theoretical Issues. Prigatano G P, Schacter D L, editors. New York: Oxford Univ. Press; 1991. pp. 176–197. ISBN 0195059417.

Johnson SC, Baxter LC, Susskind-Wilder L, Connor DJ, Sabbagh MN, Caselli RJ. Hippocampal adaptation to face repetition in healthy elderly and mild cognitive impairment. Neuropsychologia. 2004;42:980–989.

Johnson SC, Schmitz TW, Moritz CH, Meyerand ME, Rowley HA, Alexander AL, Hansen KW, Gleason CE, Carlsson CM, Ries ML, Asthana S, Chen K, et al. Activation of brain regions vulnerable to Alzheimer's disease: The effect of mild cognitive impairment. Neurobiol Aging. 2006;27:1604–1612.

Kalpouzos G, Eustache F, Desgranges B. Cognitive reserve and neural networks in normal aging and Alzheimer's disease. Psychol Neuropsychiatr Vieil. 2008 Jun;6(2):97-105.

Kircher TT, Weis S, Freymann K, Erb M, Jessen F, Grodd W, Heun R, Leube DT. Hippocampal activation in patients with mild cognitive impairment is necessary for successful memory encoding. J Neurol Neurosurg Psychiatry. 2007;78:812–818.

Mandzia JL, McAndrews MP, Grady CL, Graham SJ, Black SE. Neural correlates of incidental memory in mild cognitive impairment: An fMRI study. Neurobiol Aging. 2009;30:717–730.

Markowitsch HJ. Organic and psychogenic retrograde amnesia: two sides of the same coin? Neurocase 2 (1996), pp. 357–371.

Markowitsch HJ. Functional neuroimaging correlates of functional amnesia. Memory 7 (1999), pp. 561–583.

Markowitsch HJ. Psychogenic amnesia. Neuroimage. 2003;20 Suppl 1:S132-8.

Matsui M, Imamura T, Sakamoto S, Ishii K, Kazui H, Mori E. Transient global amnesia: increased signal intensity in the right hippocampus on diffusion-weighted magnetic resonance imaging, Neuroradiology 44 (2002), pp. 235–238.

Mazziotta JC, Phelps ME.. Human sensory stimulation and deprivation: positron emission tomographic results and strategies. Ann Neurol 1984;15:S50-S60

Moscovitch M. In: Memory Distortion: How minds, Brains, and Societies Reconstruct the Past. Schacter D L, editor. Cambridge, MA: Harvard Univ. Press; 1997. pp. 226–254. ISBN 0674566769.

Miller SL, Fenstermacher E, Bates J, Blacker D, Sperling RA, Dickerson BC. Hippocampal activation in adults with mild cognitive impairment predicts subsequent cognitive decline. J Neurol Neurosurg Psychiatry. 2008;79:630–635.

Naeser M, Palumbo C, Helm-Estabrooks N. Severe nonfluency in aphasia: role of the medial subcallosal fasciculus plus other white matter pathways in recovery of spontaneous speech. Brain 1989;112:1-38.

Nardone R, Buffone EC, Matullo MF, Tezzon F. Motor cortex excitability in transient global amnesia. J Neurol 251 (2004), pp. 42–46.

Neisser U. Cognitive Psychology. New York: Appleton-Century-Crofts; 1967, ISBN 0521485002.

Nitrini R, Buchpiguel CA, Caramelli P, Bahia VS, Mathias SC, Nascimento CM, Degenszajn J, Caixeta L. SPECT in Alzheimer's disease: features associated with bilateral parietotemporal hypoperfusion. Acta Neurol Scand. 2000 Mar;101(3):172-6.

Peres JF, McFarlane A, Nasello AG, Moores KA. Traumatic memories: bridging the gap between functional neuroimaging and psychotherapy.Aust N Z J Psychiatry. 2008;42(6):478-88.

Petersen SE, Fox PT, Posner MI, Mintun M, Raichle ME. Positron emission tomographic studies of the cortical anatomy of single word processing. Nature 1988;331:585-589.

Rajah MN, D'Esposito M. Region-specific changes in prefrontal function with age: a review of PET and fMRI studies on working and episodic memory. Brain. 2005 Sep;128 (Pt 9):1964-83.

Schacter DL, Reiman E, Curran T, Yun LS, Bandy D, McDermott KB, Roediger HL. Neuroanatomical correlates of veridical and illusory recognition memory: evidence from positon emission tomography. Neuron. 1996;17:267–274.

Schacter DL. Illusory memories: a cognitive neuroscience analysis.Proc Natl Acad Sci U S A. 1996;93(24):13527-33.

Sperling R. Functional MRI studies of associative encoding in normal aging, mild cognitive impairment, and Alzheimer's disease. Ann NY Acad Sci. 2007;1097:146–155.

Vannini P, Almkvist O, Dierks T, Lehmann C, Wahlund LO. Reduced neuronal efficacy in progressive mild cognitive impairment: A prospective fMRI study on visuospatial processing. Psychiatry Res. 2007;156:43–57.

Warren JD, Chatterton B, Thompson PD. A SPECT study of the anatomy of transient global amnesia, J Clin Neurosci 7 (2000), pp. 57–59.

# 2

# Degeneration of the Human Nervous System and Magnetic Resonance Neuroimaging

Lulé Dorothée and Ludolph Albert Christian
*Department of Neurology, University of Ulm*
*Germany*

## 1. Introduction

Neurodegenerative diseases are progressive, hereditary or sporadic diseases of the nervous system. Progressive neurodegeneration causes i.e. loss of movement ability like in motor neuron diseases or cognitive deficits like in dementia. Despite the fact that many similarities appear on the sub-cellular level that relate different neurodegenerative diseases with each other, the broad variety on the clinical level remains which causes major demands both in clinical care and daily living.

Advances in neuroimaging have led to an extensive application of this technique in clinical and scientific studies. Neuroimaging is a non-invasive approach of measuring either structural properties or activity of the brain. Activity of the brain can be investigated during defined tasks or during rest to observe functional connectivity of cortical and subcortical regions in time and space. Neuroimaging in neurodegenerative diseases has extensively increased our understanding of interaction of functional executive decline e.g. in movement and cognition and of changes in cortical pattern activity. Neuroimaging is a promising candidate for an objective marker for e.g. drug efficacy. By these means, neuroimaging as a biomarker can improve predictability of outcome in clinical trials. Furthermore, discovering patterns of vulnerability of neurons on the cortical and subcortical level helps to disentangle the course of degeneration in different diseases in vivo to support post-mortem findings. Those ex-vivo analyses had been the only means to get an understanding of disease courses before neuroimaging evolved.

The following article will give an introduction to the characteristics of the main neurodegenerative diseases and techniques that have been used in understanding pathogenesis and aetiology of neurodegenerative diseases. It encompasses main findings in structural and functional neuroimaging in Motor Neuron Diseases (MND) and in others like dementias, Parkinson's disease (PD) and Huntington's disease.

With our work we mainly focused on Motor Neuron Diseases like ALS and we provided clear evidence for pathological involvement of areas extending the motor system like emotional and sensory processing pathways. Overall, the article will highlight the capacity of neuroimaging to shed light onto aetiology and pathogenesis of neurodegeneration in the human central nervous system.

## 2. Clinical understanding and differential diagnosis among neurodegenerative diseases

Neurodegenerative diseases encompass different pathologies with the common feature of progressive loss of structure or function of neurons.

Over the last years, evidence evolved of common pathological processes in different neurodegenerative diseases like accumulation of neurofilaments, protein degradation and induced cell death. For example, accumulated TDP-43 is found in sporadic ALS cases, which links this disease to fronto-temporal dementias (FTD) (Neumann et al., 2006). Furthermore, on behavioural level there is accumulating evidence for a common cognitive decline in some ALS patients and in patients with FTD.

Genetics provide further evidence for an association between different neurodegenerative diseases like polyglutamine repeats in Huntington's disease and spinocerebellar ataxias and mutations in the alpha-synuclein in Parkinson's Disease, dementia with Lewy bodies and multiple system atrophy. Furthermore, mitochondrial dysfunction, disturbed axonal transport and endothelial dysfunction are common pathological hallmarks found in different neurodegenerative diseases. In clinical routine, differential diagnosis is usually done on clinical basis. According to clinical criteria, Amyotrophic lateral sclerosis is regarded as a disease of the peripheral and central nervous system and the other most common neurodegenerative diseases like dementias, Parkinson's disease and Huntington's disease are primarily regarded as diseases of the central nervous system (Hacke, 2007). However, evidence for overlaps in molecular or cellular pathways question this classification and suggests a major overlap of different neurodegenerative pathologies in central and peripheral nervous system (Braak et al., 2006b; Braak & Del Tredici, 2011a, 2011b; Grammas et al., 2011; Neumann et al., 2006). New imaging techniques carry the hope of revolutionizing the diagnosis of neurodegenerative disease to improve staging of patients and follow disease progression and treatment trial efficacy.

## 3. Characteristics of main neurodegenerative diseases

### 3.1 Diseases of the central and peripheral nervous system and muscles

#### 3.1.1 Motor Neuron Diseases (MND)

Motor neuron diseases describe pathologies of the motor system. The most common is Amyotrophic Lateral Sclerosis, which evolves mostly in midlife and is characterised by a fast progression of immobility and loss of verbal communication. Cognition is mostly unaffected; yet, there is an on-going debate on the proportion of patients with cognitive impairments. There are more benign forms of motor degenerative diseases e.g. affecting just the upper or just the lower motor neurons (Ludolph and Dengler, 1999). ALS, which affects upper and lower motor neurons, is usually fast progressing causing death within 3-5 years. The fatal event is usually respiratory failure. There is a gender ratio of men: women of about 1.5: 1.

The cause of ALS is mostly unknown. In the early 1990s there was evidence provided that some patients with a familial form of ALS have a defined mutation in the Superoxide-Dismutase 1 (SOD1). Since then various genetic changes have been detected as a possible cause for ALS. However, for most cases the cause is yet unknown. Riluzole as a glutamate agonist is the only applicable drug in ALS that prolongs life of ALS patients. Numerous drug trials are ongoing to provide new therapeutic targets in ALS.

## 3.2 Disease of the central nervous system

### 3.2.1 Dementias

Alzheimer's disease (AD) is the most common form of dementia. It is named after the German psychiatrist and neuropathologist Alois Alzheimer who first described the disease in the early 20th century. The other most common form of dementia is vascular dementia. Some other forms are dementia with Lewy bodies, and frontotemporal lobal degeneration, which is subdivided into the behavioural variant (fronto-temporal dementia, FTD), the semantic dementia, primary progredient aphasia, corticobasal degeneration, progressive supranuclear palsy and amyotrophic lateral sclerosis with frontotemporal dementia. Numerous other neurodegenerative illnesses have an associated dementia, including Creutzfeldt-Jakob disease, Huntington's disease, multiple system atrophy, and Parkinson's disease dementia (Tartaglia et al.,2011).

dementias are acquired diseases that clinically affect cognitive abilities and daily activities. Classification of dementias can be done according to different criteria: cortical (memory, language, thinking and social skills are affected) and subcortical pathology (emotional processing, movement and memory are primarily affected). Furthermore, it can be classified according to whether it is a progressive form (cognitive abilities worsen over time), and whether it is primary (results from a specific disease such as Alzheimer's disease) or secondary (occurs because of disease or injury like vascular dementia). Patho-anatomical hallmark is the degeneration of the brain (mainly frontal and temporal areas). Early stages of dementia are often mistakenly considered as normal aging problems like forgetfulness and memory storage problems. With the means of standardised diagnostic tools problems in memory, language (aphasia), attention, planning and concept formation, psychomotor function and personality problems can be detected.

Due to the changing demographics in western countries, the incidence of dementias constantly increases. About 5-10% of the people >65 years and 30-40% of those above 80 develop dementias. Incidence increases exponentially with age. Women are more often affected than men.

The cause of Alzheimer's disease is not fully understood. There are several hypotheses, which have different supporters. The most widely used hypothesis is the amyloid hypothesis. Amyloid beta deposits are found in the brain of AD patients preceding the onset of clinical dementia. However, amyloid beta is not pathological per se and is found in healthy aged people. Furthermore, amyloid plaque deposition do not correlate with neuron loss and also not with clinical symptoms. Abnormally phosphorylated tau protein may start quite early, i.e., before puberty or in early young adulthood and therefore decades before clinical onset of the disease (Braak & Del Tredici, 2011b).

### 3.2.2 Parkinson's Disease (PD)

Parkinson's disease is the second most common degenerative disease of the central nervous system. Pathological hallmark of the idiopathic Parkinson's syndrome are movement related symptoms like slowness of movements, rigidity and tremor. Subtypes distinguish between the predominance of symptoms in a patient. Changes in mood and cognitive deficits are described as non-motor symptoms in PD. In late stage PD dementia is a common hallmark. Like ALS, PD affects people in midlife. However, there is evidence that disease process starts early in life (Braak & Del Tredici 2011b). The disease is caused by death of dopaminergic cells in substantia nigra of the midbrain that project to the striatum. The pathological process of PD (formation of proteinaceous intraneuronal Lewy bodies and Lewy neurites) begins at two sites and continues in a topographically predictable sequence in six stages, during which components of the olfactory, autonomic, limbic, and somatomotor systems become progressively involved (Braak et al., 2006a). PD cannot be cured but dopaminergic medication is an effective treatment for the disease. However, medication may become ineffective in the cause of disease. Deep brain stimulation is an available tool in PD if no other therapy is applicable.

#### 3.2.3 Huntington's Disease

Huntington's disease (HD) is a movement disorder with inability to control movements: involuntary, sudden, fast and erratic movements of distal extremities, face, neck and trunk are seen. In early stages of HD slightly exaggerated movements might be considered as nervousness, however, in the course of the disease control of coordinated body movements are becoming more and more difficult, especially affecting walking. Men and women are similarly affected. Disease onset is usually between 30 and 50 years.

Huntington described the disease already in 1872. It has a prevalence of 2-10 per 100 000 inhabitants. It is an autosomal dominant genetic cause with full penetrance. There is a 50% chance of diseased offspring and therefore presymptomatic enrolment in clinical trials is possible.

## 4. Common neuroimaging techniques

Neuroimaging techniques in degenerative diseases are used to investigate structural or functional changes in the brain and spinal chord. Those techniques may be used to support clinical diagnosis or, as for most of the functional techniques, are used in research to enrich our understanding of pathophysiological outcomes of neurodegenerative processes.

### 4.1 Structural techniques

#### 4.1.1 Anatomical scans with CT and MRI

Conventional radiography like computerized tomography (CT) is still widely used in traumatology and other fields of medicine. For CT, x-rays pass through the body and are attenuated in the tissue. The denser a tissue is, the more the x-rays are attenuated. Detectors pick up the signals and digital geometry processing generates three-dimensional images of e.g. the brain. CT has mainly lost its importance in the clinical evaluation of neurodegenerative diseases.

With the finding of magnetic resonance imaging (MRI) in the 1970s, a new era of medical neuroimaging evolved to visualize structures of the central nervous system. MRI uses the property of magnetic resonance in atoms with uneven number of nuclei. In living organisms, protons are mostly used, but any other atom with the according properties can similarly be used. An object (e.g. a human) is placed within a permanent magnetic field. A proportion of the protons align within this field. Gradient pulses in a high radio frequency are pulsed to deflect the spins of the protons. Inbetween those pulsed gradients, spins return to their original position and emit energy. This emission can be detected in MRI.

MRI images provide images of soft tissue e.g. the brain with high contrasts and without bone artefacts. Therefore, MRI is applicable to visualize anatomical and pathological structures in the scull and in the spinal canal. Furthermore, in functional MRI it is applicable to non-invasively visualise brain function *in vivo*.

#### 4.1.2 Spectroscopy

Whereas MRI gives only information about the structure of the body like the distribution of water and fat, magnetic resonance spectroscopy is suitable to give information of property and chemical structure of tissue. MRS provides information on the nuclei of atoms, which allows deduction on the chemical properties of a tissue. It is a non-invasive technique, which is used in some clinical fields like tumour diagnostic. It can as well provide evidence of longitudinal change in cerebral function using proton-based metabolites (among others choline, creatine, lactate, N-acetylaspartate (NAA), glutamate). NAA is thought to be a marker of neuronal integrity and is therefore used as a diagnostic marker in neurodegenerative diseases. MRS has been used in research but fields of clinical application are expanding i.e. longitudinal change of metabolites in therapeutic intervention (Turner et al., 2011).

#### 4.1.3 Voxel based morphometry MRI

Voxel based morphometry (VBM) in MRI quantifies white or gray matter volume in the CNS. It is a non-invasive technique to detect brain volume changes *in vivo* and compare it between groups e.g. patients with neurodegenerative diseases and healthies. VBM registers every brain to a brain template to provide for main anatomical differences between brains. Statistical comparison of each subvolume of the brain (so called voxels) allows fast quantification of brain volume alterations.

#### 4.1.4 Diffusion tensor imaging

Diffusion tensor imaging (DTI) is based on the physics of diffusion of all molecules in e.g. the human body according to Brownian motion theory. Membranes, fibres and other molecules restrict the movement of molecules and the molecules align along barriers. The stronger the aligned diffusion, the higher is the anisotropy. In living tissue, fractional anisotropy (FA) is at its minimum (0) where there are no barriers and diffusion is not directed. FA is at its maximum (1) if alignment of diffusion is highest. DTI is applicable in white matter pathology in neurodegenerative diseases. DTI based fibre tracking gives additional information on directionality and can therefore be used to visualise e.g. direction and strength of bundles of white matter fibres within the brain. In neurodegenerative diseases it's applicable to detect white and grey matter loss.

### 4.2 Functional neuroimaging

Functional neuroimaging in neurodegenerative disease aims to explore the functional state of the brain as well as the capacity of the adult brain to functionally compensate for progressive loss of neurons. In order to map brain functions, non-invasive neuroimaging techniques have been available for almost 80 years. Since different techniques have different shortcomings, the development and implementation of new functional imaging techniques have been complementary over these years (for review see Lulé et al., 2009). Electroencephalography (EEG), already developed in the 1920s by Hans Berger, is a technique for directly measuring electrical activity of cortical neurons on the surface of the head, thus providing a high temporal but a very low spatial resolution (Berger, 1929). In

1968, the first measurements of the magnetic equivalents of EEG recordings (electrical activity of cortical neurons induce magnetic fields) signalled the beginning of magneto encephalography (MEG), which complemented the field of non-invasive imaging of neuronal activity in the brain (Cohen, 1968). However, the interpretation of signals in the spatial domain remains challenging and is not suitable for subcortical structures.

Since the mid 1970s, methods for measuring brain metabolism have been established. Changes in metabolism in the brain are a consequence of energy expenditure following neuronal activity in the brain. These data facilitate indirect measurement of overall brain activity. Accordingly, measurements of metabolism have improved spatial resolution especially for subcortical structures. Positron Emission Tomography (PET) and Single Photon Emission Computed Tomography (SPECT) record the dynamic distribution in the human brain of isotopes administered to a subject when assigned to a specific task (Phelps et al., 1975; Ter-Pogossian et al., 1975). Since metabolism is a second order effect following the electrical activity of neurons with latency, the temporal resolution of such measurements is low. Furthermore, radioactive substances have to be applied, limiting the application for scientific research.

In the 1990s, functional MRI was developed. Functional MRI can be used to measure physiological changes not only of metabolism but also of e.g. blood flow in the brain. Like metabolism, blood flow is stimulated following oxygen expenditure of the cortical substrate. Like PET and SPECT, fMRI is a second-order signal with the problem of low temporal resolution but high spatial resolution, with the potential to indirectly measure cortical and subcortical activity easily during the performance of a given task. Accordingly, fMRI combines advantages of different non-invasive functional neuroimaging techniques. However, the indirect nature by which brain activity is currently measured by fMRI continues to limit its role as a "front-line" imaging tool.

Notwithstanding, the clinical potential of a non-invasive probe of brain function with the option of repeated measures over time (e.g. due to a lack of radiation charge) in addition to the wide-spread availability of MRI scanners in many hospitals and research centres have extended its application in clinical science and contributed to an exponential increase in scientific publications on fMRI over the last decade (Jezzard & Buxton, 2006).

### 4.2.1 Principles of fMRI

Experimental work in animals first demonstrated that oxygenated blood and deoxygenated blood present different properties in a magnetic field, as noted by Linus Pauling as early as the 1930s (Pauling, 1936). Because of its unshielded iron, deoxygenated blood has paramagnetic properties whereas oxygenated blood has diamagnetic properties. Deoxyhaemoglobin as an endogenous paramagnetic contrast agent dephases nuclear spins of water protons in its vicinity with a physical effect of signal intensity change in T2*-weighted MR images (Frahms et al., 1999). Ogawa and co-workers realised that those differences in magnetic properties in blood could have implications in the visualisation of local brain function (Ogawa et al., 1990a; 1990b).

The most commonly used fMRI approach is to measure mainly blood flow changes using the blood-oxygenation-level-dependency (BOLD) effect (Kwong et al., 1992; Ogawa et al., 1992), although other parameters can also be measured. A change in neuronal activity causes a decreased local blood oxygenation and an increased demand for oxygen. The local increase in deoxygenated blood level in the corresponding brain area is followed by a rise in cerebral blood flow that at least transiently 'uncouples' from oxygen consumption (Frahms

et al., 1992). The increase in blood flow and oxygenation decreases deoxyhaemoglobin concentration and leads to an increase in the corresponding MRI signal intensity and the effective spin-spin relaxation time T2*. This can be measured as a BOLD signal change in fMRI (Kim et al., 1997a; Logothetis et al., 2004; Ogawa et al., 1990b).
The time curve of the measured BOLD signal in fMRI may be explained as follows: The local increase in deoxygenated blood level following neuronal activity in the corresponding brain area is assumed to be represented by the "initial dip" in the relevant BOLD signal. Oxygenated blood invades brain areas shortly after to compensate the increased metabolic rate in the neurons which results in a BOLD signal increase that peaks after around 6 s and returns to baseline after 20–30 s (Figure 1).

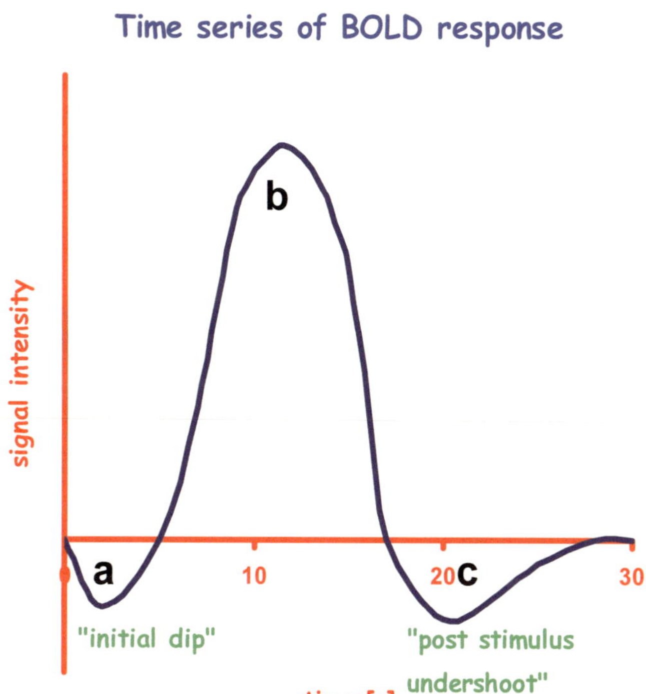


Fig. 1. Time series of BOLD response in fMRI. BOLD signal decreases as oxygen expenditure in the brain tissue (a: initial dip) increases; in the following phase extensive flow of oxygenated blood leads to increase in BOLD signal, reaching its maximum at about 6s (b). The signal returns to baseline within 20-30 s, often combined with a post-stimulus undershoot of the BOLD response (c).

The BOLD in fMRI does not directly measure neural activity but relies on a surrogate 'secondary' signal resulting from changes in oxygenation, perfusion (blood volume and flow), and metabolism (e.g. glucose and oxygen consumption) (Logothesis et al., 2004; Kim et al., 1997b; DiSalle et al., 1999). Neurovascular and metabolic correlates associated with brain activation are not yet fully understood, but there is evidence for a correlation between neuronal activity (or activation) in the brain and the fMRI signal (Logothesis et al., 2001). Functional MRI gives an approximation of neuronal activity, detecting, for example, task-induced changes in local brain function (DiSalle et al., 1999; van Geuns et al., 1999). Because the BOLD signal, however, derives from the interaction of multiple parameters (e.g. perfusion, metabolic turnover of neurons, density of venous vasculature of tissue, medication etc.) and may vary between brain areas and individuals as well as experimental and clinical settings, quantitative analysis in absolute terms is precluded (Kim et al., 1997a; Di Salle et al., 1999; Logothesis et al., 2001).

MRI sequences that are best suited for functional neuroimaging should be both fast and sensitive to changes in the deoxyhaemoglobin concentration (Frahms et al., 1999). The MRI sequence that is generally considered to be the first choice for measuring BOLD in fMRI is a T2*-weighted echo-planar imaging (EPI) sequence, with its high speed yielding imaging times which translate into a maximum temporal resolution (Edelman et al., 1994; Kwong et al., 1995; Schmitt et al., 1998; Roberts et al., 2007). Temporal and spatial parameters of MRI scanning such as repetition time (TR) or slice thickness are limited by the T2* signal decay of the MRI sequence and determined according to study-specific factors, e.g. region of interest and field strength (Schmitt et al., 1998; Turner et al., 1998; Triantafyllou et al., 2005; Norris et al., 2006; Figure 2). Other MRI sequences such as fast low angle shot (FLASH) techniques facilitate access to higher spatial resolution at the expense of temporal resolution and volume coverage of larger volumes leading to higher scanning times (Frahms et al., 1999), which is not always favourable in clinical settings.

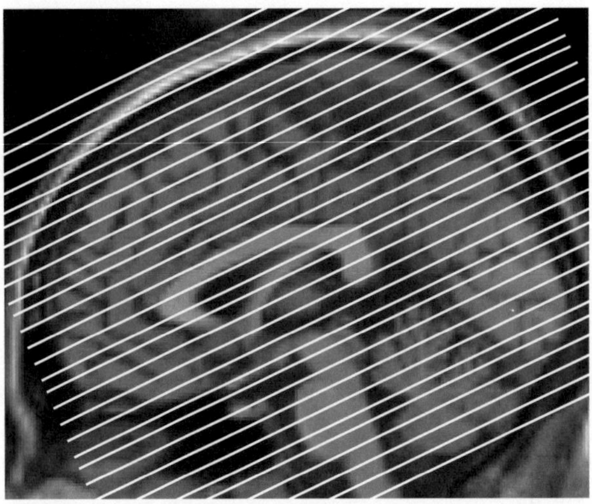

Fig. 2. Example of orientation of EPI-sequence (white lines) along the anterior-posterior commissure overlaid onto a t1 weighted image (mprage) of a head (sagittal view)

## 5. Functional neuroimaging in motor neuron diseases

### 5.1 Functional neuroimaging of motor network

In fMRI studies, ALS patients present higher volumes of activated brain areas in motor tasks compared with healthy controls, thus providing evidence for functional reorganisation and cortical plasticity in MND (Brooks et al., 2000; Lulé et al., 2009). Konrad et al. observed this in eleven ALS patients (Konrad et al., 2002) who performed a simple finger flexion task with 10% of each individual´s maximum grip force. Increased activity was found in motor areas such as the premotor area, supplementary motor area, and the cerebellum. A similarly increased activity in motor areas was observed in fifteen ALS patients compared to fifteen healthy controls during a sequential finger tapping movement task (Han et al., 2006) and in ALS patients compared both to patients with upper limb weakness due to peripheral nerve lesions and to controls during freely selected random joystick movements of the right hand (Stanton et al., 2007a). It has been proposed that these changes may represent cortical plasticity, as new synapses and pathways are developed to compensate for the selective loss of pyramidal cells in the motor cortex (Schoenfeld et al., 2005). A shift of activity to more anterior regions of the premotor cortex, i.e. Brodmann area (BA) 6, during upper limb movement has been observed in ALS patients (Konrad et al., 2002; Han et al., 2006), such findings being supported by previous functional imaging studies with PET (Kew et al., 1993a; 1994). Furthermore, there is longitudinal fMRI evidence of progressive involvement of the premotor area in upper limb motor tasks in the course of the disease (Lulé et al., 2007a). Thirteen patients with sporadic ALS and 14 healthy controls were asked to perform tasks involving a grip movement of the left, right, and both hands and to imagine the same without any overt movement of the hand. Motor imagery is known to involve similar areas as motor execution without being affected by confounding factors of effort and strain. In two consecutive fMRI measurements at a six-month interval, evidence for progressive recruitment of premotor areas in motor imagery was found in the course of the disease (Lulé et al., 2007a).

Furthermore, a changed pattern and an anterior shift of activity in ALS were also observed in further cortical areas besides the premotor cortex for various motor tasks. For instance, increased involvement of supplementary motor areas (SMA) (Konrad et al., 2002; 2006; Han et al., 2006) and sensorimotor cortices has been seen (Brooks et al., 2000; Han et al., 2006; Stanton et al., 2007a; Mohammadi et al., 2011). Activity in contralateral sensorimotor cortex activity was increased the stronger the physical impairments were in patients (Mohammadi et al., 2011). Furthermore, activity in adjacent areas such as the bilateral inferior parietal lobe (BA 40) and bilateral superior temporal gyrus (BA 22) was increased in ALS patients compared to healthy controls during upper limb motor task performance in different fMRI studies (Stanton et al., 2007a). Altered somatotopy in the sensorimotor cortices was not observed in patients with exclusive lower motor neuron involvement (Kew et al., 1994), but only in ALS patients with clinical and functional involvement of both upper and lower motor neurons (Han et al., 2006; Kew et al., 1993a; 1994) or upper motor neuron only (Stanton et al., 2007a). This suggests that this changed pattern of activity might represent the loss of the pyramidal tract (Kew et al., 1994). A similar shift of activity in motor tasks into more anterior regions of sensorimotor and premotor areas and the SMA has been demonstrated for different neuropathologies with distinct aetiology such as stroke (Weiller et al., 2006). Thus, it may be assumed that this anterior shift represents a general pattern of plasticity as a response to neuronal loss in primary motor areas as a more or less efficient way to compensate motor function rather than an ALS-specific pattern of altered motor activation (Weiller et al., 2006).

Increasing activity in ipsilateral cortical areas such as the sensorimotor cortex (Han et al., 2006; Stanton et al., 2007a) and primary motor areas (Schoenfeld et al., 2005) has been observed in ALS patients. In a motor task of upper limb movement with varying task difficulty, six ALS patients presented an increased activity in ipsilateral primary motor areas compared to six healthy controls, corresponding to the degree of difficulty (Schoenfeld et al., 2005). The fact that healthy controls recruit ipsilateral areas with increasing complexity of a task suggests that ipsilateral involvement may reflect difficulty-dependent compensation and not a pathological pattern of activation *per se*. Accordingly, ALS patients may recruit existing neuronal pathways to compensate for functional loss in primary motor cortex (Schoenfeld et al., 2005).

Furthermore, a more pronounced involvement of other motor functional areas at cortical and subcortical levels has been demonstrated in fMRI studies of motor tasks. For motor execution, a stronger involvement of areas involved in motor learning, such as the basal ganglia, cerebellum (Han et al., 2006; Konrad et al., 2006) and/or brainstem (Konrad et al., 2006) is evident. It may be assumed that alterations in functioning of basal ganglia are likely to be related to upper motor neuron pathology since they were observed in patients with exclusive upper motor neuron involvement (Tessitore et al., 2006). For motor imagery, a stronger recruitment of higher cognitive areas of motor control (frontal areas BA 9, 44, 45) and motor representation (inferior parietal activity, BA 40) in the course of the disease has been demonstrated in ALS patients compared to healthy controls (Lulé et al., 2007a). Overall, functional connectivity in the motor system network is altered in ALS (Mohammadi et al., 2009).

Moreover, an increased involvement of extra motor areas, e.g. in the anterior cingulate cortex for movements of the right hand, is evident for patients with exclusive upper motor neuron involvement by fMRI (Tessitore et al., 2006). Similarly, an increased activity in anterior insular cortex and anterior cingulate cortex has been shown in other functional studies of motor execution (Brooks et al., 2000; Kew et al., 1993a; 1994).

Whether the changed pattern of activity in other motor functional areas and higher cognitive areas during motor tasks represents the recruitment of redundant parallel motor system pathways or whether they map functional compensation or reorganisation can only be speculated upon. There is evidence that the change in cortical functioning of other motor and extramotor systems is primarily related to upper motor neuron pathology (Tessitore et al., 2006).

For motor imagery, which is known to involve similar areas as motor execution, a different pattern of cortical activity is seen in ALS compared to motor tasks. In a movement imagery task of the right hand in 16 ALS patients, there was reduced BOLD activity in the left anterior parietal lobe, the anterior cingulate, and medial pre-frontal cortex compared to 17 healthy controls (Stanton et al., 2007b). Reduced BOLD activity in the anterior cingulate cortex was also evident in a movement imagery task of both hands in the study by Lulé et al. (2007a). This reduction in cortical activation during motor imagery is at odds with the pattern observed during motor execution. This may represent the disruption of normal motor imagery networks by ALS pathology outside the primary motor cortex (Lulé et al., 2007a; Stanton et al., 2007b).

In summary, these data suggest an additional recruitment in brains of patients with ALS comprising bilateral areas in the premotor cortex in early stages along with involvement of higher order motor processing areas, determined by motor impairments (especially associated with upper motor neuron pathology) in the long run. This additional recruitment might be a (futile) way to compensate ALS-associated progressive functional loss.

The cardinal feature of ALS is the loss of giant pyramidal Betz cells in the primary motor cortex (Brownell et al., 1970). It is nowadays assumed, however, that degeneration extends beyond the motor cortex. Neurodegeneration in motor areas might lead to progressive compensation of secondary motor areas for movement representation. Compensation terminates in a non-functional distributed cortical and subcortical ALS-specific motor network. More research needs to be done on how well the ALS patients in advanced stages of the disease retain the potential for compensatory activity and how training of e.g. movement imagery might slow down the "compensatory" process. Functional MRI seems to be an appropriate way to gain more knowledge on this issue.

### 5.2 Functional imaging of extramotor paradigms in MND

The multisystemic character of ALS has been supported by various findings of functional imaging studies, although there are few fMRI studies. Involvement of sensory pathways in ALS has been reported by histopathological (Isaacs et al., 2007) and electrophysiological studies (Mai et al., 1998; Pugdahl et al., 2007). Evidence from fMRI studies for changed cortical patterns for sensory processing suggests the involvement of sensory processing areas in ALS (Lulé et al., 2010). In a visual, auditory and somatosensory stimulus paradigm, ALS patients presented reduced activity in primary and secondary sensory areas and an increased activity in higher associative areas. This increase in activity was correlated with loss of movement ability: The higher the physical restrictions were, the higher was the activity in those areas of third order sensory processing in ALS patients (Figure 3).

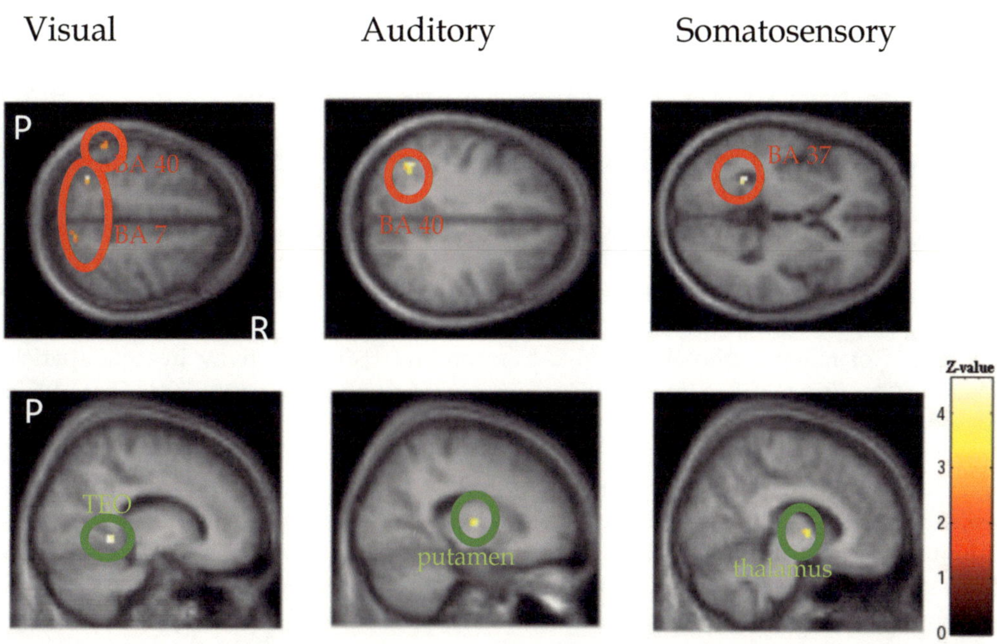


Fig. 3. Changes in brain activity associated with loss of physical function in amyotrophic lateral sclerosis (ALS). Statistical maps presenting significantly increased and decreased blood oxygen level dependent activity associated with loss of physical function (measured with ALS functional rating scale, ALS-FRS) in ALS patients for visual, auditory and somatosensory stimulation. Areas with increasing (upper row, red) and decreasing (lower row, green) activity are shown. Significant activations are overlaid onto an axial (top row) and sagittal (bottom row) mean anatomical image of all subjects. Displayed are clusters >5 voxels with uncorrected threshold $p<0.001$. P, posterior; R, right.

Structural analysis of white matter integrity in this study measured with DTI provided evidence for a disruption of sensory nerve fibres in those ALS patients (Lulé et al., 2010).

Auditory processing underlying stimulus detection measured by MEG and subsequent memory-based comparison processes were abnormal in ten ALS patients with bulbar signs (Pekkonen et al., 2004), and a reduced response to auditory and visual stimuli was observed in ALS patients compared to healthy controls using EEG (Münte et al., 1998; Vieregge et al., 1999). This finding may indicate a changed sensory processing capacity as well as reduced attention capacity (Pinkhardt et al., 2008), an ability assigned to the frontal cortex known to be involved in ALS (Ludolph et al., 1992; Kew et al., 1993b).

The association of functional cortical changes and cognitive deficits has been confirmed by an fMRI paradigm of letter fluency and confrontation naming in 28 non-demented ALS patients compared to 18 healthy controls (Abrahams et al., 2004) and had been demonstrated previously by other functional imaging techniques (Ludolph et al., 1992; Kew et al., 1993b; Abrahams et al., 2004). There is increasing evidence that not only do 2–5% of ALS patients present an ALS/dementia complex but also that patients with classical ALS without obvious clinical evidence of cognitive deficits may have subtle changes in frontal cortical function (Ludolph et al., 1992; Kew et al., 1993b; Lulé et al., 2005; Lomen-Hoerth et al., 2002). The cognitive impairment has been reported as more pronounced in ALS patients with a bulbar onset compared to patients with spinal onset (Abrahams et al., 1997; Strong et al., 1999; Lomen-Hoerth et al., 2002; Schreiber et al., 2005) and is also evident in patients with primary lateral sclerosis (PLS; Piquard et al., 2006). Longitudinal investigation of ALS patients (up to 18 months) revealed that cognitive dysfunction in ALS occurred early in the disease course and that the cognitive deficits may not progress in synchrony with motor decline, but distinctly more slowly (Schreiber et al., 2005). Functional imaging studies confirm hypoperfusion in the resting state in the frontal cortex in ALS with or without cognitive deficits (Ludolph et al., 1992; Anzai et al., 1990; Tanaka et al., 1993). Apart from the local hypometabolism, there is also evidence for decreased activity in different cortical areas during the performance of different tasks. Findings from fMRI studies support the association of reduced frontal executive function and reduced activity in fronto-parietal areas, and confirm findings from studies using other imaging techniques (Kew et al., 1993b; Abrahams et al., 1996). In non-demented ALS patients, a correlation between reduced verbal fluency and reduced activity in middle and inferior frontal gyrus, anterior cingulate cortex, and parietal and temporal lobe have been observed in an fMRI study by Abrahams et al. which included 22 non-demented ALS patients compared with 18 healthy controls (Abrahams et al., 2004). There is no evidence of additional recruitment in other areas to compensate the functional loss in the frontal cortex, as has been shown for the motor system. Cognitive functions of frontal areas do not exhibit redundancy of motor pathways, and compensation is therefore not possible. Further longitudinal fMRI studies of different cognitive functions in ALS might improve our understanding of subclinical cognitive deficits in ALS.

Further differences in cortical pattern activation were observed in ALS patients without significant cognitive impairments during processing of socio-emotional stimuli. Pictures of persons in emotional situations were presented to 13 ALS patients and 15 healthy controls at an initial measurement and to 10 of these ALS patients and 14 healthy controls at a second measurement after six months. ALS patients presented an increased activity in the right-sided supramarginal area (BA 40), which is part of the social-information processing network. This difference in social-information processing pattern increased over the course of six months (Lulé et al., 2007b). The increased activity in the social information-processing pathway might represent an altered sensitivity to social-emotional cues in ALS patients without cognitive deficits (Lulé et al., 2007b). Reduced activity in right sided frontal areas during processing of aversive emotional stimuli in ALS patients compared to controls support the assumption of an impaired processing pathway in ALS (Palmieri et al., 2010). More research is required to determine how successful and stable this compensatory recruitment is and again fMRI may be an important step.

## 6. Functional neuroimaging in other neurodegenerative diseases like dementia, Parkinson's disease, and Huntington's disease

### 6.1 Functional neuroimaging in dementia

There is the described overlap of dementia and motor neuron diseases, however, contrary to the above described prominent role in MND, the role of imaging in dementia has traditionally been directed at ruling out treatable and reversible aetiologies (Tartaglia et al., 2011). Contrary to motor neuron diseases it was rarely used to better understand the pathophysiology of the different dementias.

Structural CT and MRI scans are mainly used to assess volumetric changes in dementias with decreases in gyral and increases in sulcal size secondary to decrease in synaptic density, neuronal loss, and cell shrinkage (Tartaglia et al., 2010). The medial temporal lobes, especially the hippocampus and entorhinal cortex (ERC), are among the earliest sites of pathologic involvement in AD (Braak & Braak, 1991), and studies have repeatedly shown decreased hippocampal and ERC volumes in patients with AD compared with age-matched controls (Appel et al., 2009). Other severely affected areas include the lateral parietal and posterior superior temporal regions and medial posterior portion of the cingulate gyrus (Jones et al., 2006), but atrophy is also evident in the frontal, temporal, and occipital lobes (Rusinek et al., 1991). Recent neuropathological data provide evidence that disease pathology starts in locus coeruleus and propagates into transentorhinal region and other cerebral regions (Braak & Del Tredici, 2011a). MRI of hippocampal and cortical regions in the parietal and lateral temporal regions has been successfully used as prognostic marker in patients with mild cognitive impairment (MCI) to develop AD (Du et al., 2003; Schott et al., 2003). High field MRI provided evidence for a sensitivity of the thickness of CA1 to distinguish subjects with AD from normal controls (Kerchner et al., 2010). Like in ALS, white matter (WM) pathology was long not in focus of research. However, recent work provides evidence for WM changes in AD and MCI in association with cognitive changes (Zhang et al., 2007; Sexton et al., 2010). It might even be useful to distinguish different forms of dementia (Firbank et al., 2007; Zhang et al., 2009). NAA spectroscopy has been used as a possible diagnostic marker in dementia. NAA is consistently reported as being lower in the parietal gray matter and hippocampus of patients with AD than in cognitively normal elderly subjects (Schuff et al., 2002).

On the functional level of the brain, evidence for a reduced function of frontal areas in FTD compared to AD was seen using fMRI (Rombouts et al., 2003). Furthermore, alterations in the default mode network (areas active during rest and idling of the brain) in resting state have been found for AD and MCI patients (Tartaglia et al., 2011). In the future, the application of neuroimaging in dementia will increase, as there will be extended evidence for prognostic and clinical marker for different forms of dementia.

### 6.2 Functional neuroimaging in Parkinson's disease

Like in most neurodegenerative diseases, neuroimaging in Parkinson's disease has been challenging because the majorities of neurons are affected before clinical symptoms evolve and diagnosis is made. The clinical symptoms of PD appear when approximately 50-80% of the nigral dopamine (DA) neurons have been lost already. Consequently, structural imaging has in general been unrewarding, although some newer MRI techniques, such as diffusion tensor imaging or shape analysis, are somewhat more promising and provided evidence for a reduced volume and changed connectivity of substantia nigra (Stössl, 2011). Functional neuroimaging is a promising candidate to detect specific changes in PD. Functional connectivity measured with resting state MRI provided evidence for changed pattern in motor network (Wu et al., 2009; Helmich et al., 2010) and in the default network (Palmer et al., 2010). MRI spectroscopy may be useful in differentiating between PD and atypical parkinsonian syndromes (Firbank et al., 2002). Functional MRI in PD has been widely used and proven to be sensitive to e.g. polymorphism of catechol-O-metyltransferase (COMT) in PD. Different activation patterns in fronto-parietal areas in an fMRI task provided a clear link to genotype, dopaminergic medication and cognitive performance in PD patients (Williams-Gray et al., 2007, 2008). In the future, functional neuroimaging may be used to get a fast and objective means of functional and genetic status in advanced stage PD patients.

### 6.3 Functional neuroimaging in Huntington's disease

Among neurodegenerative disorders, HD is unique in that individuals destined to develop symptoms can be identified through genetic testing before clinical signs of the disease begin. This raises the possibility of developing therapies to prevent or delay the onset of clinical manifestations in HD gene carriers. Therefore, substantial effort has been dedicated to the characterization of quantitative descriptors of disease progression in premanifest individuals (Eidelberg & Surmeier, 2011). Neuroimaging may be used to clarify diagnosis in the pre-symptomatic stage. The idea of imaging as a preclinical marker in HD was supported by findings in a prospective observational study (Tabrizi et al., 2011).

The vast number of neuroimaging studies in HD traditionally was on single brain regions like structural and functional studies on the striatum. Several PET studies revealed association of striatal and cortical dysfunction in association with genetic alterations and cognitive function. However, with the evolvement of MRI volumetric studies with low patient load, better insight on striatal function was found in a faster and easier way. However, even with this technique, systems-level changes might not be detectable. Connectivity studies like in resting state MRI might be more susceptible and applicable in the future.

## 7. Conclusion

Despite different aetiology of neurodegenerative diseases, similar approaches have been used in diseases of the central and peripheral nervous system. MRI based neuroimaging has extended our understanding of involvement of cortical structures which by far outreach the usually described clinical changes. Different neuroimaging techniques provide limitations that can be compensated by other techniques. Structural and functional MRI has taken over radio nucleotide dependent measurements in clinical setting due to low patient load. Spectroscopy and resting state analysis will extend our understanding of molecular and functional changes of cortical structures and networks. MRI neuroimaging has the potential to fill the gap between pathogenesis and clinical outcome of neurodegenerative diseases.

## 8. Future advances of neuroimaging in neurodegeneration

### 8.1 Brain-computer interfaces

Brain computer interfaces (BCIs) are a technique, which transfers and translates brain signals to technical devices for communication, control of environment (e.g. light switches) or prosthetic devices. BCIs are the only applicable means for communication in patients with advanced neurodegenerative diseases and no voluntary muscle control like in complete locked-in patients (CLIS) at end stage of ALS. There has been the unsolved question why patients in CLIS are unable to control EEG BCIs (Kübler & Birbaumer, 2008). With the means of functional neuroimaging, the question of activity of the idling brain of CLIS patients might be solved. Neuroimaging provide essential insight into the brains of patients with neurodegenerative diseases who are unable to communicate due to the loss of motor control like in ALS or cognitive ability like in dementia.

### 8.2 Clinical implications

MRI based neuroimaging has been extensively applied in diagnosis of neurodegenerative diseases. Low patient load and high applicability are in favour for this technique. Availability of MRI scanner in many clinics has already made neuroimaging an essential key in diagnosis of neurodegenerative diseases. The value of neuroimaging techniques for biomarker is still subject to ongoing debate; yet, there is a strong need for easy to apply biomarkers. In most neurodegenerative diseases, loss and death of motor neurons occur long before onset of clinical symptoms. Diagnosis is usually based on clinical symptoms when the majority of target cells are already affected. Braak and colleagues in Alzheimer's disease have provided evidence for this. Tau tangles are found up to 30-50 years prior to onset of clinical symptoms (Braak & Braak, 1991; Braak & Del Tredici, 2011b). Effective therapeutic trials, however, ask for application as early as possible. Emergence of several disease-modifying drugs in neurodegenerative diseases has particularly highlighted the need for biomarkers of therapeutic response. Unwanted drug effects has brought additional requirement for effective biomarkers for optimal initial patient selection and timing of discontinuation (Turner et al., 2011). In the future, in search for robust biomarkes, MRI based neuroimaging techniques are a promising candidate.

## 9. Acknowledgement

Volker Diekmann, Hans-Peter Müller, Jan Kassubek and Alexander Unrath (all University of Ulm) are thankfully acknowledged for their help in the course of the fMRI and DTI experiments and data analyses. Special thanks to Sonja Fuchs and Sandra Pauli (University of Ulm) for technical assistance in MRI measurements and Johanna Heimrath for her help with the manuscript. We would like to thank Corinna Hendrich, Regina Gastl and Anne Sperfeld (all University of Ulm) for supporting us in the recruitment of patients. Special thanks to the patients and healthy subjects who participated in our studies.

## 10. References

Abrahams S, Goldstein LH, Kew JJ, Brooks DJ, Lloyd CM, Frith CD, Leigh PN. Frontal lobe dysfunction in amyotrophic lateral sclerosis. A PET study. Brain 1996;119 (6):2105-20.

Abrahams S, Goldstein LH, Al-Chalabi A, Pickering A, Morris RG, Passingham RE, Brooks DJ, Leigh PN. Relation between cognitive dysfunction and pseudobulbar palsy in amyotrophic lateral sclerosis. J Neurol Neurosurg Psychiatry 1997;62(5):464-72.

Abrahams S, Goldstein LH, Simmons A, Brammer M, Williams SC, Giampietro V, Leigh PN. Word retrieval in amyotrophic lateral sclerosis: a functional magnetic resonance imaging study. Brain 2004;127(7):1507-17.

Anzai E, Shiozawa Z, Shindo K, Tsunoda S, Koizumi K, Uchiyama G. 123I-iodoamphetamine single photon emission computed tomography in three patients with amyotrophic lateral sclerosis. Kaku Igaku 1990;27(8):863-7.

Appel J, Potter E, Shen Q, et al. A comparative analysis of structural brain MRI in the diagnosis of Alzheimer's disease. Behav Neurol 2009;21:13–19.

Berger H. Über das Elektrenkephalogramm des Menschen in: Arch f Psychiatr 1929;87:527-570.

Braak H, Bohl JR, Müller CM, Rüb U, de Vos RA, Del Tredici K.Stanley Fahn Lecture 2005: The staging procedure for the inclusion body pathology associated with sporadic Parkinson's disease reconsidered. Mov Disord. 2006a;21(12):2042-51.

Braak H, Braak E. Neuropathological stageing of Alzheimer-related changes. Acta Neuropathol (Berl) 1991;82:239–259.

Braak H, Del Tredici K. Alzheimer's pathogenesis: is there neuron-to-neuron propagation? Acta Neuropathol. 2011a;121(5):589-95.

Braak H, Del Tredici K. The pathological process underlying Alzheimer's disease in individuals under thirty. Acta Neuropathol. 2011b;121(2):171-81.

Braak H, Rüb U, Schultz C, Del Tredici K. Vulnerability of cortical neurons to Alzheimer's and Parkinson's diseases. J Alzheimers Dis. 2006b;9(3):35-44.

Brooks BR, Bushara K, Khan A, Hershberger J, Wheat JO, Belden D et al. Functional magnetic resonance imaging (fMRI) clinical studies in ALS--paradigms, problems and promises. Amyotroph Lateral Scler Other Motor Neuron Disord 2000;1(2):23-32.

Brownell B, Oppenheimer DR, Hughes JT. The central nervous system in motor neurone disease. J Neurol Neurosurg Psychiatry 1970;33:338–357.

Cohen, D. Magnetoencephalography: evidence of magnetic fields produced by alpha rhythm currents. Science 1968;161:784-786

Di Salle F, Formisano E, Linden DE, Goebel R, Bonavita S, Pepino A, Smaltino F, Tedeschi G. Exploring brain function with magnetic resonance imaging. Eur J Radiol 1999;30(2):84-94.

Du AT, Schuff N, Zhu XP, et al. Atrophy rates of entorhinal cortex in AD and normal aging. Neurology 2003;60:481–486.

Edelman RR, Wielopolski P, Schmitt F. Echo-planar MR imaging. Radiology 1994;192(3):600-12.

Eidelberg D, Surmeier DJ. Brain networks in Huntington disease. J Clin Invest. 2011;121(2):484-92.

Firbank MJ, Harrison RM, O'Brien JT. A comprehensive review of proton magnetic resonance spectroscopy studies in dementia and Parkinson's disease. Dement Geriatr Cogn Disord 2002;14:64–76.

Firbank MJ, Blamire AM, Krishnan MS, et al. Diffusion tensor imaging in dementia with Lewy bodies and Alzheimer's disease. Psychiatry Res 2007;155:135–145.

Frahms J, Fransson P, Krüger G. Magentic resonance imaging of human brain function. In Winhorst U, Johanssen H (eds.): Modern techniques in neuroscience research; Springer, Heidelberg, 1999.

Grammas P, Martinez J, Miller B. Cerebral microvascular endothelium and the pathogenesis of neurodegenerative diseases. Expert Rev Mol Med. 2011 Jun 10;13:e19.

Hacke W. Neurologie; Springer, Heidelberg, 2010.

Han J, Ma L. Functional magnetic resonance imaging study of the brain in patients with amyotrophic lateral sclerosis. Chin Med Sci J 2006;21(4):228-33

Helmich RC, Derikx LC, Bakker M, Scheeringa R, Bloem BR, Toni I. Spatial remapping of cortico-striatal connectivity in Parkinson's disease. Cereb Cortex 2010;20:1175–1186.

Isaacs JD, Dean AF, Shaw CE, Al-Chalabi A, Mills KR, Leigh PN. Amyotrophic lateral sclerosis with sensory neuropathy: part of a multisystem disorder? J Neurol Neurosurg Psychiatry 2007;78(7):750-3.

Jezzard P, Buxton RB. The clinical potential of functional magnetic resonance imaging. J Magn Reson Imaging 2006;23(6):787-93.

Jones BF, Barnes J, Uylings HB, et al. Differential regional atrophy of the cingulate gyrus in Alzheimer disease: a volumetric MRI study. Cereb Cortex 2006;16:1701–1708.

Kerchner GA, Hess, CP, Hammond-Rosenbluth KE, et al. Hippocampal CA1 apical neuropil atrophy in mild Alzheimer disease visualized with 7-T MRI. Neurology 2010;75:1381–1387

Kew JJM, Leigh PN, Playford ED, Passingham RE, Goldstein LH, Frackowiak RS, Brooks DJ. Cortical function in amyotrophic lateral sclerosis. A positron emission tomography study. Brain 1993a;116:655-680.

Kew JJ, Goldstein LH, Leigh PN, Abrahams S, Cosgrave N, Passingham RE, Frackowiak RS, Brooks DJ. The relationship between abnormalities of cognitive function and cerebral activation in amyotrophic lateral sclerosis. A neuropsychological and positron emission tomography study. Brain 1993b;116 (6):1399-423.

Kew JJM, Brooks DJ, Passingham RE, Rothwell JC, Frackowiak RS, Leigh PN. Cortical function in progressive lower motor neuron disorders and amyotrophic lateral sclerosis: A comparative PET study. Neurology 1994;44:1101-1110.

Kim SG, Ugurbil K. Functional magnetic resonance imaging of the human brain. J Neurosci Methods 1997a;74(2):229-43.

Kim SG, Uğurbil K. Comparison of blood oxygenation and cerebral blood flow effects in fMRI: estimation of relative oxygen consumption change. Magn Reson Med 1997b;38(1):59-65.

Konrad C, Henningsen H, Bremer J, , Mock B, Deppe M, Buchinger C, Turski P, Knecht S, Brooks B. Pattern of cortical reorganization in amyotrophic lateral sclerosis: a functional magnetic resonance imaging study. Exp Brain Res 2002;143(1):51-56.

Konrad C, Jansen A, Henningsen H, Sommer J, Turski PA, Brooks BR, Knecht S. Subcortical reorganization in amyotrophic lateral sclerosis. Exp Brain Res 2006;172(3):361-9.

Kübler A, Birbaumer N. Brain-computer interfaces and communication in paralysis: extinction of goal directed thinking in completely paralysed patients? Clin Neurophysiol. 2008;119(11):2658-66.

Kwong KK, Belliveau JW, Chesler DA, Goldberg IE, Weisskoff RM, Poncelet BP, Kennedy DN, Hoppel BE, Cohen MS, Turner R, et al. Dynamic magnetic resonance imaging of human brain activity during primary sensory stimulation. Proc Natl Acad Sci USA 1992;89(12):5675-9.

Kwong KK. Functional magnetic resonance imaging with echo planar imaging. Magn Reson Q 1995;11(1):1-20.

Logothetis NK, Pauls J, Augath M, Trinath T, Oeltermann A. Neurophysiological investigation of the basis of the fMRI signal. Nature 2001; 412(6843):150-7.

Logothetis NK, Pfeuffer J. On the nature of the BOLD fMRI contrast mechanism. Magn Reson Imaging 2004;22(10):1517-31.

Lomen-Hoerth C, Anderson T, Miller B. The overlap of amyotrophic lateral sclerosis and frontotemporal dementia. Neurology 2002;59(7):1077-9.

Ludolph AC, Dengler R: Geschichte, Epidemiologie und diagnostische Kriterien. In: Dengler R, Ludolph A, Zierz S. Amyotrophe Lateralsklerose. 2nd ed. Thieme, Stuttgart, 1999., pp. 1-16 (1999)

Ludolph AC, Langen KJ, Regard M, Herzog H, Kemper B, Kuwert T, Böttger IG, Feinendegen L. Frontal lobe function in amyotrophic lateral sclerosis: a neuropsychologic and positron emission tomography study. Acta Neurol Scand 1992;85(2):81-9.

Lulé D, Kurt A, Jürgens R, Kassubek J, Diekmann V, Kraft E, Neumann N, Ludolph AC, Birbaumer N, Anders S. Emotional responding in amyotrophic lateral sclerosis. J Neurol 2005;252:1517-1524.

Lulé D, Diekmann V, Kassubek J, Kurt A, Birbaumer N, Ludolph AC, Kraft E. Cortical Plasticity in Amyotrophic Lateral Sclerosis: Motor Imagery and Function. Neurorehabil Neural Repair. 2007a;21(6):518-26.

Lulé D, Diekmann V, Anders S, Kassubek J, Kubler A, Ludolph AC, Birbaumer N. Brain responses to emotional stimuli in patients with amyotrophic lateral sclerosis (ALS). J Neurol. 2007b;254(4):519-27.

Lulé D, Ludolph AC, Kassubek J. MRI-based functional neuroimaging in ALS: An update. Amyotroph Lateral Scler. 2009;10(5-6):258-68.

Lulé D, Diekmann V, Müller HP, Kassubek J, Ludolph AC, Birbaumer N. Neuroimaging of multimodal sensory stimulation in Amyotrophic Lateral Sclerosis (ALS). JNNP 2010;81(8):899-906.

Mai R, Facchetti D, Micheli A, Poloni M. Quantitative electroencephalography in amyotrophic lateral sclerosis. Electroencephalogr Clin Neurophysiol 1998;106(4): 383-6.

Mohammadi B, Kollewe K, Samii A, Krampfl K, Dengler R, Münte TF. Changes of resting state brain networks in amyotrophic lateral sclerosis. Exp Neurol. 2009;217(1):147-53.

Mohammadi B, Kollewe K, Samii A, Dengler R, Münte TF. Functional neuroimaging at different disease stages reveals distinct phases of neuroplastic changes in amyotrophic lateral sclerosis. Hum Brain Mapp. 2011;32(5):750-8.

Münte TF, Tröger MC, Nusser I, Wieringa BM, Johannes S, Matzke M, Dengler R. Alteration of early components of the visual evoked potential in amyotrophic lateral sclerosis. J Neurol 1998;245(4):206-10.

Neumann M, Sampathu DM, Kwong LK, Truax AC, Micsenyi MC, Chou TT, Bruce J, Schuck T, Grossman M, Clark CM, McCluskey LF, Miller BL, Masliah E, Mackenzie IR, Feldman H, Feiden W, Kretzschmar HA, Trojanowski JQ, Lee VM. Ubiquitinated TDP-43 in frontotemporal lobar degeneration and amyotrophic lateral sclerosis. Science. 2006;314(5796):130-3.

Norris DG. Principles of magnetic resonance assessment of brain function. J Magn Reson Imaging 2006;23(6):794-807.

Ogawa S, Lee TM, Nayak AS, Glynn P. Oxygenation-sensitive contrast in magnetic resonance image of rodent brain at high magnetic fields. Magn Reson Med 1990a;14(1):68-78.

Ogawa S, Lee TM, Kay AR, Tank DW. Brain magnetic resonance imaging with contrast dependent on blood oxygenation. Proc Natl Acad Sci USA 1990b;87(24):9868-72.

Ogawa S, Tank DW, Menon R, Ellermann JM, Kim SG, Merkle H, Ugurbil K. Intrinsic signal changes accompanying sensory stimulation: functional brain mapping with magnetic resonance imaging. Proc Natl Acad Sci USA 1992;89(13):5951-5.

Palmer SJ, Li J, Wang ZJ, McKeown MJ. Joint amplitude and connectivity compensatory mechanisms in Parkinson's disease. Neuroscience 2010;166:1110–1118.

Palmieri A, Naccarato M, Abrahams S, Bonato M, D'Ascenzo C, Balestreri S, Cima V, Querin G, Dal Borgo R, Barachino L, Volpato C, Semenza C, Pegoraro E, Angelini C, Sorarù G. Right hemisphere dysfunction and emotional processing in ALS: an fMRI study. J Neurol. 2010;257(12):1970-8.

Pauling L, Coryell CD. The Magnetic Properties and Structure of Hemoglobin, Oxyhemoglobin and Carbonmonoxyhemoglobin. Proc Natl Acad Sci USA 1936;22(4):210-6.

Pekkonen E, Osipova D, Laaksovirta H. Magnetoencephalographic evidence of abnormal auditory processing in amyotrophic lateral sclerosis with bulbar signs. Clin Neurophysiol 2004;115(2):309-15.

Phelps ME, Hoffman EJ, Mullani NA, Ter-Pogossian MM. Application of annihilation coincidence detection to transaxial reconstruction tomography. J Nucl Med 1975;16(3):210-24.

Pinkhardt EH, Jürgens R, Becker W, Mölle M, Born J, Ludolph AC, Schreiber H.Signs of impaired selective attention in patients with amyotrophic lateral sclerosis. J Neurol. 2008;255(4):532-8.

Piquard A, Le Forestier N, Baudoin-Madec V, Delgadillo D, Salachas F, Pradat PF, Derouesné C, Meininger V, Lacomblez L. Neuropsychological changes in patients with primary lateral sclerosis. Amyotroph Lateral Scler. 2006;7(3):150-60.

Pugdahl K, Fuglsang-Frederiksen A, de Carvalho M, Johnsen B, Fawcett PR, Labarre-Vila A, Liguori R, Nix WA, Schofield IS. Generalised sensory system abnormalities in amyotrophic lateral sclerosis: a European multicentre study. J Neurol Neurosurg Psychiatry 2007;78(7):746-9.

Roberts TP, Mikulis D. Neuro MR: principles. J Magn Reson Imaging 2007;26(4):823-37.

Rombouts SA, van Swieten JC, Pijnenburg YA, Goekoop R, Barkhof F, Scheltens P. Loss of frontal fMRI activation in early frontotemporal dementia compared to early AD. Neurology 2003;60:1904–1908.

Rusinek H, de Leon MJ, George AE, et al. Alzheimer disease: measuring loss of cerebral gray matter with MR imaging. Radiology 1991;178:109–114.

Schmitt F, Stehling MK, Turner R. Echo-planar imaging theory, technique and application. Berlin: Springer; 1998.

Schott JM, Fox NC, Frost C, et al. Assessing the onset of structural change in familial Alzheimer's disease. Ann Neurol 2003;53:181–188.

Schreiber H, Gaigalat T, Wiedemuth-Catrinescu U, Graf M, Uttner I, Muche R, Ludolph AC. Cognitive function in bulbar- and spinal-onset amyotrophic lateral sclerosis. A longitudinal study in 52 patients. J Neurol 2005;252(7):772-81.

Schuff N, Capizzano AA, Du AT, et al. Selective reduction of Nacetylaspartate in medial temporal and parietal lobes in AD. Neurology 2002;58:928–935.

Schoenfeld MA, Tempelmann C, Gaul C, Kühnel GR, Düzel E, Hopf JM, Feistner H, Zierz S, Heinze HJ, Vielhaber S. Functional motor compensation in amyotrophic lateral sclerosis. J Neurol 2005;252:944-952.

Sexton CE, Mackay CE, Lonie JA, et al. MRI correlates of episodic memory in Alzheimer's disease, mild cognitive impairment, and healthy aging. Psychiatry Res 2010;184:57–62.

Stanton BR, Williams VC, Leigh PN, Williams SC, Blain CR, Jarosz JM, Simmons A. Altered cortical activation during a motor task in ALS : Evidence for involvement of central pathways. J Neurol 2007a;254(9):1260-7.

Stanton BR, Williams VC, Leigh PN, Williams SC, Blain CR, Giampietro VP, Simmons A. Cortical activation during motor imagery is reduced in Amyotrophic Lateral Sclerosis. Brain Res 2007b;1172:145-51.

Stoessl AJ. Neuroimaging in Parkinson's disease. Neurotherapeutics. 2011;8(1):72-81.

Strong MJ, Grace GM, Orange JB, Leeper HA, Menon RS, Aere C. A prospective study of cognitive impairment in ALS. Neurology 1999;53(8):1665-70.

Tabrizi SJ, Scahill RI, Durr A, Roos RA, Leavitt BR, Jones R, Landwehrmeyer GB, Fox NC, Johnson H, Hicks SL, Kennard C, Craufurd D, Frost C, Langbehn DR, Reilmann R, Stout JC; TRACK-HD Investigators. Biological and clinical changes in premanifest and early stage Huntington's disease in the TRACK-HD study: the 12-month longitudinal analysis. Lancet Neurol. 2011 Jan;10(1):31-42.

Tanaka M, Kondo S, Hirai S, Sun X, Yamagishi T, Okamoto K. Cerebral blood flow and oxygen metabolism in progressive dementia associated with amyotrophic lateral sclerosis. J Neurol Sci 1993;120(1):22-8.

Tartaglia MC, Rosen HJ, Miller BL. Neuroimaging in dementia. Neurotherapeutics. 2011;8(1):82-92.

Ter-Pogossian MM, Phelps ME, Hoffman EJ, Mullani NA. A positron-emission transaxial tomograph for nuclear imaging (PETT). Radiology 1975;114(1):89-98.

Tessitore A, Esposito F, Monsurro MR, Graziano S, Panza D, Russo A, Migliaccio R, Conforti FL, Morrone R, Quattrone A, Di Salle F, Tedeschi G. Subcortical motor plasticity in patients with sporadic ALS: An fMRI study. Brain Res Bull 2006;69(5):489-94.

Triantafyllou C, Hoge RD, Kruger G, Wiggins CJ, Potthast A, Wiggins GC, Wald LL. Comparison of physiological noise at 1.5 T, 3 T and 7 T and optimization of fMRI acquisition parameters. Neuroimage 2005;26:243–250.

Turner MR, Grosskreutz J, Kassubek J, Abrahams S, Agosta F, Benatar M, Filippi M, Turner R, Howseman A, Rees GE, Josephs O, Friston K. Functional magnetic resonance imaging of the human brain: data acquisition and analysis. Exp Brain Res 1998;123:5–12.

Turner MR, Grosskreutz J, Kassubek J, Abrahams S, Agosta F, Benatar M, Filippi M, Goldstein LH, van den Heuvel M, Kalra S, Lulé D, Mohammadi B; first Neuroimaging Symosium in ALS (NISALS). Towards a neuroimaging biomarker for amyotrophic lateral sclerosis. Lancet Neurol. 2011;10(5):400-3.

van Geuns RJ, Wielopolski PA, de Bruin HG, Rensing BJ, van Ooijen PM, Hulshoff M, Oudkerk M, de Feyter PJ. Basic principles of magnetic resonance imaging. Prog Cardiovasc Dis 1999;42(2):149-56.

Vieregge P, Wauschkuhn B, Heberlein I, Hagenah J, Verleger R. Selective attention is impaired in amyotrophic lateral sclerosis--a study of event-related EEG potentials. Brain Res Cogn Brain Res 1999;8(1):27-35.

Weiller C, May A, Sach M, Buhmann C, Rijntjes M. Role of functional imaging in neurological disorders. J Magn Reson Imaging 2006;23(6):840-50.

Williams-Gray CH, Hampshire A, Robbins TW, Owen AM, Barker RA. Catechol O-methyltransferase Val158Met genotype influences frontoparietal activity during planning in patients with Parkinson's disease. J Neurosci 2007;27:4832–4838.

Williams-Gray CH, Hampshire A, Barker RA, Owen AM. Attentional control in Parkinson's disease is dependent on COMT val 158 met genotype. Brain 2008;131:397–408.

Wu T, Wang L, Chen Y, Zhao C, Li K, Chan P. Changes of functional connectivity of the motor network in the resting state in Parkinson's disease. Neurosci Lett 2009;460:6–10.

Zhang Y, Schuff N, Jahng GH, et al. Diffusion tensor imaging of cingulum fibers in mild cognitive impairment and Alzheimer disease. Neurology 2007;68:13–19.

Zhang Y, Schuff N, Du AT, et al. White matter damage in frontotemporal dementia and Alzheimer's disease measured by diffusion MRI. Brain 2009;132:2579–2592.

# 3

# Early Detection of Alzheimer's Disease with Cognitive Neuroscience Methods

Jinglong Wu, Chunlin Li and Jiajia Yang
*Biomedical Engineering Laboratory, Graduate School of Natural Science and Technology, Okayama University, Okayama, Japan*

## 1. Introduction

Recently, the exploration of human brain function was examined in cognitive neuroscience and brain science. Along with the development of engineering technology, such as measurement technology, information technology, and artificial intelligence, we can record the brain activity on the timeframe of milliseconds or at the level of a single neuron to examine basic visual function or high level brain function (e.g., memory, language, or attention). In this chapter, we introduce a new research field that combines engineering and cognitive neuroscience, which was named "Neuromedical Engineering". We focused our research on five topics: 1. tactile perception and neurology (Yang et al., 2011a, 2011b, 2011c, 2010a, 2011; Wu et al., 2010a, 2011); 2. attention and cognitive brain function (Wu & Li, 2009) and multisensory integration (Li et al, 2009a, 2010a, 2010b; Touge et al., 2008; Wu & Kakura, 2010; Wu et al., 2009); 3. basic visual cognition (Li et al., 2009b; Wu et al., 2011; Yan et al., 2011); 4. language (Cai et al., 2007; Li et al., 2011a, 2011b; Wu et al., 2007); and 5. tactile perception and rehabilitation (Bai et al., 2010). Focusing on these five topics, we provide information on human brain function and neurology. Furthermore, using these cognitive and neurological methods, we are challenging the topic of "Early Detection of Alzheimer's Disease with Cognitive Neuroscience Methods".

The earliest symptoms of Alzheimer's disease (AD) involves learning, memory or planning problems. Currently, no medical tests are available to diagnose AD conclusively pre-mortem. However, several studies have used cognitive tasks (i.e., visuospatial tasks and language tasks) to discover preclinical cognitive markers of AD. These studies demonstrated that the cognitive deficits of AD can possibly be detected during a preclinical period that spans several years. In addition, numerous neuropathological, electrophysiological and neuroimaging studies support the hypothesis that cognitive deficits in AD are related to a possible disconnection between cortical areas. In this chapter, we describe current studies and possible future experiments on the early diagnosis method using cognitive and functional imaging testing to help with the clinical diagnosis of AD.

People with AD die an average of four to six years after diagnosis, but the duration of the disease can vary from three to 20 years. As shown in Fig. 1, the rate of cognitive decline in patients with AD was faster than healthy subjects after a specific point (before diagnosis). This specific point may be detectable using memory and planning tasks, such as visuospatial and language tasks. Recent studies have demonstrated that the cognitive deficits of AD can be detected using some simplex cognitive tests.

Previous studies have suggested that both amyloid plaques and neurofibrillary tangles are clearly visible in AD brains using microscopy. The plaques and tangles spread through the cortex in a predictable pattern as AD progresses (Fig. 2). First, during the earliest AD stage, the atrophy of brain cortices occurs in the hippocampus and the surrounding areas, and the changes may begin 20 years or more before diagnosis. Second, during the mild to moderate stages, the damage to the brain cortices is found in the temporal and parietal lobes and parts of the frontal cortex and cingulate gyrus. Finally, during the advanced AD stage, the degeneration of atrophy is found in the whole brain.

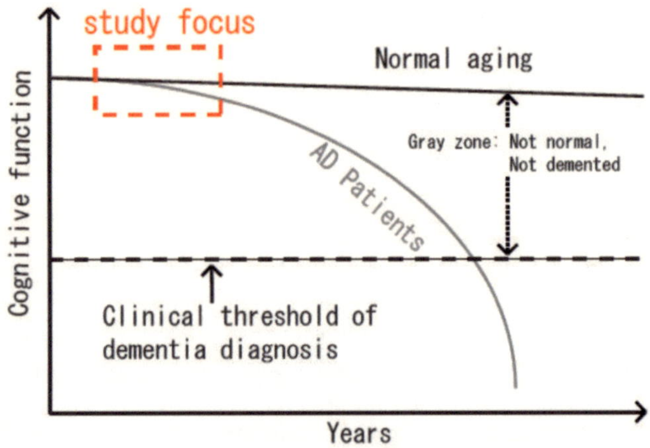


Fig. 1. The change of cognitive function deficiency model of aging healthy individuals and patients with AD.

Because the damage to the brain cortices occurs in the hippocampus, the early symptoms are mild memory loss. The first symptoms are often mistaken as related to aging or stress, but these early cognitive deficits can also be symptomatic of the early stages of AD and detected using long-term cognitive tests.

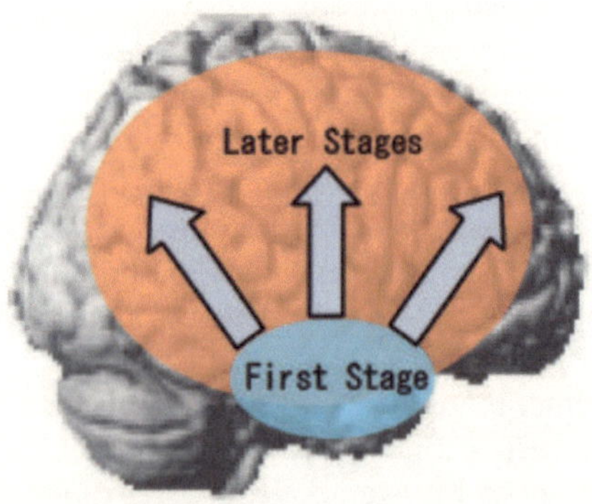


Fig. 2. The damaged cortex areas of AD patients during different stages.

Several studies have attempted to identify the preclinical cognitive markers of AD. Bäckman and Small (2007) used four episodic memory tasks on old non-dementia and incident AD subjects to investigate the cognitive deficit changes over three years. These tasks consisted of free recall of rapidly presented random words, free recall of slowly presented random words, free recall of organisable words and cued recall of organisable words. The key finding from this study suggested that although the non-dementia subjects slightly declined across the three year retest interval, the incident AD subjects showed a significant performance deficit at baseline, which was further exacerbated long-term. These findings suggest that the time of AD diagnosis is characterised by a significant decline of episodic memory. In addition, this study also indicated that a combination of global and specific cognitive measures may optimise the identification of individuals in a preclinical phase of AD.

In addition, numerous neuropathological and neuroimaging studies have suggested that the cognitive deficits in AD were related to a possible disconnection between cortical areas. The tactile and visual objects cognition are the major manual learning and memory skills of humans, which also require extensive connections between cortical areas. Thus, preclinical alterations in AD are not restricted to language tasks. There are many studies that have attempted to find cognitive markers of AD using visual, auditory or tactile tasks. This review suggested that the preclinical cognitive deficit markers of incident AD may be detectable using a combination of multisensory cognitive or functional MRI tasks.

In this chapter, we first introduce a normal study on visual and auditory orienting attention using functional magnetic resonance imaging (fMRI). Secondly, a unique tactile angle discrimination experiment was introduced, which found significant behavioural cognitive differences between normal aging and dementia.

## 2. Pilot fMRI study on spatial and temporal attention cognition of normal, young subjects

### 2.1 Introduction

The human brain is a highly efficient information processing system capable of handling a large amount of information rapidly and simultaneously. If we were able to elucidate the sophisticated mechanisms of the brain accurately, we could construct flexible, efficient, humanlike artificial systems. We would also have the capacity to assess the most relevant ways to present information and in the most appropriate manner.

Previously, we studied the human visual and auditory systems, which convey almost all external information, with an emphasis on the parallel processing of visual and auditory data. In human information processing systems, attention plays an important role in selecting and integrating information. Previous studies on attention have proposed various psychological models, which are supported by a variety of psychological and physiological evidence. The neuronal substrate of the human attention system has also been investigated using positron emission tomography (PET) and fMRI to examine visual and auditory attention in humans using audiovisual stimuli. However, the common and unique networks used by the visual and auditory attention systems remains poorly understood. Furthermore, attention to time has not been studied sufficiently compared to space, and little research has compared the differences between the visual and auditory systems regarding spatial and temporal attention.

In this study, we analysed spatial and temporal attention using both visual and auditory stimuli. To evaluate these processes behaviourally, we conducted psychological experiments where we measured the reaction times (RTs) for each task. To reveal the neuronal networks related to these attention systems, we measured the haemodynamics using fMRI.

## 2.2 Method
### 2.2.1 Subjects
The subjects were 16 healthy, right-handed students aged 21–32 years. Informed consent was obtained from each participant following a detailed explanation of the study. During fMRI scanning, visual and auditory stimuli were generated on a personal computer and presented to the subjects via a projector-screen-mirror system and headphones, respectively.

### 2.2.2 Experimental stimuli
The visual stimulus consisted of a target ("X") with a diameter of 1° eccentricity that was shown for 50 ms, 7° to the right or left of the central point on a screen located 130 cm in front of the subjects. The auditory stimulus was the sound of a 1,000 Hz sine wave presented to either ear for 50 ms. Visual and auditory experiments included space tasks (S), time tasks (T), and control tasks (N). The tasks were designed in a factorial format and are shown in Table 1.

| | Modality | |
|---|---|---|
| Task | Visual | Auditory |
| spatial | VS | AS |
| temporal | VT | AT |
| neutral | VN | AN |

Table 1. Experimental tasks

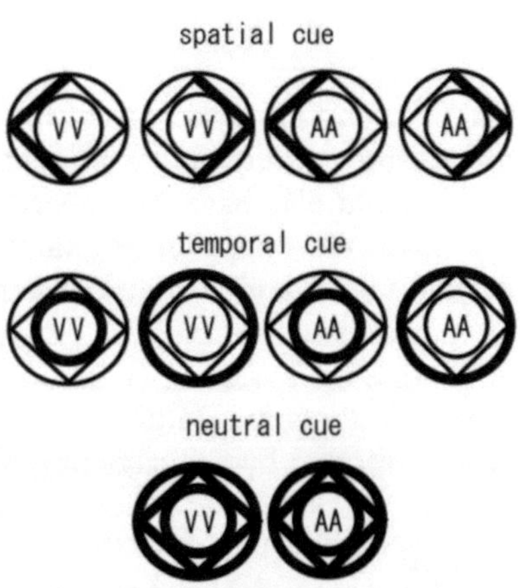


Fig. 3. Central cues used in the experimental task. The spatial cue was used in the spatial attention tasks. For the stimulus, the right or left half of the cube was lit to give the subjects information on the target location (right or left). The temporal cue was used in the temporal attention tasks. When the target came within a short cue-target interval, the inside circle was lit; and when it came after a long cue-target interval, the outside circle was lit. The neutral cue was used in the control task and gave neither spatial nor temporal information. A double 'V' in the centre of the cue indicated a visual experiment, whereas a double 'A' indicated an auditory target.

Cue stimuli (shown in fig. 3) were used to direct the subjects' attention to a particular target location or onset time. The neutral cue provided neither spatial nor temporal information; the spatial (space) cue directed the subjects' attention to the left or right; and the temporal (time) cue directed their attention to a short or long stimulus onset time. The flow chart of one trial is shown in Fig. 4. The time from the end of stimulus presentation to the onset of the next stimulus was defined as the interval of the stimuli (IOS) and was either 2,200 or 3,700 ms. We recorded the RT, the time from the presentation of a stimulus to a response indicated by a reaction key. The subjects responded to a right stimulus using the middle finger of their right hand and to a left stimulus with the forefinger of their right hand. The subjects performed 60 trials under each condition.

#### 2.2.3 fMRI scanning

We used a Philips 1.5 Tesla Magnetom Vision whole-body MRI system to measure the brain activation using a head coil. The imaging area consisted of 32 functional gradient-echo planar imaging (EPI) axial slices (voxel size 3x3x4 $mm^3$, TR=3,000 ms, TE=50 ms, FA=90°, 64x64 matrix) that were used to obtain T2*-weighted fMRI images in the axial plane. The EPI imaged the entire cortex. For each task, we obtained 124 functional volumes. Before the EPI scan, a T2-weighted volume was acquired for anatomical alignment (TR=3,500 ms, TE=100 ms, FA=90°, 256x256 matrix, voxel size=0.75x0.75x4 $mm^3$). The T2 image acquisition used the same slices as the functional image acquisition.

#### 2.2.4 Data analysis

Reaction times were used as the behavioural data. The RT data during the fMRI experiment were analysed using repeated measures analysis of variance (ANOVA; SPSS 12.0j for Windows). For each task, 60 RTs were acquired from each subject. We used the average of the RT data for the ANOVA, except for error trials (all subjects reacted with an accuracy above 90%). Therefore, we had 16 RT data for each task. Six tasks were presented in this experiment, and we compared the visual and auditory tasks separately. Between the modalities (visual and auditory), we compared VS and AS, VT and AT, and VN and AN.

For the functional images, we used MRIcro to change the DICOM files into MRIimg and MRIhdr files. In each task, the functional images of the first four volumes were not used for the data analysis. The DICOM files from the 5th through 124th scan were exported as MRIima and MRIhdr files. In addition, the DICOM files for the T2 images were exported as MRIimg and MRIhdr files.

The functional images were analysed using statistical parametric mapping (SPM5, Wellcome Department of Cognitive Neurology, London, UK). The functional images from each task were realigned using the first scan as a reference. The T2-weighted anatomical images were co-registered to the first scan in the functional images. Then, the co-registered T2-weighted anatomical images were normalised to standard T2 template images as defined by the Montreal Neurological Institute. Finally, these spatially normalised functional images were smoothed using an isotopic Gaussian kernel of 8 mm.

Statistical analyses identified the brain areas shared by visual (VS, VT) and auditory (AS, AT) attention and the brain areas that were selectively engaged by each task. To eliminate the brain activation caused by finger motion, we told the subjects to click the reaction key ten times during every rest. As a control task, we used VN for the visual attention task and AN for the auditory attention task.

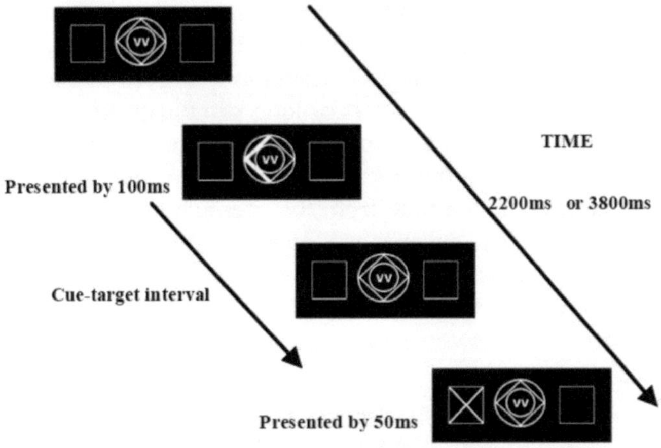


Fig. 4. Flow of a trial. The visual spatial cue indicated spatial information but provided no information about the cue-target interval. The cue was lit for 100 ms, and after the cue-target interval (300 or 1,800 ms), the target was illuminated for 50 ms.

| Task | Mean reaction time (ms) |
|---|---|
| VS | 364 (72.9) |
| VT | 373 (58.6) |
| VN | 390 (62.5) |
| AS | 394 (82.4) |
| AT | 448 (93.1) |
| AN | 460 (86.2) |

Table 2. Reaction time during each task (±SD)

## 2.3 Results

### 2.3.1 Behavioural data

Behavioural data were derived from the performance during the fMRI experiment. The reaction time for each task (Table 2) was computed from the data for the 16 subjects (the average of 16×55=880 trials).

### 2.3.2 fMRI data

From the imaging results comparing the visual tasks with the other tasks, all of the visual tasks activated the bilateral visual association cortex (BA18/19, Brodmann area). In VN, significant activation occurred only in the visual association cortex (BA18/19). From the imaging results comparing the auditory tasks with the other tasks, all of the auditory tasks activated the bilateral visual association cortex (BA18/19) because in the auditory tasks, the cues were visual as they were in the visual tasks. In addition, all of the auditory tasks activated the bilateral primary and auditory association cortex (BA41/42). In AN, significant activation occurred only in BA18/19/41/42. Therefore, as a baseline, we used VN for the visual tasks and AN for the auditory tasks.

This study focused on visual spatial attention, visual temporal attention, auditory spatial attention, and auditory temporal attention. Fig. 3 compares the activation in VS–VN, VT–VN, AS–AN, and AT–AN.

**VS-VN**

The areas of significant activation are shown in Fig. 5, and the right frontal cortex had more activations than the left. In the parietal cortex, BA7/40 was activated bilaterally, and the visual cortex had more activations on the left.

**VT-VN**

In this comparison, significant activation occurred only in the bilateral parietal cortex. In a previous study (Coull & Nobre, 1998), the medial premotor (BA6) cortex had significant activation bilaterally when the visual temporal task was compared to baseline.

**AS-AN**

More activation occurred in the left premotor (BA6) and left parietal (BA40) cortices.

**AT-AN**

Right STG was observed in this comparison.

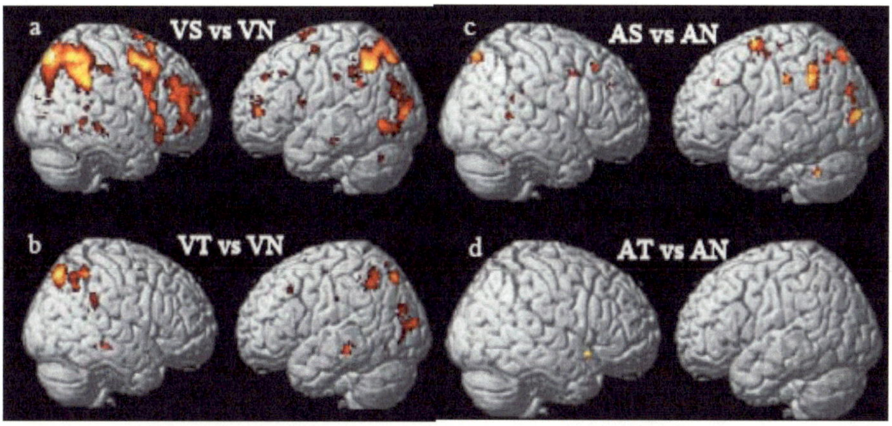


Fig. 5. Activations in visual attention and auditory attention ($p=0.001$, voxel=0). Left sides are right hemispheres in a-b, respectively.

We used SPSS for the paired t-test. The comparison of RTs across visual tasks showed a significant difference between VN and VS ($t(15)=2.53$, $p<0.05$) and between VN and VT ($t(15)=2.82$, $p<0.05$). AS and AT ($t(15)=4.86$, $p<0.001$) and AN and AS ($t(15)=6.19$, $p<0.001$) differed significantly, whereas AN and AT did not.

### 2.4 Discussion

#### 2.4.1 Baseline: At rest or during the neutral task

A previous study (Coull & Nobre, 1998) used the resting state as the baseline to be consistent with previous reports using visual fixation controls (Corbetta et al., 1993). In addition, the neutral condition engages attention and orients attention between two spatial locations and two temporal intervals.

In this study, we focused on the activation without finger movement by asking the subjects to click the reaction key ten times during rest. We compared the activation in each task with the resting state. With the exception of the visual and auditory cortices, no significant activation occurred in the N task. Therefore, we used the N task as the baseline to examine the activation that resulted from spatial or temporal cues. The activation in VS-VN in the frontal (BA4/6/47) and parietal (BA7/40) cortices was similar to previous studies (Coull & Nobre, 1998; Nobre et al., 2000). The VT-VN revealed bilateral activation in the parietal cortex (BA7) (Coull et al., 2000).

The right hemisphere bias for spatial orientation in this study was consistent with a previous report (Coull & Nobre, 1998). Therefore, we conclude that visual orienting attention uses a frontal-parietal neutral network for visual spatial orienting attention but uses the parietal cortex for visual temporal attention.

### 2.4.2 The cue used in the auditory orienting attention task

We used a visual cue in the auditory orienting attention tasks, whereas no cue was used in previous studies (Zatorre et al., 1999; Degerman et al., 2006). When comparing the activation in those studies, we found common areas in both the parietal (BA7) and frontal (BA6) cortices. In this study, the prefrontal cortex showed less activation than in previous studies (Zatorre et al., 1999; Degerman et al., 2006), and when examining the RT in the auditory orienting attention task that revealed a slow reaction, we noted that the magnetic resonance machine made a sound that drew the subjects' attention. Therefore, the AT-AN showed no activation for the same problem. One study (Schubotz et al., 2003) mentioned an auditory temporal attention task, with activation of the inferior temporal gyrus (BA20) and fusiform gyrus (BA37). In that study, only one temporal interval was used, which was different than this study.

Some studies (Loose et al., 2003; Johnson & Zatorre, 2006) used both visual and auditory stimuli to measure the attention to the stimuli feature and divided attention. Although no spatial or temporal attention task was applied using a similar task, they revealed similarities between the activation in response to visual and auditory tasks. We postulate that if the proper auditory stimulus was used in the auditory orienting attention task, neutral network activation and visual orienting attention might be demonstrated.

## 3. Tactile angle cognitive ability for distinguishing normal aging and dementia

### 3.1 Introduction

As described above, AD is a progressive neurodegenerative disease that is characterised by a loss of neurons and synapses in the cerebral cortex. Currently, many pathophysiological and molecular neurological studies (Francis et al., 1999) have focused on the cause of AD to find its clinical biomarkers, such as phosphorylated tau. In recent decades, researchers have also used PET (Huang et al., 2010) and fMRI (Delbeuck et al., 2003; Johnson et al., 2006) to assess brain functional deficits and disconnections between cerebral areas in patients with mild cognitive impairment (MCI) and AD. These studies have shown that AD brains may have different activity and connectivity patterns compared to normal brains. A few recent neuropsychological studies (Baddeley et al., 1991) have also explored the effects of disconnection between cerebral areas on cognitive functioning.

The altered cognitive symptoms in the earliest stages of AD include mild problems in learning, memory and planning (Förstl & Kurz, 1999). Unlike normally aged controls, profound impairments in working memory, episodic memory and spatial discrimination are found in patients with AD (McKhann et al., 1984). Eventually, most AD patients in the severe stages of the disease lose their ability to perform the simplest of tasks encountered in their daily routine. Mild cognitive impairment is a clinical disorder that afflicts elderly individuals and is characterised by memory impairment that does not interfere significantly with their daily living (Petersen et al., 1999). In addition, MCI is a major risk factor in the development of AD (Petersen, 2004). Currently, the mini-mental state examination (MMSE) (Folstein et al., 1975) and the clinical dementia rating (CDR) system (Morris, 1993) are used as references to help a physician determine whether a person diagnosed with memory problems has AD.

The somatosensory system is a diverse sensory system comprising the receptors and processing centres to produce the sensory modalities. Tactile spatial discrimination is one of the major manual learning and memory skills of humans. Tactile spatial acuity at the fingertips varies significantly with age (Stevens & Patterson, 1995). Previous studies have suggested two possible effects of this variation on tactile spatial discrimination: (a) differences in the central pathways of the brain leading to tactile perception and (b) differences in afferent innervation density between younger and older subjects. However, the differences in the ability to discriminate tactile angles between healthy older individuals and patients with MCI and AD has not been reported.

To differentiate two different objects by touch, humans need to store the spatial information of the first object in their working memory and then compare the spatial construction of the first object to that of the second. This procedure activates a diverse cerebral network that primarily includes areas involved with the initial processing of skin indentations (i.e., primary and secondary somatosensory cortex) (Blatow et al., 2007), the high-class areas for computation and elaborate reconstruction of shapes (i.e., part of the intraparietal sulcus) and the prefrontal cortex (Bodegård et al., 2001), which is activated for tactile working memory processing. We hypothesise that having abnormal somatosensory information processing contributes to the functional decline of tactile shape discrimination in patients with MCI and AD compared to NC individuals.

In this section from our recent study (Yang et al., 2010), we characterised tactile shape discrimination deficits in patients with MCI and AD and assessed whether tactile shape discrimination impairment could distinguish patients with MCI and AD from NC individuals. To allow a controlled study of shape, we used a restricted working definition of shape that can be applied to any object with angles (Wu et al., 2010) and to examine the ability to identify differences in raised angles in MCI and AD patients and the NC individuals. The results indicated that the decline in tactile angle discrimination in patients with MCI and AD compared to the NC group was significant.

### 3.2 Methods

#### 3.2.1 Subjects

Three groups of right-handed subjects (i.e., NC, MCI and AD) consented to participate in the study. Handedness was confirmed with the Edinburgh Handedness Inventory (EHI) (Oldfield, 1971). All MCI and AD patients were recruited from the Okayama University Hospital, Japan, and all subjects had no deficits in motor and sensory systems and deep tendon reflexes. They also reported no loss of tactile sensation or any unusual experiences with haptic input. All subjects signed informed consent forms, and the experiments were performed in accordance with a protocol approved by the Okayama University.

The NC group consisted of 14 subjects between the ages of 67 and 79, with a mean age of 71.5±3.7 years. The NC individuals were designated as "cognitively normal" when they presented no cognitively based limitations in daily living activities, and the NC was defined by an MMSE score (Folstein et al., 1975) of 27 or greater and a CDR (Hughes et al., 1982) of 0. No NC subjects had a history of neurological or psychiatric disease, and no subjects were taking any medications that affected the central nervous system at the time of testing.
The MCI group consisted of 10 subjects between the ages of 56 and 85, with a mean age of 71.3±9.4 years. Patients with amnestic MCI were diagnosed using the Petersen criteria (Petersen et al., 1999). In addition, all patients with amnestic MCI had MMSE scores of 27 or greater and CDR scale scores of 0.5. These individuals underwent magnetic resonance imaging (MRI) of the brain to confirm that they did not have a focal lesion that affected memory sensitive substrates. As assessed by the Consortium to Establish a Registry for Alzheimer's Disease cognitive battery (Morris et al., 1989), MCI patients typically show a memory performance that was 1.5 reference deviations below the age-adjusted average, which includes verbal learning, recognition and recall tests, global cognitive function and activities of daily living impairment.
The AD group consisted of 13 subjects between the ages of 57 and 83, with a mean age of 73.4±7.7 years. The diagnosis of AD was made in accordance with the National Institute of Neurological and Communicative Disorders and Stroke (NINCDS) Alzheimer's Disease and Related Disorders Association (ADRDA) criteria (Morris et al., 1989). All patients with AD had MMSE scores between 15 and 26 and a CDR score of 1 or 2, corresponding to what is known as mild to moderate AD.
In addition, all MCI and AD patients were confirmed based on a Rosen modified Hachinski ischemic score that was at least 4 (Rosen et al., 1980), and they did not show any atrophy of the somatosensory cortex on MRI. Patients were excluded if they had clinically significant neurological diseases other than MCI and AD or had a major psychiatric disorder. Psychiatric co-morbidity was excluded by history, clinical examination, and a Composite International Diagnostic Interview (Robins et al., 1988).

### 3.2.2 Apparatus and stimuli

One reference angle and eight comparison angles were used in this study. During each trial, one pair of angles consisting of the reference angle, and a comparison angle was presented to the subject. Fig. 6(a) is an illustration of the angles. In this experiment, the apex of the angles was always pointing to the right. All angles were mounted so the two arms were symmetrically placed above and below an imaginary bisector. The size of the reference angle was 60° with the eight comparison angles being larger than the reference angle by 4°, 8°, 12°, 16°, 20°, 24°, 32° and 50°. The raised angles consisted of custom-built plastic shapes that were raised 0.5 mm (Fig. 6(b)) over a 40.0 mm square base. Varying in two spatial dimensions, the angles were formed by two raised lines (i.e., the arms of the angles) at the centre of the 40.0 mm square base with an accuracy of ± 0.1°. The arms were 8.0 mm long and 1.5 mm wide.
As shown in Fig. 6(c), the two angles were clamped horizontally in the apparatus. Subjects were blindfolded and seated at a table. The right hand of the subject was fixed with tape to an immobile plastic plate with only the right index finger making contact with the angles. The apparatus consisted of an electric slide that moved the angles along the horizontal axis in the transverse plane.

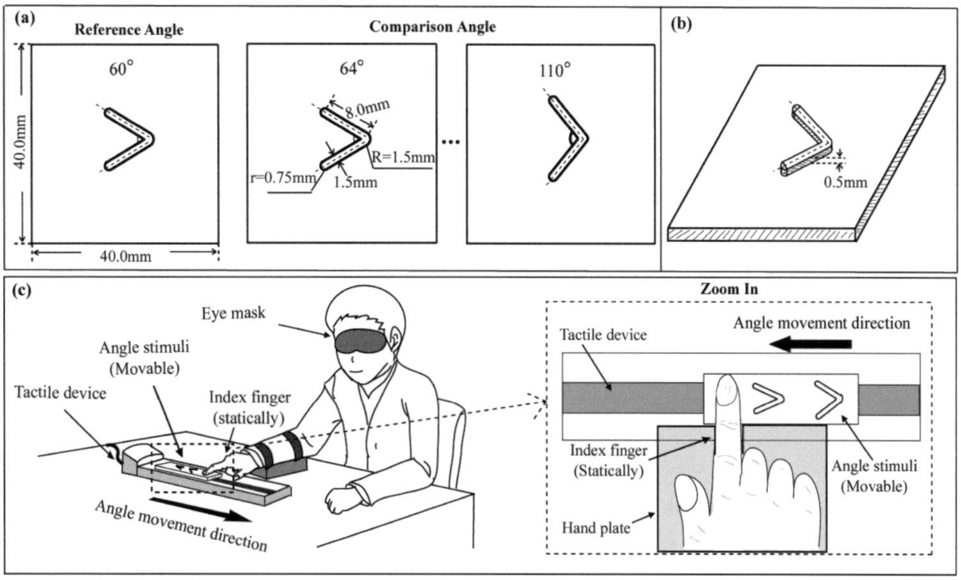


Fig. 6. Example of angle stimuli and position of subject's finger. (a) An illustration of the reference angle (60°) and two of eight comparison angles (64° and 110°) used in this experiment. (b) Three-dimensional view of an example of angle. (c) The angle movement apparatus and the subject's finger position. The reference angle and one comparison angle of a typical trial were clamped on the apparatus. These angles were moved by an electric slide on the tactile apparatus from right to left in a horizontal direction. The subject's right hand was fixed on the plate and kept static during each discrimination trial.

### 3.2.3 Procedure

We measured angle discrimination thresholds based on each subject's ability to judge the relative sizes of the reference angle and the comparison angles. All subjects were asked to place their right index fingers at the initial starting point of the plate (Fig. 6(c)). To hold the right index finger and arm in the vertical direction, the right hand was fixed to the plate, and the forearm was fixed to an immobile support stand. The subjects wore an eye mask during the task to prevent visual feedback. Moreover, all subjects were asked to keep their right hand immobile and perceive the angles passively. For AD patients, the experimenter intermittently reminded the patients of this requirement to ensure compliance with the instructions to differentiate the size of the two angles.

As shown in Fig. 6(c), the experimenter first clamped the reference angle and one of eight comparison angles on the apparatus. Then, the angles were moved under the subject's right index finger for the subject to perceive the size of the angle by following the imaginary bisector. Moreover, all angles were moved from the end points towards the apex. Each angle was scanned in succession, once per trial. The contact force was restricted, and the movement speed of the angles was maintained at 5.0 mm/s. The subject was then asked to verbally identify the larger angle in each pair of angles (2AFC: two-alternative forced choice). A pseudorandom order was used to present the reference angle and comparison angle to the subject. The reference angle was either the first or the second angle in each pair presented to the subjects who were not informed about the change in the order of angles.

Each subject underwent at least 10 practice trials prior to the start of the experiment. After the training, each pair of angles was presented 10 times in a pseudorandom order. Each subject completed 80 angle discrimination trials.

### 3.2.4 Data processing and analysis

In this study, the 2AFC technique was used to measure the angle discrimination threshold. Subjects were forced to make a choice of what they perceived was the larger of two angles even if they could not detect a difference. The logistic curve is the most common sigmoid curve used extensively in cognitive psychological experiments for measuring thresholds (Voisin et al., 2002a,b). Here, the accuracy data were applied to the following logistic function (1) (adapted from Wu et al., 2010):

$$Accuracy = \frac{1}{1 + e^{d|RA-CA|}} \quad (1)$$

In this equation, *d* represents the unique degree of freedom of the logistic curve, which was adjusted to fit the accuracy data. *RA* and *CA* represent the degree values of the reference and comparison angles, respectively.
The discrimination threshold was defined as the angle difference at an accuracy rate of 75%. Fig. 7 shows the 2AFC results of one NC subject. The discrimination threshold is indicated where the accuracy line and the 75% line (dashed line) intersect. The discrimination threshold (DT) was computed from the logistic function (2) as follows (X = 75% accuracy):

$$DT = d^{-1} Ln(\frac{1-X}{X}) \quad (2)$$

The data were incorporated into logistic functions (1) and (2). The same analyses were applied to all of the data in this experiment.

### 3.2.5 Statistics

To calculate angle discrimination thresholds, regression analysis with logistic function was performed. Differences in the accuracy and discrimination thresholds of the three subject groups were analysed using separate one-way analysis of variance (ANOVA). The level of significance was fixed at $P < 0.05$. The Bonferroni test ($\alpha = 0.05$) was performed to detect the difference between each subject group. Finally, to compare the sensitivity of angle discrimination accuracy and the MMSE score, a receiver operator characteristic (ROC) analysis was used. All analyses were performed using SPSS version 12.0j (SPSS, Tokyo, Japan).

## 3.3 Results

### 3.3.1 Accuracy

To investigate the differences in the accuracy of angle discrimination for different angle pairs, we calculated the mean accuracy for each pair of reference and comparison angles in different subject groups. The accuracy rate was defined as the number of correct trials divided by the total number of trials for each angle pair. As described above (Fig. 7), the accuracy increased with an increase in the difference between the reference angle and the comparison angle in this experiment. The regression analysis of the mean accuracy yielded significant $r^2$ values of 0.98, 0.98, and 0.67 for the NC, MCI and AD groups, respectively [NC: $F(1,6) = 323.95$, $P < 0.001$; MCI: $F(1,6) = 473.76$, $P < 0.001$; AD: $F(1,6) = 12.16$, $P = 0.013$]. The mean angle discrimination accuracy for the NC (82.1% ± 2.2%), MCI (78.6% ± 1.8%) and AD (67.9% ± 2.5%) groups is shown in Fig. 8(a). We performed a one-way ANOVA on the mean accuracy. The mean accuracy of the angle discrimination differed significantly between the three groups [$F(2,34) = 8.01$, $P = 0.001$]. A multiple comparison using the Bonferroni correction ($\alpha = 0.05$) revealed that the mean accuracy of patients with AD was significantly lower than patients with MCI ($P = 0.04$) and the NC subjects ($P = 0.001$). However, the difference in accuracy between patients with MCI and NC subjects was not significant ($P = 0.93$).

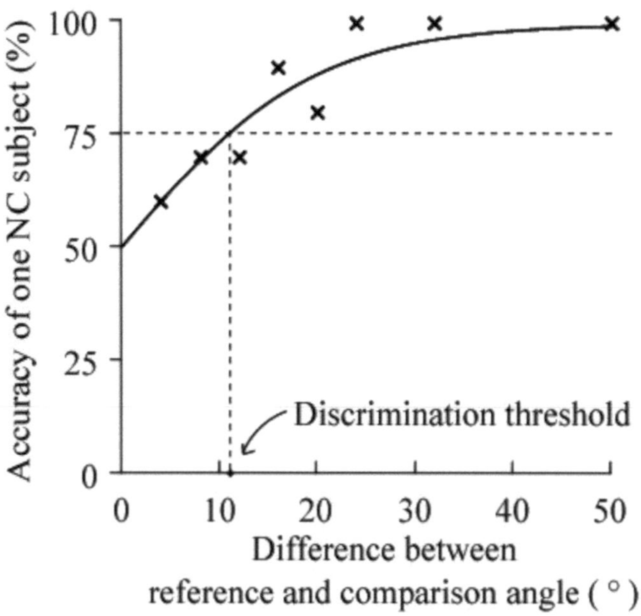


Fig. 7. Calculation method of the angle discrimination threshold. Accuracy of one NC subject is plotted as a function of the angular difference between the comparison (62°–110°) and the reference angle (60°). The solid line represents the logistic curve for threshold calculation. The horizontal dashed line indicates accuracy at 75%. The horizontal axis value of the intersection between the 75% line and logistic curve is defined as the angle discrimination threshold. For this NC subject, the threshold is 10.7°.

To examine whether the patients with MCI and AD showed any decline in angle discrimination, we further examined the angle discrimination threshold. We performed a one-way ANOVA and a multiple comparison using the Bonferroni correction ($\alpha = 0.05$) on the mean discrimination threshold. As shown in Fig. 8(b), differences in the mean discrimination thresholds among patients with AD (25.2°±4.2°) or MCI (13.8°±2.7°) and NC subjects (8.7±0.8°) were significant [$F(2,34) = 9.45$, $P < 0.001$], with a larger threshold in patients with AD compared to patients with MCI ($P = 0.036$) and NC ($P < 0.001$). In addition, the threshold in patients with MCI was also significantly larger compared to NC ($P = 0.049$). These results indicated that the decline in the ability to discriminate tactile angles in patients with MCI and AD was significant compared to the NC group.

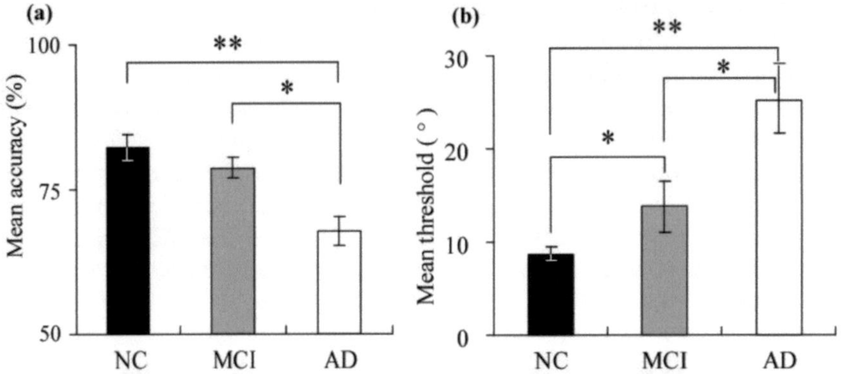


Fig. 8. Mean accuracy and discrimination threshold of MCI and AD compared to NC. (a) The mean accuracy of the three groups (NC: 82.1% ± 2.2%, MCI: 78.6% ± 1.8%, AD: 67.9% ± 2.5%). (b) The mean discrimination thresholds for the three groups are shown (NC: 8.7° ± 0.8°, MCI: 13.8° ± 2.7°, AD: 25.2° ± 4.2°). Vertical error bars represent standard error of the mean. $^*P < 0.05$, $^{**}P < 0.001$.

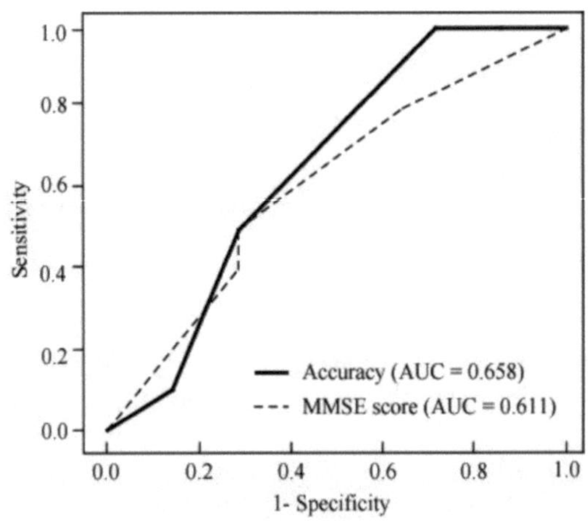


Fig. 9. Receiver operating characteristic (ROC) curves for the angle discrimination accuracy and MMSE score showing discrimination between the NC and MCI groups. The solid line represents the ROC curve of angle discrimination accuracy, and the dashed line represents the ROC curve of MMSE score. The area under the curve (AUC) of angle discrimination accuracy is larger than that of MMSE score.

### 3.3.2 Comparison between angle discrimination accuracy and MMSE score

ROC analysis is a useful tool for evaluating the performance of diagnostic tests (Mendiondo et al., 2003; Zou et al., 2007). We used a ROC analysis to compare the sensitivity of angle discrimination accuracy to that of the MMSE scores. The fundamental measures of diagnostic accuracy are sensitivity (i.e., true positive rate) and specificity (i.e., true negative rate). As described in the Subjects section, all NC and MCI patients were defined by an MMSE score of 27 or greater and the CDR score of 0 and 0.5. In contrast, all AD patients had MMSE scores between 15 and 26. Therefore, only the ROC curves for angle discrimination accuracy and MMSE score of NC and MCI subjects were compared and are presented in Fig. 8. The area under the curve (AUC, is an overall summary of diagnostic accuracy) values for the angle discrimination accuracy was 0.658, and the MMSE score was 0.611. As shown in Fig. 8, we found that the AUC of the angle discrimination accuracy was higher than the MMSE score.

### 3.4 Discussion

The present study demonstrated that patients with MCI or AD have an impaired ability to discriminate tactile angles compared to age-matched healthy subjects. The current study compared the performance of angle discrimination in three different subject groups (i.e., NC, MCI and AD). The results of this study indicated that there were significant group differences in the ability to discriminate tactile angles (NC > MCI > AD). Both the mean accuracy and threshold of angle discrimination of AD patients were significantly decreased compared to NC individuals and MCI patients. In contrast, although the mean threshold of angle discrimination of patients with MCI was significantly higher than NC individuals, the mean accuracy of the MCI group was similar to the NC group.

All subjects were asked to passively perceive the angles moved under their right index fingers and discriminate the largest of each angle pair, which consisted of a reference angle and a comparison angle. The current angle discrimination task is a commonly used procedure of tactile passive shape discrimination. The sensory feedback, which is critical for shape discrimination by passive touch, is generated by the four mechanoreceptive afferent systems (Johnson, 2001) located in the skin. Moreover, previous studies (Goodwin et al., 1997; Johnson, 2001) have suggested that tactile shape perception can be defined as the sum of the functions of cutaneous mechanoreceptors. However, there are numerous anatomical and morphological changes that develop with age and affect the hand and fingers. The density of mechanoreceptors in the skin was decreased (Wollard, 1936; Bruce, 1980), and the conduction velocity of peripheral nerves was significantly reduced with age (Peters, 2002). A decreased touch sensitivity in elderly individuals can cause many problems (Stevens & Choo, 1996; Vega-Bermudez & Johnson, 2002), including the inability to recognise objects by touch and an impaired ability to detect an object that has come into contact with the skin. Consequently, the ability of normal, older subjects to discriminate angles will be reduced compared to normal, young subjects. For example, the mean threshold of young subjects was 3.7° in our previous angle discrimination study (Wu et al., 2010), and the mean threshold of NC subjects in the present study was 8.7°, which was more than twice the previous value. However, the results of the present study indicated that the older subjects, as well as patients with MCI and AD, were able to complete the angle discrimination task. All subjects in the current experiment were able to perceive the change in size of the angle stimuli.

However, a significant deficit in angle discrimination was observed in MCI and AD patients in this study. One of the earliest symptoms of AD is impaired working memory (Baddeley et al., 1991; Bäckman & Small, 2007). In addition, previous studies have observed that patients with MCI also show impairments in memory processing compared to healthy aging subjects (Siedenberg et al., 1996; Petersen et al., 1999). In this study, all subjects were instructed to discriminate the larger of two angles by passive touch. To perform this task, the subject had to remember the composing feature of the first angle and then compare it with the second angle to make a judgment. The working memory contributed to the performance of the somatosensory discrimination (Bodegård et al., 2001; Kitada et al., 2006). Therefore, the present study suggests that the impaired working memory of MCI and AD patients is one factor that contributes to the decline of angle discrimination performance.

Moreover, we found that the mean accuracy of AD patients was significantly lower than the accuracy of the MCI and NC groups, and the mean threshold of AD patients was also reduced compared to the other two groups. Specifically, the mean threshold of AD patients was almost double the threshold of the MCI patients. However, we also found that there was a significant difference in the mean threshold between the MCI patients and the NC group, whereas the mean accuracy of the MCI patients and the NC group remained unchanged. There are two possible reasons to explain this phenomenon. First, AD is a neurodegenerative brain disease. Unlike patients with MCI, AD patients have more severe working memory impairments (Blatow et al., 2005). Second, the isolated memory impairment found in patients with MCI is more severe than the impairment observed in healthy aging individuals, whereas other cognitive functions remain normal. In contrast, AD patients have further deficits in spatial learning and memory and planning and problem solving (Kalman et al., 1995; Förstl & Kurz, 1999). These profound cognitive impairments of AD patients may explain the more severe deficits in angle discrimination found in patients with AD.

In addition, the tactile spatial discrimination procedure activates a diverse cerebral network (Bodegård et al., 2001; Kitada et al., 2006; Wu et al., 2010). The results from these neuroimaging studies also support our findings. For example, the intraparietal sulcus (located on the lateral surface of the parietal lobe) is engaged in multisensory spatial processing during the classification of grating and shape, and it has been shown that the intraparietal sulcus is a high-class area for computations and elaborates shape reconstructions (Bodegård et al., 2001). Neuroimaging studies (Delbeuck et al., 2003; Dickerson & Sperling, 2009; Huang et al., 2010) have demonstrated that abnormalities in the frontal, temporal, and parietal cortices contribute to the functional deficits in AD patients. Consequently, our results suggest that both the impairment of working memory and spatial discrimination of AD patients contribute to the lowest angle that is discernible compared to the MCI patients and the NC group.

The MMSE is a brief mental status examination designed to quantify the cognitive status in adults (Folstein et al., 1975). Recently, MMSE has been commonly used to test for complaints of memory problems or when a diagnosis of dementia is being considered. We plotted the ROC curves for the angle discrimination accuracy and MMSE score. We found that used the angle discrimination accuracy was better anbe to differentiate the MCI patients from older individuals than the MMSE score because the MMSE also has limitations. For example, previous studies (Anthony et al., 1982; Galasko et al., 1990) have suggested that the sensitivity of the MMSE has been rated at approximately 80%. Thus, the MMSE score may not represent the cognitive function deficits of all individuals. In contrast, we specifically focused on the difference in tactile angle discrimination in MCI and AD patients compared to the NC group. Although the present angle discrimination experiment examined working memory, spatial discrimination and problem-solving processes, there were limitations to this study. Despite these limitations, we have found a significant decline in tactile angle discrimination between the MCI patients and the NC group using the present tactile discrimination system. These findings may improve the sensitivity of the previous mental tests for AD diagnosis and treatment.

## 4. Conclusion

Audiovisual spatial and temporal orienting attention studies were examined in our study to further our understanding of neuroimaging studies for early detection of dementia. By using another method to compare the cognitive ability of tactile angle discrimination, we initially found that at the early stages of Alzheimer's disease, the behavioural cognition was decreased. These basic data that obtained from our studies, we consider that they are able to apply for a clinical diagnosis method of dementia early detection after enough confirm experiments.

## 5. Acknowledgment

A portion of this study was supported by a Grant-in-Aid for Scientific Research (B) 21404002, Japan and the AA Science Platform Program of the Japan Society for the Promotion of Science.

## 6. References

Anthony, J.C.; Le Resche, L.; Niaz, U.; Von Korff, M.R. & Folstein, M.F. (1982). Limits of the Mini-Mental State as screening test for demenia and delirium among hospital patients. *Pgychol Med*, Vol.12, pp. 397-408

Bäckman, L. & Small, B.J. (2007). Cognitive deficits in preclinical Alzheimer's disease and vascular dementia: Patterns of findings from the Kungsholmen Project. *Physiology & Behavior*, Vol.92, pp.80–86

Baddeley, A.D.; Bressi, S.; Della, S.S.; Logie, R. & Spinnler, H. (1991). The decline of working memory in Alzheimer's disease: A longitudinal study. *Brain*, Vol.114, pp.2521–2542

Bai, O.; Huang, D.; Lin, P.; Wu, J.; Chen, X. & Fei, D. (2010). An event-related study for dynamic analysis of corticomuscular connectivity, *Biomedical Engineering and Computational Biology*, Vol.2, p.1-10,

Blatow, M.; Nennig, E.; Durst, A.; Sartor, K. & Stippich, C. (2007). fMRI reflects functional connectivity of human somatosensory cortex. *NeuroImage* Vol.37, pp.927–936

Bodegård, A.; Geyer, S.; Grefkes, C.; Zilles, K. & Roland, P.E. (2001). Hierarchical Processing of Tactile Shape in the Human Brain. *Neuron*, Vol.31, pp.317–328

Bruce, M.F. (1980). The relation of tactile thresholds to histology in the fingers of elderly people. *Journal Neurol Neurosurg Psychiatry*, Vol.43, pp.730–734

Cai, C.; Kochiyama, T.; Osaka, K. & Wu, J. (2007). Lexical/semantic processing in dorsal left inferior frontal gyrus, *NeuroReport*, Vol. 18, No.11, pp. 1147-1151

Corbetta, M.; Miezin, F.; Shulman, G. & Petersen, S.E. (1993). A PET study of visuospatial attention. The Journal of Neuroscience, Vol.13, pp.1202–1226

Coull, J.T. & Nobre, A.C. (1998). Where and when to pay attention: the neural systems for directing attention to spatial location and to time intervals as revealed by both PET and fMRI. *The Journal of Neuroscience*, Vol.18, pp.7426–7435

Coull, J.T.; Frith, C.D.; Buèchel, C. & Nobre, A.C. (2000). Orienting attention in time: behavioural and neuroanatomical distinction between exogenous and endogenous shifts. Neuropsychologia, Vol.38, pp.808–819

Degerman, A.; Rinne, T.; Salmi, J.; Salonen, O. & Alho, K. (2006). Selective attention to sound location or pitch studied with fMRI. *Brain Research,* Vol.1077, No. 1, pp. 123–134

Delbeuck, X.; Van der Linden, M. & Collette, F. (2003). Alzheimer's disease as a disconnection syndrome? *Neuropsychology Review*, Vol.13, No.2, pp.79-92

Dickerson, B.C. & Sperling, R.A. (2009). Large-scale functional brain network abnormalities in Alzheimer's disease: insights from functional neuroimaging. *Behavioral Neurology*, Vol.21, No.1, pp.63-75

Folstein, M.F.; Folstein, S.E. & McHugh, P.R. (1975). 'Mini-mental state' A practical method for grading the cognitive state of patients for the clinician. *Journal of psychiatric research*. Vol.12, No.3, pp.189-198

Förstl, H. & Kurz, A. (1999). Clinical features of Alzheimer's disease. *European Archives of Psychiatry and Clinical Neuroscience*, Vol.249, No.6, pp.288–290

Francis, P.T.; Palmer, A.M.; Snape, M. & Wilcock, G.K. (1999). The cholinergic hypothesis of Alzheimer's disease: a review of progress. *Journal of Neurology, Neurosurgery & Psychiatry*, Vol.66, No.2, pp.137–147

Galasko, D.; Klauber, M.R.; Hofstetter, C.R.; Salmon, D.P.; Lasker, B. & Thal, L.J. (1990). The Mini-Mental State Examination in the early diagnosis of Alzheimer disease. *Archives of Neurology*, Vol.47, pp.49-52

Goodwin, A.W.; Macefield, V.G. & Bisley, J.W. (1997). Encoding of object curvature by tactile afferents from human fingers. *Journal of Neurophysiology*, Vol.78, pp.2881-2888

Huang, S.; Li, J.; Sun, L.; Ye, J.; Fleisher, A.; Wu, T.; Chen, K. & Reiman, E. Alzheimer's Disease NeuroImaging Initiative, (2010). Learning brain connectivity of Alzheimer's disease by sparse inverse covariance estimation. *Neuroimage*, Vol.50, No.3, pp.935-949

Hughes, C.P.; Berg, L.; Danziger, W.L.; Coben, L.A. & Martin, R.L. (1982). A new clinical scale for the staging of dementia. *The British Journal of Psychiatry*, Vol.140, pp.566–572

Johnson, J.A. & Zatorre, R.J. (2006). Neural substrates for dividing and focusing attention between simultaneous auditory and visual events. *NeuroImage*, Vol.31, pp.1673–1681

Johnson, K.O. (2001). The roles and functions of cutaneous mechanoreceptors. *Current Opinion in Neurobiology*, Vol.11, pp. 455-461

Johnson, S.C.; Schmitz, T.W.; Moritz, C.H.; Meyerand, M.E.; Rowley, H.A.; Alexander, A.L.; Hansen, K.W.; Gleason, C.E.; Carlsson, C.M.; Ries, M.L.; Asthana, S.; Chen, K.; Reiman, E.M. & Alexander, G.E. (2006). Activation of brain regions vulnerable to

Alzheimer's disease: the effect of mild cognitive impairment. *Neurobiology of Aging*, Vol.27, No.11, pp.1604-1612

Kalman, K.; Magloczky, E. & Janka, Z. (1995). Disturbed visuo-spatial orientation in the early stage of Alzheimer's dementia. *Archives of Gerontology and Geriatrics*, Vol.21, pp.27-34

Kitada, R.; Kito, T.; Saito, D.N.; Kochiyama, T.; Matsumura, M.; Sadato, N. & Lederman, S.J. (2006). Multisensory Activation of the Intraparietal Area When Classifying Grating Orientation: A Functional Magnetic Resonance Imaging Study. *The Journal of Neuroscience*, Vol.26, pp.7491-7501

Li, C. ; Li, X. ; Kusahara, H. & Wu, J. (2011a, accept). Neural substrates of priming effect for Japanese word and nonword when compared to figure form, *International journal of information*

Li, Q.; Yang, J.; Kakura, N. & Wu, J. (2010a). Multimodal audiovisual integration at early and late processing stages in humans: an event-related potential study, *International journal of information*, Vol.13 No.3(A), p.807-816

Li, Q.; Wu, J. & Touge, T. (2010b). Audiovisual interaction enhances auditory detection in late stage: an event-related potential study: *Neuroreport*, Vol.21 No.3, pp.173-178

Li, Q. & Wu, J. (2009). Multisenaory interactions of audiovisual stimuli presented at different location in visual-attention tasks, *International journal of information*, Vol.12 No.6, pp.1311-1320

Li, X. ; Cai, C. & Wu, J. (2009). Measurement and analysis of binocular perceptual characteristics with peripheral vision for the development of head mounted display with wide view, *International journal of information*, Vol.12, No.3

Li, X.; Wu, J.; Li, C. ; Cai, C. & Guo, Q. (2011b, accept). Different activities on Chinese character and figure processing by a visual fMRI study involving literates and illiterates，*International journal of information*

Loose, R.; Kaufmann, C.; Auer, D.P. & Lange, K.W. (2003) Human prefrontal and sensory cortical activity during divided attention tasks. *Human Brain Mapping*, Vol.18, pp.249-259

McKhann, G.; Drachman, D.; Folstein, M.; Katzman, R.; Price, D. & Stadlan, E.M. (1984). Clinical diagnosis of Alzheimer's disease: report of the NINCDS-ADRDA work group under the auspices of Department of Health and Human Services task force on Alzheimer's disease. *Neurology*, Vol.34, pp.939-344

Mendiondo, M.S.; Ashford, J.W.; Kryscio, R.J. & Schmitt, F.A. (2003). Designing a Brief Alzheimer Screen (BAS). *Journal of Alzheimer's Disease*, Vol.5, pp.391-398

Morris, J.C. (1993). The Clinical Dementia Rating (CDR): current version and scoring rules. *Neurology*, Vol.43, No.11, pp.2412-2414

Morris, J.C.; Heyman, A.; Mohs, R.C.; Hughes, J.P.; van Belle, G.; Fillenbaum, G.; Mellits, E.D. & Clark, C. (1989). The Consortium to Establish a Registry for Alzheimer's Disease (CERAD). Part I. Clinical and neuropsychological assessment of Alzheimer's disease. *Neurology*, Vol.39, No.9, pp.1159-1165

Nobre, A.C.; Gitelman, D.R.; Dias, E.C. & Mesulam, M.M. (2000). Covert visual spatial orienting and saccades: overlapping neural systems. *NeuroImage,* Vol.11, 210–216

Oldfield, R.C. (1971). The assessment and analysis of handedness: The edinburgh inventory. *Neuropsychologia,* Vol.9, pp.97-113

Peters, A. (2002). The effects of normal aging on myelin and nerve fibers: a review. *Journal of Neurocytology,* Vol.31, pp.581–593

Petersen, R.C. (2004). Mild cognitive impairment as a diagnostic entity. *Journal of Internal Medicine,* Vol.256, No.3, pp.183–194

Petersen, R.C.; Smith, G.E.; Waring, S.C.; Ivnik, R.J.; Tangalos, E.G. & Kokmen, E. (1999). Mild cognitive impairment: clinical characterization and outcome. *Archives of Neurology,* Vol.56, pp.303–308

Robins, L.N.; Wing, J.; Wittchen, H.U.; Helzer, J.E.; Babor, T.F.; Burke, J.; Farmer, A.; Jablenski, A.; Pickens, R.; Regier, D.A.; Sartorius, N. & Towle, L.H. (1988). The Composite International Diagnostic Interview. An epidemiologic Instrument suitable for use in conjunction with different diagnostic systems and in different cultures. *Archives of General Psychiatry,* Vol.45, No.12, pp.1069-1177

Rosen, W.G.; Terry, R.D.; Fuld, P.A.; Katzman, R. & Peck, A. (1980). Pathological verification of ischemic score in differentiation of dementias. *Annals of Neurology,* Vol.7, No.5, pp.486-488

Schubotz, R.I.; Yves von Cramon, D. & Lohmann, G. (2003). Auditory what, where, and, when: a sensory somatotopy in lateral premotor cortex. *NeuroImage* Vol.20, pp.173–185

Siedenberg, R.; Goodin, D.S.; Aminoff, M.J.; Rowley, H.A. & Roberts, T.P. (1996). Comparison of late components in simultaneously recorded event-related electrical potentials and event-related magnetic fields. *Electroencephalography and Clinical Neurophysiology,* Vol.99, pp.191–197

Stevens, J.C. & Choo, K.K. (1996). Spatial acuity of the body surface over the life span. *Somatosensensory & Motor Research,* Vol.13, pp.153-166

Stevens, J.C. & Patterson, M.Q. (1995). Dimension of spatial acuity in the touch sense: Changes of the life span. *Somatosensory & Motor Research,* Vol.12, pp.29-47

Touge, T.; Gonzalez, D.; Wu, J.; Deguchi, K.; Tsukaguchi, M.; Shimamura, M.; Ikeda, K. & Kuriyama, S. (2008). The interaction between somatosensory and auditory cognitive processing assessed with event-related potentials, *Journal of Clinical neurophysiology,* Vol. 25, pp.90-97

Vega-Bermudez, F. & Johnson, K.O. (2002). Spatial acuity after digit amputation. *Brain,* Vol.125, pp.1256-1264

Voisin, J.; Benoit, G. & Chapman, C.E. (2002a). Haptic discrimination of object shape in humans: two-dimensional (2-D) angle discrimination. *Experimental Brain Research,* Vol.145, pp.239-250

Voisin, J.; Lamarre, Y. & Chapman, C.E. (2002b). Haptic discrimination of object shape in humans: contribution of cutaneous and proprioceptive inputs. *Experimental Brain Research,* Vol.145, pp.251-260

Wollard, H.H. (1936), Intraepidermal nerve endings. *Journal of Anatomy*, Vol.71, pp.55-62

Wu, J.; Yang, J. & Ogasa, T. (2010). Raised angle discrimination under passive hand movement. *Perception*, Vol.39, pp.993- 1006

Wu, J.; Yan, T.; Zhang, Z.; Jin, F. & Guo., Q. (2011, accept). Retinotopic mapping of the peripheral visual field to human visual cortex by functional magnetic resonance imaging. *Human Brain Mapping*,

Wu, J.; Yang, J. & Honda, T. (2010a). Fitts' Law holds for pointing movements under conditions of restricted visual feedback, *Human Movement Science*,Vol.29 Issue.6, pp.882-892,

Wu, J. & N. Kakura (2010). Investigation on human visual and auditory calculation mechanism by event related potential: *International journal of information*, Vol.13 No.1, pp.99-109

Wu, J. ; Li, Q. ; Bai, O. & Touge, T. (2009). Multisensory interactions elicited by audiovisual stimuli presented peripherally in a visual attention task: a behavioral and event-related potential study in humans: *Journal of Clinical Neurophysilogy*, Vol.26 No.6, pp.407-413

Wu, J.; Cai, C.; Kochiyama, T. & Osaka, K. (2007). Function segregation in the left inferior frontal gyrus: a listening functional magnetic resonance imaging study, *NeuroReport*, Vol. 18, No.2, pp. 127-131

Wu, J. & Li, C. (2009). Comparison of cerebral cortex activations between visual-auditory spatial and temporal voluntary attention by using a cue stimulus: an fMRI study , *The Engineering Sciences Society* , Vol. J92-A No.9 pp.633-643 (In Japanese)

Yan, T.; Jin, F.; He, J. & Wu, J. (2011). Development of a wide-view visual presentation system for visual retinotopic mapping during fMRI. *Journal of Magnetic Resonance Imaging*, Vol.33, pp. 441-447,

Yang, J.; Ogasa, T.; Wu, J.; Y. Ohta & Abe, K. (2011a, in press).Tactile pattern delivery device to investigate cognitive mechanisms for early detection of Alzheimer's Disease. *Early Detection and Rehabilitation Technologies for Dementia: Neuroscience and Biomedical Application, IGI Global* (Chapter 11)

Yang, J.; Omodani, M. & Wu, J. (2011b, in press). Spatial attention improve performance of pointing movement, *International journal of information*,

Yang, J.; Oka, D. & Wu, J. (2011c, in press). The ebbinghaus illusion affects visual size perception but not pointing movement, *International journal of information*,

Yang, J.; Ogasa, T.; Ohta, Y.; Abe, K. & Wu, J. (2010a). Decline of human tactile angle discrimination in patients with mild cognitive impairment and Alzheimer's Disease, *Journal of Alzheimer's Disease*,Vol.22 No.1, pp.225-234

Yang, J. & Wu, J. (2010). Development and evaluation of a multi-model tactile pattern delivery device for fMRI study, *International journal of information*, Vol.13, No.5, pp.1823-1832

Zou, K.H.; O'Malley, A.J. & Mauri, L. (2007). Receiver-Operating Characteristic Analysis for Evaluating Diagnostic Tests and Predictive Models. *Circulation*, Vol.115, pp.654-657

Zatorre, R.J.; Mondor, T.A. & Evans, A.C. (1999). Auditory attention to space and frequency activates similar cerebral systems. *NeuroImage*, Vol.10, pp.544-554

4

# Staining of Amyloid Beta (Abeta) Using (Immuno) Histochemical Techniques and Abeta42 Specific Peptides

Thomas van Groen[1,2], Inga Kadish[1], Aileen Funke[3] and Dieter Willbold[3,4]
[1]*Dept. Cell Biology, University of Alabama at Birmingham, Birmingham, AL.*
[2]*Dept. Neurobiology, University of Alabama at Birmingham, Birmingham, AL,*
[3]*Forschungszentrum Jülich, ICS-6, 52425 Jülich,*
[4]*Heinrich-Heine-Universität Düsseldorf,*
*Institut für Physikalische Biologie and BMFZ, Düsseldorf,*
[1,2]*USA*
[3,4]*Germany*

## 1. Introduction

In the elderly, Alzheimer's disease (AD) is the most common form of dementia (Hebert et al., 2003). The two pathologies that characterize the disease are the presence of large numbers of intracellular neurofibrillary tangles (NFTs) and extracellular neuritic plaques in the brain (e.g., Braak and Braak, 1991; 1998; Selkoe, 2001). Neurofibrillary tangles consist of hyperphosphorylated, twisted filaments of the cytoskeletal protein tau (e.g., Duff, 2006), whereas plaques are primarily made up of amyloid β(Aβ [Selkoe, 2001; Dickson and Vickers, 2002]), a 39-43 amino acid long peptide derived from the proteolytic processing of the amyloid precursor protein (APP [Selkoe, 2001; Vetrivel and Thinakaran, 2006]). When APP is sequentially cleaved by the β-secretase and γ-secretase, one of the resulting breakdown product is Aβ, in contrast, initial cleavage by α-secretase (in the middle of the Aβ sequence) leads to production of $APP_s\alpha$ and the C83 peptide (Selkoe, 2001).
Most cases of AD are sporadic, however approximately 5 % of AD cases are familial (Price and Sisodia, 1995; Selkoe, 2001), these cases are related to mutations in the genes for APP, and presenilin 1 and 2 (PS1 and PS2 [Price and Sisodia, 1995; Hardy, 1997; Selkoe, 2001]). Transgenic mice expressing mutated human AD genes offer a powerful model to study the role of Aβ in the development of pathology (e.g., Duff and Suleman, 2004; McGowan et al, 2006). The present study employs three lines of transgenic mice expressing both human APPswe and/or PS1 mutations. These lines of mice develop elevated levels of Aβ42 at different ages, and at different locations (Van Groen et al., 2005; Wang et al., 2003).

## 2. Materials and methods

### 2.1 Animals

Two lines of APP and PS1 single and double transgenic mice (**AP/PS**) were used in the present study. The first line of mice was generated from matings between APPswe and

HuPS1-A246E transgenic mice, this mouse line was originally produced at the Johns Hopkins University (Borchelt et al., 1996), and was bred locally on a C57BL/6J background. The second line of APP/PS1 mice was the APPswe+PS1Δ9 line, originally produced at the Johns Hopkins University (Jankowsky et al., 2001), we acquired these mice from JAX at the age of six weeks. The animals were housed 4/cage in our facility; in a controlled environment (temperature 22°C, humidity 50-60%, light from 07:00-19:00), with food and water were available *ad libitum*. All procedures were conducted in accordance with the local Institutional Animal Care and Use Committee (IACUC) guidelines.

### 2.2 Peptides

In short, a mirror image phage display approach was used to identify novel and highly specific ligands for Alzheimer's disease amyloid peptide Aβ1-42 (Wiesehan et al., 2003). In short, a randomized 12-mer peptide library presented on M13 phages was screened for peptides with binding affinity for the mirror image of Aβ1-42 (Wiesehan et al., 2003). After four rounds of selection and amplification the peptides were enriched with a dominating consensus sequence. The mirror image of the most representative peptide (i.e., D1) was shown to bind Aβ1-42 with a dissociation constant in the submicromolar range (Wiesehan et al., 2003). The D2 and D3 peptides come from two other phage display selections against Aβ42. The D1 peptide has a higher affinity for Aβ42 monomers, D2 has a low specificity, whereas D3 has a high affinity for Aβ42 oligomers (Funke et al, 2010). To study the binding characteristics of the D-peptides in more detail, an L-peptide version of the D1-peptide was made, and a scrambled (sequence) peptide of similar length was also made. In the binding experiments the peptides that were used had been conjugated with a FITC molecule for visualization purposes, except in a few experiments. In those experiments D1 conjugated with other fluorophores were tested to study the interaction of the fluorescent moiety with binding characteristics of the D1 peptide.

### 2.3 Histopathological techniques

In short, mice were anesthetized, transcardially perfused with saline followed by 4% paraformaldehyde and the brains were removed from the skull. After postfixation (4h) and cryoprotection (24h in 30% sucrose), six series (1 in 6) of coronal sections were cut through the brain. The first series of sections was mounted unstained, and the second, third and fourth series were stained immunohistochemically according to published protocols (Kadish et al., 2002; Van Groen et al., 2006) the other two series were stored in at -20°C in antifreeze for future analysis. One half of the second series was stained for human Aβ using the W0-2 antibody (mouse anti-human $A\beta_{4-9}$; Ida et al., 1996), the other half of the second series was stained for mouse Aβ (rabbit anti-rodent Aβ; Covance; Van Groen et al, 2006). The first half of the third series was stained for Aβ40 (mouse anti-Aβ40, Covance) the other half for Aβ42 (mouse anti-Aβ42; Covance). In some animals, one half of the fourth series was stained for GFAP (mouse anti-GFAP; Sigma), whereas the other half was stained for CD11b (rat anti-mouseCD11b; Serotec), a marker of microglia, to analyze inflammation in the brain. Some of these sections were double stained with either Congo red, thioflavine S or thiazine red to visualise β sheets, i.e., Aβ plaque cores in our material, in a few animals methoxy-X04 (Klunk et al., 2002) was infused during the perfusion to label all Aβ in the brain. The sections destined for immunohistochemical Aβ staining were pretreated for 30 min with hot (85°C) citrate buffer. The series of sections were transferred to a solution containing the primary antibody (W0-2, mouse monoclonal), this solution consists of TBS with 0.5 % Triton X-100 added (TBS-T). Following incubation in this solution for 18 h on a shaker table at room temperature (20ºC) in the dark, the sections were rinsed three times in TBS-T and transferred to the solution containing the appropriate secondary antibody (goat anti-mouse*biotin; Sigma). After two hours, the sections were rinsed three times with TBS-T and transferred to a solution containing mouse ExtrAvidin® (Sigma), following rinsing the sections were incubated for approximately 3 min with Ni-enhanced DAB (Kadish et al., 2002). In a small number of sections, the Aβ deposits were double labeled for Aβ40 and Aβ42 using fluorescent secondary antibodies. All stained sections were mounted on slides and coverslipped.

Histochemical stains. Thioflavine-S staining (Guntern et al, 1982), sections are mounted on gelatinized slides, and air-dried. When dry the slides are immersed in distilled water for 5 min twice to rehydrate, then they are immersed in the Thioflavine-S solution (1g of Thioflavine-S in 100 ml distilled water) for 20 min. Then the slides are rinsed quickly twice in distilled water and air dried, when dry they are rinsed in xylene, and coverslipped with DPX. The staining procedure is performed in the dark, i.e., the solution of Thioflavine-S is kept in a opaque container, similarly the staining procedure is done in opaque containers. Thioflavine-T staining (Morimatsu et al, 1975), sections are mounted on gelatinized slides, and air-dried. When dry the slides are immersed in distilled water for 5 min twice to rehydrate, then they are immersed in the Thioflavine-T solution (1g of Thioflavine-T in 100 ml distilled water) for 20 min. Then the slides are rinsed quickly twice in distilled water and air dried, when dry they are coverslipped with DPX. The staining procedure is performed in the dark, i.e., the solution of Thioflavine-T is kept in a opaque container, similarly the staining procedure is done in opaque containers. Congo red staining (Glenner, 1981), slides with brain sections are put overnight in 4% paraformaldehyde solution, the next day slides are rinsed twice with distilled water for 5 min, then put in the pretreatment solution (a 80% ethanol saturated NaCl solution with 1% sodium hydroxide added [1ml per 100 ml) for 20 min. Then the slides are transferred to the Congo red staining solution (a 80% ethanol saturated NaCl solution with 0.2 g Congo red per 100 ml) for 25 min, the slides are rinsed quickly in distilled water and air dried. Thiazine red (Uchihara et al, 2000) slides with sections are rinsed in distilled water for 5 min, and put in the Thiazine red solution (0.1g Thiazine red in 300 ml 0.001 M Naphosphate buffer, pH 7.4) for 15 min. Then the slides are rinsed quickly twice in distilled water and air dried, when dry they are coverslipped with DPX. Methoxy-XO4 staining, slides with sections are rinsed in distilled water for 5 min, and put in the Methoxy-XO4 solution (3.3 mg Methoxy-XO4 in 100 ml 40% ethanol/60%distilled water at pH 10.00) for 10 min. Then the slides are rinsed quickly twice in distilled water and air dried, when dry they are coverslipped with DPX.

## 3. Results

### 3.1 In vitro staining

The staining of sections of paraformaldehyde fixed brains of **AP/PS** mice with histochemical methods revealed that all methods that are used for staining amyloid also stain amyloid β and stained all dense Aβ deposits, i.e., plaques (Figure 1). However, it should be noted that in the sections of the AP/PS mice that have large amounts of diffuse Aβ deposits, most these deposits were not stained. Staining intensity of the Aβ deposits was directly related to the method that was used, the solutions that we used contained the optimal concentrations of

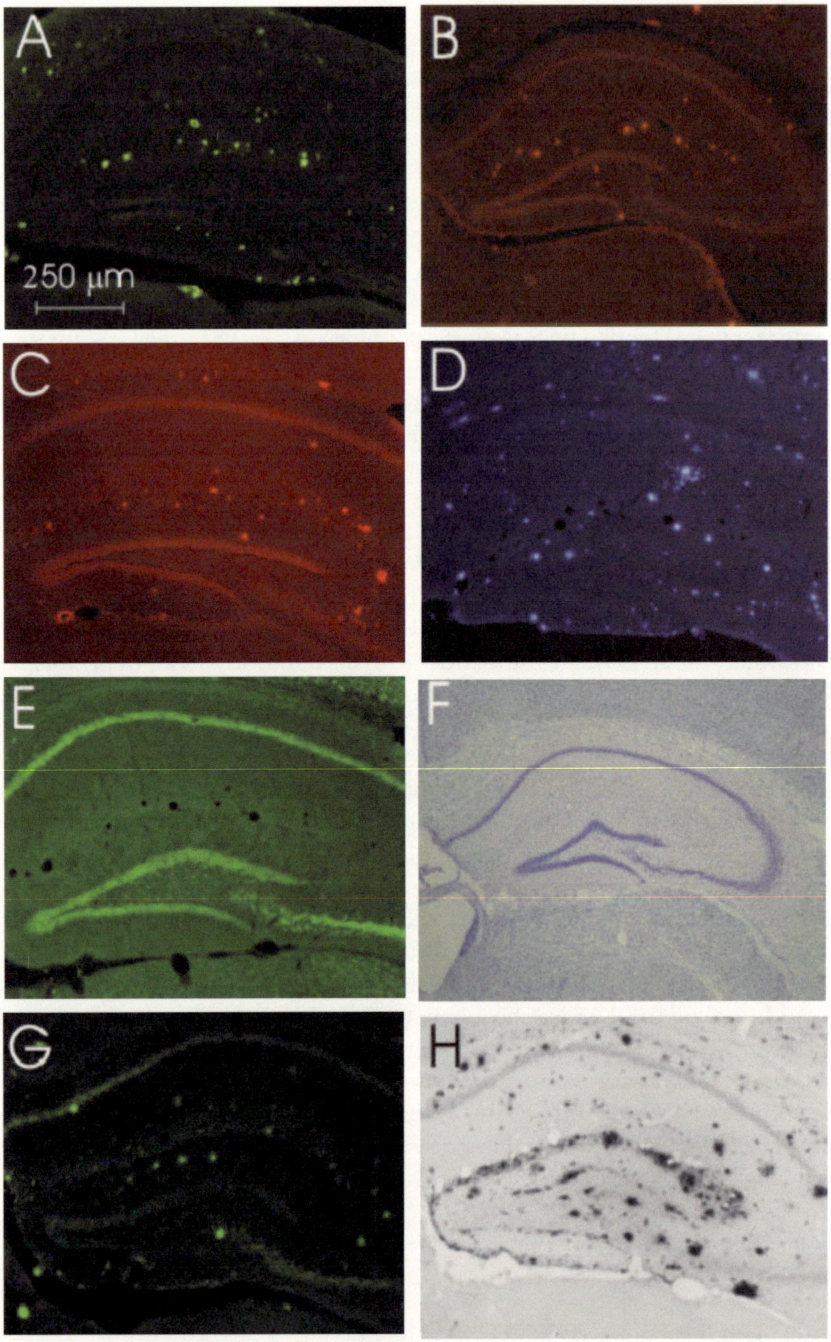


Fig. 1. Eight photomicrographs of coronal sections of the hippocampal formation of a Tg AD model mouse brain. **A**, section stained with thioflavine-S; **B**, section stained with Congo red; **C**, section stained with thiazine red; **D**, section stained with methoxy-X0; **E**, section stained with thioflavine-T; **F**, section stained with cresyl violet (Nissl stain), **G**, section stained with D3, and **H**, section stained for Aβ .

dye for these sections. They have the highest concentration that stains optimally in the shortest time. Longer time periods increased the background staining and did not improve staining quality (i.e., the signal/noise ratio; not illustrated).

The staining of sections of paraformaldehyde fixed brain sections of **AP/PS** mice with the three D-peptides revealed that all peptides (i.e., D1-D3) bound to all dense Aβ deposits, i.e., plaques (Figure 2). However, it should be noted that in the sections of the AP/PS mice that have large amounts of diffuse Aβ deposits, these deposits were not stained (Figure 1). Staining intensity of the Aβ deposits was directly related to both the D-peptide concentration that was tested (0.01, 0.001 and 0.0001 mg/ml), with the highest concentration staining optimally in the shortest time. At the highest concentration the optimal staining time was less than 5 min (i.e., with the best signal/noise ratio), whereas at the lowest

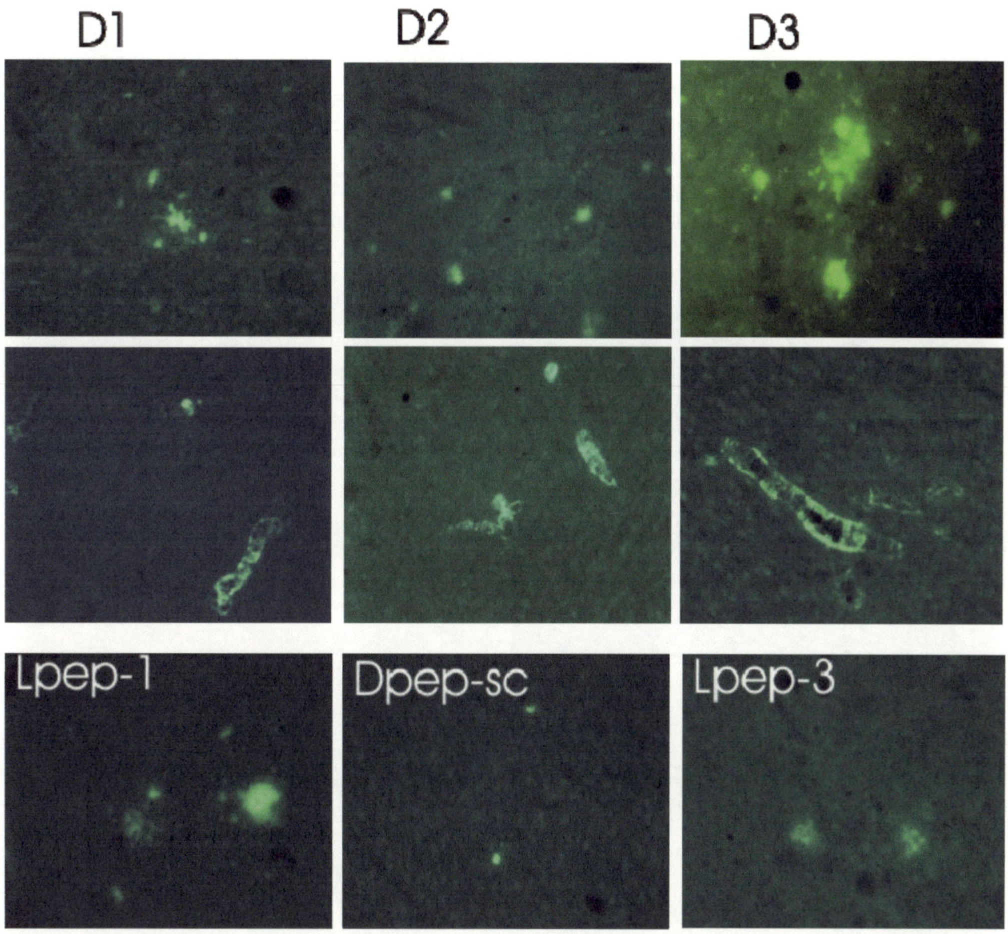


Fig. 2. Nine high power photomicrographs of adjacent coronal sections through the parietal cortex of an 18-month-old APP/PS1 mouse. The top six photomicrographs demonstrate the typical staining of plaques and blood vessels with respectively, D1, D2, and D3. The lower 3 photomicrographs show the typical staining of L-D1, sc-D1, and L3, respectively. Please note the lack of staining by the scrambled D-peptide (sc-D1), arrowhead indicates plaque core

concentration (0.0001 mg/ml) the time was more than 6 hours. Longer time periods increased the background staining and did not improve staining quality (i.e., the signal/noise ratio). It should be noted that with the lower concentrations, and appropriate longer staining time, the amount of non-specific staining (i.e., background) was significantly decreased. Similarly, post-staining rinsing of the stained sections in buffer decreased the amount of background staining, but even 24 h washing in buffer did not change the intensity of the specific binding.

Further, in general, the D3 peptide gave rise to slightly higher levels of specific staining than the D1 peptide. Further, very little Aβ was stained in the **AP** mouse brain sections, but the APP mutation in these mice is in the Aβ sequence and thus leads to Aβ proteins with a different amino acid sequence.

Comparison of the D-peptide stainings with the amyloid staining with Aβ40 and Aβ42 antibodies of sections of the **AP/PS** and **AP/PSΔ** mouse brains showed that there was nearly complete overlap between the location of Aβ42 staining (i.e., plaques) and the D-peptide binding (Figure 3; van Groen et al, 2009). Similarly, comparison of the immunohistochemical staining of the adjacent sections for human amyloid β (with the W0-2 antibody which is specific for human $A\beta_{4-10}$ sequence) showed that there was complete overlap between the location of dense Aβ staining (i.e., plaques) and the binding of the three D-peptides (D1-D3), but that the diffuse amyloid β deposits were not stained, neither in the hippocampus or in the cortex (Figure 1).

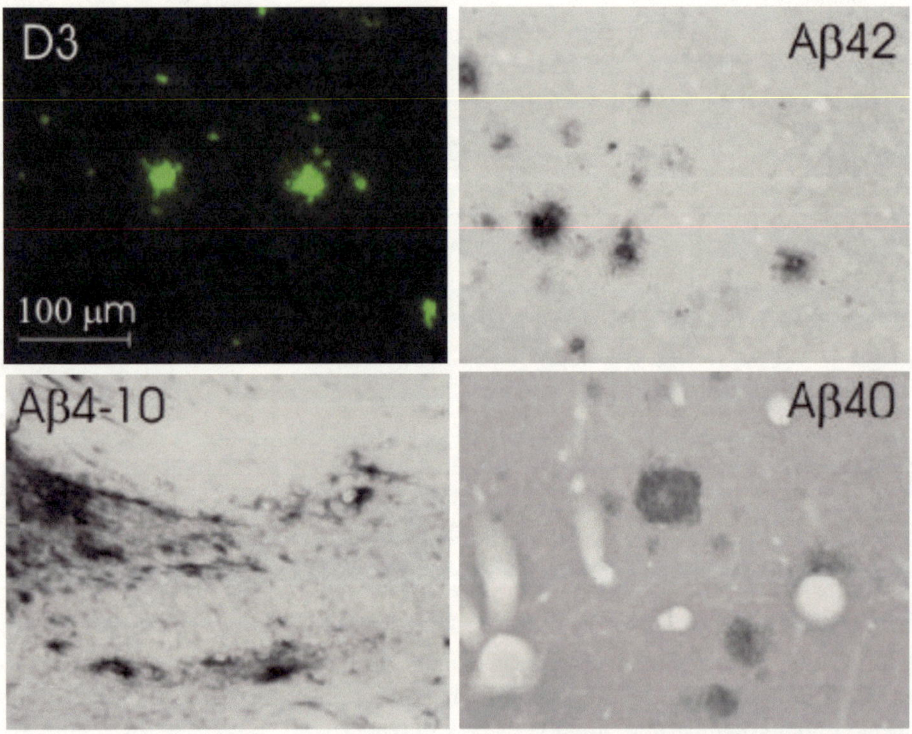


Fig. 3. Four high power photomicrographs of coronal sections through the hippocampus of a Tg AD model mouse. Sections were stained for D3, Aβ40, Aβ42, and Aβ, respectively. Please note the correspondence between D3 and Aβ42 stained sections.

Immunohistochemical staining for Aβ40 or Aβ42 of the sections that were adjacent to the sections stained with the D-peptides showed that the distribution of the D-peptides corresponded more closely to the distribution of Aβ42 than to the distribution of Aβ40 labeling (Figure 3). Both Aβ42 and D3 stain predominantly the core of the plaques, whereas Aβ40 stains mainly the outside of the plaques, i.e., the rim (Figure 3). Sections that were double-stained for both Aβ42 and the D-peptide demonstrated a total overlap between the site of dense Aβ42 deposits and the location of D1 and D3 (not illustrated). Furthermore, staining with β-sheet markers such as thioflavine-S, Congo red, or thiazine red revealed that all Aβ deposits with a β-sheet positive core also stained with the D-peptides (Figure 1). The staining of fixed brain sections of Tg AD model mice (APP-PS) from different ages revealed that in old mice (over 18 months of age), when blood vessel walls contain some Aβ42 deposits, they were stained by the D1 and D3 peptides (Figure 2), but not by the D2 peptide. It should be noted that at earlier ages only Aβ40 is found in the blood vessel wall, and that at that age no labeling with D-peptides is present. Labeling of sections of non-transgenic littermates or control animals did not show any staining at any place in the brain.

To analyze further the binding characteristics of the D-peptides in more detail, an L-peptide version of the D1-peptide (i.e., L-D1) was also tested, likewise a scrambled (sequence) peptide of similar amino acid length (i.e, sc-D1) was tested (Table 1). We used both 0.001 and 0.0001 mg/ml concentrations of L-D1 and sc-D1 on fixed brain sections of old (18 months of age) **AP/PS** mice. L-D1 bound quite similarly to Aβ deposits compared to its D-peptide analog, i.e., it labeled dense Aβ deposits, but not diffuse deposits, and it lightly labeled blood vessel walls with showed Aβ deposits. It should be noted that similar amounts of the L-peptide showed less labeling compared to the D1 peptide. Finally, in contrast to both the L- and D-peptide, the sc-D1 peptide showed significantly reduced binding to Aβ at any type of amyloid deposit (Figure 3). Further, we tested a peptide that was generated against the L-form of Aβ42, i.e., L3, this peptide showed very similar characteristics to the D3 peptide.

In these binding experiments all peptides that were used had been conjugated with a FITC molecule for visualization purposes, therefore we tested in a final set of experiments whether the D1 conjugated with different fluorophores would show distinct binding characteristics, i.e., study the interaction of the fluorescent moiety with the Aβ binding. The data show that no differences in specific binding are present at the 0.001 and 0.0001 mg/ml concentrations between these D-peptides (Figure 4). The D1 conjugated to Oregon green, which is similar in size and charge to FITC, bound Aβ42 similar to the D1*FITC, but the D1*Bodipy (Bodipy is smaller and more polar than FITC) showed significantly increased background staining (Figure 4).

| Peptide | Sequence | Description |
|---|---|---|
| D1 | qshyrhispaqv | Dominating sequence selection 1, Target: D-Aβ |
| L-D1 | QSHYRHISPAQV | L-enantiomer of D1 |
| sc-D1 | hsspqivhqayr | Scrambled D1 |
| D2 | giswqqshhlva | Dominating sequence selection 2, Target: D- Aβ |
| D3 | rprtrlhthrnr | Dominating sequence selection 3, Target: D- Aβ |
| L3 | LRMMLQIKRIPR | Dominating sequence selection 3, Target: L- Aβ |

Table 1. Showing the nomenclature and amino acid sequence of the peptides used in this study.

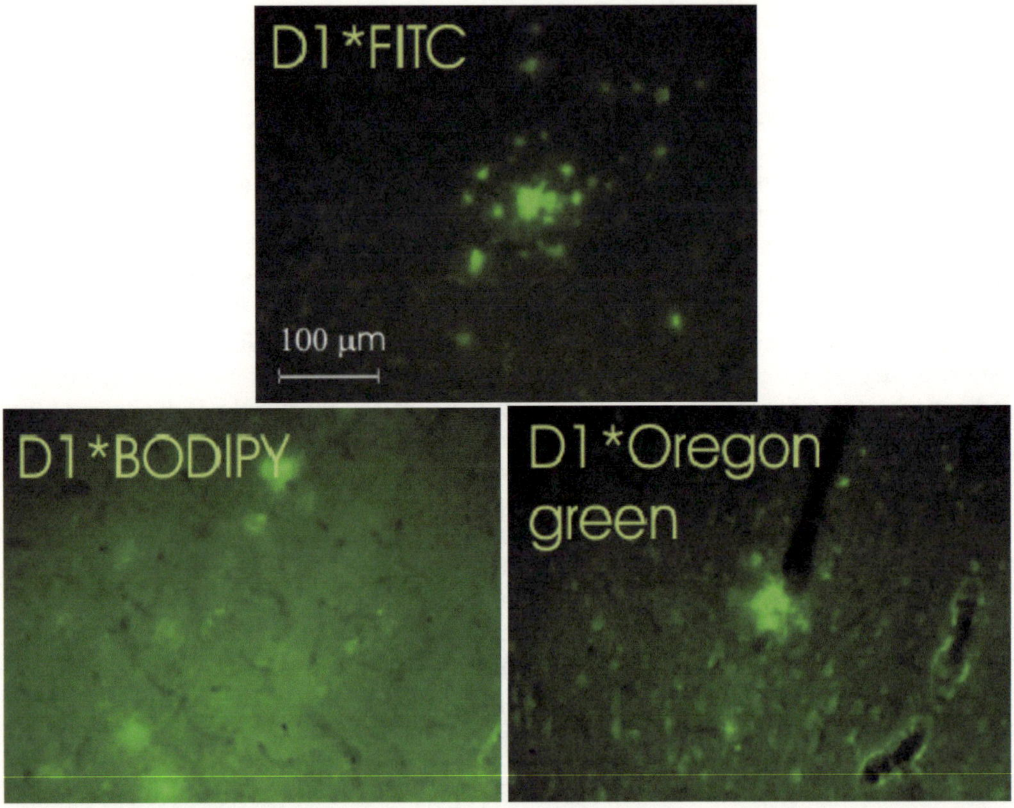


Fig. 4. Three photomicrographs of coronal sections of the parietal cortex of an 18-months-old APP/PS1 mouse stained with the D1 peptide conjugated with different fluorophores, showing staining with D1*FITC, D1*Bodipy, and D1*Oregon green, respectively. Please note the increased background staining with the D1*Bodipy, also note similarity of staining between D1*FITC and D1*Oregon green.

## 4. Discussion

In this study we compared the staining characteristics of three small D-amino acid peptides (i.e., D1, D2, and D3) that were designed to specifically bind Aβ42 (D1, Wiesehan and Willbold, 2003; Wiesehan et al., 2003; D3, ) with the two traditional histochemical methods for amyloid (thioflavine-S and Congo red) and two newer techniques. We examined the labeling of Aβ deposits in Tg AD model mouse brain, in the hippocampus, cortex and in blood vessel walls. The data demonstrate that all dense Aβ deposits (plaques) are labeled with the D-peptides, but not diffuse deposits. This corresponds to the distribution of the Aβ staining in the brain when it is labeled with Aβ42 specific antibodies. Finally, the binding of the D-peptides corresponds closely to the localization of Aβ42 in the brain, more closely than to the localization of Aβ40.

Similarly, in brain tissue sections derived from AD patients, amyloid β plaques and leptomeningeal vessels containing Aβ are stained positively with the fluorescence-labeled derivative of D1 (Wiesehan et al, 2003). In contrast, fibrillar deposits derived from other amyloidosis are not labeled by D1 (Wiesehan et al, 2003). It should be noted that none of the D-peptides showed any binding to Aβ deposits in the brains of mice which express the APPswe/dutch/iowa mutation van Groen et al, 2009). This is to be expected since the structure of the Aβ peptide with these mutations (i.e., the Dutch and Iowa mutations) is predicted to be different from the "normal" Aβ peptide (Demeester et al., 2001; Kumar-Singh et al., 2002; Tsubuki et al., 2003; Watson et al., 1999). It should be noted that these mutations are in the Aβ peptide sequence of APP, in contrast to the Swedish mutation (Selkoe, 2001).

The data demonstrate that none of the three D-peptides binds to diffuse Aβ deposits, whereas they do bind to dense Aβ deposits, i.e., plaques. Earlier we have shown that the diffuse Aβ deposits do not stain with thioflavine S, Congo red or thiazine red, whereas the core of plaques does. Furthermore, the diffuse deposits consist primarily of N-terminal fragments of Aβ, they contain some Aβ40 but do not contain stainable amounts of Aβ42 (Van Groen et al., 2003), in contrast to plaques that consist of significant amounts of both Aβ40 and Aβ42. We have suggested earlier that the diffuse deposits consist of Aβ that has a different length (and structure) from the Aβ42 and Aβ40 that is present in plaques, even if Aβ fibrils are present in the diffuse deposits (Van Groen et al., 2003). Together these data indicate that the D-peptides bind very specifically to only Aβ42.

Furthermore, it has been shown that Aβ42 is actively taken up by astrocytes and microglia (Nagele et al., 2003; Rogers and Lue, 2001. In contrast, surprisingly, no D-peptides are visible in astrocytes and microglia, the phagocytosing cells in the brain (Rogers et al, 2002). Activated microglial cells are present in the brains of AD model mice but these cells never show any presence of intracellular Aβ (e.g., Stalder et al., 2003; but see Paresce et al., 1996).

We have used these peptides to treat AD model mice and we have shown that a brain infusion with D3 significantly reduces pathology and cognitive deficits in AD model mice (van Groen et al, 2009, Funke et al, 2011). In contrast D1 infusion does not improve cognition (van Groen et al, 2009). Similarly it has been demonstrated that Congo red (Inouye and Kirschner, 2005, Lee, 2002) and thioflavine-S improve pathology (Alavez et al, 2011).

Together, we have demonstrated that 1) D-peptides that specifically bind to Aβ42 and, 2) that the D-peptides staining is similar, but more specific, to most traditional histochemical amyloid staining methods. Thus, our data strongly suggest that these novel and highly specific Abeta42 ligands have potential application(s) in the diagnosis and therapy of Alzheimer's disease (Masters and Beyreuther, 2006; Monaco et al., 2006), especially since these D-peptides are much more resistant to proteolysis than natural L-peptides.

## 5. Acknowledgements

We thank Dr. Egon von Schnier for his excellent comments on an earlier version of this manuscript, and Pasi Miettinen for his assistance with the histology. This study was partially supported by TEKES project 40043/01 and partially by NIH AG10836.

## 6. References

Alavez S, Vantipalli MC, Zucker DJ, Klang IM, Lithgow GJ. Amyloid-binding compounds maintain protein homeostasis during ageing and extend lifespan. Nature. 2011 472:226-229.

Benkirane N, Friede M, Guichard G, Briand JP, Van Regenmortel MH, Muller S, Antigenicity and immunogenicity of modified synthetic peptides containing D-amino acid residues. J Biol Chem., 1993 268:26279-26285.

Borchelt DR, Thinakaran G, Eckman CB, Lee MK, Davenport F, Ratovitsky T, Prada C-M, Kim G, Seekins S, Yager D, Slunt HH, Wang R, Seeger, M, Levey AI, Gandy SE, Copeland NG, Jenkins NA, Price DL, Younkin SG, Sisodia SS, Familial Alzheimer's disease-linked presenilin 1 variants elevate Aβ1-42/1-40 ratio in vitro and in vivo. Neuron, 1996 17:1005-1013.

Braak H, Braak E, Neuropathological stageing of Alzheimer-related changes. Acta Neuropathol. 1991 82:239-259.

Braak H, Braak E, Evolution of neuronal changes in the course of Alzheimer's disease. J. Neural. Transm., 1998 53:127-40.

D'Andrea MR, Nagele RG, Wang HY, Lee DH. Consistent immunohistochemical detection of intracellular beta-amyloid42 in pyramidal neurons of Alzheimer's disease entorhinal cortex. Neurosci Lett., 2002 333:163-166.

Demeester N, Mertens C, Caster H, Goethals M, Vandekerckhove J, Rosseneu M, Labeur C. Comparison of the aggregation properties, secondary structure and apoptotic effects of wild-type, Flemish and Dutch N-terminally truncated amyloid beta peptides. Eur J Neurosci., 2001 13:2015-2024 .

Dickson TC, Vickers JC, The morphological phenotype of beta-amyloid plaques and associated neuritic changes in Alzheimer's disease. Neuroscience 2001 105:99-107.

Duff K, Normal and abnormal tau neurobiology. Alzheimer Dis Assoc Disord., 2006 20:202-205.

Duff K, Suleman F, Transgenic mouse models of Alzheimer's disease: how useful have they been for therapeutic development? Brief Funct Genomic Proteomic. 2004 3:47-59.

Funke SA, van Groen T, Kadish I, Bartnik D, Nagel-Steger L, Brener O, Sehl T, Batra-Safferling R, Moriscot C, Schoehn G, Horn AHC, Muller-Schiffmann A, Korth C, Sticht H, Willbold D. Oral treatment with the D-enantiomeric peptide D3 improves the pathology and behavior of Alzheimer's disease transgenic mice. ACS Chemical Neuroscience 2010 1:639-648.

Glenner GG. The bases of the staining of amyloid fibers: their physico-chemical nature and the mechanism of their dye-substrate interaction. Prog Histochem Cytochem. 1981 13:1-37.

Guntern R, Bouras C, Hof PR, Vallet PG. An improved thioflavine S method for staining neurofibrillary tangles and senile plaques in Alzheimer's disease. Experientia. 1992 48:8-10.

Hebert LE, Scherr PA, Bienias JL, Bennett DA, Evans DA. Alzheimer disease in the US population: prevalence estimates using the 2000 census. Arch Neurol. 2003 60:1119-1122.

Ida N, Hartmann T, Pantel J, Schroder J, Zerfass R, Forstl H, Sandbrink R, Masters CL, Beyreuther K, Analysis of heterogeneous A4 peptides in human cerebrospinal fluid and blood by a newly developed sensitive Western blot assay. J. Biol. Chem., 1996;271:22908-14.

Inouye H, Kirschner DA. Alzheimer's beta-amyloid: insights into fibril formation and structure from Congo red binding. Subcell Biochem. 2005 38:203-224.

Jankowsky JL, Slunt HH, Ratovitski T, Jenkins NA, Copeland NG, Borchelt DR, Co-expression of multiple transgenes in mouse CNS: a comparison of strategies. Biomol Eng., 2001;17:157-65.

Kadish I, Van Groen T, Low levels of estrogen significantly diminish axonal sprouting after entorhinal cortex lesions in the mouse. J Neurosci., 2002;22:4095-102.

Klunk WE, Bacskai BJ, Mathis CA, Kajdasz ST, McLellan ME, Frosch MP, Debnath ML, Holt DP, Wang Y, Hyman BT, Imaging Abeta plaques in living transgenic mice with multiphoton microscopy and methoxy-X04, a systemically administered Congo red derivative. J Neuropathol Exp Neurol., 2002 61:797-805.

Kumar-Singh S, Julliams A, Nuydens R, Ceuterick C, Labeur C, Serneels S, Vennekens K, Van Osta P, Geerts H, De Strooper B, Van Broeckhoven C. In vitro studies of Flemish, Dutch, and wild-type beta-amyloid provide evidence for two-staged neurotoxicity. Neurobiol Dis., 2002;11:330-40.

Lazarov O, Lee M, Peterson DA, Sisodia SS, Evidence that synaptically released beta-amyloid accumulates as extracellular deposits in the hippocampus of transgenic mice. J Neurosci., 2002;22:9785-93.

Lazarov O, Morfini GA, Lee EB, Farah MH, Szodorai A, DeBoer SR, Koliatsos VE, Kins S, Lee VM, Wong PC, Price DL, Brady ST, Sisodia SS, Axonal transport, amyloid precursor protein, kinesin-1, and the processing apparatus: revisited. J Neurosci. 2005 25:2386-2395.

Lee VM. Amyloid binding ligands as Alzheimer's disease therapies. Neurobiol Aging. 2002 23:1039-1042.

Masters CL, Beyreuther K, Alzheimer's centennial legacy: prospects for rational therapeutic intervention targeting the Aβ amyloid pathway. Brain 2006;29:2823-39.

McGowan E, Eriksen J, Hutton M, A decade of modeling Alzheimer's disease in transgenic mice. Trends Genet. 2006 22:281-9.

Monaco S, Zanusso G, Mazzucco S, Rizzuto N, Cerebral amyloidoses: molecular pathways and therapeutic challenges. Curr Med Chem. 2006 13:1903-1913.

Morimatsu M, Hirai S, Muramatsu A, Yoshikawa M. Senile degenerative brain lesions and dementia. J Am Geriatr Soc. 1975 23:390-406.

Nagele RG, D'Andrea MR, Anderson WJ, Wang HY, Intracellular accumulation of beta-amyloid(1-42) in neurons is facilitated by the alpha 7 nicotinic acetylcholine receptor in Alzheimer's disease. Neuroscience. 2002 110:199-211.

Nagele RG, D'Andrea MR, Lee H, Venkataraman V, Wang HY, Astrocytes accumulate A beta 42 and give rise to astrocytic amyloid plaques in Alzheimer disease brains. Brain Res. 2003 971:197-209.

Paresce DM, Ghosh RN, Maxfield FR, Microglial cells internalize aggregates of the Alzheimer's disease amyloid beta-protein via a scavenger receptor. Neuron. 1996 17:553-565.

Radde R, Bolmont T, Kaeser SA, Coomaraswamy J, Lindau D, Stoltze L, Calhoun ME, Jaggi F, Wolburg H, Gengler S, Haass C, Ghetti B, Czech C, Holscher C, Mathews PM, Jucker M, Abeta42-driven cerebral amyloidosis in transgenic mice reveals early and robust pathology. EMBO Rep. 2006 7:940-946.

Rogers J, Lue LF, Microglial chemotaxis, activation, and phagocytosis of amyloid beta-peptide as linked phenomena in Alzheimer's disease. Neurochem. Int. 2001 39:333-340.

Rogers J, Strohmeyer R, Kovelowski CJ, Li R, Microglia and inflammatory mechanisms in the clearance of amyloid beta peptide. Glia. 2002 40:260-269.

Satpute-Krishnan P, DeGiorgis JA, Conley MP, Jang M, Bearer EL, A peptide zipcode sufficient for anterograde transport within amyloid precursor protein. Proc Natl Acad Sci U S A. 2006 103:16532-7.

Selkoe DJ, Alzheimer's disease: genes, proteins, and therapy. Physiol. Rev. 2001 81:741-66.

Sheng JG, Price DL, Koliatsos VE, Disruption of corticocortical connections ameliorates amyloid burden in terminal fields in a transgenic model of Abeta amyloidosis. J Neurosci. 2002 22:9794-9.

Stalder M, Deller T, Staufenbiel M, Jucker M, 3D-Reconstruction of microglia and amyloid in APP23 transgenic mice: no evidence of intracellular amyloid. Neurobiol. Aging. 2001 22:427-434.

Styren SD, Hamilton RL, Styren GC, Klunk WE. X-34, a fluorescent derivative of Congo red: a novel histochemical stain for Alzheimer's disease pathology. J Histochem Cytochem. 2000 48:1223-1232.

Tsubuki S, Takaki Y, Saido TC, Dutch, Flemish, Italian, and Arctic mutations of APP and resistance of Abeta to physiologically relevant proteolytic degradation. Lancet. 2003 361:1957-1958.

Uchihara T, Nakamura A, Yamazaki M, Mori O. Tau-positive neurons in corticobasal degeneration and Alzheimer's disease--distinction by thiazin red and silver impregnations. Acta Neuropathol. 2000 100:385-389.

Vallet PG, Guntern R, Hof PR, Golaz J, Delacourte A, Robakis NK, Bouras C. A comparative study of histological and immunohistochemical methods for neurofibrillary tangles and senile plaques in Alzheimer's disease. Acta Neuropathol. 1992 83:170-178.

van Groen T, Liu L, Ikonen S, Kadish I, Diffuse amyloid deposition, but not plaque number, is reduced in amyloid precursor protein/presenilin 1 double-transgenic mice by pathway lesions. Neuroscience. 2003 119:1185-97.

van Groen T, Kiliaan AJ, Kadish I, Deposition of mouse amyloid beta in human APP/PS1 double and single AD model transgenic mice. Neurobiol Dis. 2006 23:653-62.

van Groen T, Wiesehan K, Funke SA, Kadish I, Nagel-Steger L, Willbold D. Reduction of Alzheimer's disease amyloid plaque load in transgenic mice by D3, A D-enantiomeric peptide identified by mirror image phage display. ChemMedChem. 2008 3:1848-1852.

van Groen T, Kadish I, Wiesehan K, Funke SA, Willbold D. In vitro and in vivo staining characteristics of small, fluorescent, Abeta42-binding D-enantiomeric peptides in transgenic AD mouse models. ChemMedChem. 2009 4:276-282.

Van Nostrand WE, Melchor JP, Romanov G, Zeigler K, Davis J, Pathogenic effects of cerebral amyloid angiopathy mutations in the amyloid beta-protein precursor. Ann N Y Acad Sci. 2002 977:258-265.

Van Regenmortel MH, Muller S, D-peptides as immunogens and diagnostic reagents. Curr Opin Biotechnol. 1998 9:377-382.

Vetrivel KS, Thinakaran G, Amyloidogenic processing of beta-amyloid precursor protein in intracellular compartments. Neurology. 2006 66(Suppl 1):S69-73.

Wang J, Tanila H, Puolivali J, Kadish I, van Groen T, Gender differences in the amount and deposition of amyloidbeta in APPswe and PS1 double transgenic mice. Neurobiol Dis. 2003 14:318-327.

Watson DJ, Selkoe DJ, Teplow DB, Effects of the amyloid precursor protein Glu693-->Gln 'Dutch' mutation on the production and stability of amyloid beta-protein. Biochem J. 1999 340:703-709.

Wiesehan K, Buder K, Linke RP, Patt S, Stoldt M, Unger E, Schmitt B, Bucci E, Willbold D, Selection of D-amino-acid peptides that bind to Alzheimer's disease amyloid peptide abeta1-42 by mirror image phage display Chembiochem. 2003 4:748-53.

Wiesehan K, Willbold D, Mirror-image phage display: aiming at the mirror. Chembiochem. 2003 4:811-5.

Wiesehan K, Stöhr J, Nagel-Steger L, van Groen T, Riesner D, Willbold D. Inhibition of cytotoxicity and amyloid fibril formation by a D-amino acid peptide that specifically binds to Alzheimer's disease amyloid peptide. Protein Eng Des Sel. 2008 21:241-246.

# Part 2

## Sexual Disorders

# 5

# Magnetic Resonance Techniques in Study of Sexual Stimuli Processing in Paedophilia

Juan Antonio Becerra-García
*Department of Psychology, University of Jaén, Spain*

## 1. Introduction

The sexual aggression of children is a major public health and criminological issue and a paedophilic crime causes considerable public concern. Paraphilias are deviant sexual behaviors that have common clinical features: sexual fantasies leading to sexual urges and, ultimately, to the deviant sexual behavior. In these group of disorders is include the paedophilia (American Psychiatric Association [APA], 2000). Paedophilia is defined as a psychiatric disorder characterized by intense sexually arousing urges and behaviours focused on the sexual activity with a prepubescent child (APA, 2000; Fagan et al., 2002). The ICD-10 defines paedophilia as a sexual preference for children, boys or girls or both, usually of prepubertal or early pubertal age (World Health Organization [WHO], 2010).

The Diagnostic and Statistical Manual of Mental Disorders, define a paedophile as an individual who fantasizes about, is sexually aroused by, or experiences sexual urges toward prepubescent children (generally <13 years) for a period of at least 6 months. Paedophiles are either severely distressed by these sexual urges, experience interpersonal difficulties because of them, or act on them (diagnostic criteria, according to the DSM-IV-TR, are shown in Table 1), usually come to medical or legal attention by committing an act against a child because most do not find their sexual fantasies distressing or ego-dystonic enough to voluntarily seek treatment. The clinical diagnosis of paedophilia is based on a specific act, it usually is not solely the result of intoxication or caused by another state or condition (APA, 2000).

Paedophiles are subdivided into several classifications. One of the first classifications divided to the paedophiles in two groups, group "exclusively" attracted to children (exclusive paedophile) or attracted to adults as well as children (nonexclusive paedophile group) (APA, 2000). Other categorization of paedophiles is based in if they are attracted to only male children (homosexual paedophilia), female children (heterosexual paedophilia), or children from both sexes (bisexual paedophilia).

The course of paedophilia is usually long term and has yet no cure. The onset of paedophilia usually occurs during adolescence. Occasional paedophiles begin their activities during middle age but this late onset is uncommon. The frequency of behavior associated with paedophilia varies with psychosocial stress . As the paedophile's stress levels increase, the frequency of his or her acting out generally rises also. Various treatments are available. The medical treatments (medications anti-androgens, luteinizing hormone-releasing hormone agonists, female hormones, antidepressant ) and psychological treatments (aversive

behavior therapy and cognitive-behavioral therapy) are aimed at reducing or preventing the expression of paedophilic behavior and to reducing the prevalence of child sexual abuse (Drapeau et al., 2005; Rosler & Witztum, 2000; Schober et al., 2005). The prognosis of successfully ending paedophilic habits among persons who practice paedophilia is not favorable. Paedophiles have a high rate of recidivism; that is, they tend to repeat their acts often over time. Paedophiles offer rationalizations or excuses that enable them to avoid assuming responsibility for their actions. They may blame the children for being too attractive or sexually provocative. They may also maintain that they are "teaching" the child about "the facts of life" or "love". This cognitive distortions made that paedophile behavior is maintained (Mihailides et al., 2004; Ward et al., 1997).
Paedophiles may engage in a wide range of sexual acts with children. These activities range from exposing themselves to children (exhibitionism), undressing a child, looking at naked children (voyeurism), or masturbating in the presence of children to more intrusive physical contact, such as rubbing their genitalia against a child (frotteurism), fondling a child, engaging in oral sex, or penetration of the mouth, anus, and/or vagina (APA, 2000; Cohen & Galinker, 2002).

---

A. Over a period of at least six months, recurrent and highly arousing sexual fantasies, sexual urges or behaviors that involve sexual activity with prepubertal children or children somewhat older (generally 13 years old or under).

B. The fantasies, the sexual urges or the behaviors produce clinically significant unease or deterioration on the social or professional level or in other important areas of the activity of the individual.

C. The person is at least 16 years old and is at least five years older than the child or children referred to in criterion A.

Note: Individuals in the final stages of adolescence who have contact with 12 or 13-year-olds should not be included.

Specify whether:
There is sexual attraction to males.
There is sexual attraction to females.
There is sexual attraction to both sexes.

Specify whether:
The type is exclusive (attraction only to children).
The type is not exclusive.

---

Table 1. DSM-IV-TR criteria for the diagnosis of paedophilia.

In relation to sex preference of the victims, the ratio of girls to boys is 11:1 among (male) paedophiles in contrast to 20:1 among (male) adults committing sex crimes like rape. The homosexual attraction is greater in paedophiles than in other adults involved with sexual crimes with nearly a 2:1 difference (Freund & Watson, 1992). With respect to the choice of children as the object of sexual desire, the distinction has been made between paedophiles and hebephiles, depending on the age of the children. Individuals who engage in sexual activities with pubescent teenagers under the legal age of consent (ages 13-16 years) are known as hebophiles (attracted to females) or ephebophiles (attracted to males) (Blanchard

& Barbaree, 2005; Stone et al., 2000) The term hebophilia or hebephilia is generic term to describe sexual interest in either male or female pubescent children ((Blanchard & Barbaree, 2005; Blanchard et al., 2000; Danni & Hampe, 2000; Stone et al., 2000). The hebophiles tend to be more interested in having reciprocal sexual affairs or relationships with children, are more opportunistic when engaging in sexual acts, have better social functioning, and have a better posttreatment prognosis than paedophiles (Danni & Hampe, 2000; Stone et al., 2000). Other subclassification of paedophilia known as infantophilia, which describes individuals interested in children younger than 5 years (Greenberg et al., 1995). These distinctions are important in understanding current research about paraphilias, selection criteria for studies of sexual behavior and for future diagnosis criteria of paedophilia or pedohebephilic disorders (table 2 shown the future diagnosis criterias of this disorder, where are included criteria of paedophilia and hebephilia).

---

A. Over a period of at least six months, one or both of the following, as manifested by fantasies, urges, or behaviors:
1. Recurrent and intense sexual arousal from prepubescent or pubescent children.
2. Equal or greater arousal from such children than from physically mature individuals.

B. One or more of the following signs or symptoms:
1. The person has clinically significant distress or impairment in important areas of functioning from sexual attraction to children.
2. The person has sought sexual stimulation, on separate occasions, from either of the following:
a. Two or more different children, if both are prepubescent.
b. Three or more different children, if one or more are pubescent.
3. Repeated use of , and greater arousal from, pornography depicting prepubescent or pubescent children than from pornography depicting physically mature persons, for a period of six months or longer.

C. The person is at least age 18 years and at least five years older than the children in Criterion A or Criterion B.

Specify type:
Pedophilic type: sexually attracted to prepubescent children (generally younger than 11).
Hebephilic type: sexually attracted to pubescent children (generally age 11 through 14).
Pedohebephilic type: sexually attracted to both.

Specify type:
Sexually attracted to males.
Sexually attracted to females.
Sexually attracted to both.

Specify if:
In remission (no distress, impairment, or recurring behavior and in an uncontrolled environment): state duration of remission in months: ____.
In a controlled environment.

---

Table 2. Futures DSM-V criteria for the diagnosis of Pedohebephilic Disorder (Recommendation of American Psychiatric Association for to rename Paedophilia to Pedohebephilic Disorder; APA, 2011).

In the field of personality, individuals with this disorder generally experience feelings of inferiority, isolation or loneliness, low self-esteem, internal dysphoria, and emotional immaturity. They have difficulty with mature age-appropriate interpersonal interactions, particularly because of their reduced assertiveness, elevated levels of passive-aggressivity, and increased anger or hostility (Egan et al., 2005; Huprich et al., 2004; Vandiver, 2006; Vandiver & Kercher, 2004). Finally, has been found other differences between paedophilia and control groups. This differences shown that paedophiles presented: a lower intelligence (an area of controversy), a slight increase in the prominence of left-handed individuals, impaired cognitive abilities, neuroendocrine differences, and brain abnormalities, particularly frontocortical irregularities and/or differences (Blanchard & Barbaree, 2005; Bogaert, 2001; Cantor et al., 2005; Tost et al., 2004).

### 1.2 Neuroanatomic theories in paedophilia: brief description

The role of neurological factors and neuropsychological functioning are being integrated in theories of sexual offending (Ward & Beech, 2006). In this disorder, from a neuropsychiatric and neuropsychological perspective, different neuroanatomic theories exist that involve to different cerebral regions in paedophilia.

a. On one hand, the Frontal-Dysexecutive Theories associate sexual offending with dysfunction of frontal cortex and behavioural disinhibition. Proponents of this theory cite studies that show that heterogeneous groups of sexual offenders perform poorly on tests that assess executive functioning, tests as for example: Verbal Fluency, Digit Span, Tower of London, Porteus Mazes, Stroop, Trail-Making, and Wisconsin Card Sort (Dolan et al., 2002; Kelly et al., 2002; Stone & Thompson, 2001; Valliant et al., 2000).
b. Other group is of the Temporal-Limbic Theories that implicate in the regulation of sexual behaviour to temporal lobe structures or give a role to these structures in behavioural disinhibition. The theorists of this point of view cite the associations between temporal lobe epilepsy and paraphilia and between temporal lobe lesions and the hypersexuality exhibited in Kluver-Bucy Syndrome (Hucker et al., 1986; Lilly et al., 1983; Mendez et al., 2000).
c. These two previous approximations have joined in the Dual Dysfunction Theories, in which is defends that the paedophilic men suffer from dysfunction both in temporal regions (causing sexual urges) and in frontal regions (causing behavioural disinhibition) (Cohen et al., 2002).

### 1.3 Justification and objective

Human sexual arousal is a multidimensional experience comprising physiological and psychological processes. Is known that in normal sexual functioning the frontal and temporal cortices are involved in the modulation of drive, initiation, and sexual activation, subcortical structures including the hippocampus, the amygdala, the septal complex and the hypothalamus are implicated in the modulation of sexual behaviours and genital responses. Modern imaging techniques allow the in vivo observation of brain activation correlated with sensory or cognitive processing and emotional states (Krueger et al., 2005) Today the neuroimaging studies in normal sexual functioning confirmed the involvement of inferior temporal cortex, the orbitofrontal cortex, the inferior and superior parietal lobules, the cingulate cortex, the anterior cingulated cortex, the insula, and the hypothalamus in the processing of visual sexual stimuli (Arnow et al., 2002; Bocher et al., 2001; Ferrettiet al., 2005;

Hamann et al., 2004; Holstege et al., 2003; Karama et al., 2002; Mouras et al., 2003; Redoute et al., 2000).In summary, that the cortical and subcortical structures are implicated in the regulation of sexual arousal and in the processing of visual sexual stimuli.

Currently the available data concerning the links between brain anomalies and deviant sexuality, between them the paedophilia has been obtained by means of four main approaches:

1. Neuropsychiatry, the study of acquired psychiatric disorders following brain damage.
2. Structural neuroimaging.
3. Neuropsychological assessments.
4. Functional neuroimaging of sexual offenders compared with nonsexual offenders and the general population.

Of this four approaches, especially the neuroimaging studies have a great potential to identify relevant brain networks and affected structures and for to estimate the brain activation and functioning during the processing of visual information in paedophilia. Previous studies with computed tomography find that the child molesters have less dense skulls and lower cerebral blood flow values (Hendricks et al., 1988). Recent studies show that the functional response patterns of the brain to sexual stimuli contain sufficient information to predict individual sexual orientation with high accuracy, and suggest that the neuroimaging techniques could be a good methods for the diagnosis of the paraphilic disorders, for example paedophilia (Ponseti et al., 2009). Though the neuroimaging studies are very small and very recent in this disorder and the application of these technologies in paedophilia has lagged behind in comparison with others psychopathologies. For what little is known about brain function in paedophilia, the structures involved in sexual behaviour and in the sex stimuli processing in this disorder. For this reason, from a neurological perspective, the aims of this review are to summarize the findings from structural and functional magnetic resonance studies in paedophilia realized up to the date and to present a summary of how is the neurological activation during sex images processing in people with this disorder.

## 2. Selection methods of magnetic resonance studies

### 2.1 Methods of literature review

The search of works was performed in different databases. The databases used were Pubmed, PsycINFO, Scopus and Cochrane. There has been no restriction in the years to search or on the type of document sought. The terms used for search were: "pedophilia" and "paedophilia" searched in conjunction with the terms "brain" and "neuroimaging". The search terms were limited to title, abstract and keywords.

### 2.2 Inclusion criteria

1. Works in which they studied people with diagnosis of paedophilia, according to the diagnostic criteria of the DSM.
2. Works in which they studied the structure or function of the brain in paedophilia by neuroimaging techniques, specifically by structural and functional Magnetic Resonance Image. This criterion allowed to reject works that used other types of techniques that were not specifically neuroimaging techniques.

3. Works that were using as variable of interest the results of the structural and functional techniques to compare paedophiles with other groups (group of control or groups of other sexual aggressors and delinquents in general).
4. Works that were contributing empirical original information published in English, rejecting theoretical previous works, neuropsychological studies and studies of clinical case.

### 2.3 Procedure

The search was realized during September, 2010. Once recovered all the works was reviewed with the aim to analyze if they are complying with the criteria of incorporation. They were checked also by the aim to extract the pertinent information.

### 2.4 Codification of the results

From each of the works the following information was extracted:

1. Authors and year of publication.
2. Sample and Groups. From that was extracted the number of participants, sex and groups in which was divided the sample (in case such that division is existing).
3. Magnetic renonance technique used. It was gathered information about the technique of neuroimage used in the study.
4. Type of design used for the study. It was gathered information about the type of design used in the study, for example if they were experimental, quasi-experimental, and descriptive, among others.
5. Principal obtained findings. Were extracted the principal results contributed by the work.

## 3. Results

### 3.1 Findings of magnetic resonance studies applied to sex stimuli processing in paedophilia

The detailed procedure gave a total of only 7 documents that were complying with the criteria of incorporation. All the documents were articles published in scientific journals. All these works was gathered in two different principal subject matters:

1. Structural or functional studies.
2. Works that study regions of interest or brain in total.

The structural studies were 3 and functional studies 4. The works that study regions of interest was 6 and works that study of the brain in total was 1. Respect to the design, the total of the studies have an experimental design. The type of sample has been organized on the basis of a two category:

1. The type of groups that they include.
2. The sexual orientation of the people included in the sample.

In all the works the sex of the participants was masculine. The works that include group control (of healthy controls and not offenders) was 6 and the works that include other groups of delinquents (non sex offenders) was 1. On the other hand, the works that included homosexuals sample was 1, heterosexuals 2 and both (homosexuals and heterosexuals) was 4. The principal results obtained in every work are described of general form immediately afterwards (a brief summary of the same ones can observe in the table 3).

| | | Number of studies | % of the Review |
|---|---|---|---|
| Brain Study | | | |
| | Total Brain | 1 | 14.29 |
| | Region of Interest | 6 | 85.71 |
| Technique | | | |
| | MR functional | 4 | 57.14 |
| | MR Structural | 3 | 42.86 |
| Design | | | |
| | Experimental | 7 | 100 |
| | Others | 0 | 0 |
| Sample | | | |
| | Control Group: | 7 | 100 |
| | Healthy Control | 6 | 85.71 |
| | Others (non sex offenders) | 1 | 14.29 |

Table 3. Brief description and % of the studies included in the review.

### 3.2 Structural magnetic resonance studies

The results of the structural magnetic resonance studies that study regions of interest, as frontal and temporo-limbic structures, showed that paedophiles had a lesser volume of gray matter in the frontostriatal circuits and the ventral striatum, which extended into the nucleus accumbens and orbitofrontal cortex (Schiffer et al., 2007).

| Authors-year | N Groups (n) | Sex orientation | Study | Findings in paedophiles |
|---|---|---|---|---|
| Schiffer *et al.* (2007) | 42 P (18), HC (24) | Hetero and homosexuals | sMRI of ROI | Lesser volume of gray matter in ventral striatum, OFC and cerebellum |
| Schiltz *et al.* (2007) | 30 P (15), HC (15) | Hetero and homosexuals | sMRI of ROI | Lesser volume of gray matter in subcortical regions (amygdala, hypothalamus and septal regions) |
| Cantor *et al.* (2008) | 130 P(65), NO (65) | Hetero and homosexuals | sMRI of TB | Lesser volume of white matter in parietal and temporal lobes |

HC = Healthy Controls Group, N = Total Sample, NO = Nonsexual Offenders Group, OFC = Orbitofrontal Cortex, P = Paedophiles Group, ROI = Regions of Interest, TB = Total Brain.

Table 4. Brief summary of the different sMRI studies in paedophilia.

Another study also looks for differences in specific areas. This investigation study portions of the limbic system, such as the amygdala, and in the gray matter of structures related to the development of sexual behaviour, such as the hypothalamus. In paedophiles, there was a significant decrease in the volume of the right amygdala and a bilateral reduction of the gray matter of the hypothalamus, septal regions, substantia innominata and bed nucleus of the stria terminalis (Schiltz et al., 2007) (A brief summary of this studies can be seen in table 4).
The study with more statistical power realized up to the date, and that compares the brain in your totality; find negative associations between paedophilia and the volumes of bilateral white matter of the parietal and temporal lobes. The regions with the lowest volume of white matter were adjacent to two major groups of fibres: the superior frontooccipital fasciculus and the right arcuate fasciculus. No difference was observed in the gray matter or in the volume of cerebrospinal fluid (Cantor et al., 2008) (Figure 1 shown a schema of brain white matters tracts. In this figure can observed the tracts of white matters affected in paedophilia, according to the Cantor et al., 2008).

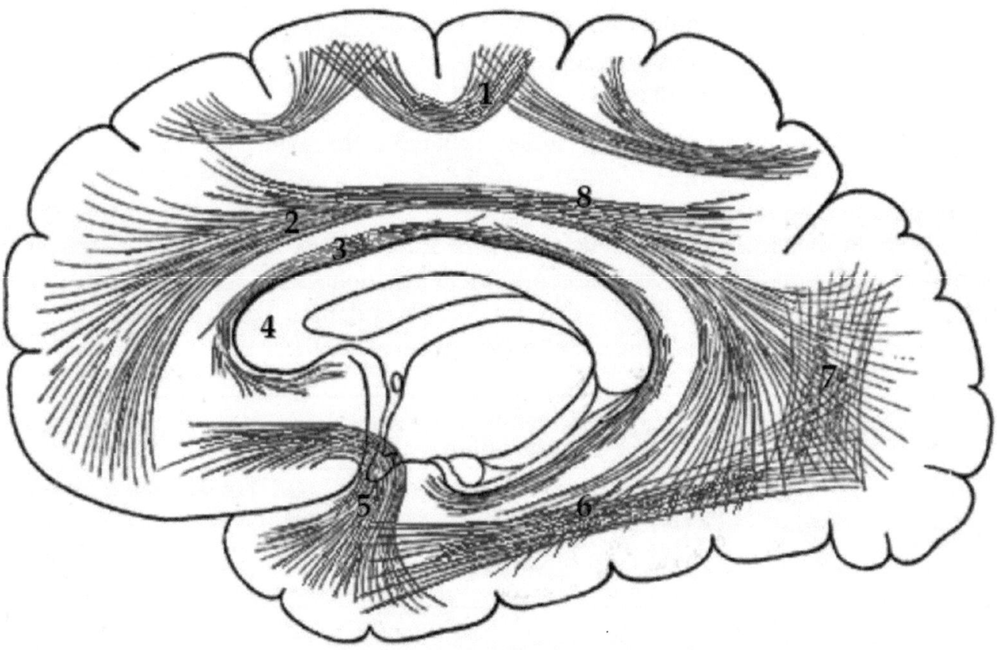


Brain White Matter Tracts: 1) Arcuate Fasciculus (Short Fibres), 2) Superior Fronto-Occipital Fasciculus, 3) Cingulum, 4) Corpus Callosum, 5) Uncinate Fasciculus, 6) Inferior Longitudinal Fasciculus, 7) Perpendicular Fasciculus and 8) Superior Longitudinal Fasciculus. The white matter fibres affected in paedophilia are structures 1 and 2 (Cantor et al., 2008).

Fig. 1. Brain White Matter Tracts.

### 3.3 Functional magnetic resonance studies

On the other hand the functional neuroimaging studies during emotional and erotic stimulation find the following results. In a one o this studies is compared a group of paedophiles and a control group using emotional and erotic pictures. It was observed that the paedophiles responded less to visual erotic stimulation in three regions: dorsolateral prefrontal cortex, hypothalamus and periaqueductal gray matter. However, in no erotic emotional processing, they exhibited a less marked functional response in structures such as the amygdala, hippocampus and dorsomedial prefrontal cortex (Walter et al., 2007). A later research studies specifically the amygdale. Since the amygdala activation is central for emotional valuation, arousal, and salience this study investigate the amygdala activation, with functional magnetic resonance, in response to pictures of adults and children in paedophiles (exclusively attracted to boys) and in a control group (heterosexual). The controls showed less amygdala activation to pictures of children compared to adults. The activation profile was reversed in subjects with paedophilia, who exhibited significantly more activation to children than adults (Sartorius et al., 2008).

Another research compare if the cerebral response of the heterosexual paedophiles to heteropaedophilic visual stimuli are comparable to the cerebral response of heterosexual men to heterosexual stimuli. This response included the activation of different limbic structures (amygdala, cingulated gyrus and hippocampus), substantia nigra, caudate nucleus, anterior cingulated cortex, different thalamic nuclei and association cortex. However, heterosexual men of the control group exhibited a cerebral response in the orbitofrontal cortex during visual sexual stimulation; this frontal response was not similar in the paedophiles that showed an abnormally reduced activity in the dorsolateral prefrontal cortex (Schiffer, Paul et al., 2008). Finally, other research studied of the pattern of cerebral activation in homosexual paedophiles and homosexual controls, during visual sexual stimulation. For this purpose was using photographs that are sexually stimulating and emotionally neutral to the two groups. In both groups finding that the sexually arousing images activated cerebral areas involved in the visual processing of emotional stimuli (occipitotemporal and prefrontal cortexes), but during the presentation of these images, there was a significant activation of areas such as the thalamus, globus pallidus and striata only in the group of paedophiles (Schiffer, Krueger et al., 2008).

| Authors-year | N Groups (n) | Sex orientation | MRI Study | Findings in paedophiles |
|---|---|---|---|---|
| Walter *et al.* (2007) | 27 P (13), HC (14) | Heterosexuals | fMRI of ROI | Reduced activation in hypothalamus and lateral PFC |
| Sartorius *et al.* (2008) | 20 P (10), HC (10) | Hetero (HC) Homosexuals (P) | fMRI of ROI | Increased activation in amygdala |
| Schiffer, Paul *et al.* (2008) | 20 P (8), HC (12) | Heterosexuals | fMRI of ROI | Reduced activation of OFC and dorsolateral PFC |
| Schiffer, Krueger *et al.* (2008) | 23 P (11), HC (12) | Homosexuals | fMRI of ROI | Increased activation of thalamus, globus pallidus and striatum |

HC = Healthy Controls Group, N = Total Sample, NO = Nonsexual Offenders Group, OFC = Orbitofrontal Cortex, P = Paedophiles Group, PFC = Prefrontal Cortex, ROI = Regions of Interest.

Table 1. Brief summary of the different fMRI studies in paedophilia.

## 4. Discussion

Paedophilic and non paedophilic men exhibit a frontal and subcortical activation during processing of sexually relevant stimuli. The paedophiles show more activation in subcortical regions during sex relevant images processing (in hippocampus, amygdala, thalamus, septal areas), regions that are implicated in the modulation of sexual behaviours and genital responses. The activation of these subcortical areas is more intense in paedophiles in comparison to controls that exhibit more activation of prefrontal cortex, the essential structure in the control of the information processing and to co-ordinate behaviour and inhibition of urges impulses.

The findings of the neuroimaging studies in paedophilia suggest that paedophilic and no paedophilic men may differ more fundamentally in the brain function during processing of sexually relevant stimuli. They differ in the brain areas that are activated and not in the brain areas that are implied. In paedophilia this different neural activation in comparison with healthy controls men (without paedophilia) could be owe principally to an alterations in the association fibres of brain that connect different cortical and subcortical areas that realize visual processing or to a structural alteration in neural areas that are important in the development of sexual behaviour (for example in the frontal cortex, amygdala, hypothalamus and septal regions). Too the data of the structural studies could indicate an atypical brain development in paedophiles that could lead to an atypical processing in relation to sexual stimuli and sexual behaviour. But it is necessary to be cautious in the interpretation of the results of these studies. Since some of these works, as the study of Walter et al. (2007) finds a differential activation of subcortical regions in relation to other works that find different evidence. For what it is very necessary to increase the knowledge in this field with new studies.

The results of these studies offer a new perspective on paedophilia and can provide the bases for the development of more sophisticated diagnostic tools and new therapeutic approaches to the treatment of this disorder. Although in relation with the methodology of the works realized up to the date, will be of importance that future studies include a more number of persons with diagnosis of paedophilia, for what works with greater statistical power would be desirable to observe if the findings continue being after of to increase the sample. Also future researchs with a larger sample size would aid in the discovery of other possible differences.

Regarding the groups to include in later studies, would be suitable the incorporation of different groups as sexual non-paedophile aggressors group and of other groups of offenders for if there is some type of alteration that can be due to the sexual aggression or the delinquency in general. Finally, the study of the entire brain might be a method of study more succeeded to try to discover possible differences that the studies that have centred on regions of interest could have overlooked. It is necessary to bear in mind that the area of study, for the social repercussions that carries among other things, is a difficult area for planning some type of study and especially for obtaining the necessary sample.

## 5. Conclusion

In conclusion and although are necessary more studies in this area; people with this disorder seem to show an atypical brain development and respect to your brain function in comparison with control subjects, the results of these latter studies appear to demonstrate that, in the presence of stimuli that are sexually relevant for each group, the central processing of these stimuli is comparable in the two groups, while the pattern of cerebral activation exhibited differs.

## 6. References

American Psychiatric Association, APA (Ed.). (2000). *Diagnostic and Statistical Manual of Mental Disorders. Revised 4th ed.* American Psychiatric Association, Washington, D.C.

American Psychiatric Association, APA. (2011). Sexual and Gender Identity, In: *Disorders Proposed draft revisions to DSM disorders and criteria,* April 5, 2011. Available from: <www.dsm5.org>

Arnow ,B.A., Desmond, J.E., Banner, L.L., et al. (2002). Brain activation and sexual arousal in healthy heterosexual males. *Brain,* Vol. 125, pp. 1014-1023.

Blanchard, R., & Barbaree, H.E. (2005). The strength of sexual arousal as a function of the age of the sex offender: comparisons among pedophiles, hebephiles, and teleiophiles. *Sex Abuse.,* Vol. 17, pp. 441-456.

Blanchard, R., Barbaree, H.E., Bogaert, A.F., et al. (2000). Fraternal birth order and sexual orientation in pedophiles. *Arch Sex Behav.,* Vol. 29, 463-478.

Bocher, M., Chisin, R., Parag, Y., et al. (2001). Cerebral activation associated with sexual arousal in response to a pornographic clip: A 15O-H2O PET study in heterosexual men. *Neuroimage,* Vol. 14, pp. 105-117.

Bogaert, A.F. (2001). Handedness, criminality, and sexual offending. *Neuropsychologia.,* Vol. 39, pp. 465-469.

Cantor, J.M., Kabani, N., Christensen, B.K., et al. (2008). Cerebral white matter deficiencies in pedophilic men. *J. Psychiatr. Res.,* Vol. 42, pp. 167-183.

Cantor, J.M., Klassen, P.E., Dickey, R., et al. (2005). Handedness in pedophilia and hebephilia. *Arch. Sex. Behav.,* Vol. 34, pp. 447-459.

Cohen, L.J., & Galynker, I.I. (2002) Clinical features of pedophilia and implications for treatment. *J Psychiatr Pract.,* Vol. 8, pp. 276-289.

Cohen, L.J., Nikiforov, K., Gans, S., et al. (2002). Heterosexual male perpetrators of childhood sexual abuse: a preliminary neuropsychiatric model. *Psychiatr. Q.,* Vol. 73, pp. 313-336.

Danni, K., & Hampe, G.D. (2000). An analysis of predictors of child sex offender types using presentence investigation reports. *Int J Offender Ther Comp Criminol.,* Vol. 44, pp. 490-504.

Dolan, M., Millington, J., & Park, I. (2002). Personality and neuropsychological function in violent, sexual, and arson offenders. *Med. Sci. Law,* Vol. 42, pp. 34-43.

Drapeau, M., Körner, A., Granger, L., et al. (2005). A plan analysis of pedophile sexual abusers' motivations for treatment: a qualitative pilot study. *Int. J. Offender Ther. Comp. Criminol.,* Vol. 49, pp. 308-324.

Egan, V., Kavanagh, B., & Blair, M. (2005). Sexual offenders against children: the influence of personality and obsessionality on cognitive distortions. *Sex Abuse.*, Vol. 17, pp. 223-240.

Fagan, P.J., Wise, T.N., Schmidt, C.W., et al. (2002). Pedophilia. *JAMA*. Vol. 228, pp. 2458-2465.

Ferretti, A., Caulo, M., Del Gratta, C., et al. (2005). Dynamics of male sexual arousal: distinct components of brain activation revealed by fMRI. *Neuroimage*, Vol. 26, pp. 1086-1096.

Freund, K., & Watson, R.J. (1992). The proportions of heterosexual and homosexual pedophiles among sex offenders against children: an exploratory study. *J Sex Marital Ther.*, Vol. 18, pp. 34-43.

Greenberg, D.M., Bradford, J., Curry, S. (1995). Infantophilia-a new subcategory of pedophilia? a preliminary study. *Bull Am Acad Psychiatry Law.*, Vol. 23, pp. 63-71.

Hamann, S., Herman, R.A., Nolan, C.L., et al. (2004). Men and women differ in amygdala response to visual sexual stimuli. *Nat. Neurosci.*, Vol. 7, pp. 411-416.

Hendricks, S.E., Fitzpatrick, D.F., Hartmann, K., et al. (1988). Brain structure and function in sexual molesters of children and adolescents. *J. Clin. Psychiatry*, Vol. 49, pp. 108-112.

Holstege, G., Georgiadis, J.R., Paans, A.M., et al. (2003). Brain activation during human male ejaculation. *J. Neurosci.*, Vol. 23, pp. 9185-9193.

Hucker, S., Langevin, R., Wortzman G., et al. (1986). Neuropsychological impairment in pedophiles. *Can. J. Behav. Sci.*, Vol. 18, pp. 440-448.

Huprich, S.K., Gacono, C.B., Schneider, R.B., et al. (2004). Rorschach oral dependency in psychopaths, sexual homicide perpetrators, and nonviolent pedophiles. *Behav Sci Law.*, Vol. 22, pp. 345-356.

Karama, S., Lecours, A.R., Leroux, J.M. et al. (2002). Areas of brain activation in males and females during viewing of erotic film excerpts. *Hum. Brain Mapp.*, Vol. 16, pp. 1-13.

Kelly, T., Richardson, G., Hunter, R., et al. (2002). Attention and executive function deficits in adolescent sex offenders. *Child Neuropsychol.*, Vol. 8, pp. 138-143.

Krueger, T.H., Hartmann, U., & Schedlowski, M. (2005). Prolactinergic and dopaminergic mechanisms underlying sexual arousal and orgasm in humans. *World J. Urol.*, Vol. 23, pp. 130–138.

Lilly, R., Cummings, J.L., Benson, D.F., et al. (1983). The human Kluver-Bucy syndrome. *Neurology*, Vol. 33, pp. 1141-1145.

Mendez, M.F., Chow, T., Ringman, J., et al. (2000). Pedophilia and temporal lobe disturbances. *J. Neuropsychiatry Clin. Neurosci.*, Vol. 12, pp. 71-76.

Mihailides, S., Devilly, G.J., & Ward, T. (2004). Implicit cognitive distortions and sexual offending. *Sex. Abuse*, Vol. 16, pp. 333-350.

Mouras, H., Stoleru, S., Bittoun, J., *et al.* (2003). Brain processing of visual sexual stimuli in healthy men: a functional magnetic resonance imaging study. *Neuroimage*, Vol. 20, pp. 855-869.

Ponseti, J., Granert, O., Jansen, O., *et al.* (2009). Assessment of sexual orientation using the hemodynamic brain response to visual sexual stimuli. *J. Sex. Med.*, Vol. 6, pp. 1628-1634.

Redoute, J., Stoleru, S., Gregoire, M.C., et al. (2000). Brain processing of visual sexual stimuli in human males. *Hum. Brain Mapp.*, Vol. 11, pp. 162-177.

Rosler, A., & Witztum, E. (2000). Pharmacotherapy of paraphilias in the next millennium. *Behav. Sci. Law.*, Vol. 18, pp. 43-56.

Sartorius, A., Ruf, M., Kief, C., et al. (2008). Abnormal amygdala activation profile in pedophilia. *Eur. Arch. Psychiatry Clin. Neurosci.*, Vol. 258, pp. 271-277.

Schiffer, B., Paul, T., Gizewski, E., et al. (2008). Functional brain correlates of heterosexual paedophilia. *Neuroimage*, Vol. 41, pp. 80-91.

Schiffer, B., Peschel, T., Paul, T., et al. (2007). Structural brain abnormalities in the frontostriatal system and cerebellum in pedophilia. *J. Psychiatr. Res.*, Vol. 41, pp. 753-762.

Schiffer, B., Krueger, T.H., Paul, T., et al. (2008). Brain response to visual sexual stimuli in homosexual pedophiles. *J. Psychiatry Neurosci.*, Vol. 33, pp. 23-33.

Schiltz, K., Witzel, J., Northoff, G., et al. (2007). Brain pathology in pedophilic offenders: evidence of volume reduction in the right amygdala and related diencephalic structures. *Arch. Gen. Psychiatry*, Vol. 64, pp. 737-746.

Schober, J.M., Kuhn, P.J., Kovacs, P.G., et al. (2005). Leuprolide acetate suppresses pedophilic urges and arousability. *Arch. Sex. Behav.*, Vol. 34, pp. 691-705.

Stone, M.H., & Thompson, E.H. (2001). Executive function impairment in sexual offenders. *J. Individ. Psychol.*, Vol. 57, pp. 51-59.

Stone, T.H., Winslade, W.J., & Klugman, C.M. (2000). Sex offenders, sentencing laws and pharmaceutical treatment: a prescription for failure. *Behav Sci Law.*, Vol. 18, pp. 83-110.

Tost, H., Vollmert, C., Brassen, S., et al. (2004). Pedophilia: neuropsychological evidence encouraging a brain network perspective. *Med. Hypotheses.*, Vol. 63, pp. 528-531.

Valliant, P.M., Gauthier, T., Pottier, D., et al. (2000). Moral reasoning, interpersonal skills, and cognition of rapists, child molesters, and incest offenders. *Psychol. Rep.*, Vol. 86, pp. 67-75.

Vandiver, D.M. (2006). Female sex offenders: a comparison of solo offenders and co-offenders. *Violence Vict.*, Vol. 21, pp. 339-354.

Vandiver, D.M., & Kercher, G. (2004). Offender and victim characteristics of registered female sexual offenders in Texas: a proposed typology of female sexual offenders. *Sex Abuse.*, Vol. 16, pp. 121-137.

Walter, M., Witzel, J., Wiebking, C., et al. (2007). Pedophilia is linked to reduced activation in hypothalamus and lateral prefrontal cortex during visual erotic stimulation. *Biol. Psychiatry*, Vol. 62, pp. 698-701.

Ward, T., & Beech, A. (2006). An integrated theory of sexual offending. *Aggress. Violent. Behav.*, Vol. 11, pp. 44-63.

Ward, T., Hudson, S.M., Johnston, L., et al. (1997). Cognitive distortions in sex offenders: An integrative review. *Clin. Psychol. Rev.*, Vol. 17, pp. 479-507.

World Health Organization, WHO. (2010). International Statistical Classification of Diseases: ICD-10, In: *World Health Organization*, December 15, 2010. Available from: <www.who.int>

# Part 3

## Systems & Networks

6

# Functional Anatomy, Physiology and Clinical Aspects of Basal Ganglia

Edward Jacek Gorzelańczyk
*Polish Academy of Sciences Sue Ryder Home in Bydgoszcz*
*Poland*

## 1. Introduction

Ensuring coordination of the nervous system functioning, communication between various structures, adjusting the functions to the changes in internal and external environment depends on processing of substantial amount of information (Groenewegen, 2007; Groenewegen & van Dongen, 2007).

The concept of cortico-subcortical loops is one of the explanations of the physiological control of the majority of motor, emotional and cognitive functions.

The most important elements are striatum and cerebral cortex. Especially in the pyramidal cells of the cerebral cortex and medium spiny neurons of the striatum there is capacity for plastic changes relating to the control of broadly defined mental functions (motor, emotional, cognitive).

The cerebral cortex is linked to the striatum via cortico-subcortical pathways, from where information is transmitted to the globus pallidus pars internalis or the substantia nigra pars reticulata (which physiologically and anatomically constitute one structure) or via the ventral globus pallidus reach the thalamus and the cerebral cortex subsequently.

The evidence of the anatomical and physiological brain research supported by clinical data and theoretical models suggests there are at least five loops (also called circuits) related to motor, emotional and cognitive functioning control (Alexander et all., 1986; DeLong et all., 1998). The loops division as well as the control of functions assigned to these loops has more model and didactic character rather than it reflects the real character and complexity of the functions controlling these loops.

The following cortico-subcortical loops have been described: 1. motor - between additional motor area of the cerebral cortex and the lateral part of dorsal striatum – putamen; 2. oculomotor - between the frontal visual eye field of the cerebral cortex and the corpus of the caudate (nucleus caudatus) belonging to the medial part of dorsal striatum; 3. prefrontal (associative) - between dorso-lateral prefrontal cortex and the dorso-lateral part of the head of caudate (nucleus caudatus) (the frontal part of the medial part of dorsal striatum); 4. latero-orbito-frontal - between lateral orbito-frontal cerebral cortex and the ventromedial part of the head of caudate (medial part of the dorsal striatum); 5. limbic (circuit of the anterior part of the cingular gyrus) - between the anterior part of the anterior cingulate gyrus and the ventral striatum (of which the main part is the nucleus accumbens).

According to the classic description (Alexander et all., 1986) these circuits pass through various areas of cerebral cortex and subcortical structures and they have similar principles of connections (Royall et all., 2002). As shown in Fig. 1, it was conventionally assumed that individual circuits pass through particular areas of the cerebral cortex, dorsal and abdominal striatum and thalamic nuclei, from where the information reaches the cerebral cortex. Moreover, structurally and functionally related areas of the anterior cerebral cortex and striatum are linked to the posterior parts of the cerebral cortex, e. g. the associative circuit processes information from the dorso-lateral prefrontal cortex and from premotor and posterior part of the parietal cerebral cortex (ibid.) (the areas responsible for the control of motor and spatial functions (ibid.). The fronto-subcortical loops leaving various, distantly located from one other, regions of the cerebral cortex converge in relatively small, limited areas of the target basal ganglia, thalamic nuclei and frontal cerebral cortex (ibid.). Classic hypothesis that individual cortico-subcortical circuits are functionally separated and act simultaneously and independently (Alexander et all., 1986), does not explain the complexity of the nervous system functioning and is not confirmed by the results of investigations and clinical observations of the nervous system damages and disturbances in the loop functioning caused by mental disorders. The complex nature of cortico-subcortical loops functioning is most likely the result of functional connections between the loops. This would explain the control of functions related to integration and convergence of the information processed (Percheron & Filion, 1991; Joel & Weiner, 1994; Parent & Hazrati, 1995).

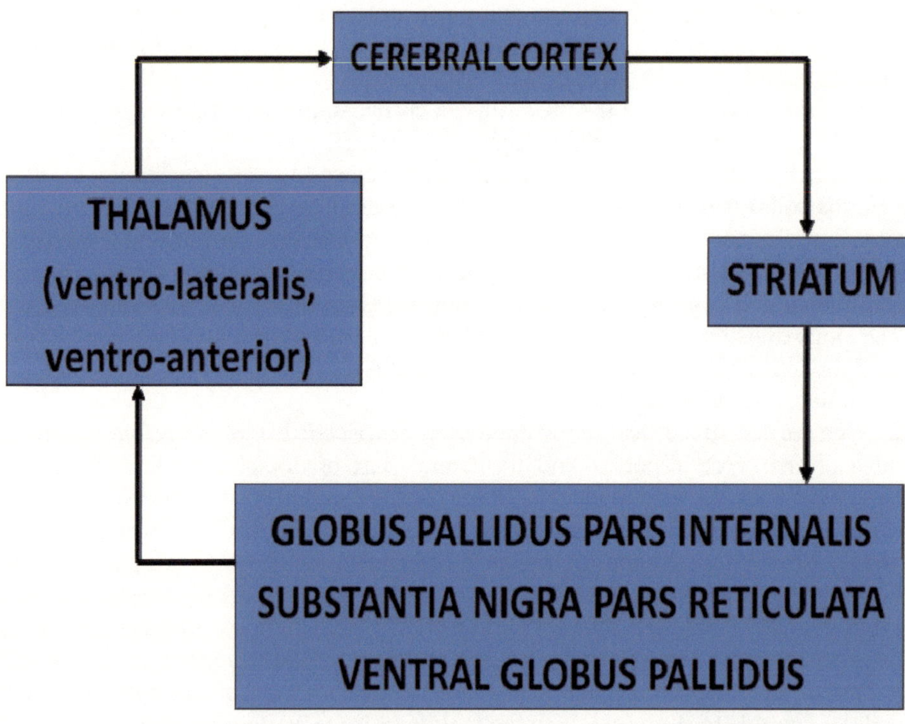


Fig. 1. General scheme of cortico-subcortical loops.

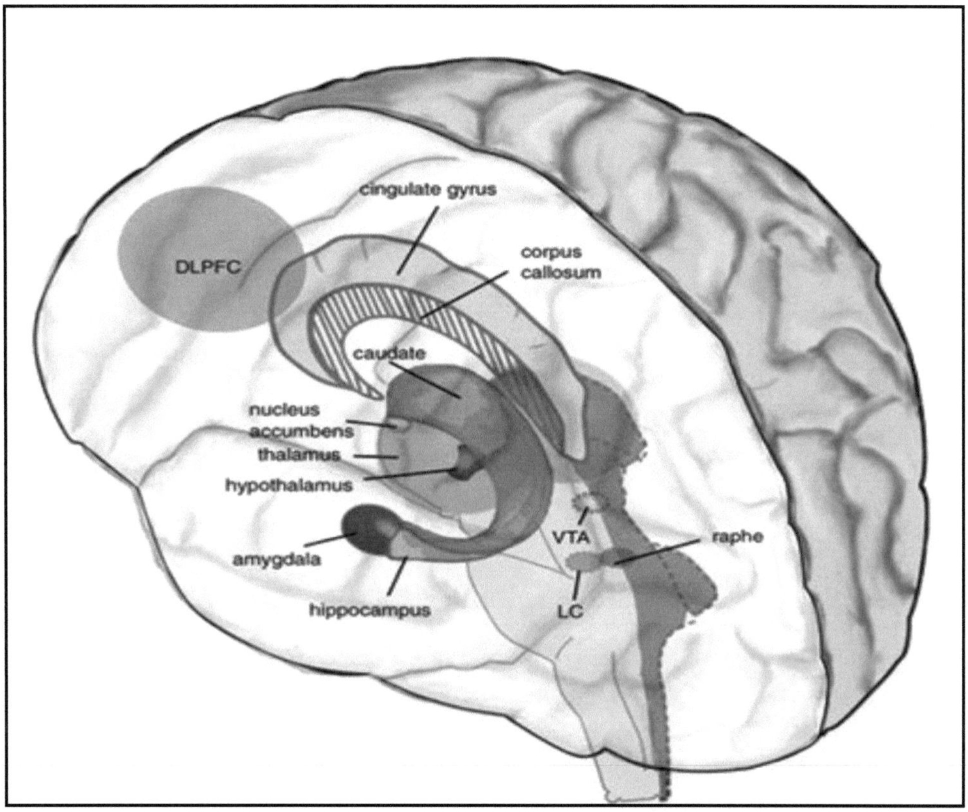


Fig. 2. The circuits connecting the basal ganglia with the cerebral cortex (Stahl, 2008).

The basal ganglia are connected not only with the motor areas of the cerebral cortex but they also influence the areas that are responsible for operating memory and executive functions (dorso-lateral prefrontal cortex and the anterior part of the gyrus cinguli) (Alexander et all., 1986; Middleton & Strick, 1994; Smith & Jonides, 1999; Hartley & Speer, 2000; Elliott, 2003). Prefrontal (associative), latero-orbito-frontal and limbic loops are particularly essential in the control of executive functions (Alexander et all., 1986; Royall et all., 2002; Haber, 2003).

Impairment of prefrontal loop functioning causes disturbances of verbal and spatial operating memory and executive functions (the choice of the aim, planning, accepting and changing of cognitive attitude, self-control and metacognition), involve, in particular, difficulties in executing tests such as Wisconsin Card Sorting Test, WCST) (Fuster, 1980; Cummings, 1995; Fuster, 1995; Goldman-Rakic, 1995a; Milner, 1995; Truelle et all., 1995).

The orbito-frontal circuit is most probably responsible for socially adjusted behaviour and hampering not socially accepted one (Cummings, 1995; Truelle et all., 1995). Efficient functioning of this circuit is of importance for the estimation of the risk of the behaviour chosen (Rogers et all., 1999; Schiffer & Schubotz, 2011). The choice between behaviour in which the probability of a reward is large though the reward is small and behaviour in which the probability of a reward is small but the reward is significant depends on the activity of the inferior and preorbital areas of the prefrontal cortex. The damage to the orbital areas of the prefrontal cortex impairs *"go/do not go"* type tasks execution of in animals (Thorpe et all., 1983) and people (Drewe, 1975; Bunzeck et all., 2011).

| | | | | | | |
|---|---|---|---|---|---|---|
| | | LOOPS | | | | |
| loop unit | | MOTOR | OCULOMOTOR | DORSO-LATERAL PREFRONTAL | LATERAL ORBITO-FRONTAL | LIMBIC (anterior cingulate) |
| cerebral cortex | | premotor area primary motor cortex somatosensory cortex additional motor area | dorsolateral prefrontal cortex posterior parietal cortex frontal oculomotor area | posterior parietal cortex premotor area dorsolateral prefrontal cortex | superior and inferior temporal gyrus anterior part of the gyrus cinguli lateral orbitofrontal cortex | hippocampal cortex entorhinal cortex superior and interior temporal gyrus |
| | | | CAUDATE (caudate nucleus) | | | |
| striatum | | PUTAMEN | body | head | | ventral striatum |
| | | | middle part | dorso-lateral part | ventro-medial part | |
| pallia-dum | globus pallidus pars internalis | ventro-lateral | dorso-medial (posterior part) | dorso-medial (lateral part) | dorso-medial (middle part) | anterio-lateral |
| | substantia nigra pars reticularis | postero-lateral | ventro-lateral | anterio-lateral | anterior-medial | anterio-lateral |
| | ventral globus pallidus | | | | | ventral globus pallidus |
| thalamus | nucleus | | | | | |
| | nucleus ventralis anterior [2] | | pars magnocellularis (lateral part)[6] | pars parvocellularis | pars magnocellularis (medial part) | |
| | nucleus ventralis lateralis [1] | anterior part (rostral)[4] medial part[5] | | | | |
| | anteriors (group) | | | | | |
| | nucleus medialis dorsalis [3] | | pars paralamellaris[7] | pars parvocellularis | pars magnocellularis | postero-medial part |

[1](nucleus ventralis lateralis) = (nucleus ventralis intermedius)
[2](nucleus ventralis anterior) = (nucleus ventralis anteromedialis)
[3](nucleus medialis dorsalis) = (nucleus medialis)
[4](nucleus ventralis lateralis (medial part (rostral) = (nucleus ventrolateralis pars oralis)
[5](nucleus ventralis lateralis - medial part) = (nucleus ventrodorsalis pars medialis)
[6](nucleus ventralis anterior pars magnocellularis) = (nucleus anterior pars magnocellularis)
[7](nucleus medialis dorsalis pars paralamellaris (most lateral) = (nucleus medialis dorsalis pars paralamellaris)

Table 1. Five basalo-thalamo-cortical loop (Mink 1999; Smith et all., 2004; Bochenek & Reicher 2006; Laskowska et all., 2008, Laskowska & Gorzelańczyk, 2009).

It was shown that the anterior cingulate loop is responsible for correcting behaviour following a mistake (Peterson et all., 1999). During the Stroop Interference Color Test, which consists of inhibition of answers learned while choosing opposing answers, the activity of the anterior part of cingulate gyrus and its connections with the central part of the frontal cerebral cortex increases (ibid.).

Motor, emotional and cognitive functions are controlled by two neuronal pathways, being the part of cortico-subcortical loops: direct and indirect (Fig 1). These pathways are under control of connections of the nigrostriatal system of zona compacta nigra (Mandir & Lenz, 1998). The striatum is connected with the thalamus by pathways going through the internal part of the globus pallidus and the reticular part of the substantia nigra. The direct pathway runs from the striatum through the medial part of the globus pallidus, the reticular part of the substantia nigra and the ventral part of the globus pallidus to the thalamus (this causes activation of inhibitory neurons of the thalamus and in consequence activates the cerebral cortex) and further to the cortex of the brain (Longstaff, 2003; Morgane et all., 2005). The indirect pathway runs through the lateral part of the globus pallidus and reaches the subthalamic nucleus (inhibiting glutaminergic transmission of the subthalamic nucleus), from where axons reach the medial part of the globus pallidus and further the thalamus and the brain cortex (ibid.). Control of the stimulation of the cerebral cortex is held, among the others, by striatal neurons (medium spiny neurons) (ibid.). The axons of glutaminergic neurons from the cerebral cortex reach the medium spiny neurons (cortico-striatal pathway) (ibid.). The axons of striatal medium spiny neurons release gamma-aminobutyric acid (GABA) inhibiting activity of the globus pallidus (both: internal and external). Striatal spiny neurons, which are morphologically indistinguishable, can be divided into two populations: 1) medium spiny neurons with D1 receptors containing P substance (SP) and dynorphin (DYN) (GABA/D1/SP/DYN), reach the internal part of the globus pallidus (direct pathway) (Mink, 1999; Longstaff, 2003). 2) medium spiny neurons with D2 containing enkephalin (ENK) (GABA/D2/ENK), reach the external part of the globus pallidus (indirect pathway). Stimuli from the substantia nigra pars compacta neurons of nigrostriatal pathway are transmitted to both populations of the striatal medium spiny neurons. The nigro-striatal pathway increases the activity of the direct pathway and inhibits the activity of the indirect pathway (Mink, 1999; Groenewegen, 2003; Longstaff, 2003; Morgane et all., 2005). Dopamine released in the axon terminals of the nigro-striatal pathway causes in GABA /D1/SP/ DYN striatal medium spiny cells an increase, and in GABA/D2/ENK cells a decrease, in the concentration of the second transmitter: 3'5' - cyclic adenosine monophosphate (cAMP) (ibid.). The activity of the cerebral cortex is proportional to the concentration of cAMP (ibid.).

Glutaminergic neurons of the subthalamic nucleus (indirect pathway) stimulate the external part of the globus pallidus, simultaneously reducing activity of the thalamus and cerebral cortex neurons. The striatum inhibits the neurons of the lateral part of the globus pallidus, what leads to disinhibition of glutaminergic cells of the subthalamic nucleus and stimulation of the globus pallidus pars interna. Dynamic changes of the activity of direct and indirect pathway make it possible to stimulate well defined areas of the cerebral cortex with simultaneous inhibition of the areas, which do not take part in execution of particular movement or mental action (Mink, 1999; Groenewegen; 2003).

The damage of various structures of basalo-thalamo-cortical loop can manifest with symptoms related to a definite loop (Alexander, 1986; Royall et all., 2002). According to this argumentation it can be assumed that pathology of the basal ganglia can cause symptoms typical for the damage of a particular loop or cause typical symptoms for the damage of several of them (ibid.). The symptoms, being the consequence of, definitely localized in the brain, damages of the particular structures of cortico-subcortical loops, can overlap with the symptoms from different areas of encephalon connected with a specific functional system, which is not a part of this system (ibid.). The conceptual model of basalo-thalamo-cortical connections can be helpful in interpretations of the symptoms of mental disorders relating to basal ganglia pathologies, for example in Parkinson's disease (Tröster & Arnett, 2005).

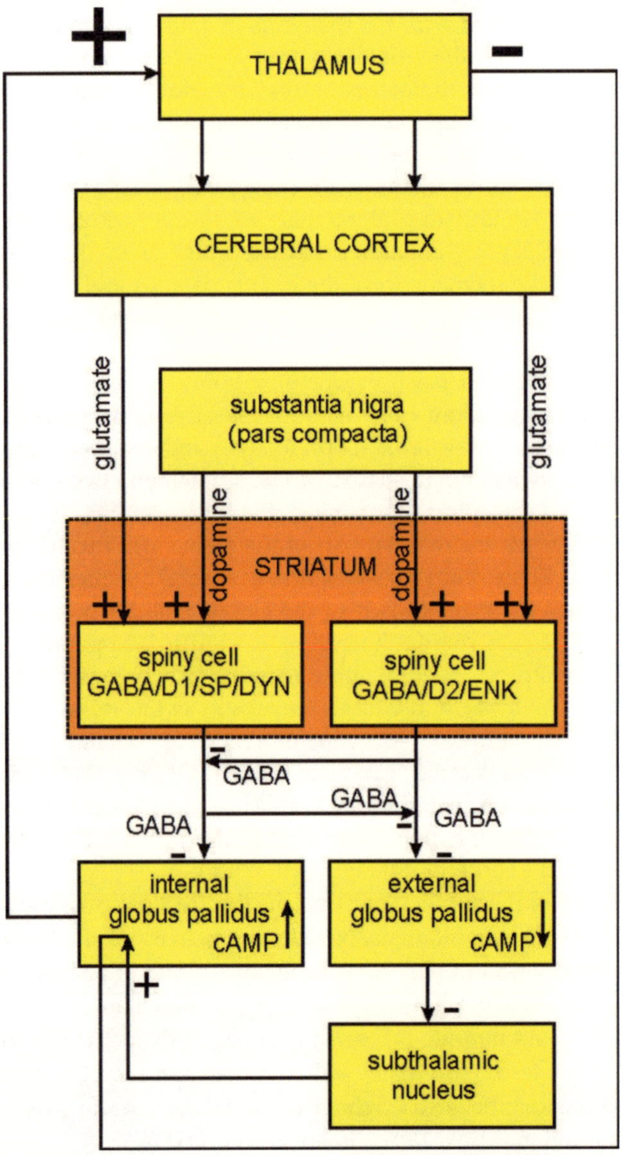


Fig. 3. The original conceptual model of the neuronal loop connecting the internal globus pallidus (GPI), subthalamic nucleus (STN) and thalamus with the cerebral cortex compiled on the basis of the literature (Fix, 1997; Longstaff, 2003; Groenewegen, 2003).

## 2. Motor loops (motor and oculomotor)

Motor control of skeletal muscles relates to the motor loop (motor circuit) and the oculomotor loop (oculomotor circuit) (ibid.). The dorso-medial prefrontal loop, orbito-frontal loop and the anterior part of the cingular gyrus loop are associated with the control of cognitive and emotional functions (ibid.).

The motor circuit is responsible, inter alia, for automatic motor activity connected with maintenance of body posture and reflexes (Fix, 1997), as well as for the control of muscular tension. The motor loop plays an essential role in initiating and fluent performing of motor actions executed by skeletal muscles especially during will dependent movements. The disorders of this loop can cause muscular stiffness, bradykinesia, akinesia and hipokinesia (e.g. in Parkinson's disease and parkinsonian syndrome) or excessively large and uncontrolled movements of limbs (e.g. Huntington's chorea, balism) (Fix, 1997).

The oculomotor loop participates in the control of saccadic eyeball movements. Efferent connections to the superior colliculus (Sc) from the cortical areas of the brain and subcortical nuclei, especially the reticular part of substantia nigra (SNr) make it possible to control rapid eyeball movements through the inhibition of movements disturbing the execution of a task (Hikosaka, 2000). Pressumably the neurons of ventro-lateral part of substantia nigra pars reticularis and caudate nucleus play essential role in external eyeball muscles movements, both through the neurons in which information on previously executed movements is remembered (memory-guided saccades), as well as neurons reacting on currently incoming visual stimuli (visually-guided saccades) (ibid.). In the result of oculomotor loop damage visual fixation can be impaired, and unilateral neglect syndrome, as well as attention deficits can be observed especially in the tasks requiring rapid movements targeted at stimuli (Hikosaka, 2000). The shortage of functions of external eyeball muscles caused by damages of basal ganglia (e.g. in Parkinson's disease, Huntington's disease) can impair saccadic movements of eyeballs depending on previously remembered information. In persons with basal ganglia disorders dysfunctions in intentional inhibition of eye movements, triggered by visual stimuli (ibid.), were observed.

## 3. Dorsolateral prefrontal loop

The dorsolateral prefrontal loop is responsible for the choice of aims, planning, programming of the sequence of mental actions and behaviours, switching between sentences (the ability to change attitude flexibly), verbal and spatial working memory, self-control and metacognition (self-consciousness) (Royall et all., 2002). The disorders of the loop functions can lead to incorrect order of linguistic behaviours what results in verbal fluency reduction (DeLong & Wichmann, 2007).

## 4. Lateral orbitofrontal loop

The lateral orbitofrontal circuit takes part in initiating social behaviours motivated by an award and in inhibiting behaviours, which can trigger punishment (Royall et all., 2002). Incorrect functioning of this circuit may result in disinhibition of behaviours, personality changes, lack of control and emotional liability, as well as irritability and gaiety (DeLong & Wichmann, 2007). The damage of this loop can cause perseverations, which make it difficult to process information from external environment and adaptation of behaviours to a particular situation (Royall et all., 2002).

## 5. Anterior cingulate circuit

The anterior cingulate circuit (limbic loop) is important in behavior control and adaptation of behaviours after making a mistake (ibid.). The damage of this circuit results in emotional disorders especially deep apathy and lack of spontaneity. Lowered mood is accompanied by weakening of affect and motor adynamy (ibid.).

On the basis of a pattern of basal ganglia connections, being a part of particular loops with cerebral cortex, similarity of motor and emotional functions can be deducted (Alexander et all., 1990). Information processed by various loops partly overlap in the striatum (ibid.). In the globus pallidus pars internalis and the substantia nigra pars reticularis and subsequently in the thalamus pieces of information from various circuits converge. Pieces of information from the thalamus reach limited areas of the cerebral cortex, which control motor, emotional and cognitive functions (ibid). Such functional organization makes it possible to select motor and mental actions depending on information incoming from external and internal environment (Mink, 1999; Morgane et all., 2005; Groenewegen & Dongen, 2007).

The circuits, described above, functionally connect the basal ganglia with the cerebral cortex (Alexander et all., 1986; DeLong et all., 1998; Elliot, 2003; Haber, 2003; Saint-Cyr et all., 2003; Morgane et all., 2005; Olzak & Gorzelańczyk, 2005; Groenewegen & van Dongen, 2007; Laskowska et all., 2008; Haber et all., 2009). The assumption that the circuits connecting the cerebral cortex with the basal ganglia work independently and in a parallel way (Alexander et all., 1986, 1990; DeLong et all., 1998) has expired. Various consequences of the damages of particular loops activity depend on the cerebral cortex areas with which they connect and on the circumstances in which they are activated. The degree of co-operation of particular basalo-thalamo-cortical loops is not known (Longstaff, 2006; Laskowska et all., 2008; Haber et all., 2009; Sadikot et all., 2009), however more and more data indicate that the exchange of information between particular circuits takes place (McFarland et all., 2002; Groenewegen & van Dongen, 2007; Laskowska et all., 2008; Haber & et all., 2009; Sadikot et all., 2009).

Subcortical nuclei relate not only to motor control, but also to the processes of reminding as well as executive functions processes, short-term memory, the analysis of mutual setting of objects and to undertaking actions (Sławek et all., 2001; Frank et all., 2001; Royall et all., 2002; Elliot, 2003; Haber, 2003; Laskowska et all., 2008; McNab et all., 2008; Haber et all., 2009).

The basal ganglia take part in the control of motor, emotional and cognitive behaviours by two pathways (indirect and direct) exerting contradictory effect on the stimulation of the thalamus and the cerebral cortex. (Albin et all., 1989; DeLong, 1990; Obeso et all, 1997, 2000b; Sławek, 2003; Sobstyl et all., 2003; Groenewegen, 2003; Longstaff, 2006; DeLong & Wichmann, 2007; Groenewegen & van Dongen, 2007; Szołna, 2007). In the nigrostriatal pathway there are two kinds of dopaminergic receptors relating to striatal medium spiny neurons: D1, which activate GABA-ergic neurons of the putamen in the direct pathway; and D2, whose stimulation inhibits GABA-ergic neurons of the putamen in the indirect pathway (ibid.).

The direct pathway relates to striatal medium spiny neurons (SP/DYN) releasing GABA and inhibiting GABA-ergic neurons running from GPi and SNpr to the thalamus. Cortical stimulation of this pathway causes activation of thalamus neurons (Groenewegen, 2003; Sobstyl et all., 2003; Longstaff, 2006; Groenewegen & van Dongen, 2007; Szołna, 2007). The direct pathway connects the putamen, where the connections from the cerebral cortex and the substantia nigra (SNpc) meet, with the exit structures - the internal part of the globus pallidus and reticular part of substantia nigra pars reticulata – (SNpr) (ibid.).

The direct pathway is connected with striatal medium spiny neurons (ENK) secreting GABA and it leads through the external part of the globus pallidus (GPe) to STN, which stimulates inhibitory neurons in GPi and SNr structures. Cortico-striatal stimulation of the indirect pathway decreases thalamus stimulations and inhibits motor cerebral cortex (Albin et all., 1989; DeLong, 1990; Obeso et all., 1997, 2000b; Herrero et all., 2002; Sobstyl et all., 2003; Longstaff, 2006; Groenewegen & van Dongen, 2007).

Dopamine is a neurotransmitter in SNc neurons (Groenewegen, 2003; Sobstyl et all., 2003; Groenewegen & van Dongen, 2007). During repose occasional discharges of small frequency, which do not affect movement, appear in these neurons (Longstaff, 2006). The frequency of neurons firing changes when a stimulus rewarding a movement is present (ibid.). They influence the reply of striatal medium spiny neurons to the stimulation from the cerebral cortex. GABA/SP/DYN neurons increase responsiveness in the direct pathway, however GABA/ENK neurons reduce responsiveness in the indirect pathway due to the SNc influence. As a result, the nigro-striatal connection increases the activity of the direct pathway, inhibiting the indirect pathway (ibid.).

The basal ganglia are responsible, inter alia, for executing motor sequences (Alexander et all., 1990; Mink, 1999; Sadowski, 2001; Herrero et all., 2002; McFarland et all., 2002; Longstaff, 2006; Haber et all., 2009). Each sequence is represented by striatal medium spiny neurons creating motor or oculomotor microloops in the cortico-subcortical circuit, which can be activated or inhibited (Alexander et all., 1986; Longstaff, 2006). A considerable part of striatal medium spiny neurons has low frequency of electric discharge at rest (0,1-1Hz). In other subcortical nuclei - GPi and SNr, the frequency of electric discharge at rest is considerably higher and it amounts to about 100*Hz* (ibid.). According to a contemporary model of motor control carried out by the basal ganglia, movements are initiated by activation of the motor cerebral cortex, which consequently activates the striatum (Groenewegen, 2003; Sobstyl et all., 2003; Longstaff, 2006; Groenewegen & van Dongen, 2007; Sadikot et all., 2009). The activity of striatal medium spiny neurons increases during the execution of movements being a result of functioning of cortico-striatal neurons (Longstaff, 2006). When a discharge frequency of GPi and SNr decreases, a reduction in the thalamus inhibition follows making it possible to execute a movement or other mental action (Albin et all., 1989; DeLong et all., 1990; Obeso et all., 1997, 2000; Sobstyl et all., 2003; Longstaff, 2006).

Motor, emotional and cognitive functions are controlled by the system of structures and connections of the central nervous system, among which three levels of co-operation were distinguished: lower, middle and upper (Schotland & Rymer, 1993; Longstaff, 2006). Experimentally induced damages of the nervous system centers in animals result in the lack of the function subjected to the place of the damage and the appearance of new or enhancement of until now executed actions. A damage of the motor center of the cerebral cortex causes limbs paresis, an increase in muscles tension, intensification of tendinous reflexes in these limbs as well as appearance of Babiński's reflex (Babinski, 1986). The occurrence of such symptoms indicates that lower in hierarchy structures are inhibited by higher ones and that the lack of this inhibition causes unblocking of the physiologically inhibited centre. Clinical observations of persons with the basal ganglia damages indicate that these structures do not initiate movements, but they control the course of skilled sequence of movements (ibid.). An increase in the activity of the direct pathway increases, and of the indirect pathway decreases, stimulation of particular areas of the cerebral cortex (Groenewegen, 2003; Longstaff, 2006; Groenewegen & van Dongen, 2007; Szołna, 2007).

Cooperation between the direct and indirect pathways changes the activity of the cerebral cortex in such a way that the activity increases in the areas which control execution of a particular motor action and inhibits the areas which are not involved in the executed activity (ibid.). Planning of motor activity relates to the functioning of the cerebral prefrontal cortex controlling the process of scheduling and execution of a particular sequence of movements (LeDoux, 1996; Groenewegen, 2003; Longstaff, 2006; Groenewegen & van Dongen, 2007). The control of implementation of the actions scheduled is possible when the the centers of the cerebral cortex and basal ganglia (especially the caudate) cooperate properly (Alexander et all., 1986, LeDoux, 1996; Herrero et all., 2002; Groenewegen & van Dongen, 2007). The nucleus caudatus - a part of the ventral striatum is connected with a substantial part of the frontal, mainly with the associative cerebral cortex (ibid.). Pieces of information incoming from the cerebral cortex to the caudate make it possible to control and implement a particular sequence of movements (ibid.). A program relating to the implementation of a specific sequence of movements is sent from the caudate through the thalamus to the premotor prefrontal cerebral cortex, which controls voluntary movements (ibid.). The basal ganglia in connection with ventral nuclei of the thalamus and frontal areas of the cerebral cortex play an essential role in instrumental conditioning (Petri et all., 1994; Smith's Petri et all., 2006; Rueda-Orozco et all., 2008). The results obtained in investigations on animals confirm the meaning of the basal ganglia in the procedural memory (Petri et all., 1994; Akhmetelashvili et all., 2007; Hartman et all., 2008; Rueda-Orozco et all., 2008).

The pattern of basal-thalamic-cortical connections carrying out motor, emotional and cognitive functions is mutual for these functions (Alexander et all., 1996; DeLong et all., 1998; Herrero et all., 2002; Groenewegen, 2003; Saint-Cyr, 2003; Groenewegen & van Dongen, 2007; Laskowska et all., 2008), and the control of these functions consists in the choice of the sequence of behaviours adapted to a particular situational context (Heilman et all., 1993; Royall et all., 2002; Longstaff, 2006).

The control of motor, emotional and cognitive functions is hierarchical and the processing of information connected with these functions can be executed sequentially or simultaneously in various structures of the brain. Clinical observations and the results of the investigations carried out in persons with a damage of the basal ganglia confirm the participation of subcortical structures not only in motor but also cognitive functions (Oberg and Divac, 1979; Berns and Sejnowski, 1995; Frank et all., 2001). Also the results of computer simulations of cognitive actions such as: maintenance of information in operating memory, remembering, planning of sequences of behaviors and making decisions indicate a participation of the basal ganglia in the control of cognitive functions (Prescott et all., 2002; Jessup et all., 2011). The function of the basal ganglia in the control of motor, emotional and cognitive functions relates to cooperation with frontal cerebral cortex areas (Brown et all., 1997). The basal ganglia cooperating with the prefrontal cerebral cortex make it possible to initiate motor, emotional and cognitive actions. A complex system of stimulations (inhibition and disinhibition) limits the flow of excessive information which disables the initiation of an activity. A complex choice mechanism makes it possible to initiate a particular kind of movement without detailed determination of the whole sequence of the movements executed (Bullock & Grosberg, 1988; Hikosaka, 1989; Chevalier & Deniau, 1990; Passingham, 1993).

According to the concept of mental (motor, emotional, cognitive) functions control carried out by cortico-subcortical loops a proper action of all the structures of these loops is a condition necessary for their efficient functioning (Brown et all., 1997). Mental processes, such as for example: making decisions, the choice of motor action, the change of behavior, working memory can be disturbed in a similar degree, independently from which structure of a particular loop is damaged (ibid.). Because of a specific structure of striatal medium spiny neurons (having a very large quantity of synaptic connections) and synaptic processes like long-term synaptic potentiation (LTP) and long-lasting synaptic depression (LTD), similar to those carried out in the cerebral cortex, the striatum (including the ventral striatum) is functionally the main structure of cortico-subcortical loops (Picconi et all., 2005) that controls motor, emotional and cognitive functions. Due to numerous inter-striatal and cortico-striatal connections and described above plastic mechanisms enabling enhancement or reduction of stimulations, the striatum together with the cerebral cortex controls the functions of particular cortico-subcortical loops, substantially influencing mental processes (Brown et all., 1997; Prescott et all., 2002).

The results obtained from the experiments on a model of shoulder movement simulation indicate that the higher dopamine concentration is in the striatum the shorter is the time necessary to initiate a movement (ibid.). This means that the time necessary to initiate a movement becomes shorter simultaneously with an increase of the striatum stimulation (ibid.). Moreover, the simulation of a decrease in dopamine concentration in the striatum in the same model causes bradykinesia and akinesia, similar to that observed in the Parkinson's disease (Prescott et all., 2002). The key function of the striatum is to produce signals which reach, through the thalamus, the cerebral cortex (ibid.). It was suggested that the choice of a particular pattern of action takes place in the striatum due to so called gating mechanism. Activation of the neurons responsible for processing of a particular pattern leads to inhibition of other striatal neurons. The mechanism makes it possible e.g. to process efficiently information introduced to the working memory with simultaneous inhibition of the inflow of new information before completing a presently executed task (Frank et all., 2001). If the gate is closed, new information does not influence the memory essentially and that is why it allows a stable maintenance of information being processed (ibid.). Opening of the gate enables data updating (ibid.). The inhibition of new information inflow prevents their interference with previously gathered data (ibid.). This mechanism enables continuous selection of the processed information optimizing in this way execution of mental actions (ibid.). The disturbance of the mechanism of selective actualization of data in proper time (both too frequent and too rare data updating) increases the number of errors made in various tasks. This disorder relates to initiation of both movement and thought processes. A confirmation of the concept equity is psychic akinesia observed in persons with a damage of the striatum (Brown and Marsden, 1990). However, inhibition of the internal part of the globus pallidus leads to disinhibition of frontal loops activity, which results in continuous updating of data. Continuous updating of data is caused by the lack of blocking in access to the working memory (Frank et all., 2001). Results of these disorders can be Absent-mindedness, impulsivity and hyperactivity (occurings in the disorders such as: Huntington's disease, Tourette syndrome, attention deficit hyperactivity disorder) can be the results of the above mentioned disorders (ibid.). Diminishing of dopamine concentration in the striatum causes that the gate regulating the access to the working memory is opened and closed in the wrong time, and in permanent inhibition of the internal part of the globus pallidus it is opened all the time (ibid.).

The gating model does not fully explain the selection of data, which arises from the fact that dopamine is secreted in large areas of the prefrontal cortex. In this model, different areas of the prefrontal cortex are activated simultaneously, making it impossible to select one particular piece of information (ibid.). This mechanism does not meet the functional requirements of selective updating of data, which is, as explained above, a simultaneous updating of certain information and maintaining the remaining data unaltered (ibid.).

The gating model is complemented by the concept of selective gating mechanism based on the functioning of parallel basal-thalamic-cortical loops (Frank et all., 2001). Inhibitory nature of the connections leading from the striatum to the internal part of the globus pallidus (GPi), the reticular part of the substantia nigra (SNr) and the thalamus has a decisive influence on the processes of gating. For this reason, the activity of neurons in the striatum causes the stimulation of neurons in the thalamus (via dual inhibition) (Deniau & Chevalier, 1985, Chevalier & Deniau, 1990). Disinhibition of the thalamus evokes gating function that enables emergence of other functions, although it does not induce them directly.

Selective gating mechanism explains the role of the basal ganglia in the initiation of the process of collecting new information in the working memory and the possibility of its inflow of new information before completing a presently executed task (Frank et all., 2001). If the fast update (Frank et all., 2001). In the absence of stimulation of striatal neurons the gate remains closed and the frontal cerebral cortex maintains the information currently being processed. This is possible due to existence of multiple parallel loops (ibid.).

In a classical division five parallel basal-thalamic-cortical loops were proposed (Alexander, 1986). However, on the basis of anatomical characteristics, existence of many subloops inside this five basic circuits was assumed. Due to this a relatively precise control of the working memory is possible (Beiser & Houk, 1998). It was assumed that control of the working memory depends on maintaining constant stimulation of neurons of the prefrontal cortex (Frank et al, 2001), which is the result of a continuous self-stimulation via a feedback loop (ibid.). Maintaining of this state is possible due to active feedback connections between the neurons of the frontal cerebral cortex and the thalamus. (ibid.).

The importance of the basal ganglia in senso-motor processes consists in the fact that they decide on the choice of a particular activity (Prescott et all., 2002). In the computational model, which was based on the observation of two different, competing with each other behaviors, it is assumed that coded is only one of them (i.e. the one whose execution by the motor system is being currently more important) (Redgrave et all., 1999). At the cellular level, a complex choice mechanism that allows solving a conflict between competing behaviors through fast and decisive switch between pre-selected actions, may be related to the degree of polarization of the neuron cell membrane. Resting membrane potential of striatal spiny neurons fluctuate from the values close to depolarization state so-called "up" state to hyperpolarization - "down" state (Calabresi et all., 2007). The selection mechanism consists of four steps: 1) selection of the cells in "up" state and exclusion of the cells in "down" state; 2) local inhibition within the striatum, which selectively increases the probability of stimulation of some spiny neurons and decreases the probability of stimulation of the other ones (accordingly to the cognitive model it increases the probability of the flow of information through specific channels (perceived as groups of spiny cells) (Redgrave et all., 1999); 3) localized inhibition induced by striatal medium spiny neurons (D1) together with dispersed stimulating impulses, incoming from the subthalamic nucleus, which act like a feed- forward loop, controlling the information coming out of the basal ganglia (from the internal globus pallidus and the substantia nigra reticularis); 4) local mutual inhibition occurring in the output basal ganglia (thalamus), which additionally restricts the selection criteria (ibid.).

According to the described above hypothesis on action selection, an alternative explanation for the functional organization of the basal ganglia was proposed. Instead of traditionally selected pathways (*direct* and *indirect)* the existence of neuronal circuits responsible for the choice (called selection circuit) and control (control circuit) of the activities undertaken is postulated. The selection circuit (traditionally called: direct pathway), leading from D1 dopamine receptors of striatal medium spiny neurons to the entopeduncular nucleus (EP) (or internal globus pallidus in primates) and a reticular part of the substantia nigra pars reticularis (SNR), receiving also the stimulation from the subthalamic nucleus reaching the EP and SNr, creates a selection mechanism acting as the feedforward selection circuit, which allows, on the basis of information coming into the system, the choice of motor or cognitive schema, before it starts to be executed. In this perspective, the neural connections of the striatum with the globus pallidus (Gp) and the nucleus subthalamicus (traditionally called indirect pathway) are included in the loop responsible for the choice control (control circuit) (Gurney et all., 1998, Prescott et all., 2002). Based on the analysis of the results of the experiments simulating the described above way of the striatum function regulation, two functions of the control loop were distinguished: 1) inhibition of STN by the GP using negative feedback allows to regulate the number of impulses outgoing from STN through the channels of information flow (associated with the activity of striatal medium spiny cells) (ibid.); 2) inhibition of EP/SNr by the GP as a part of a selection support mechanism. The increase in concentration of dopamine in the striatum facilitates the choice of information channels, which will be disinhibited, while the decrease in concentration of dopamine hinders the choice (ibid.). The reason of errors occurring in the selection of behaviors adjusted to a particular situation or difficulties in completing already chosen behaviors in the Parkinson's disease, in which concentration of dopamine in the nigrostriatal pathway is decreased, are tried to be explained with the above presented model (Prescott et all., 2002).

## 6. References

Akhmetelashvili O.K., Melkadze I.A., Davitashvili M.T. & Oniani T.I. Effects of electric stimulation and destruction of caudate nucleus on short-term memory. *Bull Exp. Biol. Med.* 2007, 143 (3): 302-304.

Alexander G. E., DeLong M. & Strick P. L. Parallel organization of functionally segregated circuits linking basal ganglia and Cortex *Ann. Rev. Neurosci.* 1986, 9, 357-381.

Albin R. L., Young A. B. & Penney J. B. The functional anatomy of basal ganglia disorders. *Trends. Neurosci.* 1989, 12, 366-375.

Alexander G.E., Crutcher M.D. & DeLong M.R. Basal ganglia-thalamocortical circuits: parallel substrates for motor, oculomotor, "prefrontal" and "limbic" functions. *Progress in Brain Research,* 1990, 85, 119-46.

Babinski J. Sur le réflexe cutané plantaire dans certaines affections du systeme nerveux central. *Comptes rendus des Séances et Mémoires de la Société de Biologie* 1896, 207-208.

Beiser D.G., Houk J.C. Model of cortical-basal ganglionic processing: encoding the serial order of sensory events. *The Journal of Neurophysiology,* 1998, 79 (6), 3168-3188.

Berns G.S,. Sejnowski T.J. How the basal ganglia make decisions. W: Damasio A., Damasio H., Christen Y., red. *The Neurobiology of Decision Making*. Berlin, Springer-Verlag, 1995, 101-113.

Bochenek A., Reicher M. *Anatomia człowieka*. Wyd. lek. PZWL, Warsaw 2006.

Brown R.G., Marsden C.D. Cognitive function in Parkinson's disease: from description to theory. *Trends in Neurosciences,* 1990, 13, 21-29.

Brown L.L., Schneider J.S. & Lidsky T.I. Sensory and cognitive functions of the basal ganglia. *Cur. Opinion. Neurobiol.* 1997, 7, 157-163.

Bullock D., Grossberg S. Neural dynamics of planned arm movement: Emergent invariants and speed-accuracy properties during trajectory information. *Psychological Review,* 1988, 95, 49-90.

Bunzeck N., Doeller C.F., Dolan R.J. & Duzel E. Contextual interaction between novelty and reward processing within the mesolimbic system. Hum Brain Mapp. 2011 Apr 21. doi: 10.1002/hbm.21288.

Calabresi P, Picconi B., Tozzi A. & Di Filippo M. Dopamine-mediated regulation of corticostriatal synaptic plasticity. *Trends in Neurosciences,* 2007, 30 (5), 211-219.

Chevalier G., Deniau J.M. Disinhibition as a basic process in the expression of striatal functions. *Trends in Neurosciences,* 1990, 13, 277-280.

Cummings J. L. Anatomic and behavioral aspects of frontalsubcortical circuits. W: Grafman J., Holyoak K. J., Boller F., red. *Structure and Functions of the Human Prefrontal Cortex.* Annals of the New York Academy of Sciences, vol. 769, 1995, 1–13.

DeLong M.R., Primate models of movement disorders of basal ganglia origin. Trends Neurosci., 1990 Jul; 13 (7), 281-5.

DeLong M., Wichmann T. & Vitek J.L. (1998) Pathophysiological basis of neurosurgical treatment of Parkinson's disease, In: *Srereotactic and Functional Neurosurgery,* Gildenberg, Tasker, pp. (1139-1146), The McGraw-Hill Comp. Inc, New York.

DeLong M.R., Wichmann T. Circuits and circuit disorders of the Basal Ganglia. *Archives of Neurology,* 2007, 64 (1), 20-24.

Deniau J.M., Chevalier G. Disinhibition as a basic process in the expression of striatal functions: II. The striato-nigral influence on thalamocortical cells of ventromedial thalamic nucleus. *Brain Research,* 1985, 334, 227-233.

Drewe E. A. Go no-go learning after frontal lobe lesions in humans. *Cortex.* 1975, 11, 8 –16.

Elliott R. Executive functions and their disorders. *Br. Med. Bull.* 2003, 65, 49-59.

Fix J.D. *Neuroanatomia.* 1997, Urban & Partner, Wrocław.

Fuster J. M. *The Prefrontal Cortex.* 1980, Raven, New York.

Fuster J. M. Memory and planning: two temporal perspectives of frontal lobe function. In: Jasper H. H., Riggio S., Goldman-Rakic P. S., red. *Epilepsy and the Functional Anatomy of the Frontal Lobe.* 1995, New York, Raven, 9–18.

Frank M.J., Loughry B. & O'Reilly R.C. Interactions between frontal cortex and basal ganglia in working memory A computational model Cognitive, Affective & Behavioral, *Neuroscience.* 2001, 1 (2), 137-160.

Friedman A. Epidemiologia, etiopatogeneza, rozpoznawanie i leczenie choroby Parkinsona. In: Friedman A., red. *Choroba Parkinsona.* Bielsko-Biała, α-Medica Press, 1999.

Goldman-Rakic P. S. Anatomical and functional circuits in prefrontal cortex of non-human primates: relevance to epilepsy. In: Jasper H. H., Riggio S., Goldman-Rakic P. S., edit. *Epilepsy and the Functional Anatomy of the Frontal Lobe.* 1995a, New York, Raven, 85–96.

Gołąb B.K. *Anatomia czynnościowa ośrodkowego układu nerwowego.* 2000, Wydawnictwo Lekarskie PZWL, Warsaw.

Groenewegen H. J. The basal ganglia and motor control. *Neural. Plast.* 2003, 10 (1-2), 107-120.

Groenewegen H.J. The ventral striatum as an interface between the limbic and motor systems. *CNS Spectr.* 2007, 12 (12): 887-892.

Groenewegen H.J., van Dongen Y.C. *Role of the basal ganglia.* W: W. van Laar (red.) *Parkinsonism and related disorders.* VU University Press Amsterdam 2007, 21-54.

Gurney K.N., Prescott J. & Redgrave P. The basal ganglia viewed as an action. 1998

Haber S. N. The primate basal ganglia: parallel and integrative networks. *J. Chem. Neuroanat.* 2003, 26 (4), 317-330.

Haber S.N., Calzavara R. The cortico-basal ganglia integrative network The role of the thalamus. *Brain Res. Bull.* 2009, 78 (2-3), 69-74.

Hartley A. A., Speer N. K. Locating and fractionating working memory using functional neuroimaging: storage, maintenance and executive functions. *Microsc. Res. Tech.* 2000, 51(1), 45-53.

Hartman R.E., Rojas H., Tang J. & Zhang J. Long-term behavioral characterization of a rat model of intracerebral hemorrhage. *Acta. Neurochir. Suppl.* 2008, 105, 125-126.

Heilman K.M., Bowers D. & Valenstein E. *Emotional disorders associated with neurological disease.* In: K.M Heilman, E. Valenstein (edit.) *Clinical Neuropsychology* Oxford University Press, New York 1993.

Herrero M. T., Barcia C. & Navarro J. M. Functional anatomy of thalamus and basal ganglia. *Childs. Nerv. Syst.* 2002, 18 (8), 386-404.

Hikosaka O. Role of basal ganglia in intiation of voluntary movements. W: Arbib M.A., Amari S., red. *Dynamic interaction in neural networks: models and data.* Berlin, Springer-Verlag, 1989, 153-167.

Hikosaka O., Takikawa Y. & Kawagoe R. Role of the basal ganglia in the control of purposive saccadic eye movements. *Physiological Revievs,* 2000, 80 (3), 953-978.

Jessup R.K., O'Doherty J.P. Human Dorsal Striatal Activity during Choice Discriminates Reinforcement Learning Behavior from the Gambler's Fallacy. J Neurosci. 2011, 31(17), 6296-304.

Joel D., Weiner I. The organization of the basal ganglia-thalamocortical circuits: Open interconnected rather than closed segregated. *Neuroscience.* 1994, 63, 363-79.

Kostowski W. Zaburzenia procesów neuroprzekaźnictwa w chorobie Parkinsona. In: Friedman A., red. *Choroba Parkinsona.,* Bielsko-Biała, α-Medica Press, 1999, 18.

Kowalska D.M., Kuśmierek P. *Anatomiczne Podstawy Pamięci.* In: T. Górska, A. Grabowska, J. Zagrodzka (Edit.) *Mózg a zachowanie.* Wydawnictwo Naukowe PWN, Warsaw 2006, 349-374.

Kozubski W., Paweł P. & Liberski P.P. (edit.) *Neurologia. Podręcznik dla studentów Medycyny.* Warsaw, Wydaw. Lekarskie PZWL. 2006, 84-85.

Laskowska I., Ciesielski M. Gorzelańczyk E.J. Udział jąder podstawy w regulacji funkcji emocjonalnych. *Neuropsych. Neuropsychol.* 2008, 3 (3-4), 107-115.

Laskowska I., Gorzelańczyk E.J. Rola jąder podstawy w regulacji funkcji poznawczych. *Neuropsych. Neuropsychol.* 2009, 4, 1, 26-35.

*LeDoux* J.E. *The Emotional Brain.* Simon & Schuster, New York 1996.

L'Hermitte F. 'Utilization behaviour' and its relation to lesions of the frontal lobes. *Brain.* 1983, 106 (Pt 2), 237-255.

L'Hermitte F. Human autonomy and the frontal lobes, part II: patient behavior in complex and social situations: the environmental dependency syndrome. *Ann. Neurol.* 1986, 19, 335–343.

Longstaff A., *Krótkie wykłady. Neurobiologia.* 2003, Wydawnictwo Naukowe PWN, Warsaw.
Longstaff A., Instant Notes in Neuroscience. BIOS Scientific Publ, 2006.
Mandir A. S., Lenz F. A. Clinical pathophysiology in Parkinson's Disease. In: Gildenberg Ph.L., Tasker R.R., edit. *Textbook of Stereotactic and Functional Neurosurgery.* New York, McGraw-Hill, 1998, 1133 - 1137.
McFarland N.R., Haber S.N. Thalamic relay nuclei of the basal ganglia form both reciprocal and nonreciprocal cortical connections, linking multiple frontal cortical areas. *J. Neurosci.* 2002, 22(18), 8117-8132.
McNab F., Klingberg T. Prefrontal cortex and basal ganglia control access to working memory. *Nature Neurosci.* 2008, 11, 103-107.
Middleton F. A., Strick P. L. Anatomical evidence for cerebellar and basal ganglia involvement in higher cognitive function. *Science.* 1994, 266, 458–461.
Milner B. Aspects of human frontal lobe function. W: Jasper H. H., Riggio S., Goldman-Rakic P. S. *Epilepsy and the Functional Anatomy of the Frontal Lobe.* 1995, New York, Raven, 67–81.
Mink J. W. The basal ganglia: focused selection and inhibition of competing motor programs. *Prog. Neurobiol.* 1996, 50, 381–425.
Mink J.W. Basal ganglia. In: Zigmond M.J., Bloom F.E., Landis S.C., Roberts J.L., Squire L.R., red. *Fundamental Neuroscience.* San Diego, Academic Press, 1999, 951-972.
Morgane P.J., Galler J.R. & Mokler D.J. A review of systems and networks of the limbic forebrain/limbic midbrain. *Progress in Neurobiology,* 2005, 75 (2), 143-160.
Oberg R.G.E., Divac I. (1979). Cognitive functions of the neostriatum. In: *The Neostriatum.* Divac, Oberg, pp. (291-312), Pergamon Press, New York.
Obeso J.A., Rodriguez M.C. & DeLong M.R. Basal ganglia pathophysiology. A critical review. *Adv. Neurol.* 1997, 74, 3- 18.
Obeso J. A., Rodriguez- Oroz M. C., Rodriguez M. Lanciego J.L., Artieda J., Gonzalo N. & Olanow C.W. Pathophysiology of the basal ganglia in Parkinson's disease. *Trends Neurosci.* 2000b, 47(10), 8-19.
Olié J.P., Costa e Silva J.A. & Marcher J.P. (2004). Interpretacja kliniczna danych biologicznych dotyczących neuroplastyczności. In: *Neuroplastyczność. Patofizjologia depresji w nowym ujęciu.* Olié, Costa e Silva, Marcher, pp. 72, Gdańsk, Wydawnictwo Via Medica.
Olzak M., Gorzelańczyk E. J. Zwoje podstawy i wzgórze a pamięć operacyjna i funkcje wykonawcze: przegląd badań. *Aktualn. Neurol.* 2005, 4(5), 282-289.
Parent A., Hazrati L. Functional anatomy of the basal ganglia. I. The cortico-basal ganglia-thalamo-cortical loop. *Brain Res. Rev.* 1995, 20, 91-127.
Passingham R.E. *Frontal lobes and voluntary action.* 1993, Oxford University Press, Oxford.
Percheron G., Filion M. Parallel processing in the basal ganglia: up to a point. *Trends. Neurosci.* 1991, 14 (2): 55-59.
Peterson B. S., Skudlarski P., Gatenby J. C., Zhang H., Anderson A. W & Gore J. C. An fMRI study of Stroop Word-Color Interference: evidence for anterior cingulate subregions subserving multiple distributed attentional systems. *Biol. Psychiatry.* 1999, 45, 1237–1258.
Petri H.L., Mishkin M. Behaviorism, cognitivism and the neuropsychology of memory. *Am. Sci.* 1994, 82, 30-37.

Picconi B., Pisani A. , Barone I., Bonsi P., Centonze D., Bernardi G. & Calabresi P. Pathological synaptic plasticity in the striatum: implications for Parkinson's disease. *Movement Disorders,* 2005,20 (4), 395-402.

Prescott T.J., Gurney, K. & Redgrave, P. Basal ganglia. W: Arbib M. A., red., *The Handbook of Brain Theory and Neural Networks,* Cambridge, MA, MIT Press, 2002, 147-151.

Redgrave P., Prescott T. & Gurney K. Basal ganglia: A vertebrate solution to the selection in problem? *Neuroscience,* 1999, 89, 1009-1023.

Rogers R. D., Own A. M., Middleton H. C., Williams E. J., Pickard J. D., Sahaklan B. J. & Robbins T. W. Choosing between small, likely rewards and large, unlikely rewards activates inferior and orbital prefrontal cortex. *J. Neurosci.* 1999, 19, 9029- 9038.

Royall D. R., Lauterbach E. C., Cummings J. L., Reeve A., Rummans T. A., Kaufer D. I., LaFrance W. C. & Jr, Coffey C. E. Executive control function: a review of its promise and challenges for clinical research. A report from the Committee on Research of the American Neuropsychiatric Association. *J. Neuropsychiatry Clin. Neurosci.* 2002, 14 (4), 377-405.

Rueda-Orozco P.E., Montes-Rodriguez C.J., Soria-Gomez E., Méndez-Díaz M. & Prospéro-García O. Impairment of endocannabinoids activity in the dorsolateral striatum delays extinction of behavior in a procedural memory task in rats. *Neuropharmacolog.* 2008, 55(1), 55-62.

Sadikot A. F., Rymar V.V. The primate centromedian-parafascicular complex anatomical organization with a note on neuromodulation. *Brain Res. Bull.* 2009, 78 (2-3), 122-130.

Sadowski B. *Biologiczne mechanizmy zachowania się ludzi i zwierząt.* Wydawnictwo Naukowe PWN, Warsaw 2001.

Saint-Cyr J.A. Frontal-striatal circuit functions context, sequence, and consequence. *J. Int. Neuropsych. Soc.* 2003, 9, 103-127.

Schotland J.L., Rymer W. Z. Wipe and flexion reflexion reflexes of the frog, II. Response to perturbation. *J. Neurophysiol.* 1993, 69, 1736-1748.

Schiffer A.M., Schubotz R.I. Caudate nucleus signals for breaches of expectation in a movement observation paradigm. Front Hum Neurosci. 2011, 5, 38.

Sławek J., Bojko E. & Szady J. Częstość występowania otępienia u chorych z chorobą Parkinsona. *Neurol. Neurochir. Pol.* 2001, 35, 569-581.

Sławek J. Zabiegi stereotaktyczne w chorobie Parkinsona - zasady kwalifikacji chorych w świetle dotychczasowych badań. *Neurol. Neurochir. Pol.* 2003, 1, 215-227.

Smith E. E., Jonides J. Storage and executive processes in the frontal lobes. *Science.* 1999, 283 (5408): 1657-1661.

Smith Y., Raju D.V., Pare J.F. & Sidibe M. The thalamostriatal system: a highly specific network of the basal ganglia circuitry. *Trends Neurosci.* 2004, 27(9), 520–527.

Sobstyl M., Ząbek M. & Koziara H. Patofizjologiczne podstawy operacyjnego leczenia choroby Parkinsona. *Neurol. Neurochir. Pol.* 2003, 37 (1), 203-213.

Stahl S.M. Stahl's essentials phychopharmacology. Neuroscientific basis and practical applications. University of California, San Diego, 2008.

Szołna A. *Historia stereotaksji i neurochirurgii czynnościowej. Leczenie operacyjne zaburzeń ruchu: choroba Parkinsona* In: M. Harat (edit.). *Neurochirurgia czynnościowa.* TOM, Bydgoszcz 2007, 9-19.

Thorpe S. J., Rolls E. T., Maddison S. The orbitofrontal cortex: neuronal activity in the behaving monkey. *Exp Brain Res.* 1983, 49, 93–115.

Truelle J. L., Le Gall D., Joseph P. A., Aubin G., Derouesne C. & Lezak M. D. Movement disturbances following frontal lobe lesions: qualitative analysis of gesture and motor programming. *Neuropsychiatry Neuropsychol. Behav. Neurol.* 1995, 8, 14–19.

Tröster A.I., Arnett P.A. Assessment of movement and demyelinating disorders. In: *Clinical neuropsychology: A pocket handbook for assessment.* Snyder, Nussbaum, Washington D.C. The American Psychological Association, 2005, 243-293.

Wu Y., Richard S., Parent A. The organization of the striatal output system: a single-cell juxtacellular labeling study in the rat. *Neuroscience Research,* 2000, 38 (1), 49-62.

# 7

# Cognitive Integration in the Human Primary Sensory and Motor Areas: An Overview

Jozina B. De Graaf[1] and Mireille Bonnard[2]
[1]*Institute of Movement Sciences*
[2]*Mediterranean Institute for Cognitive Neuroscience*
*CNRS – Aix-Marseille University, Marseille, France*

## 1. Introduction

Although many different definitions of cognition exist, there is a general acceptance that cognition can be defined as a higher function with respect to both the primary stages of sensory information processing and the final stage of motor output. This idea has been the basis of many well known psychological models where one can identify "input boxes" (i.e., visual, auditory, somatosensory information), and "output boxes" (i.e., motor commands), with, intermediate, high level (attention, language, memory, ...) and low-level (motor intention, preparation) cognitive functions (see, for instance, the information processing model of Smidt and Lee (2005), or the model for central representation of goal-directed movements of Jeannerod (1990)).

Although these models are, without doubt, well suited to the study of cognitive processes from a psychological standpoint, they are not very helpful from a neuroscientific point of view. Indeed, ever since the very first investigations into the functioning of the living brain, the main aim has been to localize cognitive functions into the cortical structures of the brain. There exist at least **two** problems related to this approach. Firstly, and this is not a recent objection (e.g., Posner and Raichle (1998) page 16), it is doubtful whether the cognitive functions as presently conceived have a meaning for the brain. Let us take for example the so-called "eye-hand coordination". This "function" is much studied today and many publications report attempts to localize it in the brain. But, for a normally developed brain, this is not a specific function which is needed at specific moments and which is necessarily implemented in a specific brain structure. All input is continuously put in relation with each other as a function of the particular output. It seems more likely that eye-hand coordination is controlled in a continuous, implicit and distributed way. It is pertinent here to mention the ecological approach of perception (Gibson, 1986). This approach is based on the concept of "affordance" that characterizes the object of perception as a whole of many possible actions and interactions, and is in rupture with the cognitive approach. Indeed, according to the latter approach, the brain organizes the perception of the world, whereas in the ecological approach, the world organizes the perception: The role of the brain is to extract the information presented by the world. This theory suggests that the traditional approach of studying cerebral functioning is not very appropriate: the cognitive functions that we define do not have much sense for the brain and, what's more, we generally put subjects in environments which are too artificial in order to study brain functioning. However, since in their opinion perception is "direct", Gibson and his successors have largely ignored the brain and have, therefore, not contributed to the understanding of brain functioning. Although there is much more to say on this subject, we will not develop this point any further in the present chapter.

The second drawback with the cognitive approach is the fact that cognition has mainly been sought outside the primary cortical areas. Indeed, since the above-mentioned cognitive models localize cognition between the input and the output, cognition is necessarily located in the secondary and associative cortical areas. For a long time, the primary motor area has been considered as a simple "execution area" of which the neuronal activity reflects the immediate output to the muscles. In the same way, the primary sensory areas are often presumed to simply transfer sensory information to higher order cognitive systems. For the same reason, studies concerned with the functioning of the secondary and associative areas do not really take into account the direct projections of the nervous system to peripheral structures.

In this chapter, we aim to show that the hierarchical and modular vision of brain functioning is no longer defendable. Cognition emerges from the interaction between regions that are distributed over the whole brain, including the primary cortical areas. After a brief review of the anatomy of the primary somatosensory (S1) and motor (M1) areas, we will develop arguments in favor of this hypothesis. We will mention the highly flexible functional organization of the primary sensorimotor cortical areas. We will show that the neuronal activity of S1 depends on the environmental and cognitive context, i.e., on the value of the stimulus at a given moment. Then, we will show that M1 is much more than a simple transmission area between the non-primary motor areas and the spinal cord. Indeed, M1 is active in tasks without any motor output and the M1 neuronal activity depends on the context in which a motor output is produced and can be adapted and modified in real time. We will end with an example of a clinical implication of this hypothesis, concerning phantom limb sensations in patients with upper limb amputations.

## 2. Primary cortical areas

### 2.1 Anatomical organization of the primary areas

What makes a primary cortical area "primary" is that it is, either, the first cortical structure receiving the sub-cortical projections transporting visual, auditory or somatosensory information, or the last cortical stage before the motor commands descend to sub-cortical structures. The cortex of each hemisphere contains one primary motor area (M1) and three primary sensory areas. M1 is localized on the pre-central wall at the depth of the central sulcus. The post-central gyrus contains the primary somatosensory area (S1), extending from the posterior wall of the central sulcus to the depth of the anterior wall of the post-central sulcus. The primary auditory area (A1) is situated in the superior temporal gyrus on the dorso-postero-medial part of the transverse gyri of Heschl (Liégeois-Chauvel et al., 1991). Finally, the primary visual area (V1) is located at the posterior poles of the occipital lobes in the calcarian sulcus.

Broadly speaking, the cortex contains at least 6 well defined neural layers that can often even be sub-dived into sub-layers. The cellular organization differs sufficiently between the different cortical regions that we can use it as a criterion to delimitate *functional* cortical areas. This was first done by Korbinian Brodmann at the beginning of the twentieth century who established the well-known cerebral map based on the cytoarchitecture of the different regions of the cortex. Each region of the cortex containing the same cellular organization was attributed the same number, ranging from 1 to 52. Brodmann's assumption was that a given anatomical organization must correspond to a particular function. For instance, Brodmann's area 17, which receives information from a thalamic nucleus which in turn receives projections from the retina, is called the primary visual cortex; Brodmann's areas 41 and 42 form the primary auditory cortex; Brodmann's areas 1 to 3 form the primary somatosensory cortex; Brodmann's area 4 globally corresponds to the primary motor cortex. It is important to note that the Brodmann classification is based on adult brains and so were anatomically and neurophysiologically fully developed. It has been shown that the cytoarchitecture of the sensorimotor cortex is subject to considerable modifications from birth (or even before) until the age of 20 (Shumeiko, 1998). Today, it is not clear how the cytoarchitecture of the cortex depends on its *functional* development.

The primary sensory areas differ from other cortical areas mainly by the thickness of layer 4. Whatever the cortical structure, this layer receives sensory information. For instance, the axons from the optical radiation primarily project onto neurons of the fourth layer of V1. M1 has a fourth layer that is clearly thinner than S1, indicating that it receives less sensory information. However, M1 does receive some sensory input in layers 1 to 4, not only from cortical sensory areas but also directly from the thalamus. Also, several secondary motor areas, such as the premotor (PM), supplementary motor (SMA) and cingular motor areas, project directly onto M1 (Dum & Strick, 2002). Concerning the efferent fibers of M1, layer 5 contains the so-called "Cells of Betz" (large pyramidal neurons), visible with only little optical enlargement. Part of the corticospinal tract finds its origin in these pyramidal neurons. This tract consists of well myelinated axons which directly descend into the spinal cord. Some of these axons even project directly onto the motoneurons of the distal muscles without passing by interneurons (Maier et al., 2002). M1 also sends small efferent axons from layers 5 and 6 to other cortical areas.

### 2.2 Flexibility and plasticity of the primary cortical areas

The primary cortical areas represent the information coming from (or going to) the periphery according to a topological principle, i.e., retinotopic for V1, tonotopic for A1, and somatotopic for S1 and M1. These "maps" were long considered as stable and definitive once the neural functions are fully developed. We now know that this is not correct. Without elaborating on this huge research domain, we will give some examples involving M1 and S1 which show that these topologic maps are highly flexible and constantly re-actualized.

We begin with some basic details concerning the somatotopy of M1. In a normal subject, M1 shows a rather global somatotopic organization in a medial-lateral direction, representing the leg, back, arm, hand and face (Penfield & Boldrey, 1937). This rather fine somatotopic organization seems to reflect a "basic" organization that exists when the subject is passive. However, when engaged in a task, within each sub-area, we can identify a distributed representation adapted to the requirements of the task. This has been shown by Sanes and colleagues (1995) in an fMRI study. They asked subjects to make flexion/extension movements with different fingers (one at a time) or with the wrist. For each movement, they found multiple activation sites in the arm area of M1. Moreover, these sites showed an important overlap. These results, which have since been confirmed by other studies (see

Indovina et Sanes, 2001; for a review Sanes & Donoghue, 2000), strongly suggest that the neurons within the arm area of M1 form a distributed network controlling ensembles of arm muscles as a function of how they are implicated in the particular movement. Pascual-Leone and colleagues (1995), in a transcranial magnetic stimulation (TMS) study, confirmed this by showing a modification of the hand representation in M1 in subjects learning a 5-finger piano exercise. During a training period of 2 hours a day over 5 consecutive days, the cortical area targeting the muscles implicated in the task enlarged. Moreover, the activation threshold decreased. This modification was limited to the implicated hand. Similarly, again using TMS, it has been shown that the cortical area targeting an immobilized part of the body is diminished after immobilization, the reduction being correlated to the duration of the immobilization (Liepert et al., 1995).

Several animal studies have also shown a reorganization of S1 after tactile stimulation. For example, when monkeys are trained to get food out of holes of different diameters, the representation of the hand surface in area 3b of S1 shows less overlap of receptive fields for the trained fingers than for the control fingers (Xerri et al., 1999). Also, rats exposed to an environment rich in tactile stimulation, show an enlarged tactile representation of their paws with a higher spatial resolution in S1 (Xerri et al., 1996). It is interesting to note that this reorganization of S1 can be produced at all ages (Coq & Xerri, 2001).

In an extensive review, Xerri (1998) reported on the plasticity of the primary somatosensory and motor areas after either a peripheral or central lesion. A temporary anesthesia of the dorsal roots of the spinal cord related to the fingers gives rise very rapidly (i.e., within some minutes) to both an enlargement of the receptive fields close to the anesthetized fingers, and the appearance of new receptive fields. At the cortical level, this means that the cortical zone corresponding to the anesthetized fingers is invaded by the representation of the hand surface adjacent to the anesthetized fingers. This reorganization is reversible and disappears after dissipation of the anaesthesia. Contrary to the expanded zones seen immediately after denervation, those observed later on show a clear somatotopic organization. This means that there is an organized spatial redistribution of a large number of cortical input fibers. After amputation of the hand or forearm, the territories of the cortical representation of the lost body part are reoccupied by the afferent information from the adjacent body part and from the face (e.g., Florence & Kaas, 1995). This reorganization is known to be (at least partly) reversible. This has been confirmed in an fMRI study before and after a transplantation of both hands in an adult human subject (Giraux et al., 2001). This particular patient had had a traumatic amputation of both hands 4 years earlier. After the bilateral transplantation of the hands and an extensive rehabilitation, the centre of activity evoked by movements of the elbow and the hand was modified in such a manner that the cortical organization became similar to that before amputation of the hands. After six months, the transplanted hands were recognized and could be used quasi-normally. These examples show the important flexibility and plasticity at the level of the primary sensorimotor areas as a function of the afferent information and the task in which the subject is engaged.

### 2.3 Functional activity of the primary sensory areas

As mentioned before, the primary cortical areas have been long considered as a simple information transmission area between the outside world and the associative and cognitive areas. We now know that the activity of the primary areas is, on the one hand, not simply related to the input or output of information of the concerned modality, and, on the other hand, a complex function of the sensory information and the cognitive context in which the activity is evoked. In this section, we will give several examples concerning the primary sensory areas to justify this hypothesis. We will then elaborate on the functioning of the primary motor area in section 2.4.

### 2.3.1 Multimodality

Several recent neurophysiologic studies have shown that the activity of the primary sensory areas can be influenced by the sensory information of another modality. This has long been established in blind or deaf subjects (e.g., Finney et al., 2001; Hunt et al., 2006; Théoret et al., 2004), but it has also been identified in normal subjects. Non-invasive neuroimaging studies in human subject have shown a cross-modal modulation of evoked activity in primary sensory areas. For example, when both the face and voice of a speaking person were presented, the BOLD level in A1 and V1 was increased compared to when only the face or only the voice was presented (Calvert et al., 1999; Clavagnier et al., 2004). Interestingly, lip reading (with no sound) evokes an increase of BOLD level in the auditory cortex (Calvert et al., 1997). Also, a vibrotactile stimulation of the fingers evokes a response in the auditory cortex (Caetano & Jousmäki, 2006), and tactile exploration without visual information increases the BOLD level in V1 (Merabet et al., 2007).

Unitary recording in monkeys has shown that the eye position in the head influences the activity of neurons in A1 (Fu et al., 2004). Not only is the sound-response of these neurons affected but also their spontaneous activity (Werner-Reiss et al., 2003). Broche and colleagues (2005) recently found neurons in A1 of the monkey whose activity was related to non-auditory but relevant-to-the-task events. The monkeys performed a difficult auditory categorization task: After the appearance of a light, the monkey had to initiate a sound sequence by pushing a lever, and subsequently release the lever only when the frequency envelop of the sound sequence was diminishing. The authors found neurons whose activity was synchronized either with the appearance of the light, or with the start or end of lever pushing. This activity in A1 did not exist when the same monkeys performed a visual discrimination task.

All these results suggest the existence of corticocortical projections binding cortical areas of different modalities. Indeed, direct projections from the auditory cortex on V1 have been identified (Falchier et al., 2002), as well as bidirectional projections between S1 and A1 (Budinger et al., 2006) and between the visual cortex and S1 (Cappe & Barone, 2005). This shows that part of the activity of the primary sensory areas can be due to information coming from other modalities. In other words, the primary sensory areas cannot be considered as isolated centres for unimodal information processing.

### 2.3.2 Influence of the cognitive context

First of all, S1 can be active before the arrival of the sensory information. For example, when one is anticipating being tickled, S1 is already active before the real tickling starts in a similar way to when the tickling is actually happening (Carlsson et al., 2000). Moreover, the level of S1 activity during the anticipation of a painful stimulus seems to be correlated to the level of temporal predictability of the stimulus, i.e., the activity is higher when one knows exactly the moment of arrival of the stimulus (Carlsson et al., 2006). In a similar way, we recently showed an increase in BOLD level in S1 during the anticipation of a motor perturbation to which the subject had to react, i.e., well before the arrival of the proprioceptive information evoked by the perturbation (De Graaf et al., 2009). These examples clearly show that the activity of S1 is not only found following a somatosensory stimulus but that is can precede it. Maybe even more surprising, the simple observation of another person being touched evokes an activity in S1 of the observer which has a somatotopy corresponding to the part of the body of the person who is being touched (among others, Blakemore et al., 2005). In this case, there is no corresponding somatosensory stimulus of the observer's own body at all.

Secondly, the activity in the primary sensory areas appears to depend in an important way on the cognitive context in which the activity is evoked. This is already clear from the above-mentioned study from Broche and colleagues (2005) showing that as a function of the task the activity can be multimodal, but there are other examples. For instance, Molchan and colleagues (1994) presented pairs of sounds and air puffs in the right eye (evoking an eye blink) and measured the metabolic cerebral response by PET. After the initial learning process, they found not only that the sound alone evoked an eye blink, but also that the same sound evoked a higher activity an A1 compared to the activity level before learning. This implies that the activity of A1 depends on the "associative value" of the sound. Another example is the long established fact that electrophysiological responses depend on the level of the attention we give to a signal (Hillyard et al., 1973). More recently, it has been shown that this attention level dependant activity can be localized in the primary areas. Indeed, Woldorff and colleagues (1993), in an auditory dichotic listening task, found increased short-latency neuromagnetic responses (20-50 ms) for the sound presented in the attended ear. Localization techniques placed the neural generator of these short-latency responses in A1. This suggests that auditory attention can selectively modulate early sensory processes, i.e., before or at the onset of the cortical processing. Another example is the observation that the somatotopic organization of S1 is modulated as a function of the cognitive context of the task in which the subject is engaged. Schaefer and colleagues (2005) analysed the functional organization of S1 of subjects performing a "Tower of Hanoi" task, and compared this to the organization of S1 in the same subjects performing the same movements but without the cognitive demands of the puzzle. The results clearly showed that the representation of the fingers implied a larger neural population in S1 during the Tower of Hanoi task than during the control task, although the executed movements (and thus the somatosensory information) were the same. This does not only confirm the flexibility in real time of S1, but also, and more importantly, shows that the functional organisation of S1 depends on the cognitive context.

In two reviews concerning unitary recording in A1, Weinberger (2007a, b) has shown how neuronal activity in A1 of animals depends on the behavioural context. The optimal frequency of the receptive field of different cells was determined in several Guinea pigs. The animals were then presented with 30-45 sound/shock pairs, the sound having a frequency different from the optimal frequency. After the experimental session, the optimal frequency of the cells was found to be modified, approaching the frequency of the sound used in the experimental session, whereas the response to the prior optimal frequency was reduced. This modification of the response in A1 develops very fast (detectable after only 5 trials, like cardiac and behavioural responses). It was also found to be stable in time after 8 weeks, even without further training (Weinberger 2004). It is worth noting that these characteristics are one of the most important features of the associative memory. This implies that not only the frequency response in A1 depends on the environmental context of the animal, but also a neurophysiologic trace of memory might exist in a primary sensory area.

The neuronal activity of V1 also depends on the context. It has been shown that the spatial and temporal contexts of the visual stimulus can influence cellular responses to the stimulus. For instance, when a stimulus with an optimal orientation for a given cell is presented at the same time as other stimuli with orthogonal orientations, the cell response increases, whereas when the same optimal stimulus is presented at the same time as other stimuli with the *same* orientation, the cell response decreases (Gilbert and Wiesel, 1990). Also, when monkeys are trained in visual discrimination tasks with the same stimuli at the same position in the visual field, the neuronal response characteristics depend on the task (Li et al., 2004). Another example is the fact that the evoked activity of neurons in V1 significantly depends on the location to which the spatial attention is directed without changing the gaze direction: When the attention is directed to the location of the receptive field, the cellular response increases (Motter, 1993).

All these examples strongly suggest that the primary sensory cortical areas do more than simply transmit peripheral sensory information. The neuronal activity depends strongly on the environmental context (i.e., other sensory information) as well as the cognitive context (i.e., the task in which the subject is engaged), in other words, on the value that we give to a stimulus at a given moment. A too restricted vision of the functioning of the primary sensory areas would lead to a loss of important information and would impede a full understanding of the functioning of these areas.

### 2.4 Functional activity of the primary motor area

At the cortical level, voluntary motor control is well-known to involve several areas: M1, and three non-primary motor areas (the pre-motor cortex, the supplementary motor area and the cingular motor cortex) (e.g., Rouiller, 1996). Concerning the functional role of area M1 within this network, the most classical view suggests that the primary motor cortex is the final output of a complex network in which the most cognitive aspects of movement control (e.g. action preparation and/or planning) are processed upstream within the non-primary motor areas. This model supports a hierarchical organization of the cortical control of movement. Alternatively, some recent physiological findings suggest that area M1 is itself involved in important movement-related cognitive functions (see Requin et al., 1991; Georgopoulos, 2000; Bonnard et al., 2004 for reviews), arguing in favor of a more distributed model.

#### 2.4.1 M1 activity without motor production

M1 can be active during the preparation of an action, i.e., well before the motor production. Indeed, in several human EEG and fMRI studies it has been shown that M1 is active during the preparation phase of a voluntary movement, either just before the execution (Ball et al., 1999; Cunnington et al., 2003; Toro et al., 1993; Wildgruber et al., 1997), or from the very beginning of the preparation phase in the case of sequential movements (see Zang et al., 2003). In a different context, we recently reported an important activity in M1 during the whole duration of the preparation of a reaction to a motor perturbation (De Graaf et al., 2009). Similarly, unitary recordings in monkeys have also shown active neurons in M1 during the preparation without any accompanying muscular activity (see Riehle (2005) for a review). Moreover, Lu and Ashe (2005) found neurons in M1 with an anticipatory activity that was exclusively related to a specific movement sequence. These neurons showed an interaction between the temporal order of the movement and the associated direction, i.e., their sensitivity to movement direction depended on the movement sequence to prepare. This suggests that M1 activity is not limited to "simply" coding the next movement direction (Bremmer, 2005).

In these examples, although the activity of M1 is observed *before* the movement, it still involved preparation of a real movement. Recently, it has been shown that M1 is also active during motor imagery which is not followed by an action. Indeed, when imagining performing a movement, the blood flow in M1 increases, even without any muscular activity (Porro et al., 1996; Roth et al., 1996; see Grèzes and Decety, 2000, for a review). Moreover, through TMS, it has been shown that the corticospinal excitability (reflected by the amplitude of the motor evoked potentials recorded for the muscles that would be implicated in overt movement execution), depends on the content of the motor image (Yahagi and Kasai, 1998). The temporal dynamics of the corticospinal excitability during imagery is similar to that found during overt movement execution (Hashimoto and Rothwell, 1999). Another example is the implication of M1 during the observation of another person's movements (e.g., Fadiga et al., 1995; 2005; Raos et al., 2004). A Bereitshafts potential has even been found while observing predictable movements (Kilner et al., 2004). Also, a movement illusion, evoked by muscular vibration (without any associated movement), evokes an activity in M1 (Casini et al., 2006). Morover, the increase of the BOLD level in M1 during the illusion is correlated with the force of the illusion (Romaiguère et al., 2003). Longcamp and colleagues (2006) found M1 to be implicated in passive reading of hand written texts. Very interestingly, Hauk and colleagues (2004) published a study concerning the passive reading of words that represented actions of the tongue, the arm or the leg (for example "lick", "pick", kick"). Although no muscular activity could be found, the BOLD level in M1 was increased following the somatotopic organization of this area. In other words, they found an activity in the arm area of M1 for words concerning actions of the arm, in the tongue area for tongue words, etc. All of these examples clearly show that M1 is active in circumstances where, although there is some sort of "motricity", it is not necessary to have an actual motor output: The simple reading of verbs representing an action can evoke an activity in that area that is classically accepted as the area of motor production.

### 2.4.2 Influence of the context on M1 activity

Several results in the literature show that, for a given motor output, the activity of M1 can strongly depend on the context. One example is the result of our fMRI study on the awareness of muscular force (De Graaf et al., 2004). In a reference condition, subjects made rhythmical hand movements and they were informed that, in a subsequent condition in which the resistance to the movement would be increased, they had to either reproduce their initial muscular forces or reproduce the movement kinematics (Fig. 1B). To vary the external force, the subject had a manipulandum attached to the right forearm and hand over the wrist joint (Fig. 1A). This manipulandum was an fMRI-compatible mechanically jointed arm, only allowing flexion and extension movements at the wrist. A laterally attached lever allowed the internal friction of the manipulandum to be varied. The lever had two possible positions: High and low internal friction. During the experiment, the subjects easily changed the lever position themselves in response to an instruction given on a screen. A potentiometer was fixed on the rotation axis of the manipulandum to record the subjects' wrist movements.

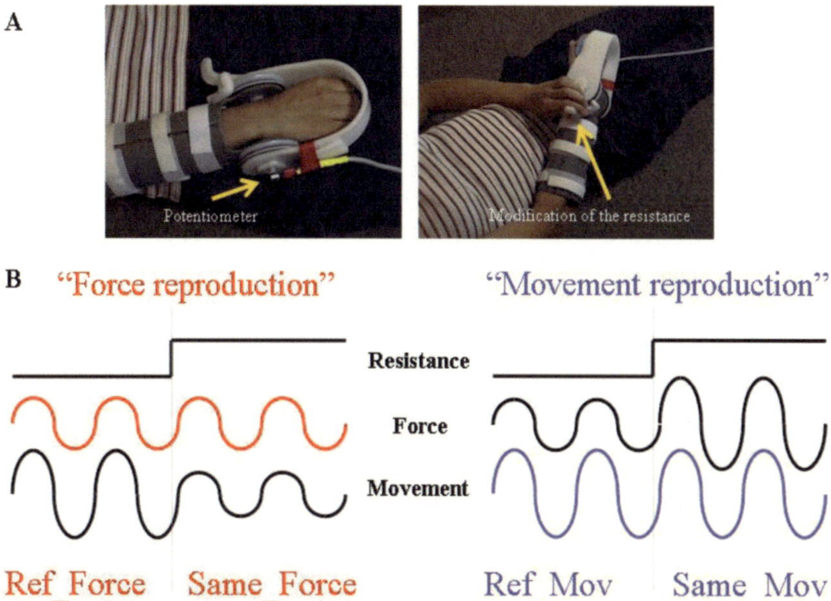


Fig. 1. Manipulandum used to measure the rhythmical wrist extension/flexion, as well as to vary the resistance to the movement (A). Schematical representation of the protocol (B). Note that during the reference conditions (Ref_Force and Ref_Mov), the actual motor output was the same.

The contrast in M1 activity between the condition during which the subjects had to pay attention to their muscular forces (Ref_Force) and the condition during which they had to pay attention to their kinematics (Ref_Mov) (conditions in which the actual motor output was equivalent!) suggests that obtaining awareness of muscular forces exerted during movement execution makes much higher demands on many brain structures, in particular the primary sensorimotor areas (Fig. 2). Interestingly, for the contrast between Same_Force and Same_Mov, conditions for which the actual muscle forces were very different, we did not find any difference in BOLD level. This clearly suggests, on the one hand, that for a similar motor output the BOLD level of M1 can vary with the specific attention the subject gives to the task, and, on the other hand, that different levels of force production do not necessarily imply different levels of BOLD activity in the primary sensorimotor areas. In a subsequent study (Bonnard et al., 2007), we showed an increase in BOLD level as well as corticospinal excitability of M1 when subjects were required to produce forces with higher precision, although the actual force level was the same. So, as a function of the attention the subject gives to certain aspects of the task, the global level of activity of M1 can vary for the same motor output.

At a unitary neuronal level, Hepp-Reymond and colleagues (1999) gave a very powerful demonstration of the dependence of the coding of the force production on the context. Several monkeys were trained to finely control their force production with a precision grip in a visuomotor force pursuit task: The monkeys had to follow a rectangle presented on a screen with a cursor by exerting pressure on a force transducer held between their thumb and index. They were presented with either two or three different force levels in a trial.

Importantly, the monkeys knew in advance which trial type was going to be presented by means of a colour coding of the rectangle. The discharge frequency of M1 neurones for a given force level appeared to vary with the *total* force the monkeys had to produce during the trial, i.e., the discharge frequency was lower for the second force level when the monkeys also had to produce the third force level during the trial than when the second force level was the maximum force level of the trial. This clearly shows that the coding of force in M1 neuronal population depends on the context of the task, in this case the total force range. Moreover, this adaptation to context is achieved in real time (here, trial per trial), suggesting an important flexibility at the level of functioning of the neuronal network within M1.

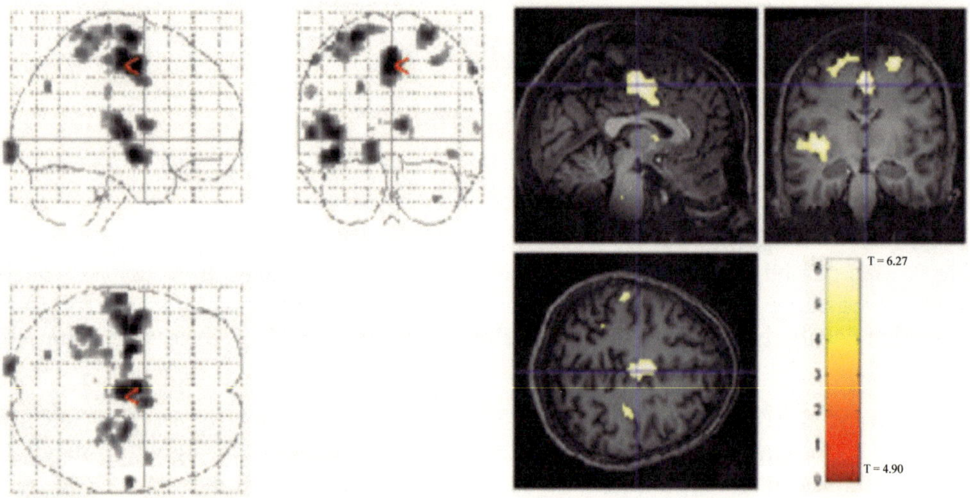


Fig. 2. Result of the t-contrast Ref_Force– Ref_Mov. Height threshold of significance: corrected P<0.01 (T = 4.90). Voxel extent threshold: 20 voxels. The voxels, all seen in the glass brain representation, are superimposed on the spm single subject canonical brain on the anatomical slices passing through Talairach coordinates [-2 -13 47].

All of the above-mentioned results concerning the neuronal activity of M1 clearly show that M1 is not a simple transmission relay between the non-primary motor areas (that anticipate, prepare) and the spinal cord, but rather a real crossroad playing an important role in cognitive motor integration. Indeed, M1 is implicated in tasks without any motor output. Moreover, the functioning of M1 depends on the cognitive context in which a motor output will be or is produced: Its functioning is modulated in real time.

## 3. Secondary cortical areas

It is important to remember that M1 is not the only origin of the corticospinal tract. In monkeys, the topographical distribution of these projections has been studied by isolating the corticospinal neurons projecting on the spinal cord between the cervical and thoracic level (C5-T1), using an injection of a retrograde marker in the region of the motoneurons in the spinal cord (Dum and Strick, 1991; Maier et al., 2002). Is has been shown that half of the fibers of the pyramidal tract find their origin in M1, the other half comes from non primary motor areas, i.e., SMA proper (12-19%), premotor area (21%), and cingular motor area (17-21%). Also, a large number of unitary recording studies in cortical neurons in awake monkeys have shown that neurons presenting particular parametric relations with different phases of movement execution can be found in all structures of the cortical motor network, i.e., in M1, premotor cortex and the supplementary motor cortex (for reviews see Porter and Lemon, 1993; Requin et al., 1991; Georgopoulos, 2000). This strongly suggests that these non primary cortical regions can also send motor commands directly to motoneurons. We have already seen that M1 is not uniquely a "motor execution area", and now we can add that premotor areas, classically regarded as "preparation centres", can also have executive functions.

In a similar way, direct projections from the thalamus to non-primary visual areas have been found. For example, there exists a direct projection from the lateral geniculate nucleus onto MT (V5) without passing by V1. These projections represent about 10% of those coming from V1 (Sincich et al., 2004). Also, direct thalamo-cortical projections on secondary auditory areas (Barth et al., 1995; Di and Barth, 1992) and on secondary somatosensory areas (Hiraga et al., 2005; Stevens et al., 1993) have been identified.

Since the topic of this chapter is the primary cortical areas, we will not elaborate on the possible function of these direct projections onto and from secondary cortical areas. However, it was important to mention this since the existence of these direct projections confirms that the segmental and hierarchic vision of brain functioning is no longer defendable. Indeed, the primary cortical areas are an integral part of a cortical network underlying cognitive integration, and, whatsmore, the secondary motor areas have executive functions.

## 4. A clinical implication

An important implication of this conception of cerebral functioning is that the whole cortex should be considered when studying, for instance, the consequences of cortical plasticity following central or peripheral lesions. In this last section of the chapter, we will use as example the amputation of the hand and/or forearm.

As already mentioned in section 2.2, after amputation of the hand or forearm, the territories of the representation of the lost body part in S1 seem rapidly occupied by afferent information from adjacent body parts (e.g., Florence & Kaas, 1995; Gagné et al., 2011; Vandermeeren et al., 2003). The same reorganization is known to hold for M1, i.e., neurons originally sending motor commands to hand muscles pre-amputation send them to stump muscles post-amputation. Indeed, TMS on this reorganized part of M1 evoked MEPs in the stump muscles (Mercier et al., 2006).

This reorganization, however, is very complex and appears to be incomplete. Indeed, after amputation, patients very often report a vivid perception of presence of their lost limb. This "phantom limb" can be the object of mechanical, thermal and even painful sensations (Kooijman et al., 2000). Even more surprisingly is that the phantom limb can often be "moved" at will (Kooijman et al., 2000; Reilly et al., 2006). Although these voluntary phantom movements are slow and more effortful than movements of the intact limb, the patients feel these movements to be "executed" corresponding to their will (e.g., Reilly et al., 2006), and they are able to imitate with their intact arm the movements they execute with their phantom limb. Some results in the literature suggest that the sending of motor commands is necessary in order to "perform" voluntary phantom limb movements. These motor commands, as they cannot arrive on the muscles of the lost limb, arrive on the muscles of the stump instead. Indeed, during voluntary phantom limb movements, the EMG pattern found on the stump muscles correspond to neither the EMG patterns for real movements of the stump, nor to the EMG patterns found on the corresponding muscles of the intact arm during imitation of the phantom limb movements (Reilly et al., 2006; Gagné et al., 2009). This strongly suggests that specific motor commands are sent from M1 when "executing" a specific phantom limb movement. Moreover, when the hand area of M1 in an amputated patient is stimulated with TMS, a phantom limb movement is evoked (Mercier et al., 2006). So, there exists a reorganization of the primary somatosensory and motor areas, leading to new relations between body parts and neuronal populations, where motor commands to the missing limb can still be sent.

There seems to exist a relation between the degree of cortical reorganization and the degree of phantom limb pain. Lotze and colleagues (2001), in a fMRI study, reported that patients without phantom limb pain showed significantly less reorganization of the primary sensorimotor areas than patients with phantom limb pain. This raises the question whether cortical reorganization should be avoided, and, if so, how.

Currently, it is not known what exactly underlies the appearance of phantom limb sensations such as movements or pain, but it seems likely that it is, at least partly, related to the complex cortical reorganization following amputation. The search for answers to questions such as "What causes phantom limb pain and how can we avoid it?", "Why are phantom limb movements slow and effortful?", and "Can we use phantom limb movements to increase control of prostheses?", must take into account that the primary cortical areas are an integral part of a cortical network underlying cognitive (motor) functioning, and the secondary motor areas can have an executive function. With respect to this latter point, a possible reorganization of the secondary motor areas following amputation has not yet been investigated.

## 5. Acknowledgement

The authors warmly thank Thelma Coyle for correcting de English language of the chapter.

## 6. References

Ball T, Schreiber A, Feige B, Wagner M, Lücking CH & Kristeva-Feige R (1999). The role of higher-order motor areas in voluntary movement as revealed by high-resolution EEG and fMRI. *Neuroimage* Vol 10: 682-694

Barth DS, Goldberg N, Brett B & Di S (1995) The spatiotemporal organization of auditory, visual, and auditory-visual evoked potentials in rat cortex. *Brain Res* Vol 678: 177-190

Blakemore SJ, Bristow D, Bird G, Frith C & Ward J (2005). Somatosensory activations during the observation of touch and a case of vision-touch synaesthesia. *Brain.* Vol 128: 1571-1583

Bonnard M, De Graaf JB & Pailhous J (2004). Interactions between cognitive and sensorimotor functions in the motor cortex. Evidence from the preparatory motor sets anticipating a perturbation. *Rev Neurosci* Vol 15: 371-382

Bonnard M, Galléa C, De Graaf JB & Pailhous J (2007). Corticospinal control of the thumb-index grip depends on precision of force control: A TMS and fMRI study in humans. *Eur J Neurosci* Vol 25: 872-880

Bremmer F (2005). What's next? Sequential movement encoding in primary motor cortex. *Neuron* Vol 3: 819-821

Broche M, Selezneva E & Scheich H (2005). Nonauditory events of a behavioral procedure activate auditory cortex of highly trained monkeys. *J Neurosci* Vol 25: 6797-6806

Budinger E, Heil P, Hess A & Scheich H (2006). Multisensory processing via early cortical stages: Connections of the primary auditory cortical field with other sensory systems. *Neurosci* Vol 143: 1065-1083

Caetano G & Jousmäki V (2006). Evidence of vibrotactile input to human auditory cortex. *Neuroimage* Vol 29: 15-28

Calvert GA, Brammer MJ, Bullmore ET, Campbell R, Iversen SD & David AS (1999). Response amplification in sensory-specific cortices during crossmodal binding. *NeuroReport* Vol 10: 2619-2623

Calvert GA, Bullmore ET, Brammer MJ, Campbell R, Williams SC, McGuire PK, Woodruff PW, Iversen SD & David AS (1997). Activation of auditory cortex during silent lipreading. *Science* Vol 276: 593-596

Cappe C & Barone P (2005). Heteromodal connections supporting multisensory integration at low levels of cortical processing in the monkey. *Eur J Neurosci* Vol 22: 2886-2902

Carlsson K, Andersson J, Petrovic P, Petersson KM, Öhman A & Ingvar M (2006). Predicability modulates the affective and sensory-discriminative neural processing of pain. *NeuroImage* Vol 32: 1804-1814

Carlsson K, Petrovic P, Skare S, Petersson KM & Ingvar M (2000). Tickling expectations: neural processing in anticipation of a sensory stimulus. *J Cogn Neurosci* Vol 12: 691-703

Casini L, Romaiguère P, Ducorps A, Schwartz D, Anton, J-L & Roll J-P (2006). Cortical correlates of illusory hand movement perception in humans: a MEG study. *Brain Res* Vol 1121: 200-206

Clavagnier S, Falchier A & Kennedy H (2004). Long-distance feedback projections to area V1: implications for multisensory integration, spatial awareness, and visual consciousness. *Cogn Affect Behav Neurosci* Vol 4: 117-126

Coq JO & Xerri C (2001). Sensorimotor experience modulates age-dependent alterations of the forepaw representation in the rat primary somatosensory cortex. *Neuroscience* Vol 104: 705-15

Cunnington R, Windischberger C, Deecke L & Moser E (2003). The preparation and readiness for voluntary movement: a high-field event-related fMRI study of the Bereitschafts-BOLD response. *NeuroImage* Vol 20: 404-412

De Graaf JB, Galléa C, Pailhous J, Anton J-L, Roth M & Bonnard M (2004). Awareness of muscular force during movement production. An fMRI study. *Neuroimage* Vol 21: 1357-1367

De Graaf JB, Frolov A, Nazarian B, Fiocchi M, Pailhous J & Bonnard M (2009). Preparing for a motor perturbation: Early implication of primary motor and somatosensory cortices. *Human Brain Mapping* Vol 30: 575–587

Di S & Barth DS (1992). The functional anatomy of middle-latency auditory evoked potentials: thalamocortical connections. *J Neurophysiol* Vol 68: 425-31

Dum RP & Strick PL (1991). The origin of corticospinal projections from the premotor areas in the frontal lobe. *J Neurosci* Vol 11: 667-689

Dum RP & Strick PL (2002). Motor areas in the frontal lobe of the primate. *Physiol Behav* Vol 77: 677-682

Fadiga L, Fogassi L, Pavesi G & Rizzolatti G (1995). Motor facilitation during action observation: A magnetic stimulation study. *J Neurophysiol* Vol 73: 2608-2611

Fadiga L, Craighero L & Olivier E (2005). Human motor cortex excitability during the perception of others' action. *Curr Opin Neurobiol* Vol 15: 213-218

Fago J, Hopkins WD & Vauclair J (1993). Hand movements and hemispheric specialization in dichhaptic explorations. *Perception* Vol 22: 897-853

Falchier A, Clavagnier S, Barone P & Kennedy H (2002). Anatomical envidence of multimodal integration in primate striate cortex. *J Neurosci* Vol 22: 5749-5759

Finney EM, Fine I & Dobkins KR (2001). Visual stimuli activate auditory cortex in the deaf. *Nature Neuroscience* Vol 4: 1171-1173

Florence SI & Kaas JH (1995). Large-scale reorganization at multiple levels of the somatosensory pathway follows therapeutic amputation of the hand in monkeys. *J Neurosci* Vol 15: 8083-8095

Fu K-MG, Shah AS, O'Connell MN, McGinnis T, Eckholdt H, Lakatos P, Smiley J & Schroeder CE (2004). Timing and laminar profile of eye position effects on auditory responses in primate auditory cortex. *J Neurophysiol* Vol 92: 3522-3531

Gagné M, Reilly KT, Hétu S & Mercier C (2009). Motor control over the phantom limb in above-elbow amputees and its relationship with phantom limb pain. *Neuroscience* Vol 162: 78–86

Gagné M, Hétu S, Reilly KT & Mercier C (2011). The map is not the territory : motor system reorganization in upper limb amputees. *Human Brain Mapping* Vol 32: 509–519

Georgopoulos AP (2000).Neural aspects of cognitive motor control. *Curr Opin Neurobiol* Vol 10: 238-241

Georgopoulos AP, Ashe J, Smyrnis N & Taira M (1992). The motor cortex and the coding of force. *Science* Vol 256: 1692-1695

Gibson JJ (1986). *The ecological approach to visual perception*. Lawrence Erlbaum Associates, publishers, ISBN 0-89859-959-8, Hillsdale, New Jersey, London

Gilbert CD & Wiesel TN (1990). The influence of contextual stimuli on the orientation selectivity of cells in primary visual cortex of the cat. *Vision Res* Vol 30: 1689-1701

Giraux P, Sirigu A, Schneider F & Dubernard J-M (2001). Cortical reorganization in motor cortex after graft of both hands. *Nature Neurosci* Vol 4: 691-692

Grèzes J & Decety J (2001). Functional anatomy of execution, mental simulation, observation, and verb generation of actions: a meta-analysis. *Human Brain Mapping* Vol 12: 1-19

Hashimoto R & Rothwell JC (1999). Dynamic changes in corticospinal excitability during motor imagery. *Exp Brain Res* Vol 125: 75-81

Hauk O, Johnsrude I & Pulvermüller F (2004). Somatotopic representation of action words in human motor and premotor cortex. *Neuron* Vol 41: 301-307

Hepp-Reymond M-C, Kirkpatrick-Tanner M, Gabernet L, Qi H-X & Weber B (1999). Context-dependent force coding in motor and premotor cortical areas. *Exp Brain Res* Vol 128: 123-133

Hillyard SA, Hink RF, Schwent VL & Picton TW (1973). Electrical signs of selective attention in the human brain. *Science* Vol 182: 177-180

Hiraga A, Sakakibara R, Mizobuchi K, Asahina M, Kuwabara S, Hayashi Y & Hattori T (2005). Putaminal hemorrhage disrupts thalomocortical projection to secondary somatosensory cortex: case report. *J Neurol Sci* Vol 231: 81-83

Hunt DL, Yamoah EN & Krubitzer L (2006). Multisensory plasticity in congenitally deaf mice: how are cortical areas functionally specified? *Neuroscience* Vol 139: 1507-1524

Indovina I & Sanes JN (2001). On somatotopic representation centers for finger movements in human primary motor cortex and supplementary motor area. *Neuroimage* Vol 13: 1027-1034

Jeannerod M (1990). The representation of the goal of an action and its role in the control of goal-directed movements. In: *Computational neuroscience,* EL Schwartz, MIT Press, ISBN-13: 978-0-262-69164-2 , Cambridge, Mass., pp 352-368

Kalaska JF, Cohen DA, Hyde ML & Prud'homme M (1989). A comparison of movement direction-related versus load direction-related activity in primate motor cortex, using a two-dimensional reaching task. *J Neurosci* Vol 9: 2080-2102

Killner JM, Vargas C, Duval S, Blakemore S-J & Sirigu A (2004). Motor activation prior to observation of a predicted movement. *Nature Neurosci* Vol 7: 1299-1301

Kooijman CM, Dijkstra PU, Geertzen JHB, Elzinga A & Van der Schans CP (2000). Phantom pain and phantom sensations in upper limb amputees: an epidemiological study. *Pain* Vol 87: 33-41

Li W, Piëch V & Gilbert CD (2004). Perceptual learning and top-down influences in primary visual cortex. *Nat Neurosci* Vol 7: 651-657

Liégeois-Chauvel C, Musolino A & Chauvel P (1991). Localization of primary auditory area in man. *Brain* Vol 107: 115-131.

Liepert J, Tegenthoff M & Malin J-P (1995). Changes of cortical motor area size during immobilization. *Electroencephal Clin Neurophysiol* Vol 97: 382-386

Longcamp M, Tanskanen T & Hari R (2006). The imprint of action: motor cortex involvement in visual perception of handwritten letters. *Neuroimage* Vol 33: 681-688

Lotze M, Flor H, Grodd W, Larbig W & Birbaumer N (2001). Phantom movements and pain. An fMRI study in upper limb amputees. *Brain* Vol 124: 2268-2277

Lu X & Ashe J (2005). Anticipatory activity in primary motor cortex codes memorized movement sequences. *Neuron* Vol 45: 967-973

Maier MA, Armand J, Kirkwood PA, Yang HW, Davis JN & Lemon RN (2002). Differences in the corticospinal projection from primary motor cortex and supplementary motor area to macaque upper limb motoneurons: an anatomical and electrophysiological study. *Cereb Cortex* Vol 12: 281-296

Merabet LB, Swisher JD, McMains SA, Halko MA, Amedi A, Pascual-Leone A & Somers DC (2007). Combined activation and deactivation of visual cortex during tactile sensory processing. *J Neurophysiol* Vol 97: 1633-1641

Mercier C, Reilly KT, Vargas CD, Alallea A & Sirigu A (2006). Mapping phantom movement representations in the motor cortex of amputees. *Brain* Vol 129: 2202-2210

Molchan SE, Sunderland T, McIntosh AR, Herscovitch P & Schreurs BG (1994). A functional anatomical study of associative learning in humans. *Proc Natl Acad Sci* Vol 91: 8122-8126

Motter BC (1993). Focal attention produces spatially selective processing in the visual cortical areas V1, V2, and V4 in the presence of competing stimuli. *J Neurophysiol* Vol 70: 909-919

Pascual-Leone A, Nguyet D, Cohen LG, Brasil-Neto JP, Cammarota A & Hallett M (1995). Modulation of muscle responses evoked by transcranial magnetic stimulation during the acquisition of new fine motor skills. *J Neurophysiol* Vol 74: 1037-1045

Penfield W & Boldrey E (1937). Somatic motor and sensory representation in the cerebral cortex of man as studied by electrical stimulation. *Brain* Vol 60: 389-443

Porro CA, Francescato MP, Cettolo V, Diamond ME, Baraldi P, Zuiani C, Bazzocchi M & Di Prampero PE (1996). Primary motor and sensory motor cortex activation during motor performance and motor imagery : A fMRI study. *J Neurosci* Vol 16: 7688-7698

Porter R & Lemon R (1993). Corticospinal function and voluntary movement. Clarendon, Oxford University Press, ISBN 0198577451, Oxford, New-York.

Posner MI & Raichle ME (1998). *L'esprit en images*. Collection Neurosciences & Cognition. Translation of *Images of mind*. De Boeck Université, Paris, Bruxelles

Raos V, Evangeliou MN & Savaki HE (2004). Observation of action : grasping with the mind's hand. *NeuroImage* Vol 23: 193-201

Reilly KT, Mercier C, Schieber MH & Sirigu A (2006). Persistent hand motor commands in the amputees' brain. *Brain* Vol 129: 2211-2223

Requin J, Brener J & Ring C (1991). Preparation for action. In: *Handbook of cognitive psychophysiology: central and autonomic nervous system approaches*. Jennings JR & Coles MG. John Wiley & Sons, ISBN: 0471916137, New York, pp 357-448

Riehle A (2005). Preparation for action: one of the key functions of motor cortex. In: *Motor cortex in voluntary movements: a distributed system for distributed functions*. Riehle A & Vaadia E, CRC Press, ISBN 0-8493-1287-0, Boca Raton, pp 213-240

Romaiguère P, Anton J-L, Roth M, Casini L & Roll J-P (2003). Motor and parietal cortical areas both underlie kinaestesia. *Cog Brain Res* Vol 16: 74-82

Roth M, Decety J, Raybaudi M, Massarelli R, Delon-Martin C, Segebarth C, Morand S, Gemignani A, Décorps M & Jeannerod M (1996). Possible involvement of primary motor cortex in mentally simulated movement: a functional magnetic resonance imaging study. *NeuroReport* Vol 7: 1280-1284

Sanes JN & Donoghue JP (2000). Plasticity and primary motor cortex. *Annu Rev Neurosci* Vol 23: 393-415

Sanes JN, Donoghue JP, Thangaraj V, Edelman RR & Warach S (1995). Shared neural substrates controlling hand movements in human motor cortex. *Science* Vol 268: 1775-1777

Schaefer M, Heinze HJ & Rotte M (2005). Task-relevant modulation of primary somatosensory cortex suggests a prefrontal-cortical sensory gating system. *Neuroimage* Vol 27: 130-135

Shumeiko NS (1998). Age-related changes in the cytoarchitectonics of the human sensorimotor cortex. *Neurosci Behav Physiol* Vol 28: 345-348

Sincich LC, Park KF, Wohlgemuth MJ & Horton JC (2004). Bypassing V1: a direct geniculate input to area MT. *Nature Neurosci* Vol 7: 1123-1128

Smidt RA & Lee TD (2005). *Motor control and learning: A behavioral emphasis* ($4^{th}$ edition), Human Kinetics. ISBN 0-7360-4258-X.

Stevens RT, London SM & Apkarian AV (1993). Spinothalamocortical projections to the secondary somatosensory cortex (SII) in squirrel monkey. *Brain Res* Vol 631: 241-246

Théoret H, Merabet L & Pascual-Leone (2004). Behavioral and neuroplastic changes in the blind: evidence for functionally relevant cross-modal interactions. *J Physiol Paris* Vol 98: 221-233

Toro C, Matsumoto J, Deuschl G, Roth BJ & Hallett M (1993). Source analysis of scalp-recorded movement-related electrical potentials. *Electroencephalogr Clin Neurophysiol* Vol 86: 167-175

Vandermeeren Y, Bastings E, Good D, Rouiller E & Olivier E (2003). Plasticité des aires motrices corticales : progrès récents et perspectives thérapeutiques. *Revue Neurologique (Paris)* Vol 159: 259-275

Weinberger NM (2007a). Associative representational plasticity in the auditory cortex: A synthesis of two disciplines. *Learn Mem* Vol 14: 1-16

Weinberger NM (2007b). Auditory associative memory and representational plasticity in the primary auditory cortex. *Hear Res* Vol 229: 54-68

Werner-Reis U, Kelly KA, Trause AS, Underhill A & Groh JM (2003). Eye position affects activity in primary auditory cortex of primates. *Curr Biol* Vol 13: 554-562

Wildgruber D, Erb M, Klose U & Grodd W (1997). Sequential activation of supplementary motor area and primary motor cortex during self-paced finger movement in human evaluated by functional MRI. *Neurosci Lett* Vol 227: 161-164

Woldorff MG, Gallen CC, Hampson SA, Hillyard SA, Pantev C, Sobel D & Bloom FE (1993). Modulation of early sensory processing in human auditory cortex during auditory selective attention. *Proc Natl Acad Sci* Vol 90: 8722-8726

Xerri C (1998). Plasticité post-lésionnelle des cartes corticales somatosensorielles: une revue. *CR Acad Sci Paris* Vol 321 : 135-151

Xerri C, Coq JO, Merzenich MM & Jenkins WM (1996). Experience-induced plasticity of cutaneous maps in the primary somatosensory cortex of adult monkey and rats. *J Physiol Paris* Vol 90: 277-287

Xerri C, Merzenich MM, Jenkins W & Santucci S (1999). Representational plasticity in cortical area 3b paralleling tactile-motor skill acquisition in adult monkeys. *Cerebral Cortex* Vol 9: 264-276

Yahagi S & Kasai T (1998). Facilitation of motor evoked potentials (MEPs) in first dorsal interosseous (FDI) muscle is dependent on different motor images. *Electroencephalogr Clin Neurophysiol* Vol 109: 409-417

Zang Y, Jia F, Weng X, Li E, Cui S, Wang Y, Hazeltine E & Ivry R (2003). Functional organization of the primary motor cortex characterized by event-related fMRI during movement preparation and execution. *Neurosci Lett* Vol 337: 69-72

# 8

# Ciliopathies: Primary Cilia and Signaling Pathways in Mammalian Development

Carmen Carrascosa Romero[1], José Luis Guerrero Solano[2] and Carlos De Cabo De La Vega[3]
*[1]Neuropediatrics,*
*[2]Neurophsyology and*
*[3]Neuropsychopharmacology Units, Albacete General Hospital*
*Spain*

## 1. Introduction

### 1.1 Ciliopathies, an emerging class of human genetic diseases

The physiological role of motile cilia or flagella in cell locomotion, sexual reproduction and fluid movements is well known. In 1898, the Swiss anatomist KW Zimmerman first described cilia on the surface of mammalian cells, for which he suggested a sensory role. His findings were largely ignored until the late 1960s, when Wheatley, using the electron microscope, stumbled upon a properly sized bubble in his histological preparation, verifying it as the cilium described by Zimmerman 63 years earlier[1]. Although it became known that all cells, from green alga Chlamydomonas to human cells - especially kidney cells- possessed a nonmotile cilium, it was initially considered a vestigial structure with no clear function.

Recent discoveries have assigned novel functions to primary (nonmotile) cilia, ranging from mechanosensory in maintaining cellular homeostasis, to participation in signal transduction pathways that regulate intracellular $Ca2+$levels. Furthermore, the cilium is now emerging as an essential organelle in morphogenesis, important to key developmental pathways such as Sonic Hedgehog (Shh) and Wnt (planar cell polarity (PCP) pathways). The function of nodal cilia, for example, is vital for breaking early embryonic symmetry, Shh signaling is important for tissue morphogenesis and successful Wnt signaling for organ growth and differentiation. Defects in cilia formation or function have profound effects on anatomical development and the physiology of multiple organ systems such as death of photoreceptors, kidney tubule cysts, extra limb digits and brain malformation [2, 3]. Alterations in ciliary function also play a role in specific organ diseases (polycystic kidney disease, pigmentosa retinitis...) and pleiotropic phenotypes (Bardet-Bield Syndrome, Alstrom S., Meckel-Gruber S., Oro-Facio-Digital S...), until recently of unknown origin. Our greater knowledge of genetics and the recognized role of cilium in morphogenetic signaling pathways, especially in neurogenesis, bring Bronowski's phrase "All science is the search for unity in hidden likenesses" to life [4].

## 2. Histology

### 2.1 Cilium structure

The cilia are organelles extending from the eukaryotic cell surface, similar to hair. The cilia are short and flagella are long, yet they share the same structure in all eukaryotes [5,6]. The primary cilium emerges from one of the centrioles, a *basal body* (a modified centriole) formed by 9 triplets of microtubules. The basal body is the microtubule organizing center derived from the oldest of the pair of centrioles and controls the movement of cilia and flagella. During interphase the distal end of the older centriole in the centrosome attaches to and becomes enclosed by a membrane vesicle. The microtubule core of the cilium (the axoneme) then assembles directly onto the microtubules of the centriole. As the axoneme lengthens, the primary ciliary vesicle enlarges and becomes a sheath. With time, the sheath (ciliary membrane) fuses with the cytoplasmic membrane and the primary cilium protrudes from the cell surface.

Microtubules are double and parallel (A complete, B incomplete), and are linked by nexin bridges. Some cilia also contain a pair of central single microtubules, called the central pair, involved in regulating motility, surrounded by a sheath and linked by bridges. Thus the types of cilia are classified as follows (TABLE 1):

- Motile: Axonemes: the 9 + 2 Pattern (with central pair).
- Sensory, primary or immotile: Axonemes 9+0 Pattern (no central pair).

Defects in any of these structures can lead to ciliary diseases, and symptoms depend on the target structure.

Ciliary motility is accomplished by dynein motor activity, which slides the microtubule doublets relative to one another. At its base, the ciliary axoneme extends from the nine triplet microtubules of the basal body. Motility is provided by two sets of dynein arms, internal and external, emerging from a doublet of the *A microtubule* and going to the *B microtubule* of the following doublet. It is regulated by a 9-spoke (radial spoke) interacting with the central pair from the *A microtubule.* [7].

Hundreds of proteins are required for cilia formation and function, which is essential for Hh signaling in mammals, therefore these proteins could influence the Hh signal transduction. If this is proven, the challenge will be to understand the physical relationships between components and the Hh pathway that allow efficient ciliary Hh signaling [8, 9]. Ciliary abnormalities fall into four major categories: 1) cilia with abnormal axial microtubules; 2) compound cilia; 3) swollen cilia; and 4) cilia with dynein arm defects.

### 2.2 Cilium functions: The role of cilia in cell physiology

The different functions of cilia are a reflection of their structural diversity, even within the same body. These functions are involved in regulating critical cellular processes:

1. Motility.
2. Polarization of cell division: Cell cycle and cytoskeletal organization.
3. Intraflagelar transport (IFT).
4. Reception and transduction of extracellular signals: These sensory organelles act as *cellular signaling systems:* as antenna for reception and transduction of extracellular molecular signals [10], and as physiological ligands into the cell [11]. They have crucial roles in several signal transduction pathways such as: Hedgehog (Hh) signaling in gene transcription (morphogenic signal) and cell differentiation regulation; Wnt *(canonical*

*Wnt and noncanonical Wnt)*, planar cell polarity (PCP) and platelet-derived growth factor (PDGF) pathways.

| | MOTILE CICLIA | PRIMARY CILIA |
|---|---|---|
| AMOUNT | 1 to billions per cm2* | 1 |
| ESTRUCTURE | 9+2<br>a) respiratory epithelium | 9+0<br>-motile: b)nodal cells.<br>-non motile:<br>c) renal cells<br>d) olfactory cells<br>e) connecting segment, photoreceptor<br>f) balance system kinocilia with the stereocilia. |
| MOTILITY | MOTILE | NON MOTILE |
| FUNCTION | CELL MOTION OR EXTRACELULLAR FLUIDS. | SENSORY |
| | "SWEEP" | "ANTENNAE" |
| DISEASE | Early embyo death.<br>Respiratory dysfunction (bronchiectasis, sinusitis).<br>Situs inversus. Reproductive sterility. Hydrocephalus. | LIMB DEVELOPMENT: morphogenetic signals: polydactyly<br>NEURALTUBE: Gastrulation and Neurulation movements<br>RETINA: retinitis pigmentosa<br>KIDNEY: PDK, nephronophthisis.<br>PDK and retinal degeneration.<br>COGNITIVE IMPAIRMENT<br><br>CILIA GLOBAL DISFUNCTION, PLEIOTROPIC HUMAN DISEASES:<br>-Z-BIEDL SYNDROME (BBS)<br>-ALSTRÖM SYNDROME (ALMS)<br>-OROFACIODIGITAL 1 SYNDROME<br>-MECKEL-GRUBER SYNDROME<br>-JOUBERT SYNDROME<br>-ELLIS-VAN CREVELD SYNDROME<br>-ASPHYXIATING THORACIC DYSTROPHY, JEUNE SYNDROME |

Table 1. Cilia types

## 3. Motility: Agents of cellular movement

Cilia also generate mucus flow and cerebrospinal fluid [12], and can act as mechanosensors and flow meters. Many studies have demonstrated motility as one of the main functions of cilia, and its impairment may cause severe phenotypes such as decreased ciliary beat frequency in the respiratory epithelium [13]. Ciliary motility is also required for brain development and function. The ependymal motile 9+2 cilia are responsible for ependymal flow; ciliary motility loss leads to reduced fluid flow in brain ventricles, resulting in hydrocephalus [14, 15, 16]

Motility is the main feature of the unique 9+0 primary cilium at the embryonic node, which is essential for correct embryonic development. Impairment of these cilia result in embryos showing randomized left-right asymmetry and randomized turning and heart looping [17

## 4. Cell cycle: Centriole union link

Polarization of cell division: Recent advances have demonstrated that ciliary proteins are involved in the regulation of the cell cycle. Centrioles play a dual role in the cell. They form the centrosomes that can interconvert with basal bodies upon ciliation. At the same time, they also give rise to the poles of the mitotic spindle. Centrioles may function as a signaling platform, through proteins that promote the transition from one phase to another in mitosis [18].

- Apc2, anaphase promoting complex protein 2
- *Platelet-derived growth factor receptors (Pdgfr)*

The Centrosome is an organelle located in the center of eukaryotic cells, and acts as an organizing center rather than a microtubule [19]. The centrosome is known as the cytoskeleton's microtubule organizing center of the eukaryotic cell animal, that radiates in a star way or ASTER during mitosis. Experiments show that centrosome absence prevents the cytogenesis process; the cycle does not progress beyond G1.

The centrosome consists of: a) the *Diplosome,* two cylindrical centrioles arranged perpendicularly, located near the nucleus (9 groups of 3 microtubules in cylindrical provision, diameter of 200 nm and 400 nm long). The centrioles of the centrosome are distinguished by a Mother centriole (mature) and a Daughter one; the *Mother* centriole is associated with proteins forming appendices: distal (related to cilia and flagella; a centriole at the base of each cilium or flagellum) and subdistal, involved in microtubule nucleation. b) the *pericentriolar material,* the dense part of the cytosol (amorphous-looking material) and c) the *aster fibers* (microtubules organized in rays).

The centrosome´s main function is to form and organize the microtubules that comprise the achromatic spindle in division of the cell nucleus. The paternal centrosome plays the motor role in meiosis, while the maternal centrosome disappears. Only the mature mother centriole, likely due to the existence of subdistal appendages, transforms into the peculiar structure at the distal end, the basal body, which gives rise to the cilia and flagella of eukaryotic cells. If certain factors are absent (the ODF2 in mice), the cells are unable to organize cilia or flagella [20].

The centrioles are surrounded by an electron-dense matrix called the pericentriolar material (PCM), composed of sets of proteins that modulate or assist in centrosome involving processes. To this day, genome sequencing and comparison has detected and described about 300 proteins that most likely work with the centrosome, although few of them are well known.

Mutations in intraflagellar transport (IFT) genes have clearly demonstrated a correlation between primary cilia and cell cycle control. The basal body-centrosome complex also plays a crucial role in coordinating IFT and the formation of cilia. The centrosome is surrounded by pericentriolar material (PCM), which serves as a nucleation site for microtubules. In mammalian cells, RNAi knockdown of a protein important for PCM organization, pericentrin, inhibits ciliogenesis and reduces the abundance of IFT components near the centrioles [21]. Mutations in a *Drosophila* pericentrin-like homolog also cause malformations in sensory neuron cilia and sperm, indicating that the pericentrin-mediated interaction between centrosomal and IFT proteins is evolutionarily conserved [22]. Misregulation of cell cycle control is at the basis of oncogenesis. The cancer-promoting proteins Aurora A and HEF1/NEDD9/CAS-L play a role in primary cilium stabilization. Loss of cilia in cancer may contribute to the insensitivity of cancer cells to environmental repressive signals [23].

## 5. Intraflagellar transport protein system (IFT)

During ciliogenesis, cilia elongate from the basal body by the addition of new axonemal subunits to the distal tip. As protein synthesis does not occur in cilia, axonemal and membrane components are conveyed in non-membrane-bound macromolecular particles by intraflagellar transport (IFT) along the axonemal microtubule doublets [24].
The proteins are transported as convoys, bringing together several proteins called "*IFT particles*". IFT have 2 transport routes [25, 26]:

- anterograde transport, from the cytoplasm to the outside and
- retrograde transport, from the tip of the cilium to the interior.

At the tip of the cilium there is a particular structure where there is a change in intraciliar transport direction [27 a 29]. Large IFT particles move between the axoneme microtubule doublets and ciliary membrane, transported by specific Golgi vesicles directed toward the ciliary pore complex using cytoplasmic dynein. These vesicles exocyst at the base of the cilium, where kinesin II transports the particles up to the tip. By shortening or recycling of the cilium, the IFT descend to the base by means of dynein 2 for recycling [31]. IFT play a key role in ciliogenesis, taking axoneme components synthesized in the cytoplasm to the tip of the cilium.
Intraciliar or intraflagellar transport is responsible for cilia growth, for renewal of its components and for the particular formation of the cilium membrane that distinguishes it from the rest of the plasma membrane [30].

## 6. Hedgehog pathway

The process and transfer of information signals to the cell are mediated by specialized proteins [3]:

- Cationic channels compounds by *polycystin proteins Pc1 and Pc2* in the ciliary membrane are sensitive to mechanical stimuli.
- *Platelet-derived growth factor receptors (Pdgfr)*, sensitive to extracellular ligands.
- Smoothened Receptors (Smo) [32]: The nodal point of life.
- Several microtubule-associated protein complexes that include proteins associated with nephronophthisis [NPHP, investment (Invs)], and with Bardet-Biedl syndrome (BBS).

Hedgehog proteins (Hh) are a group of signaling proteins generating extracellular ligands that play an important role in regulating cell differentiation. In humans, there are three known Hedgehog proteins: Sonic Hh (Shh), Indian Hh and Desert Hh. When these ligands bind to various specific receptors, they trigger a signaling cascade resulting in activation of transcription factors of the Gli family that regulate the transcription of effector genes. The Hh receptors in vertebrates are the integral membrane "Patched" proteins Ptc1 and Ptc2 .

The 1st step in the Hh signaling process is the physical union with Ptc, activating the pathway and producing internalization by endocytosis of the Hh-Ptc complex and its subsequent lysosomal degradation. This eliminates the extracellular morphogen and sets the concentration gradient.

- The transduction system involves Smoothened (Smo), a transmembrane protein. The Hh to Ptc union begins its internalization and releases Smo that, from intracellular vesicles, shifts and accumulates on the cell surface where it is translocated to the cilia, initiating the signaling cascade that culminates in the modulation of the transcription factors Ci / Gli (Gli protein 1, 2 and 3) [33, 34]

### 6.1 Embryonic development

The Hedgehog (Hh) pathway determines growth patterns and embryonic differentiation in a large number of organs. Approximately half of all mutations affect the initial establishment of the body plan, and several of these produce phenotypes that have not been described previously. A large fraction of the genes identified affect cell migration, cellular organization, and cell structure. Findings indicate that phenotype-based genetic screens provide a direct and unbiased method for identifying essential regulators of mammalian development [35]. The mutant cilia are short, with a specific defect in the structure of the ciliary axoneme [36].

- The Hh signaling pathway is essential in embryogenesis due to its involvement in the development of multiple organs where it controls such important aspects as specification of different kinds of cells, cell proliferation and cell survival (apoptosis control).
- The ligand Shh (Sonic hh) is responsible for the functions of the best characterized development signaling centers such as the notochord and the zone of polarizing activity (ZPA) of the tip [37].
- The morphogen concentration provides cells with *positional value* commensurate with gradient position, determining cell destiny, generating an appropriate pattern or morphology, and foreshadowing the final organ or tissue pattern. Hh proteins act as morphogens in the development of the central nervous system, limbs, heart, blood vessels, gonads, intestine and kidney. In vertebrates, cilia also function in the Shh-dependent patterning of the developing neural tube and limb [38]. Mutant mice with defects in ciliogenesis resulting from mutations in IFT protein-encoding genes, such as polaris, wimple (Ift172), Ngd5 (Ift52) and the gene encoding the retrograde motor Dnchc2, have neural tube defects and preaxial polydactyly phenotypes similar to mutants with defects in Shh pathway proteins [33, 39 a 42].

#### 6.1.1 Hh and limb development

Cilia are present in the forebrain neurectoderm and in ectodermal and mesenchymal cells of the limb, but are aberrant or absent from these tissues in IFT mutants [33, 41, 42]. The zone of polarizing activity (ZPA), a small cluster of mesodermal cells located at the rear edge of the developing limb, is responsible for the anteroposterior pattern of the limb by secreting Shh, the morphogen controlling the number and identity of the fingers plus antero-posterior specification. The normal expression of Shh in chicken wing ZPA is accompanied by its diffusion gradient model scheme along the anteroposterior axis. Normal skeletal pattern of the chicken wing consists of 3 digits known as 2 (d2), 3 (d3) and 4 (d4).

Formation of finger-type depends on morphogen levels to which precursor cells were subjected during development. When another source of Shh is introduced at previous levels, either naturally or through experimental means, two gradients are generated in the outline of the limb which, depending on their geometry, may overlap with each other in the central area of the limb. This configuration leads to mirror duplications of the digits (d4-d3-d2-d3-d4) [41].

### 6.1.2 Hh and central nervous system development

In the developing mammalian ventral spinal cord, five different neuronal cell types, comprising the motoneuron (MN) and four different interneurons (V0-V3), are generated from their respective neural progenitors (pMN, pV0-pV3) under the influence of signals from the notochord [43]. Shh, one of the Hedgehog (Hh) family of proteins, is strongly expressed in the notochord and later in the floor plate, and is able to mimic the ability of the notochord for inducing different ventral spinal cord cell types. In response to Shh signaling, neural progenitors activate or suppress the expression of several homeobox and basic helix-loop-helix (bHLH) transcription factors. The combinatorial expression of these transcription factors defines the fate of the neural progenitor cells [44].

Although Shh has been shown to be sufficient for the induction of distinct ventral spinal cord neurons, recent studies have suggested an alternative derepression mechanism whereby many neuronal cell types could be generated in the absence of Shh signaling. For example, although most of the ventral cell types are absent from Shh or Smo mutants because of the ectopic production of Gli3 repressor, most of the ventral neurons are generated in Shh; Gli3 and Smo;Gli3 double mutants [45,46]. Similarly, in embryos that lack all Gli transcription factors and cannot respond to Hh signaling, many of the ventral neurons are also present [47, 48]. These results suggest that perhaps the primary role of Hh signaling is to repress excess Gli3 repressor in the ventral spinal cord so that progenitors can respond to other signals. An additional role for Shh signaling is to organize the formation of distinct progenitor domains, as different cell types intermix in the absence of Shh signaling [49].

The mouse mutation, hennin (hnn), causes coupled defects in cilia structure and Sonic hedgehog (Shh) signaling. Gli3 repressor activity is normal in hnn embryos, but Gli activators are constitutively active at low levels. The hnn phenotypes are whole e10.5 wild-type (A) and hnn (B and C) embryos, which show exencephaly and spina bifida. As a result, IFT mutants display a loss of Hh signaling phenotype in the neural tube, where Gli activators play the major role in pattern formation, and a gain of Hh signaling phenotype in the limb, where Gli3 repressor plays the major role. Because both anterograde and retrograde IFT are essential for positive and negative responses to Hh, and because cilia are present on Hh responsive cells, it is likely that cilia act as organelles that are required for all activity of the mouse Hh pathway [50].

During development of the central nervous system, *Shh secreted* in the prechordal plate, notochord and floor plate, disseminates and establishes a concentration gradient across the dorsal ventral axis of the neural tube, with maximum levels at the ventral side, forming an appropriate dorsoventral pattern of cell differentiation. Finally, mediated by the three Gli transcription factors′ combined activity, Shh, in the neural tube, not only controls the specification but also regulates cell proliferation and survival through cell cycle regulation and expression of antiapoptotic genes. Moreover, the neocortex, cerebellum and tectum growth also depend on the mitogenic activity of Shh [51 a 55]. Recently, it has been attributed a role in axonal growth [56], and in maintaining stem cell niches in the adult.

### 6.2 Stem cell proliferation and differentiation: neurogenesis

In adults, the Hh signal is involved in maintaining stem cell and tissue homeostasis. In neurogenesis, the brain's mature CM receives signals to divide and differentiate into neurons. The primary cilium plays a key role in the CM receiving orders to divide by the uptake of cell growth factors through the route called "Sonic hedgehog".

Degenerative defects:

Neural stem cells (NSCs) are present in the mammalian brain from embryo to adult. It has been shown that these cells are a significant source of new neurons, and promise to be the origin of a new central nervous system restorative therapy: Hedgehog (Hh) signaling is involved in a wide range of important biological activities. Within the vertebrate central nervous system, Sonic Hedgehog (Shh) can act as a morphogen or mitogen that regulates the patterning, proliferation, and survival of neural stem cells (NSCs). However, its role in embryonic stem cell (ESC) neurogenesis has not been explored in detail. Hh signaling is required for ESC neurogenesis; in order to elucidate the underlying mechanism, Cai C. et al [57] utilized the Sox1-GFP ESC line, which has a green fluorescent protein (GFP) reporter under the control of the Sox1 gene promoter, providing an easy means of detecting NSCs in live cell culture. That ESC differentiation in adherent culture follows the ESC--> primitive ectoderm --> neurectoderm transitions observed in vivo. Selective death of the Sox1-GFP-negative cells contributes to the enrichment of Sox1-GFP-positive NSCs. Interestingly, Shh is expressed exclusively by the NSCs themselves and elicits distinct downstream gene expression in Sox1-GFP-positive and -negative cells. Suppression of Hh signaling by antagonist treatment leads to different responses from these two populations as well: increased apoptosis in Sox1-GFP-positive NSCs and decreased proliferation in Sox1-GFP-negative primitive ectoderm cells. Hedgehog agonist treatment, in contrast, inhibits apoptosis and promotes proliferation of Sox1-GFP-positive NSCs. These results suggest that Hh acts as a mitogen and survival factor during early ESC neurogenesis, and evidence is presented to support a novel autocrine mechanism for Hh-mediated effects on NSC survival and proliferation.

An intravenous Hh agonist at doses that upregulate spinal cord Gli1 transcription also increases the population of neural precursor cells after spinal cord injury in adult rats. These data support previous findings based on injections of Shh protein directly into the spinal cord [58].

A common feature of embryonic and adult NSCs is that they have a primary cilium emerging from a mother centriole, and through its receptors Sonic Hedgehog (Shh) is involved in cell specification and neurogenesis with neural progenitors´ expansion in brain development [59]. Shh is active in some groups of cells in mature organs which seem to be involved in maintaining stem cell numbers.

In mammalian telencephalon, two postnatal neurogenesis areas are known: the hippocampus dentate gyrus and the telencephalic ventricles´ subventricular zone. Quiescent cells express low levels of Gli1, a marker of responding Shh cells, but the Shh/Gli pathway is activated to regulate the generation of new neurons [60]. The Shh signaling cascade is also involved in the maintenance of other types of adult stem cells such as hematopoietic cells [61].

### 6.3 Oncology and carcinogenicity

Recently, many vertebrate-specific components have been identified that act between the GOS and Gli. These include intraflagellar transport proteins which link vertebrate Hh signaling to cilia. Because abnormal Hh signaling can cause birth defects and cancer, these vertebrate-specific components may play a role in human health. Hh signaling has been involved in development of several human cancers including small cell lung carcinoma, medulloblastoma, basal cell carcinomas, digestive tract (pancreas) tumors, brain, prostate, skin, etc. [62 a 67].

PTC has been considered a tumor suppressor gene: Ptc inhibits the signaling pathway, so the loss of activity results in activation of the Shh pathway.

Many oncogenic factors may converge on Gli activity to promote tumor progression, thus pointing towards the Hh signaling cascade as a phenomenon to be considered in potential treatments for many different types of cancer. For example, Gorlin syndrome or nevoid basal cell carcinoma syndrome is caused by a disorder of chromosome 9 (q22.3 and q31) and 1 (p32), leading to mutations in the PTCH tumor suppressor gene, a human homologue of *Drosophila melanogaster patched* gene. The PTCH gene encodes the signal's Sonic Hedgehog (Shh) transmembrane protein receptor, a regulatory molecule in embryogenesis and carcinogenesis [68].

## 7. Wnt Signaling pathways

There are 3 known pathways, activated after docking of Wnt to its "Frizzle" family receptors (FZD) (*See Gerdes JM y Katsanis N. 2008* review[69]):

### 7.1 Canonical wnt pathway

It acts through β-catenina/Arm and specifies different cell types, controlling proliferation and apoptosis depending on the development context. It is activated in virtually all tumors. Induces stabilization and accumulation in the cytoplasm of ß-catenin and its subsequent translocation to the cell nucleus where it affects transcription of target genes [2, 3, 70, 71].

a. When the Wnt signal is not activated, ß-catenin binds to the degradation complex consisting of APC axin and the serine/threonine kinases CK1 and GSK3. The degradation complex´s main role is to phosphorylate ß-catenin, guiding it to its degradation through addition of multiple ubiquitins and its enzymatic process in the proteasome. There are several negative regulators operating at the ligand receptor-like level, such as Cer1, DKK, and sFRP, whose function is to modulate Wnt-induced positive signals.
b. Wnt contact with its receptors leads to stabilization of ß-catenin and its accumulation in the cytoplasm. ß-catenin displaces Groucho transcriptional repression from the complex formed by LEF/TCF, leading to activation of target genes such as C-MYC and CCND1, which are involved in cell cycle progression and proliferation.
c. *Canonical Wnt signaling is involved in the* generation of different cell types in the ventral spinal cord: The identity of distinct cell types in the ventral neural tube is generally believed to be specified by sonic hedgehog (Shh) in a concentration-dependent manner. However, recent studies have questioned whether Shh is the sole signaling molecule determining the fate of ventral neuronal cells. There is evidence showing that canonical Wnt signaling is involved in the generation of different cell types in the ventral spinal

cord. Wnt signaling is active in the mouse ventral spinal cord at the time when ventral cell types are specified. Furthermore, using an approach that stabilizes beta-catenin protein in small patches of ventral spinal cord cells at different stages, Wnt signaling activates different subsets of target genes depending on the time when Wnt signaling is amplified. Moreover, disruption of Wnt signaling results in the expansion of ventrally located progenitors. Finally, Wnt signaling interacts with Hh signaling at least in part through regulating the transcription of Gli3. Yu W. et al [72] reveal a novel mechanism by which ventral patterning is achieved through coordination of Wnt and Shh signaling.

### 7.2 The planar cell polarity pathway (PCP)

Sets the polarization of the cells along the plane of a tissue membrane. This pathway is important for neural tube closure and cochlear extension of the inner ear. Is involved in cell polarity, tissue and cell movement processes.

### 7.3 WNT/CA+2 OR "Non-canonical" pathway

Regulates cell adhesion and motility mediated by Wnt-5a, triggers intracellular Ca2+ release to activate Ca2+-sensitive enzymes such as protein kinase C (PKC ), calmodulin-dependent kinase II and Ca2+ (CaMKII) without ß-catenin pathway activation.

## 8. Ciliary dysfunction: Human phenotypes

Given the multiple roles of cilia in development and physiology, it is not surprising that defects in cilia cause multiple human diseases (reviews see Afzelius, 2004 [73]; Badano et al., 2006 [74]; Fliegauf et al., 2007 [75]; Quinlan RJ et al, 2008 [2]; D'Angelo A. et al, 2009 [76])
Perhaps the most puzzling aspect of ciliopathies is that different ciliary diseases involve different, often partially overlapping sets of symptoms. For instance, Bardet-Biedl patients suffer from obesity, retinal degeneration, and cystic kidneys, whereas Oral-Facial-Digital syndrome patients suffer from polydactyly and cystic kidneys. However, both types of diseases result from defects in genes whose protein products localize to the ciliary basal body. Why don´t all ciliary defects produce the same set of symptoms? The key to this question is to realize that despite the growing wealth of genomic and proteomic data on cilia composition [77], cilia are not just lists of genes but complex organelles with variable ultrastructures that must assemble and function in different tissue contexts. Why might defects in two cilia-related genes lead to distinct diseases? There are several ways this can happen: (1) some ciliary genes may have additional cilia-unrelated gene functions; (2) some mutations may affect the ciliogenesis of only a subset of all cilia in the body; and (3) genetic defects may affect different ultrastructural modules of cilia and, thus, only influence a subset of ciliary functions [78].

### 8.1 Cilia motility dysfunction

- Major clinical features:
  - Early embryo death.
  - Respiratory dysfunction (bronchiectasis, sinusitis).
  - Reproductive sterility.
  - Hydrocephalus

- Embryo symmetry. Nodal cilia: It has been proven that nodal ciliary flow is required to generate the right/left symmetry axis. Between days 10 and 25 of embryonic development, a sophisticated biochemical reaction cascade determines that the human body will be: asymmetrical inside -with the heart on the left and liver on the right; and symmetrical outside -with two hands, two feet and the navel in the middle. Stem cells that become different body tissues enter the node (cells that direct embryo growth). The node has hundreds of cilia (nodal cilia) that guide each cell to its destination in the embryo. Nodal cilia run in subtle circular motion, creating convection currents in the fluid where the embryo is immersed (nodal flow). These currents help to carry the cells to their proper place. FoxJ1 transcription factor is the master key to the formation of nodal cilia, which are responsible for left-right asymmetry [79 a 81].
- Primary ciliary dyskinesia (PCD): is a rare autosomal recessive disease (GENE: DNAHC11, locus:7p21), characterized by abnormal ciliary structure and function. The ciliary defect is a result of absence or anomalies of dynein arms and pairs of microtubule structures responsible for movement. Patients show recurrent lung, sinus and middle ear infections. Male infertility may be present, due to immotile sperm. Female fertility is also affected, given the presence of cilia in the fallopian tubes and fimbriae. Kartagener syndrome (50%) is associated with situs inversus [82 a 85].
- Hydrocephalus appears to be specifically associated with defects in the central pair of microtubules as typified by the mouse hydin mutant, which has hydrocephalus and lacks the central pair. Ciliary motility is necessary for brain development and function; the "ependymal flow" is required to maintain an open aqueduct [86, 87].

### 8.2 Sensory cilia dysfunction (cilium)

Given the many roles of cilia in physiology and development, it is not surprising that its defects cause multiple human diseases. Perhaps cilia´s most enigmatic aspect is that only one defect involves different diseases, often with a partially overlapping set of symptoms [2]. High ranked phenotypes by: 1° the necessary ubiquitous presence in each of the cell types of the human body, and 2° the emerging role in morphogenetic signal transduction. (TABLE 2).

- Development of limbs: morphogenetic signals: Polydactyly
- Neural tube: movements during gastrulation and neurulation
- Retina: Retinitis Pigmentosa, retinal blindness
- Kidney: PKD y Nephronophthisis.
- PKD and retinal degeneration (Senior-Loken Syndrome)
- Cognitive impairment

Retina: photo-receptors: have a primary cilium (9+0) that connects the outer segment (rhodopsin disks) to the inner segment where rhodopsin is synthesized. Molecules that detect light are synthesized in the inner segment and must be transported to the outer segment by intraciliar transport. Mutations in a gene involved in transport of these molecules needed for seeing or outer segment maintenance result in degeneration of photoreceptors leading to blindness such as in retinitis pigmentosa. Dysfunction of primary cilia due to mutations in cilia-centrosomal proteins is associated with pleiotropic disorders. The primary (or sensory) cilium of photoreceptors mediates polarized trafficking of proteins for efficient phototransduction. Retinitis pigmentosa GTPase regulator (RPGR) is a cilia-centrosomal protein mutated in >70% of X-linked RP cases and 10%-20% of simplex RP males. Accumulating evidence indicates that RPGR may facilitate the orchestration of multiple ciliary protein complexes. Disruption of these complexes due to mutations in component proteins is an underlying cause of associated photoreceptor degeneration. Here, we highlight the recent developments in understanding the mechanism of cilia-dependent photoreceptor degeneration due to mutations in RPGR and PGR-interacting proteins in severe genetic diseases, including retinitis pigmentosa, Leber congenital amaurosis (LCA), Joubert syndrome, and Senior-Loken syndrome. Additionally, we explore the physiological relevance of photoreceptor ciliary protein complexes [88, 89].

| | |
|---|---|
| 1 | Dandy-Walker Syndrome |
| 2 | Corpus callosum agenesis |
| 3 | Situs inversus |
| 4 | Posterior Encephalocele |
| 5 | Renal cystic disease |
| 6 | Postaxial polydactyly |
| 7 | Liver disease |
| 8 | Retinitis Pigmentosa |
| 9 | Mental retardation |

Table 2. Clinical features that may predict cilia involvement (listed by relevance) From: Badano JL, et al [74]

RENAL: Polycystic kidney disease (PKD) [90], and Nephronophthisis [91]. PKD is the most common inherited disease in the United States. Current estimates are that 600 000 patients have PKD in the US, with 12.5 million cases worldwide (for a recent, comprehensive review on PKD see [90]. The inherited PKDs include autosomal dominant type (ADPKD), autosomal recessive (ARPKD), and nephronophthisis. ADPKD, the most common form, occurs in 1 amongst 600–800 live births and affects 500 000 persons in the US. The disease occurs during adult life and is characterized by extensive cystic enlargement of both kidneys. Of the two types of ADPKD, type I is caused by a mutation in the PKD1 gene, and type II by a mutation in the PKD2 gene [92]. The proteins encoded by both genes are transmembrane proteins. Polycystin 1 is proposed to be a cell–cell and cell– matrix adhesion receptor [93] and polycystin 2 is thought to act as a calcium-permeable membrane channel [94]. Polycystic kidney is the result of altered intraciliar transport of non-motile primary cilia of the renal tubule epithelial cells [95]. In PKD, cyst formation is associated with increased numbers of cells in the circumference of renal tubules. In mice with renal-specific inactivation of Tcf2, and in the *pck* rat, which has reduced expression of *Pkd2* and/or *Pkhd1*, mitotic alignments along the axis of the tubules are significantly distorted, indicating a loss of PCP [96].

**Cognitive impairment**

Patients with ciliary dysfunction disorders display variably expressive brain dysgenesis as well as neurocognitive impairments. Joubert syndrome is a ciliopathy defined by cerebellar vermis hypoplasia, oculomotor apraxia, intermittent hyperventilation, and mental retardation. Recent evidence suggests important roles for the primary cilium in mediating a host of extracellular signaling events such as morphogen, mitogen, homeostatic and polarity signals. Based upon the clinical features of ciliopathies and cilia mediated signaling pathways, the data support a role for the primary cilium in modulating neurogenesis, cell polarity, axonal guidance and possibly adult neuronal function [97,98].

## 9. Global ciliary dysfunction in pleiotropic human diseases

- BARDET-BIEDL (BBS) / OMIM: 209900
- ALSTRÖM (ALMS) / OMIM: 203800
- OROFACIODIGITAL TYPE 1/ OMIM: 311200
- JOUBERT SYNDROME / OMIM: 213300
- MECKEL-GRUBER / OMIM: 249000
- ELLIS - VAN CREVELD SYNDROME / OMIM: 225500
- ASPHYXIATING THORACIC DYSTROPHY, JEUNE SYNDROME /OMIM 208500.

**Bardet-Biedl syndrome (BBS) or Laurence Moon-Biedl syndrome [99].**

Retinal dystrophy, obesity, and polydactyly.
INHERITANCE: RA. Genes:12 BBS genes. Locus:11q13; 16q21; 3p12-q13; 15q22.3; 2q31; 20p12; 4q27; 14q32.11; 7p14; 12q; 9q33.1; 4q27.
PHENOTYPE: Obesity (83%). Polydactyly, syndactyly, or both (75%). Mental Retardation (80%), spinocerebellar degeneration. Retinal degeneration: Retinitis pigmentosa (68%) with night vision problems, loss of peripheric-central vision. By the age of 20, 73% are blind. Genital hypoplasia, hypogonadism (60%). Renal cystic disease. Other: nystagmus, anosmia, asthma, diabetes insipidus, cardiac malformations and situs inversus.

**Alström (Alms) Syndrome**

INHERITANCE: RA; GENE: ALMS1; Locus:2P13. Protein: Alström syndrome protein 1.
PHENOTYPE: Obesity. Type 2 diabetes mellitus. Sensorineural hearing loss (cochlear neuronal degeneration). Photophobia and nystagmus (degeneration of photoreceptor cone cells). Others: short stature, cardiomyopathy, liver and renal failure, hypogonadism.

**Meckel-Gruber Syndrome**

INHERITANCE: RA. Genetic heterogeneity. 3 loci: *MKS1* on 17q23, *MKS2* on 11q13, *MKS3* on 8q21.13-q22.1
PHENOTYPE: A fatal disease, characterized by: occipital encephalocele, bilateral renal cystic dysplasia, hepatic ductal dysplasia and cysts, and polydactyly.

**Orofaciodigital syndrome 1**

INHERITANCE: X-linked Dominant (fatal in males). GENE: OFD1; Locus: Xp22.3-p22.2. PROTEIN: Oral-facial-digital syndrome 1 protein.
PHENOTYPE: ORAL: Membrane between oral mucosa and alveolar bone. Partial clefts: upper lip, tongue, alveolar, palate. FACIAL: alar cartilage hypoplasia, short filter, hypertelorism with lateral location of inner edges. DIGITAL: asymmetric shortening of fingers (polydactyly / syndactyly). RENAL: renal microcysts. OTHER: Mental retardation (IQ 70), agenesis of the corpus callosum, cerebellar abnormalities and hydrocephalus, alopecia ...

**Joubert syndrome (JBTS)**

INHERITANCE: RA. 3genes: (AHI1, NPHP1, CEP290). Incidence: 1x100.000 NB. Affects the cerebellum (vermis hypoplasia) and brainstem; appears in neonatal period with a characteristic breathing pattern of tachypnea/apnea.

PHENOTYPE: Head: macrocephaly, prominent forehead. Eyes: coloboma, nystagmus, strabismus, ptosis. Ears: low-set and thick. Nose: broad nasal bridge, epicanthus, anteverted nostrils. Open mouth, tongue protusion with rhythmic tongue movements. Neurological: generalized hypotonia, frog posture, hyperpnea followed by apnea. Ataxia. Other: polydactyly, seizures, scoliosis, congenital heart disease, pigmented retina. MRI: molar sign: There are 4 specific abnormalities: 1) Increased posterior interpeduncular fossa and decreased length of the isthmus. 2) Thick and elongated superior cerebellar peduncles in greater perpendicular orientation towards brainstem compared with normal orientation. 3) Hypoplastic or aplastic superior cerebellar vermis.4) Sagittal vermian cleft.

**Ellis-Van Creveld syndrome**

INHERITANCE: AR. GEN: two genes (EVC y ECV2). LOCUS:14p16. Protein: EVCS protein. Condroectodermal dysplasia, Mesoectodermal dysplasia. Incidence: 0.5x100.000. 30% consanguineous. Common among the Pennsylvania Amish population.
PHENOTYPE: Acromesomelic dwarfism resulting in disproportionately short limbs, predominantly in the lower limbs and most striking distally (farthest from central trunk or midline). Final height reached is between 109 to 155cm. Postaxial polydactyly in hands and, occasionally, feet. Carpal and pastern bones fusion. Cleft lip at the junction of the upper hemi-lips, and labiogingival frenulum hypertrophy.
Congenital heart disease (50-60%), septal defects, single atrium. Differential diagnosis with short rib-polydactyly syndromes: Jeune syndrome or asphyxiating thoracic dystrophy and oro-facio-digital syndrome.

**Asphyxiating Thoracic Dystrophy, Jeune Syndrome.**

INHERITANCE: RA. GENES: 2 (JATD1,JATD2). LOCI :15q13, 3q24-26. Protein: intraflagellar transport protein 80 homolog
PHENOTYPE: Retinal degeneration, kidney cysts, hepatic portal fibrosis, affecting infants who die of asphyxia in the neonatal period secondary to small chest with short ribs. Skeletal: Chondrodysplasia; shortness of long bones, hypoplastic iliac wings, conical epiphysis and phalangeal fusion. Polydactyly. OTHER: impaired pancreatic ...

## 10. Conclusion

Recent studies provide evidence for novel functions of primary cilia ranging from mechanosensory and cellular homeostasis, to signal transduction pathways that regulate intracellular $Ca^{2+}$levels. Their importance in key developmental pathways such as Sonic Hedgehog and Wnt is beginning to emerge. Defects in cilia formation or function have profound effects on the development of body pattern and the physiology of multiple organ systems. Thus, impairment of ciliar function is involved in organ specific diseases (e.g. polycystic kidney disease, retinitis pigmentosa) as well as pleiotropic syndromes (e.g. Bardet-Biedl, Alstrom, Meckel-Gruber and orofaciodigital syndromes) of unknown origin until recently. Increasing knowledge of the ciliar role in morphogenesis pathways in conjunction with genetic studies is helping to characterize a new group of diseases, previously unconnected to each other.

## 11. References

[1] Wheatley DN. Landmarks in the first hundred years of primary (9+0) cilium research. Cell Biol Int. 2005; 29: 333-9.

[2] Quinlan RJ, Tobin JL, Beales PL: Modeling Ciliopathies: Primary Cilia in Development and Disease. Current Topics in Developmental Biology, 2008; 84: 250-282
[3] BW, Yost HJ: The roles of cilia in developmental disorders and disease. Development. 2006; 133, 4131-4143
[4] Bronowski J. Science and human values (New York: Harper & Row. 1965).
[5] Haimo LT, Rosenbaum JL: Cilia, flagella, and microtubules. The journal of cell biology. 1981; 91 n°. 3 pt :125s-130s
[6] Afzelius B A: Cilia-related diseases. J. Pathol. 2004; 204: 470-477
[7] Sloboda R D: Intraflagellar transport and the flagellar tip complex. J. Cell Biochem. 2005; 94: 266-272
[8] Avidor-Reiss T. Maer A.M. Koundakjian E. Polyanovsky A. Keil T. Subramaniam S. et al.: Decoding cilia function; defining specialized genes required for compartmentalized cilia biogenesis. Cell. 2004; 117:527 -539.
[9] Li J. B. Gerdes J. M. Haycraft C. J., Fan Y. Teslovich, T. M. May-Simera et al: Comparative Genomics Identifies a Flagellar and Basal Body Proteome that Includes the BBS5 Human Disease Gene. Cell. 2004; 117: 541 -552
[10] Praetoriu H.A. and Spring K.R.: The renal cell primary cilium functions as a fl ow sensor. Curr. Opin. Nephrol. Hypertens. 2003; 12 : 517 - 520
[11] Christensen S.T. Pedersen L.B. Schneider L. Satir P: Sensory cilia and integration of signal transduction in human health and disease. Traffi c . 2007; 8 : 97 - 100
[12] Eggenschwiler J.T. Anderson K.V: Cilia and developmental signaling.Annu. Rev. Cell Dev. Biol. 2007; 23 : 345 - 373 .
[13] Fernandez-Gonzalez A. Kourembanas S. Wyatt TA. Mitsialis SA: Mutation of murine adenylate kinase 7 underlies a primary ciliary dyskinesia phenotype. Am J Respir Cell Mol Biol. 2008; 40:305-313.
[14] Banizs B, Pike MM, Millican CL, Ferguson WB, Komlosi P, Sheetz J, Bell PD, Schwiebert EM, Yoder BK: Dysfunctional cilia lead to altered ependyma and choroid plexus function, and result in the formation of hydrocephalus. Development. 2005; 132:5329-5339.
[15] Ibanez-Tallon I, Pagenstecher A, Fliegauf M, Olbrich H, Kispert A, Ketelsen UP, North A, Heintz N, Omran H: Dysfunction of axonemal dynein heavy chain Mdnah5 inhibits ependymal flow and reveals a novel mechanism for hydrocephalus formation. Hum Mol Genet. 2004; 13:2133-2141.
[16] Eley L, Yates LM, Goodship JA: Cilia and disease. Curr Opin Genet Dev 2005; 15: 308-314.
[17] Nonaka S, Tanaka Y, Okada Y, Takeda S, Harada A, Kanai Y, Kido M, Hirokawa N: Randomization of left-right asymmetry due to loss of nodal cilia generating leftward flow of extraembryonic fluid in mice lacking KIF3B motor protein. Cell 1998; 95:829-837.
[18] Linck R.W, Stephens R.W: Functional protofi lament numbering of ciliary, fl agellar, and centriolar microtubules. Cell Motil. Cytoskeleton. 2007; 64: 489-495
[19] Rieder CL, Faruki S, Khodjakov A. The centrosome in vertebrates: more than a microtubule-organizing center. Trends Cell Biol 2001; 11: 413–419.
[20] Dirksen, E.R. Centriole and basal body formation during ciliogenesis revisited. Biol. Cell. 1991; 72: 31 - 38 .

[21] Jurczyk A, Gromley A, Redick S. San Agustin J, Witman G, Pazour G.J. et al: Pericentrin forms a complex with intraflagellar transport proteins and polycystin-2 and is required for primary cilia assembly. J. Cell Biol. 2004; 166, 637-643
[22] Martinez-Campos M, Basto R, Baker J, Kernan M, Raff J. W: The Drosophila pericentrin-like protein is essential for cilia/flagella function, but appears to be dispensable for mitosis. J. Cell Biol. 2004; 165, 673-683
[23] Plotnikova OV, Golemis EA, Pugacheva EN: Cell cycle-dependent ciliogenesis and cancer. Cancer Res 2008; 68: 2058-2061
[24] Kozminski KG, Johnson KA, Forscher P, Rosenbaum J L: A motility in the eukaryotic flagellum unrelated to flagellar beating. Proc. Natl.Acad. Sci. USA.1993; 90: 5519-5523
[25] Pazour GJ, Dickert BL, Witman GB. The DHC1b (DHC2) isoform of cytoplasmic dynein is required for flagellar assembly. J. Cell Biol. 1999; 144: 473-481
[26] Signor D, Wedaman K P, Orozco JT, Dwyer N D, Bargmann C I, Rose L S, et al: Role of a class DHC1b dynein in retrograde transport of IFT motors and IFT raft particles along cilia, but not dendrites, in chemosensory neurons of living Caenorhabditis elegans. J. Cell Biol. 1999; 147: 519-530
[27] Qin H, Burnette D T, Bae Y K, Forscher P, Barr M M, Rosenbaum JL: Intraflagellar transport is required for the vectorial movement of TRPV channels in the ciliary membrane. Curr. Biol. 2005; 15, 1695-1699
[28] Wang Q, Pan J, Snell WJ.: Intraflagellar transport particles participate directly in cilium-generated signaling in Chlamydomonas. Cell 2006; 125: 549-562
[29] Pedersen LB, Geimer S, Sloboda R D, Rosenbaum J L: The Microtubule plus end-tracking protein EB1 is localized to the flagellar tip and basal bodies in Chlamydomonas reinhardtii. Curr. Biol. 2003; 13: 1969-1974
[30] Rosenbaum JL, WitmanGB: Intraflagellar transporte. Nat. Rev. Mol Cell Biol. 2002; Nov; 3 (11) :813-25
[31] Scholey JM. Intraflagellar transport motors in cilia: moving along the cell's antenna. J. Cell. Biol . 2008; 180: 23-29
[32] Corbit K C, Aanstad P, Singla V, Norman A.R, Stainier D Y, Reiter JF: Vertebrate Smoothened functions at the primary cilium. Nature 2005; 437: 1018 -1021
[33] Haycraft C J, Banizs B, Aydin-Son Y, Zhang Q, Michaud E J, Yoder B: KGli2 and Gli3 localize to cilia and require the intraflagellar transport protein polaris for processing and function. PLoS Genet. 2005; 1, e53.
[34] Dai P, Akimaru, H, Tanaka Y, Maekawa T, Nakafuku M, Ishii S: Sonic Hedgehog-induced activation of the Gli1 promoter is mediated by GLI3. J. Biol. Chem. 1999; 274: 8143 -8152
[35] García-García MJ, Eggenschwiler JT, Caspary T, Alcorn HL, Wyler MR, Huangfu D, Rakeman AS, Lee JD, Feinberg EH, Timmer JR, Anderson KVAnalysis of mouse embryonic patterning and morphogenesis by forward genetics. Proc Natl Acad Sci U S A. 2005 Apr 26; 102(17): 5913-9
[36] Huangfu D, Anderson KV. Cilia and Hedgehog responsiveness in the mouse. Proc Natl Acad Sci U S A. 2005; Aug 9; 102(32):11325-30
[37] Echelard Y, Epstein D J, St-Jacques B, Shen L, Mohler J., McMahon J A. et al: Sonic hedgehog, a member of a family of putative signaling molecules, is implicated in the regulation of CNS polarity. Cell 1993; 75: 1417 -1430

[38] Huangfu D, Anderson K V: Signaling from Smo to Ci/Gli: conservation and divergence of Hedgehog pathways from Drosophila to vertebrates. Development. 2006; 133: 3-14

[39] Huangfu D, Liu A, Rakeman A S, Murcia N S, Niswander L, Anderson K V: Hedgehog signalling in the mouse requires intraflagellar transport proteins. Nature 2003; 426: 83-87.

[40] Liu A, Wang B, Niswander LA: Mouse intraflagellar transport proteins regulate both the activator and repressor functions of Gli transcription factors. Development. 2005; 132: 3103-3111

[41] May S R, Ashique A M, Karlen M, Wang B, Shen Y, Zarbalis K, et al.: Loss of the retrograde motor for IFT disrupts localization of Smo to cilia and prevents the expression of both activator and repressor functions of Gli. Dev. Biol. 2005; 287: 378-389.

[42] Zhang Q, Murcia N S, Chittenden L R, Richards W G, Michaud E J, Woychik R P, et al.: Loss of the Tg737 protein results in skeletal patterning defects. Dev. Dyn. 2003; 227: 78-90.

[43] Tanabe Y, Jessell T M: Diversity and pattern in the developing spinal cord. Science 1996; 274:1115 -1123.

[44] Briscoe J, Pierani A, Jessell T M, Ericson J: A homeodomain protein code specifies progenitor cell identity and neuronal fate in the ventral neural tube. Cell 2000; 101: 435 -445.

[45] Litingtung Y, Chiang C: Specification of ventral neuron types is mediated by an antagonistic interaction between Shh and Gli3. Nat. Neurosci 2000; 3: 979-985.

[46] Wijgerde M, McMahon J A, Rule M, McMahon A P: A direct requirement for Hedgehog signaling for normal specification of all ventral progenitor domains in the presumptive mammalian spinal cord. Genes Dev. 2002; 16: 2849 -2864.

[47] Bai C B, Stephen D, Joyner A L: All mouse ventral spinal cord patterning by hedgehog is Gli dependent and involves an activator function of Gli3. Dev. Cell 2004; 6:103 - 115.

[48] Lei Q, Jeong Y, Misra K, L, S, Zelman A K, Epstein D J, Matise M P: Wnt signaling inhibitors regulate the transcriptional response to morphogenetic Shh-Gli signaling in the neural tube. Dev. Cell 2006); 11:325 -337

[49] Fuccillo M, Joyner A L, Fishell G: Morphogen to mitogen: the multiple roles of hedgehog signalling in vertebrate neural development. Nat. Rev. Neurosci. 2006; 7: 772 -783

[50] Huangfu D, Anderson KV. Cilia and Hedgehog responsiveness in the mouse. Proc Natl Acad Sci U S A. 2005 Aug 9;102 (32):11325-30.

[51] Buxton P, Francis-West P H, Davey M G, Tickle C, Paton I R, Morrice D R, et al: Craniofacial development in the talpid3 chicken mutant. Differentiation 2004; 72: 348 -362

[52] Chiang C, Litingtung Y, Lee E, Young K E, Corden J L, Westphal H, et al: Cyclopia and defective axial patterning in mice lacking Sonic hedgehog gene function. Nature 1996; 383,407 -413.

[53] Cole F, Krauss R S: Microform holoprosencephaly in mice that lack the Ig superfamily member Cdon. Curr. Biol. 2003; 13: 411 -415

[54] Concordet J P, Lewis K E, Moore J W, Goodrich L V, Johnson R L, Scott M P, et al: Spatial regulation of a zebrafish patched homologue reflects the roles of sonic hedgehog and protein kinase A in neural tube and somite patterning. Development. 1996; 122: 2835 -2846
[55] Cooper A F, Yu K P, Brueckner M, Brailey L L, Johnson L, McGrath J M, et al. Cardiac and CNS defects in a mouse with targeted disruption of suppressor of fused. Development. 2005; 132: 4407 -4417 .
[56] Kondo S, Sato-Yoshitake R, Noda Y, Aizawa H, Nakata T, Matsuura Y, et al: KIF3A is a new microtubule-based anterograde motor in the nerve axon. J. Cell Biol. 1994; 125 : 1095 - 1107
[57] Cai C, Thorne J, Grabel L.: Hedgehog serves as a mitogen and survival factor during embryonic stem cell neurogenesis. Stem Cells.2008 May; 6(5):1097-108.
[58] Bambakidis NC, Horn EM, Nakaji P, Theodore N, Bless E, Dellovade T, et al: Endogenous stem cell proliferation induced by intravenous hedgehog agonist administration after contusion in the adult rat spinal cord. J Neurosurg Spine. 2009 Feb; 10(2):171-6.
[59] Han Y-G, Spassky N, Romaguera Rosa M, Garcia-Verdugo JM, Aguilar A, Schneider-Maunoury S, et al.: Hedgehog signaling and primary cilia are required for the formation of adult neural stem cells. Nat Neurosci. 2008; 11(3):277-84.
[60] Ekker S C, Ungar A R, Greenstein P, von Kessler D P, Porter J A, Moon R T, et al: Patterning activities of vertebrate hedgehog proteins in the developing eye and brain. Curr. Biol. 1995; 5: 944-955
[61] Spassky N, Han Y-G, Aguilar A, Strehl L, Besse L, Laclef C, et al: A Primary Cilia are required for cerebellar development and Shh-dependent expansion of progenitor pool Dev Biol. 2008; 317(1): 246-59
[62] Savage JJ, Casey JN, McNeill IT, Sherman JH. Neurenteric cysts of the spine. J. Craniovertebr Junction Spine. 2010 Jan; 1(1): 58-63
[63] Huangfu D, Anderson KV: Signaling from Smo to Ci/Gli: conservation and divergence of Hedgehog pathways from Drosophila to vertebrates. Development. 2006 Jan; 133(1):3-14.
[64] Schermer B, Ghenious C, Bartram M, Mueller RU, Kotsis F, Hoehne M, et al: The von Hippel- Lindau tumor suppressor protein controls ciliogenesis by orienting microtubule growth. J. Cell Biol. 2006;175 : 547 - 554
[65] Saran A. Basal cell carcinoma and the carcinogenic role of aberrant Hedgehog signaling. Future Oncol. 2010 Jun; 6(6):1003-14
[66] Romé P, Prigent C, Giet R. Centrosomes, mitotic spindle and cancer: find the odd one out! Med Sci (Paris). 2010 Apr; 26(4): 377-83.
[67] Saqui-Salces M, Merchant JL. Hedgehog signaling and gastrointestinal cancer. Biochim Biophys Acta. 2010 Jul; 1803(7):786-95.
[68] Yagyuu T, Kirita T, Sasahira T, Moriwaka Y, Yamamoto K, Kuniyasu H. Recurrence of keratocystic odontogenic tumor: clinicopathological features and immunohistochemical study of the Hedgehog signaling pathway. Pathobiology. 2008; 75(3):171-6.
[69] Gerdes JM, Katsanis N. Ciliary Function and Wnt Signal Modulation. Current Topics in Developmental Biology 2008; Volume 85:176-191

[70] Dejana E. The role of wnt signaling in physiological and pathological angiogenesis. Circ Res. 2010 Oct 15;107(8):943-52
[71] Rao TP, Kühl M. An updated overview on Wnt signaling pathways: a prelude for more. Circ Res. 2010 Jun 25;106 (12):1798-806.
[72] Yu W, McDonnell K, Taketo MM, Bai CB. Wnt signaling determines ventral spinal cord cell fates in a time-dependent manner. Development. 2008 Nov; 135(22):3 687-96
[73] Afzelius BA. Cilia-related diseases. J. Pathol. 2004; 204 : 470- 477 .
[74] Badano JL, Mitsuma N, Beales PL, Katsanis N. The ciliopathies: an emerging class of human genetic disorders. Annu. Rev. Genomics Hum. Genet. 2006; 7: 125-148.
[75] Fliegauf M, Benzig T, Omran H. When cilia go bad: cilia defects and ciliopathies. Nat. Rev. Mol. Cell Biol. 2007; 8 : 880 - 893 .
[76] D'Angelo A, Franco B. The dynamic cilium in human diseases. PathoGenetics 2009, 2:3:1-15
[77] Inglis P, Noroevich KA, Leroux MR. Piecing together a ciliome. Trends Genet. 2006; 22 : 491- 500.
[78] Marshall WF: The cell biological basis of ciliary disease. The Journal of Cell Biology, 2008; Vol. 180, No. 1, January 14, 17-21
[79] McGrath J, Brueckner M. Cilia are at the heart of vertebrate left-right asymmetry. Curr Opin Genet Dev 2003; 13:385-392
[80] McGrath J, Somlo S, Makova S, et al. Two populations of node monocilia initiate left-right asymmetry in the mouse. Cell 2003; 114:61-73.
[81] Nonaka S, Shiratori H, Saijoh Y, et al. Determination of left-right patterning of the mouse embryo by artificial nodal flow. Nature 2002; 418: 96-99
[82] Berdon WE, Willi U. Situs inversus, bronchiectasis, and sinusitis and its relation to immotile cilia: history of the diseases and their discoverers-Manes Kartagener and Bjorn Afzelius. Pediatr Radiol 2004; 34:38-42
[83] Afzelius BA: A human syndrome caused by immotile cilia. Science 1976, 193:317-319.
[84] Zariwala MA, Knowles MR, Omran H: Genetic defects in ciliary structure and function. Annu Rev Physiol 2007; 69: 423-450.
[85] Bartoloni L, Dombi V, O'Rawe A, Walne A, Chung E, Afzelius BA, et al. Primary ciliary dyskinesia: a genome-wide linkage analysis reveals extensive locus heterogeneity. Eur J Hum Genet 2000; 8: 109-118
[86] Davy BE, Robinson M.L. Congenital hydrocephalus in hy3 mice is caused by a frameshift mutation in Hydin, a large novel gene. Hum. Mol. Genet. 2003; 12 : 1163 - 1170
[87] Lechtreck KF, Witman GB. Chlamydomonas reinhardtii hydin is a central pair protein required for fl agellar motility. J. Cell Biol. 2007; 176 : 473 - 482
[88] Murga-Zamalloa CA, Swaroop A, Khanna H. RPGR-containing protein complexes in syndromic and non-syndromic retinal degeneration due to ciliary dysfunction. J Genet. 2009 Dec; 88(4): 399-407.
[89] Fain GL, Hardie R, Laughlin SB. Phototransduction and the evolution of photoreceptors. Curr Biol. 2010 Feb 9; 20(3): R114-24.
[90] Wilson PD. Polycystic kidney disease. N Engl J Med 2004; 350: 151-164.
[91] Simons M, Gloy J, Ganner A, Bullerkotte A, Bashkurov M, Kronig C, et al. Inversin, the gene product mutated in nephronophthisis type II, functions as a molecular switch between Wnt signaling pathways. Nat. Genet. 2005; 37: 537-543.

[92] Barr MM, DeModena J, Braun D, Nguyen CQ, Hall D.H, Sternberg P.W . The Caenorhabditis elegans autosomal dominant polycystic kidney disease gene homologs lov-1 and pkd-2 act in the same pathway. Curr. Biol. 2001; 11 : 1341 - 1346.
[93] Hughes J, Ward CJ, Peral B, et al. The polycystic kidney disease 1 (PKD1) gene encodes a novel protein with multiple cell recognition domains. Nat Genet 1995; 10:151-160
[94] Mochizuki T, Wu G, Hayashi T, et al. PKD2, a gene for polycystic kidney disease that encodes an integral membrane protein. Science 1996; 272: 1339-1342
[95] Yoder BK,. Hou X, Guay-Woodford LM. The polycystic kidney disease proteins, polycystin-1, polycystin-2, polaris, and cystin, are colocalized in renal cilia. J. Am. Soc. Nephrol. 2002; 13 : 2508 - 2516
[96] Fischer E, Legue E, Doyen A, Nato F, Nicolas J F, Torres V, et al: Defective planar cell polarity in polycystic kidney disease. Nat. Genet. 2006; 38, 21-23.
[97] Lee JH, Gleeson JG: The role of primary cilia in neuronal function. Neurobiol Dis. 2010 May; 38(2):167-72
[98] Green JA, Mykytyn K. Neuronal ciliary signaling in homeostasis and disease. Cell Mol Life Sci. 2010 Oct; 67(19): 3287-97
[99] Nachury MV, Loktev AV, Zhang Q, Westlake CJ, Peranen J, Merdes A, et al.: A core complex of BBS proteins cooperates with the GTPase Rab8 to promote ciliary membrane biogenesis. Cell. 2007; 129 : 1201 - 1213

# 9

# Review of Printed and Electronic Stereotactic Atlases of the Human Brain

Eduardo Joaquim Lopes Alho[1,2], Lea Grinberg[2], Helmut Heinsen[1] and Erich Talamoni Fonoff[1]
[1]*Julius-Maximilian University of Würzburg*
[2]*University of São Paulo*
[1]*Germany*
[2]*Brazil*

## 1. Introduction

The scientific developments of the latter half of the 19th century and the beginning of the 20th century supplied comprehensive data and insight on brain structure and function. Knowledge on structure and function provided strategies and tools for the management of previously lethal or highly incapacitating diseases, e.g. Parkinson's disease (PD) and tremor. A major challenge for neurosurgery was the endeavor to reach some deep and hitherto hidden regions inside the brain without damaging the surrounding tissue, since most of these small regions are vital and not directly visible *in situ*. Using the Cartesian coordinate system based on cranial landmarks, Victor Horsley and Robert Clarke introduced in 1908 a new apparatus that allowed them to accurately target subcortical nuclei of monkeys (Horsley & Clarke, 1908) with quasi-mathematical precision. A modified version of this device was adopted by Spiegel and Wycsis (1947) for human intracerebral interventions. Nevertheless, the space in which these mechanical devices were navigating still remained obscure and perilous. Almost four decades later, the parallel progress of neuroimaging shed light into the hitherto hidden structures and regions of the human brain. However, in order to find out appropriate pathways to specific functional units within clinically relevant targets the necessity of detailed brain maps was mandatory. Even with the great advance in neuroimaging in the last twenty to thirty years, it is still not possible to unequivocally delineate closely related subcortical structures by means of high-resolution computed tomography (CT) or in magnetic resonance image (MRI) (Coffey, 2009). For this reason, brain atlases derived from appropriate histological, histochemical, or immunohistochemical techniques on post-mortem human brain tissue continue to represent an important tool for functional neurosurgeons and brain researchers. To supplement the post-mortem anatomic maps, electrophysiologic in vivo recording of neuronal activity was added to neurosurgeries. This technique is intended to be an ancillary method to assist neurosurgeons in verifying their targets. In this chapter we will summarize and critically review the merits and the shortcomings of the most frequently consulted atlases. Some ideas on scope, form, and presentation of future atlases will be forwarded.

## 2. Printed stereotactic atlases

The history of human brain atlases begins in 1947, when the surgeons noticed that it was possible to adapt mechanical devices used in animals to navigate precisely the human brain. Therefore, it was mandatory to generate maps with coordinates of the uncertain territory in order to plan the best routes to avoid even minimal collateral damage and to focus the targets with high precision. Printed stereotactic atlases were considered to supply blueprints to neurosurgeons for intracerebral navigation.

### 2.1 Stereoencephalotomy ( thalamotomy and related procedures), part I: methods and stereotaxic atlas of the human brain (Spiegel & Wycsis, 1952)

The first stereotactic human brain atlas was entitled *Stereoencephalotomy.* It was developed to solve the lack of accuracy of referenced systems based on cranial references and to allow the stereotaxic surgery to be performed in humans. It should be noted that since 1973 the term "stereotactic" is used for surgery in humans, whereas "stereotaxic" is used exclusively for neurosurgery in animals.

In 1947, Spiegel and Wycsis described the first human stereotactic instrument used routinely in subcortical surgery. It is based on the use of intraoperative radiographs, allowing the visualization of cerebral references. After the emergence of the technique of interventricular instillation of air (ventriculography), anatomical structures including the foramen of Monro (FM) and the calcification of the pineal gland could be used for localization of intracranial targets. With the advent of new contrast media it was possible to use new landmarks in the brain, such as the anterior commissure (AC), the posterior commissure (PC) and the intercommissural line (ICL).These new references are much more reliable than the former ones, as verified by Talairach (Talairach et al., 1957).With these new reference points at hand, the indication for neurosurgical interventions could be extended, since new targets appear within the coordinates of the stereotactic apparatus. Spiegel and Wycsis' (1952) atlas consisted of photographs of a series of coronal brain, sliced at regular intervals in relation to the posterior commissure and the midline, with a reference graph located at the edges of each section. Using this parameter, the surgeon was able to assess distances in millimeters in depth and laterality of subcortical targets with a known distance of the posterior commissure. Coordinates for many targets were derived from this concept, and neuroablative procedures became reality. These studies were the basic guidelines for targets used in pallidotomy for treatment of abnormal movements and mesencephalotomy for treatment of refractory chronic pain, published in 1950 by Spiegel and Wycis.

Prefrontal lobotomies were frequently performed in the days before the emergence of appropriate psychotropic medication. At the time of the development of stereotactic surgery, Spiegel hoped to refine this procedure to avoid the unwanted complications and deficits frequently associated with these procedures. With this in mind, the first use of the stereotactic apparatus was the coagulation of the dorsal median nucleus of the thalamus in patients with severe psychiatric disorders, seeking a less traumatic intervention than a lobotomy. Around the same time the use of stereotaxy for interruption of pain pathways, surgical treatment of abnormal movements, and drainage of fluid from pathological cavities, - , for instance, cystic tumors -, had also been proposed.

Initially, their reference coordinate system was the Cp-PO line (posterior commissure-pons line). This coordinate system was not simple and was not widely used. In their next work in 1962, Spiegel and Wycsis (Spiegel & Wycsis, 1962) assumed the intercommissural line as standard reference system. The second part was a textbook and revised atlas updated from the first version. This atlas is currently out of print (Coffey, 2009).

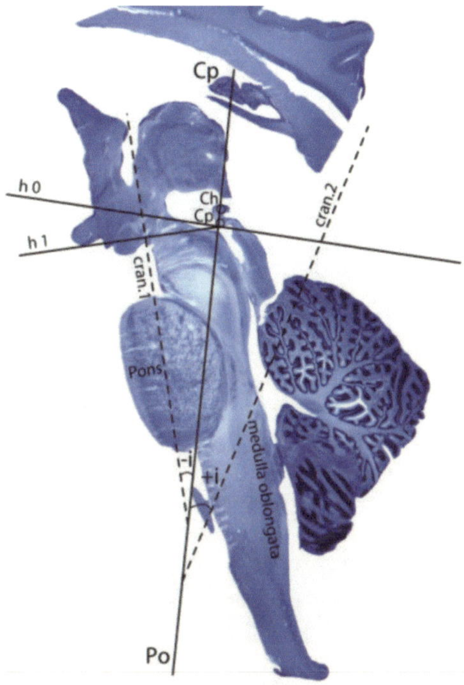


*Main lines for spatial orientation are the mediosagittal Cp-Po line that connects the posterior commissure (Cp) with the bulbopontine sulcus. The h 0, a horizontal line (perpendicular to the Cp-Po-line) which crosses the Cp-Po-line at the level of the posterior commissure. The h1 line emerges in an acute angle at the crossing point of the Ch and the Cp and runs in a rostral direction. Cran.1 and cran.2 can be considered as ancillary lines. Cran.1 is perpendicular to h1 and forms an acute angle of 4° (-i) with the CP-PO-line, cran.2 like cran.1 leaves the Cp-Po-line with an inclination of 4°, however, posterior to the Cp-Po-line (+i).*

Fig. 1. First intracerebral reference system proposed by Spiegel & Wycsis in 1952.

### 2.2 Atlas d'anatomie stéréotaxique: Repérage radiologique indirect des noyaux gris centraux des regions mésencéphalo-sous-optique et hypothalamique de l'homme (Talairach et al., 1957)

The most important contribution of this publication is the use of AC and PC as reliable intracerebral stereotactic markers and their stable relationship to deep brain structures. From this work, came the concept of Talairach's space. The Talairach's space is a coordinate system based on AC and PC as pivotal landmarks. Using the distance between them and the orthogonal plans erected, it is possible to compare the location of brain structures in two different brains, independent from individual differences. Because of the individual variations in the three dimensions of human brains, the distances measured in millimeters are applicable only to one individual. This becomes increasingly true with greater distance from the basal lines. Talairach concluded that dimensions given in millimeters can apply only in a general population to the gray central nuclei, whose dimensional variations remain moderate. For this reason they presented later the three-dimensional proportional grid system ( Talairach & Tournoux, 1988).

Several brains were studied, but the atlas was based on a single specimen. Talairach used his double-grid stereotactic instrument to create perforations in the craniocerebral specimen filled with air in the ventricular system. It was mounted on a stereotactic apparatus and metal probes were introduced. Radiographs were taken in profile and the brain was then removed and sectioned. The paths of the probes in the brain were used to establish the directional planes. Accurate coordinate measurements and profiles were derived for deep cerebral nuclei, subnuclei, and tracts.The stereotactically marked brains were cut in either parasagittal or frontal sections along Talairach's standard planes.

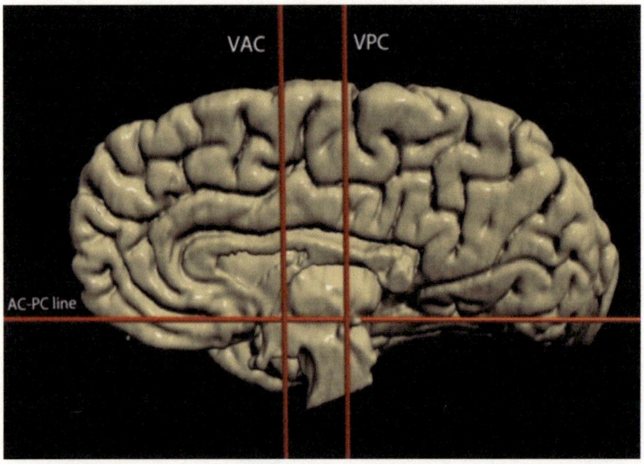


*The principal line for intracerebral orientation is the AC-PC line (also called the intercommissural line or ICL) that connects the superior edge of the anterior commissure with the inferior edge of the posterior commissure. Two perpendicular lines cut the AC-PC-line, the VAC, that runs through the center of the anterior commissure and the VPC, that runs through the center of the posterior commissure. Transformation of the ICL, VAC and VPC lines into planes yield the intercommissural plane (ICP), the anterior verticofrontal plane (VACp) and the posterior the verticofrontal plane, (VPCp) respectively.*

Fig. 2. Talairach's stereotactic references.

The three-dimensional profiles of the thalamic nuclei and other structures were mapped on millimeter-ruled diagrams. The reference line was the intercommissural line. This line is widely used even to the present day. This atlas is currently out of print.

### 2.3 Introduction to stereotaxis with an atlas of the human brain (Schaltenbrand & Bailey, 1959 )

Schaltenbrand and Bailey published the most comprehensive and detailed stereotactic atlas. They studied 111 brains that were sectioned in the coronal, sagittal, and horizontal planes. Variability diagrams were based on seven specimens. Hassler and Wahren completed profound studies of nuclear structures in coronal and parasagittal sections. Akert, Bucy, Walker, Snider, and Hassler contributed with detailed chapters on the physiology and pathophysiology of deep structures of the human brain. Nearly forty years later, this atlas also contributes immensely to functional neurosurgeons, and it could be the most used atlas in the pre-CT era. Even today, the expanded 1977 edition with the most useful features of this work is used world-wide. Their coordinate system appears to be derived from Talairach's space, but shows slight differences.

## 2.4 A stereotaxic atlas of the human thalamus and adjacent structures: A variability study (Andrew et al.,1969)

Since the beginning of stereotactic surgery, the main concern of the neurosurgeons was precision. The authors noted that all the previously presented atlases were based on very few specimens and even in the Schaltenbrand's atlas, despite the high total number of brains, only 7 out 111 were comprehensively studied. It was concluded that the stereotactic coordinates of subcortical nuclei were inadequately established, and that the variations would be so great that the procedures could not be reliably done with these coordinates.

The authors thus presented a variability study, aiming to compensate for this lack of precision. They studied nineteen brains, and focused on thalamic nuclei variability. Besides the thalamus, the atlas includes adjacent basal ganglia, and medial temporal lobe structures. It consists of statistical analysis of the data, with probability tables and distances to important ventricular reference points such as the foramen of Monro (FM), PC and midcommisural plane. It was surely an important work to define variability patterns in pre-CT/MRI era.

They used the FM-PC line and the total thalamic length (TthL) as reference system instead of the Talairach's space, although they have measured the AC-PC distance as well.

## 2.5 Variations and connections of the human thalamus (Van Buren & Borke,1972)

These authors, together with Schaltenbrand and Talairach, published one of the most important atlases of that time. The atlas is the result of a meticulous work on this challenging structure of the human brain, and it comprises a detailed cytoarchitectonic description of the individual thalamic nuclei. The literature on the connections of each nucleus is also reviewed. A special section of the book is dedicated to present the primary lesions (intervention) and secondary thalamic degeneration in fifty-four patients due to stereotactic procedures. The authors care about questions such as correcting differential shrinkage with computational tools, and variation of the position of thalamic nuclei in relation to midline, anterior, and posterior commissures.

## 2.6 The human somesthetic thalamus with maps for physiological target localization during stereotactic neurosurgery (Emmers & Tasker, 1975)

In this work Tasker and Emmers have presented a detailed map for electrical stimulation of the thalamus, with 2mm interval stimulation. During stereotactic procedures performed with awake patients, the distribution of somesthetic responses elicited by electrical stimuli was projected into the templates and used to build a three-dimensional homunculus of the somesthetic thalamus. Tasker emphasized that physiologically defined anatomy rather than blind obedience to atlas coordinates should determine how to conduct functional stereotactic operations.

## 2.7 Atlas for stereotaxy of the human brain with accompanying guide (Schaltenbrand & Wahren,1977)

According to the preface of the second edition of their atlas the first one was "an exploration of a new field of clinical anatomy." The latest edition concentrates on clinically relevant issues. The authors emphasized the importance of the myelin sections and reduced the number of macroscopical sections that proved to be of less interest. Thus the material could be condensed into a single and more practical volume. Some of the modifications took into account promising procedures at that time, such as operations on the small nuclei of the hypothalamus to treat deviant sexual behavior and vegetative disorders. They also added electroanatomical observations on the localization of important trigger points and radioanatomical observations in more than 300 patients.

The 111 brains, ranging in age from neonate to 86 years used in the preparation of this atlas were collected at the University of Würzburg, University of Lund (Germany) and the Sodersjuhuset in Stockholm (Sweden). They have considered to use Reid's plane (the plane that extends from the lower margin of the orbit to the center of the external acustic foramen) as reference, however the examination of the macroscopic series did not reveal consistent spatial relations between points on the outer surface of the skull and the subcortical structures, and they chose the AC-PC axis and the perpendicular line erected on the middle point of the two commissures as the basis for their system of reference.

The extremely careful work with great histological sections through the most clinically relevant structures inserted in a consensual reference system made this atlas one of the most consulted until the present day. This atlas is still in print, due to its practical value and use in functional neurosurgical procedures. Many other authors used this work to construct a computational tool for stereotactic surgery.

### 2.8 Stereotaxic atlas of the human brainstem and cerebellar nuclei: A variability study (Afshar et al., 1978)

In the early '70s, strategies for the treatment of spasticity due to cerebral palsy and other disturbances of muscle tone and posture by ablation of the dentate nucleus of the cerebellum were developed. In this context, Afshar focused on the cerebellar nuclei and brainstem structures involved in muscle tone disturbances and pain.

Thirty brains were studied using positive-contrast ventriculography and stereotactic marking of the specimens *in situ*. Their atlas comprises a variability and probabilistic study comparable to their previous study in 1969. They present a coordinate system based on the fastigium-floor line (FFL), and orthogonal to the ventricular-floor plane.

### 2.9 Co-planar stereotaxic atlas of the human brain: Three-dimensional proportional system: An approach to cerebral imaging (Talairach & Tournoux, 1988)

This work can be considered one of the most important in the field of brain mapping. Its focus is less on histology and architectonic and more on presenting the concept of proportionality and a new coordinate system, the so called Talairach space.

The Talairach's proportional grid system is based on the three dimensions (length, height, and width) of the human brain. The reference planes are defined as: the midline, defining the sagittal plane; the intercommissural plane that is obtained from the line that passes through the superior edge of the AC and inferior edge of PC, defining the horizontal plane; and two verticofrontal planes that intersect the anterior and posterior commissures (named VACp and VPCp). The authors state that direct distance coordinates vary widely from one brain to another and the variation is greater considering points far from the midline.

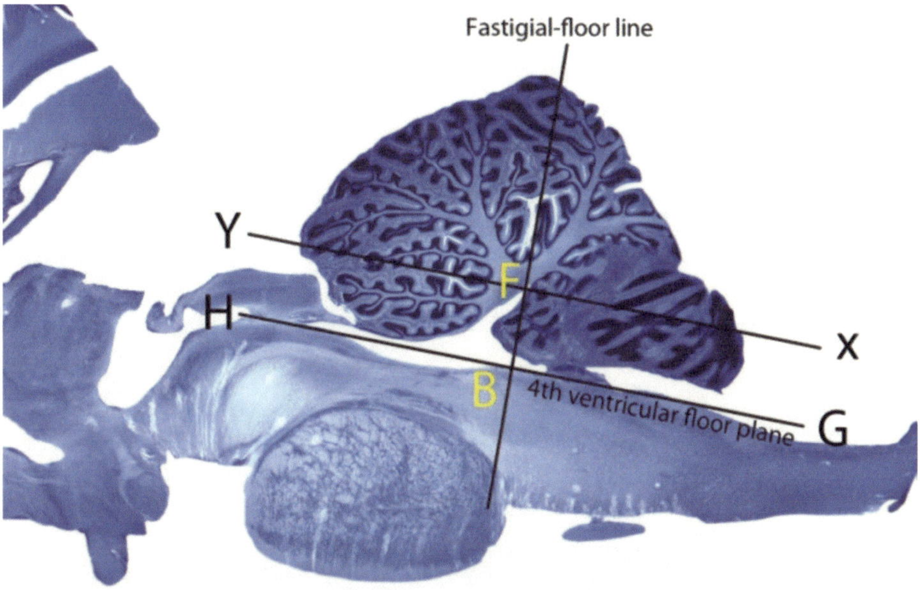


*The reference lines of Afshar et al. are confined to brainstem and cerebellar structures. The ventral HBG line runs in a rostro-caudal direction tangentially to the floor of the IVth ventricle. The parallel dorsal YFX line passes the tip of the fastigium. A line perpendicular to YX and HG goes likewise through the tip of the fastigium. Its intersection with YX defines F ; the one with HG defines B.*

Fig. 3. Coordinate system proposed by Afshar et. al., 1978.

However this variation is proportional for each brain, and they propose to divide the brain in proportional voxels or "orthogonal parallelograms."

Each hemisphere is divided in twelve parts (1-12) in its supero-inferior (z) axis, in nine parts (A-I) in its anteroposterior (y) axis and in four parts (a-d) in the laterolateral (x) axis. Each voxel has the following dimensions: x: one-fourth of the distance between midline and the most lateral point of the parietotemporal cortex, named a-d ; y: The voxels located anterior to AC have ¼ from the distance from AC to the frontal pole(named A-D). The voxels located posterior to PC have ¼ of the distance from PC to the occipital pole (named F-I), and finally the AC/PC distance is the 9$^{th}$ voxel (named E) and can be divided in thirds, called "mini-voxels"; z: the voxels located above the IC line have 1/8 of the distance between IC line and the highest point of the parietal cortex (called 1-8) and the voxels located below the IC line have ¼ of the distance between the IC line and the most inferior point of the temporal cortex (named 9-12). This voxels are fixed for every brain, allowing the normalization between two different subjects having in mind these proportions and not absolute distances in millimeters. The proportional grid system is the greatest contribution given by this work.It allows us to warp our atlases to the patient's MRI using this proportionality. The term "warping" is used in neuroimaging to describe the process of distorting an image (e.g.,

atlases) to fit other similar images (e.g. MRI). When two brains are normalized using this proportional system a " Talairach transformation" is performed.
Even with some known disadvantages, such as inter-slice distances variable between 2 and 5 mm, inconsistencies of orthogonal planes and assuming left/right symmetry, this atlas is widely used by neurosurgeons while planning interventions.

### 2.10 Multiarchitectonic and stereotactic atlas of the human thalamus (Morel et al., 1997)

Morel's et al. (1997) atlas is based on standard as well as histochemical and immuniohistochemical methods. Advanced neurochemical markers were used to further characterize thalamic nuclei and delimit subterritories of functional significance for stereotactic explorations. The objective was to improve the anatomical definition and precision of thalamic targets.

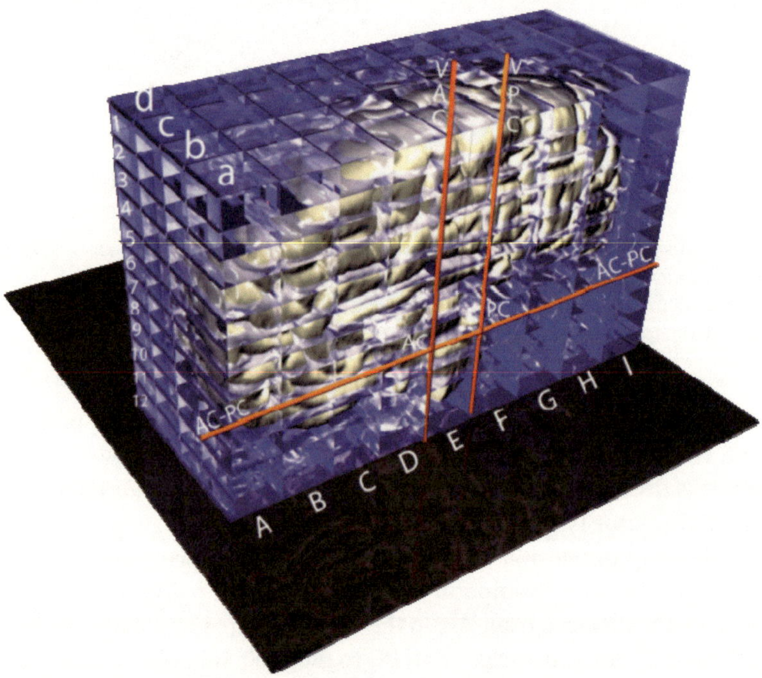


*The principal Talairach planes (ICp, VACp, VPCp) can be further parcelated by nine coronal planes (A-I), by four sagittal planes (a-d), and by twelve horizontal planes (1-12). Independent of individual hemispheric sizes, each hemisphere will consist of a total of 9x12x4 = 432 voxels. The coronal plane E, based on the AC-PC distance, represents a kind of core structure. Its dimensions are directly measured from the MRIs. The relative voxel sizes of A to D, F to I, a-d and 1-12 are a matter of convenience. They are derived from the maximal lobar extensions rostral, caudal, and lateral from VAC and VPC, and ventral from the AC-PC plane. They are expressed as fractions of the respective plane (1/4 in the coronal plane rostral and caudal to E, ¼ in the sagittal plane corresponding to a – d, 1/8 in horizontal planes dorsal to the AC-PC plane, and ¼ in horizontal planes ventral to the AC-PC plane).*

Fig. 4. Hemisphere inserted in Talairach's space

They could observe the distribution of immunostaining among the thalamic groups and correlate specific markers to functional units.
One interesting technical aspect of this atlas is the correction for shrinkage factors. It was done by means of preoperative MRI from two patients who underwent medial thalamotomy for cancer-related neurogenic pain and who died later from their disease. Intercommissural distances were measured post-mortem at the end of histological processing, and an additional distortion factor was taken into account for coordinates between sections, by measuring the distance between two coronal sections intersecting the centers of the two commissures. The most valuable contribution of this atlas is though the presentation of a chemoarchitectonic organization of the human thalamus.

### 2.11 Atlas of the human brain (Mai et al.,1998, 2003)

This atlas consists of printed sections and digital media, making it especially easy to use. The first section is a topographic and topometric atlas, in which *in vivo* and *in vitro* MRI scans are compared to whole head sections in horizontal, coronal and sagittal plans. The myeloarchitectonic atlas is based on serial coronal sections through a single hemisphere from a 24-year-old male. Although the templates give detailed information about cytoarchitectonic fields, it is hard to imagine how they could have been segmented from the sections presented on the book, since the staining allows very good contrast between gray and white matter; however, it is hard to define cytoarchitectonic borders with this method. It is a comprehensive study, and its most interesting features are the *in vivo* and *in vitro* MRI comparison to the cadaveric slices, and the user-friendly interface in the digital version.

### 2.12 Stereotactic atlas of the human thalamus and basal ganglia ( Morel, 2007)

In 2007, Morel presented this atlas with the main objective to combine high anatomical resolution (taking advantage of new staining methods) and stereotactic precision. This paper presents a collection of diagrams of the human thalamus, basal ganglia, and adjoining structures, consisting of a series of maps in the three stereotactic planes, and comparisons between brains with similar and differing intercommissural distances. This work, like the previously presented one ten years before, examines the distribution of different neurochemical markers in the thalamus and basal ganglia for comparison with non-human primate data.
Fiber tracts leading to the thalamus are also described, and there is a correlation between histological maps with MRI images. They compare also the individual representations, giving an idea of variability.
This atlas is especially useful in functional neurosurgery for research purposes to those who want to understand the connections and plan new targets for neurosurgical interventions in diseases involving the thalamus and basal ganglia.

### 2.13 Summary of materials and methods used in the preceding publications

To give a better overview of various details, ranging from the number of cases studied to the reference coordinate systems, a table will summarize the salient features concerning materials and methods applied.

| Reference | Nr. of brains and sections | Staining and other investigative tissue methods | Orientation of sections and interval | Range of Slices | Coordinate System | MRI |
|---|---|---|---|---|---|---|
| Spiegel & Wycsis,1952 | 1 brain (30 sections) | Unstained (1) and myelin-stained (2) | (1)cor.,sag., horiz.and oblique through brainstem (5mm int.) (2)cor. (2-4 mm) and oblique through brainstem (5mm) | | PC-PO line MSP | No |
| Talairach et al., 1957 | 1 brain | Unstained and Myelin-stained | | | ICP, MSP, VACp , VPCp | No |
| Schaltenbrand & Bailey,1959 | 111 brains (7 brains for variability study) | Unstained (1) and myelin – stained (2) | (1)16 coronal (1- 4 mm) and 18 sagittal (0.5 to 2.5 mm);(2)20 horizontal | 16.5 mm ant. to AC and 16.5 mm post.to PC;2.0 - 27.5mm lat. to midline;16mm above to 9.5mm below midcom. pt. | ICP MSP McomP | No |
| Andrew et al., 1969 | 19 brains | Nissl and myelin stained from 1 brain | 21 coronal (1 mm) and 17 sagittal (1mm) | 1-21 mm behind FM;3-20 mm from midline; includes thalamus, basal ganglia, and medial temporal lobes. | FM-PC line TthL | No |
| Van Buren &Borke, 1972 | 6 brains individual profiles and 25 hemisph. for gross anatomy variability | Cresyl-violet, myelin and Golgi preparations | 10 sagittal (0.5 to 4mm); 8 horizontal (3.5mm) ; 10 coronal sections | 2-25mm lat.to midline parallel to ICP; 17mm above to 8.1 mm below IC; 23.4 mm ant. PC - 47mm post. PC | ICP MSP VAC | No |
| Emmers& Tasker, 1975 | 2 brains: 1 for macrose-ries 1 for microseries | Electrical stimulation at 2mm intervals and mapping of the somesthetic responses elicited in awake patients; results projected into the templates | 5 sag. and 5 cor. plates; 10 sag. and cor. whole brain sections | Cut at 9, 11,13.5,16 and 18 mm lat. to midline; 8.5, 10 , 11, 12.5 mm post. to the midcom. point | ICP MSP VAC | No |

| Reference | Nr. of brains and sections | Staining and other investigative tissue methods | Orientation of sections and interval | Range of Slices | Coordinate System | MRI |
|---|---|---|---|---|---|---|
| Schaltenbrand &Wahren, 1977 | 34 sec. for macro and 57 sec.for microseries (frozen sec. 30μm) Paraffin used to brainstem and cerebellum | Unstained(1), myelin-stained and Nissl (2) | (1)19 cor.,5 sag., 6 horiz.from 1 brain, and 4 from another; (2) 20 cor., 17 sag.and20 horiz. | (1)57 mm ant. - 44 mm post. to AC; 0 - 22mm from midline; 18 above-20mm below ICL; 5-28mm below ICL; (2)16.5 mm ant.-16.5mm post midcom. line 1.5-27.5 mm lat. Midline 16.0mm above to 9.5mm below ICL | ICP MSP McomP | No |
| Afshar et al.,1978 | 30 brains | Myelin-stained | (1)54 plates, 1mm thick ;(2) 12 cerebellar plates | (1)23mm rostral to 30mm caudal to FFL; 1mm rostral to 10mm caudal to FFL | VFP FFL Fastigial point | No |
| Talairach& Tournoux,1988 | 1 brain cut sagittaly, frontal and horizontal sections were interpola-ted | Anatomic sections, that are drawn as a result of tracing the sections | 36 sagittal (1-4mm int.); 38 frontal (5mm int); 27 horizontal (5mm int) | Right: 18 sec 0-62mm ;Left:18 sec 0-61mm ;0-65mm ant. To VAC; 0-100mm post VAC;0-6.5 mm above ICL;0-4.1mmbelow ICL | ICP MSP VAC | Yes |
| Morel et al.,1997 | 9 thalamic frozen blocks cut in 40μm thick slices from 5 brains | Nissl, myelin and Immunohystoc hemestry parvalbumin (PV), calbindinD-28K (CB), and calretinin (CR) | 3 blocks sagittal, 4 horizontal and 2 coronal | Region of interest: thalamus | ICP MSP VAC | Preopera tive MRI of 2 patients |
| Mai et al.,1998,2003 | 6 brains – macrose-ries (frozen, 1 cm thick) and 1 hemisphere for Microseries (paraffin) | (1)Sudan red or Sudan Black B (2)Hematoxyli n- or sudan black B for myelinated fibers | 17 horizontal;15 coronal and 8 sagittal; (2) 69 coronal sections | (2) 60mm ant.AC-100 mm post. AC (100μm) | ICP MSP VAC | Yes for the macroser ies |

| Reference | Nr. of brains and sections | Staining and other investigative tissue methods | Orientation of sections and interval | Range of Slices | Coordinate System | MRI |
|---|---|---|---|---|---|---|
| Morel, 2007 | 7 brains, frozen, cut 40-50μm thick | Nissl and cresyl violet, myelin;parvalbumin (PV), calbindinD-28K (CB), and calretinin (CR) ;antibodies anti tyrosine hydroxylase (TH), Acetylcholinesterase (AChE) or immunore-acted with SMI-32 | Thalamus : 26 horizontal,24 sagittal Basal ganglia: 25 sagittal and coronal | 14 mm superior to 8.1 mm inferior to ICL;4.6 to 25.8 mm from midline; 3 to 41.5 mm anterior to PC; 3 to 27mm lateral to midline | ICP MSP VAC | Yes, from 2 brains, obtained 10 days and 1 year after fixation in formalin |

*Definitions: PC-PO line: connects the center of posterior commissure (PC) to the ponto-medullary sulcus (posterior border of the pons) and the midsagittal plane (MSP); ICL- intercommissural line: line that passes through the superior edge of the anterior commissure (AC) and inferior edge of PC; ICP- intercommissural plane: plane obtained from the ICL, defines the horizontal plane; MSP-Midsagittal plane: obtained from midline; VACp:Verticofrontal plane is formed by VAC line, that is a vertical line traversing the posterior margin of the AC: VPCp is the verticofrontal plane perpendicular ICL crossing it at PC; MComP: Midcommissural plane is erected from the midcommissural point, that is the midpoint of the ICL;The FM-PC line is the distance between the posterior inferior margin of the foramen of Monro (FM) to the midpoint of the ventricular surface of PC;The total thalamic length (TthL) is the distance between the FM and the top of the pulvinar;The ventricular-floor plane (VFP) is the plane defined by the floor of the fourth ventricle. Perpendicular to this plane and reaching the fastigium (apex of the roof of the fourth ventricle) is the fastigium-floor line(FFL).*

Table 1. Printed stereotactic atlases based on number of cases studied, histological protocols, planes of section, coordinate systems, and reference to neuroimaging.

## 3. Three-dimensional electronic atlases based on printed two-dimensional stereotactic atlases

Printed stereotactic atlases have an intrinsic limitation due to the fact that they consist of a two-dimensional representation of the brain, which is a three-dimensional structure (Yelnik et al., 2009).The first solution encountered in literature to overcome this problem was simply to scan the previously published 2D templates into a computer and delineate 3D volumes on them. This was the beginning of the development of deformation algorithms and volumetric visualization of anatomical structures that would change the standard on neurosurgical planning.

### 3.1 Creation of a three-dimensional atlas by interpolation from Schaltenbrand-Bailey's atlas (Yoshida, 1987)

In 1987 Yoshida proposed the creation of a 3D atlas of the human brain based on the interpolation of the 2D templates of the Schaltenbrand-Bailey's atlas. Although the rendering resulted in great three-dimensional incoherency due to the lack of correction of the linear and non-linear tissue distortions present at the original sections, this atlas is important as the first of its kind and of the concept of referring to a volume instead of confining exclusively on two-dimensional representations of the neural tissue.

### 3.2 Multiple brain atlas database and atlas-based neuroimaging system (Nowinski et al., 1997)

Nowinski and his collaborators started in 1997 a project in which four previously published atlases were digitized, enhanced, segmented (color coded or contoured), labeled, aligned, and organized into volumes for the purpose of developing an atlas-based neuroimaging system for analysis, quantification, and real-time manipulation of cerebral structures in two and three dimensions. A software was developed that is available in a CD-ROM called "Electronic Clinical Brain Atlas-ECBA." It is impressive in terms of three-dimensional visualization of the structures; however, due to some inaccuracies inherent in the original print atlases, three dimensional structures reconstructed from Schaltenbrand & Wahren atlas are often convoluted and displayed in unrealistic shapes. As noticed and discussed by the authors in this paper, a given point in the stereotactic space may have up to three different labels on the Talairach & Tournox atlas, due to inconsistent orthogonal plates. Nevertheless, important questions about the 3D accuracy of the most-used atlases were evidenced.

### 3.3 Automated atlas integration and interactive three-dimensional visualization tools for planning and guidance in functional neurosurgery (St-Jean et al., 1998)

The authors created a deformable volumetric atlas of the basal ganglia and thalamus from the Schaltenbrand and Wahren atlas (SW atlas) to help neurosurgeons navigate through MRI-invisible structures. They developed also a visualization platform that permits manipulation of the merged atlas and MRI data set in two- and three-dimensional views. A really interesting and new method of correction of errors was developed by this group. After digitizing the sections and the transparent overlays from the SW atlas, they aligned and segmented the nuclear contours based on the overlays and performed an interpolation to create a 3D volume. The alignment was based on the original grid, and they noted that the grid structure present in the atlas was placed on the cryotome images subsequent to photography, and so even precise alignment with respect to the grid is no guarantee that the underlying slices were not themselves distorted during the slicing process. However, they developed a methodology for matching automatically the slices with the 3D model. The atlas is registered point-to-point (250 homologous landmarks identified by a neuroanatomist) to a model MRI or standard reference volume. Even though any MRI could be chosen, they opted by the Colin27 that is the result of an average of 27 MRI scans of the same subject. As they have a labeled MRI based on the SW atlas, an algorithm called ANIMAL (Automated Nonlinear Image Matching and Anatomical Labeling) computes a nonlinear transformation to register the patient's MRI with the pre-labeled

Colin27.The most important contribution from this work was the use of a special algorithm to align and segment the images and the use as reference a MRI standard volume, the Colin27.

| References | Original Atlas | Method | Correction of distortions of the original atlas and segmentation | Registration and atlas-to-patient normalization |
|---|---|---|---|---|
| Yoshida, 1987 | Schaltenbrand& Bailey,1959 | A 0.5-mm step atlas was interpolated from the original atlas | | |
| Nowinski et al.,1997 | Talairach& Tournoux,1988, 1993; Schaltenbrand& Wahren,1977; Ono et al.,1990 | The print atlases listed were digitized, enhanced, segmented , labeled, aligned, and organized into volumes | Manual correction of rotation and overlay-plate misregistrations. Some of the sources of errors cannot not be corrected | Registration based on max.dimensions of the brain and head of caudate, optic tract or putamen used as landmarks.Talairach's Transformation is applied |
| St-Jean et al.,1998 | Schaltenbrand& Wahren,1977 | Digit.sec. and transp. overlay, aligned and extracted 2D surfaces based on it and interpolated sec. | Slice-to-slice spatial inconsistencies in structure contours were considered to be small, and thus not accounted for. ANIMAL algorithm warps atlas to Colin27 | ANIMAL algorithm warps the pre-labeled Colin27 to patient's MRI |
| Nowinski and Belov, 2003 | Talairach& Tournoux, 1988 | Digitized and processed the original print plates | Added structures to original templates to improve 3D consistency; developed algorithms to reformat the atlas to ICP | Talairach landmarks are set and then Talairach's Transformation is applied |
| Ganser et al, 2004 | Talairach& Tournoux, 1988 | Digitized and used only the 38 coronal plates | Interpolated additional cross-sections and applied algorithms to enhance the 3D coherence | Correspondences between the atlas and the patient are established in an automatic fashion nonrigid approach; |

*At variance with Table 2 data and 3D reconstructions were generated by the authors from new series of brains and details on histological procedures and data manipulation are listed.*

Table 2. Electronic atlases derived from previously printed 2D stereotactic atlases Authors, sources, digital manipulation, and registration are listed.

### 3.4 The cerefy neuroradiology atlas: A talairach–tournoux atlas-based tool for analysis of neuroimages available over the internet (Nowinski & Belov, 2003)

The article published in 2003 introduces an atlas-assisted method and a tool called the Cerefy Neuroradiology Atlas (CNA), available over the internet for neuroradiology and human brain mapping. The Talairach & Tounoux atlas is presented in digital format and can be warped to the patient's MRI scan by means of a Talairach transformation. The Talairach landmarks (AC, PC, the most lateral point of the parietotemporal cortex, the most anterior point of the frontal cortex, the most posterior point of the occipital cortex, the most superior point of the parietal cortex, and the most inferior point of the temporal cortex) are set manually or semi-automatically and a linear transformation is performed. The great achievements of this atlas are the ease of use, new atlas-user interface, and availability over the internet.

### 3.5 A deformable digital brain atlas system according to talairach and tournoux (Ganser et al., 2004)

The authors have developed a digital version of the Talairach &Tournoux atlas. The main goal is to assist neurosurgical planning rather than brain mapping. They present a 3D representation of most of the brain structures contained in the Talairach atlas. They have also developed a tool which has a non-rigid matching capability, allowing the standard atlas structure to be warped to an individual brain MRI, even when lesions such as tumors are present. The great contribution of this work is the development of the nonlinear algorithm used to warp the atlas to the patient's MRI, despite the need for substantial nonlinear transformations.

## 4. Three-dimensional electronic atlases based on histological data

The digitization of previous published atlas led to problems in accuracy due to errors inherent in the technique used to construct them. In order to achieve better precision and accuracy in the 3D atlases, three groups have proposed to generate their electronic three-dimensional reconstructions based on own histological sections instead of aligning and trying to correct previous published templates.

### 4.1 The creation of a brain atlas for image guided neurosurgery using serial histological data (Chakravarty et al, 2006)

Until 2006, the group from MNI (Montreal Neurological Institute, Canada) used the atlas developed by St-Jean et al., 1998 to program neurosurgical interventions. However, some shortcomings were recognized, including limited inherent resolution in the slice direction, limited number of structures, and some small mis-registrations between the digital atlas and the Colin27 MRI average that are propagated to patient MRI data during the atlas customization procedure. In this manuscript, the authors addressed these limitations and presented a technique for the creation of a brain atlas of the basal ganglia and thalamus derived from serial histological data. The technique used was identical to the one used in St-Jean's (1998) atlas. However, in the latter instance own histological preparations were available instead of scanned figures from the Schaltenbrand & Wahren atlas. The authors digitized coronal histological sections and delineated 105 anatomical structures in them. A slice-to-slice nonlinear registration technique to correct for spatial distortions was introduced into the histological data set at the time of acquisition. Since the histological data were acquired without any anatomical reference, this registration technique was optimized to use an error metric which calculates a nonlinear transformation minimizing the mean distance between the segmented contours between adjacent pairs of slices in the data set. To register the atlas to Colin27, a pseudo-MRI was created by setting the intensity of each anatomical region defined in the geometric atlas to match the intensity of the corresponding region of the reference MRI volume. This allowed the estimation of a 3D nonlinear transformation using a correlation-based registration scheme to fit the atlas to the reference MRI. The result of this procedure was a contiguous 3D histological volume, a set of 3D objects defining the basal ganglia and thalamus, both of which are registered to a standard MRI data set, to be used for neurosurgical planning.

### 4.2 A three-dimensional, histological and deformable atlas of the human basal ganglia. I. Atlas construction based on immunohistochemical and MRI data (Yelnik et al., 2007)

The French group describes in detail the construction of an atlas of the human basal ganglia. One brain was selected for reconstruction, and prior to the removal from the skull it was subject to MRI acquisition and then cryosectioned. The MRI was used for the coregistration of the atlas and permitted the production of more consistent 3D surfaces. Three different software tools were used in this study. A Threedimensional Tracing Software application (TTS) was developed for the purpose of digitization and processing of serial cerebral contours. The second tool is called Yav++ and its principal features include comparison and fusion of 3D images in multiplanar viewers as well as a 3D camera allowing visualization of serial contours, 3D surfaces, and 3D images in the same image. The last software tool is called BALADIN software, and it is an automatic image registration algorithm that allows registration of 2D or 3D images through an intensity-based block-matching approach. The novelty of this atlas is the MRI acquisition, which represents the core data element of the study.

### 4.3 A mean three-dimensional atlas of the human thalamus: Generation from multiple histological data (Krauth et al., 2010)

The stereotactic anatomical atlas under consideration consists of a three-dimensional thalamic model derived of a mean from six series of histologically processed brain sections. Postmortem MRIs are available for three of the stacks. The authors recommend that atlases should be based on a population instead of individuals. Therefore, previously studied stacks (Morel, 2007) were reconstructed based on multiarchitectonic criteria and integrated by an iterative algorithm -the so called bootstrap approach- to result in a three-dimensional average from three brains. The authors contend that their atlas improves the previous work on thalamic model reconstruction in several aspects. Firstly, while those models are based on the geometry seen in a single stack, their model incorporates topological and geometric details from different stacks and different stereotactic directions. Secondly, it would represent the average anatomy of several specimens instead of a single one, which would remove the bias towards a specific individual. This paper describes mainly how previous stacks can be used to build an average model of the human thalamus and the advantages of this kind of approach.

| Reference | Nr of brains and Sections | Methods | Staining and other methods | Orientation and interval of sections | Range of Slices | Coordinate System | Correction of tissue deformation | Registration and atlas-to-patient normalization |
|---|---|---|---|---|---|---|---|---|
| Chakravarty et al., 2006 | 1 block from the left hemisphere (86 pairs of slices) | Mounted on paraffin; 105 anatomical structures manually delineated | Luxol Blue (myelin)<br>Nissl(cell Bodies) | Coronal sections (0.70 mm interval) | Thalamus, hypothalamus, basal ganglia amygdala and hippocampus | ICP MSP VAC | The ANIMAL slice-to-slice registration procedure is applied | 2 Steps ANIMAL application |
| Yelnik et al, 2007 | 1 Brain<br>800 sections | Frozen sections, 70µm thick; Post mortem MRI | 80 sections Nissl-stained ; 80 sections immunostaining for calbindin | coronal sections | Basal ganglia | ICP MSP | Automated Processing for data coregistration and semi-automatic processing | BALADIN algorithm |
| Krauth et al.,2010 | 3 Brains (6 stacks), frozen, cut at 40-50 µm | Postmortem MRI (3 stacks);algorithm "bootstrap approach" was used to construct an 3D average | Nissl ; Myelin; Calcium-binding proteins(non-phosphorylated neurofilament protein and Acetylcholinesterase | (0.9 or 1.0 mm) intervals | Thalamus, basal ganglia, subthalamic fiber tracts | ICP MSP VPC | Calculated distortion factors from ICL mesurement | Not described |

Table 3. Three-dimensional electronic atlases based on histological data

### 4.4 The São Paulo-Würzburg electronic atlas of the human brain initiative

Since 2005, the Brain Bank of the Brazilian Aging Brain Research Group (BBBABSG) of the University of São Paulo Medical School (USPMS) collaborates with researchers interested in neuroimaging-neuropathological correlation studies including dementias, white matter hyperintensities, and epilepsy. As a particularity, the BBBABSG is linked to the MRI section of the USPMS, so the brains can be scanned postmortem in-situ within a short postmortem interval.

At the Julius-Maximilian University of Würzburg (Germany), a fast, reliable, and easy to use celloidin method for serial sections of the human brain has been developed (Heinsen et al., 2000).

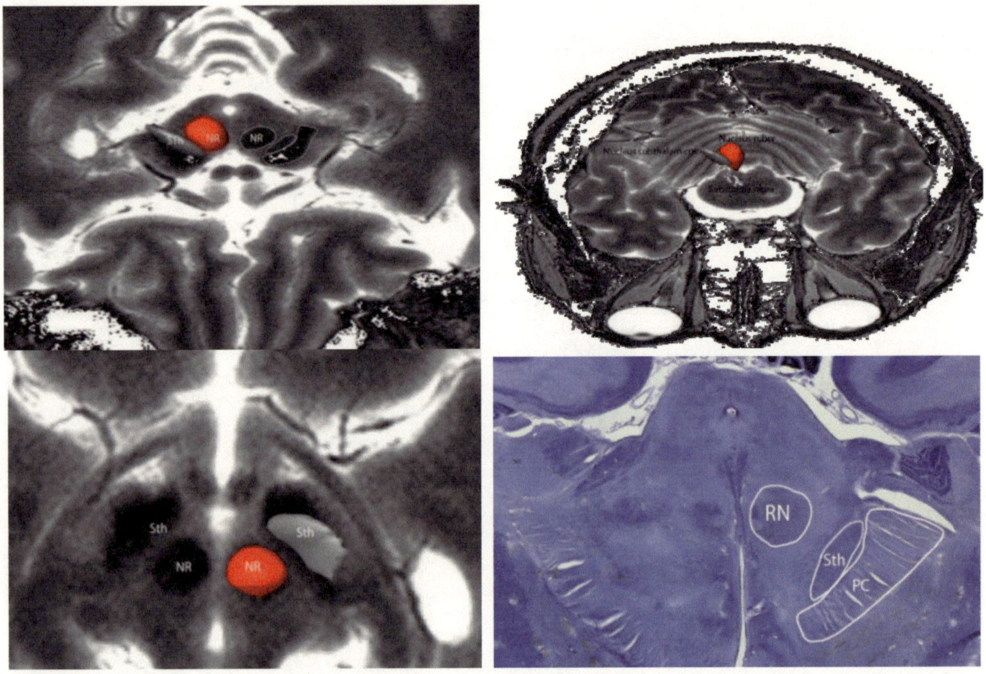


*Cytoarchitectonic 3D contours of red nucleus (NR or RN, in red), subthalamic nucleus (STh in gray), and substantia nigra (in white) merged to the MRI from the same brain. PC in this case is the abbreviation for pedunculi cerebri. The question concerning the hypointense region in MRI antero-lateral to red nucleus is presently being studied in detail, applying this method to additional cases*

Fig. 5. Cytoarchitecture x MRI

By combining both technologies, fundamental questions on post-mortem delay, appropriate fixation and neuroimagaing/neuropathological correlations could be addressed (Grinberg et al., 2008, 2009; Teipel et al. 2008).

The salient feature of this methodological approach to an atlas on the human basal ganglia is the post-mortem in situ MRI-scanning of the brain and the histological processing of the brain to generate serial 400 µm thick Nissl-stained sections. This protocol greatly facilitates cytoarchitectonic delineation of cortical and subcortical grey matter, compensation for shrinkage, and deformation and co-registration of high-resolution Nissl-stained sections with MRI scans.

Compelling results of match (red nucleus) and mismatch (subthalamic nucleus) of Nissl-stained sections with the MRI-boundaries are depicted in Fig. 5.

The images are imported to software tools and warped to the original MRI scans, following nonlinear and linear correction protocols developed by the team and yet to be published. Three-dimensional cytoarchitectonic contours can then be compared to the original scans.All the illustrations presented in this chapter were made using our own material and techniques.

## 5. Probabilistic atlases

Probabilistic atlases depict the normal range in size, shape, and topographical location of individual cortical or subcortical structures from many subjects. The rationale behind the idea is that the neuroanatomy of a select single subject's brain cannot cover the pronounced anatomic variability. Consequently, errors in diagnosis and neurosurgical interventions impend on generalizing interrelationships of a single brain. Probabilistic maps can include features such as cytoarchitecture, chemoarchitecture, blood flow distributions, metabolic rates, behavioral and pathologic correlates, electrophysiologic tissue characteristics and others (Mazziota, 1995). Some previously described atlases list probabilistic features (Andrew et al., 1969; Afshar et al., 1978; Krauth et al., 2010). In this paragraph, special focus will be on probabilistic atlases not classified in previous sections.

### 5.1 A probabilistic atlas and reference system for the human brain: International consortium for Brain Mapping (ICBM)(Mazziotta et al., 2001)

Through an International Consortium for Brain Mapping (ICBM) a data set that includes 7000 subjects between the ages of eighteen and ninety years and including 342 mono- and dizygotic twins has been collected.

Data on each subject include detailed demographic, clinical, behavioral, and imaging information. DNA has been collected for genotyping from 5800 subjects. A component of the program uses post-mortem tissue to determine the probabilistic distribution of microscopic cyto- and chemoarchitectural regions in the human brain. This can be combined with macroscopic information about structure and function derived from subjects *in vivo*, providing the an opportunity to gain meaningful insights into the concordance or discordance in micro- and macroscopic structure and function (Mazziota et al., 2001).

### 5.2 A probabilistic functional atlas of the human subthalamic nucleus (Nowinski et al., 2004)

The concept of probabilistic functional atlas (PFA) was introduced by Nowinski. His idea is to overcome limitations of the current electronic stereotactic brain atlases, such as anatomical nature, spatial sparseness, inconsistency, and lack of population information. The PFA is an algorithm that converts the coordinates of the neurologically most effective contacts into probabilistic functional maps, taking into account the geometry of a stimulating electrode and the patient's anatomy. Nowinski published the use of this algorithm to build an atlas of the subthalamic nucleus and of the ventrointermediate thalamic nucleus (VIM) (Nowinski et al., 2004, 2006).

This paper introduces a method for generation and validation of a probabilistic functional brain atlas of subcortical structures from electrophysiological and neuroimaging data. The method contains three major steps: (1) acquisition of pre-, intra-, and postoperative multimodal data; (2) selection of an accurate data set for atlas generation; and (3) generation of the atlas from the selected data set. The method is here applied to construct the probabilistic functional atlas of the human subthalamic nucleus from data collected during surgical treatment of 184 patients with Parkinson's disease. It is based on preoperative X-ray ventriculography imaging, intraoperative electrophysiological measurements and X-ray imaging, and postoperative neurological assessment. This method can be used to build PFAs from other regions, as the next work from 2006 did.

### 5.3 A probabilistic functional atlas of the VIM nucleus constructed from pre-, intra- and postoperative electrophysiological and neuroimaging data acquired during the surgical treatment of Parkinson's disease patients (Nowinski et al, 2006)

This work addresses construction of the PFA for the ventrointermediate nucleus (PFA-VIM). The PFA-VIM is constructed from pre-, intra- and postoperative electrophysiological and neuroimaging data acquired during the surgical treatment of Parkinson's disease patients. The data contains the positions of the chronically implanted electrodes and their best contacts. For each patient, the intercommissural distance, height of the thalamus, and width of the third ventricle were measured. An algorithm was developed to convert these data into the PFA-VIM, and to present them on axial, coronal, and sagittal planes and in 3D. The PFA-VIM gives a spatial distribution of the best contacts, and its probability is proportional to best contact concentration in a given location. The region with the highest probability corresponds to the best target. The authors content that the PFA-VIM atlas overcomes several limitations of the current anatomical atlases, and can improve targeting of thalamotomies and thalamic stimulations.

## 6. Discussion

Inserting electrodes and needles without direct visual control into a hermetically closed space, filled with complex and vital structures, sounds at the first sight at least dangerous. Stereotactic interventions allow a tiny margin of error, since coagulation of the wrong nucleus or finding a big vessel inadvertently with a small opening on the skull may result in immediate death or irreparable neurological damage. Mechanical devices were developed (Horsley & Clarke, 1908) to give the neurosurgeons the precision that their hands will never achieve. A version of the stereotaxic apparatus created by Horsley and Clarke was adapted by Spiegel and Wycsis to perform such procedures in humans. At that time, they realized that safe intracerebral navigation with minor side effects necessitates a precise brain map. In 1952 these authors published the first stereotactic atlas of the human brain, objecting that functional stereotactic neurosurgery "requires an exact preoperative calculation of the electrode position, and such a calculation depends on two conditions: (1) determination of a reference point by means of an X-ray picture taken under definite standard conditions, and (2) an exact knowledge of the position of the area to be destroyed in relation to the reference point. Thus . . . a stereotaxic atlas of the human brain is presented" (Spiegel &Wycis, 1952).Today, high-resolution images from the brain are possible; however, some important target regions are still hidden, and others are so far not subject to a precise morpho-functional delineation.

### 6.1 Correcting tissue processing-induced errors

The rationale for a stereotactic atlas is to unravel the position of certain brain regions that we cannot directly see with the current image technologies from the patient's cerebrum. In 1952, Spiegel and Wycis had to project their atlas into an X-ray picture. Today, we can count on much more refined images of the human central nervous system, like 3.0T MRI. As we will discuss later, even this detailed picture is not enough to show all the structures we are aiming to reach.

Histological methods still supply the standard tools for identification of deep brain structures, be they neurons or fiber tracts. Conventional histology is applied to thin slices of brain tissue obtained from a diseased subject. The tissue is most often submitted to a formalin fixation (Yelnik et al., 2009).The processing of the nervous system leads to transformations in its size and form since the moment of death. Formalin fixation and other chemical reactions cause several volumetric changes in the nervous tissue. The changes in cerebral tissue due to fixation have been studied since the late 1960s (Bauchot, 1967) and the reliability of dimensions of formalin-fixed brains as well (Small & Peterson, 1982). The effects of formaldehyde on the human cerebrum have been described to result in a maximum increase in weight and volume between the first and fifth day, which decreases during the following weeks and months

(Fischer et al., 1973; Kato, 1939; Lagerlöf & Torgersruud, 1934; Stevenson, 1923; Treff & Kraus, 1960; Tutsch-Bauer, 1979 as cited in Quester & Schröder, 1997). This "positive formalin effect" (Schremmer, 1967 as cited in Quester & Schröder, 1997) is higher for lower formalin concentrations (Flatau, 1897; Treff and Kraus, 1960 as cited in Quester & Schröder, 1997).The results from Quester and Schröder (1997) confirm that local shrinkage and correction factors have to be determined for each area of interest owing to the heterogeneous constitution of the individual cerebral structures.

Embedding, sectioning, staining and mounting are likewise sources of tissue distortion. Each of these factors deforms the histological slice either in a homogeneous (linear distortion) or heterogeneous (nonlinear distortion) fashion. For example, the gray and the white matter have a differential staining shrinkage (Simmons & Swanson 2009; Kretschmann et al., 1982). In Schaltenbrand's study from 1977 (Schaltenbrand &Wahren, 1977) the average shrinkage rate for different applied methods was variable. Embedding in paraffin led to an average shrinkage of 30%, while celloidin shrank the tissue in 20%, wax in 5% and freezing in 1%. For this reason they chose freezing as method, but they noticed that when freezing is used there is no embedding material to hold the tissue together, causing parts to become dislodged and float around, especially those close to the surface.

In order to correct all these confounding factors, it is mandatory to know the precise volume and shape of the tissue prior to processing. Spiegel and Wycis used fiducial markers to guide them. Many years later, the fiducial concept was resumed by Yelnik et al. (2007), but with the great technological improvement of having the specimen scanned in a MRI scanner before the brain was removed. High-resolution post-mortem imaging provides important information about the volume and form of the brain before being processed (Pfefferbaum et.al, 2004) and it can be used to correct and align histological slices. In 1952 these corrections were performed by photographic manipulation, and within the following years this was the standard procedure. In 1987 Yoshida (Yoshida, 1987) focused on extracting a three-dimensional volume from the great histological slices obtained by Schaltenbrand and Bailey (Schaltenbrand & Bailey, 1959). In the following years, other authors created three-dimensional atlases based on the most-consulted printed atlases, using computational technology (Nowinski et al.,1997; St-Jean et al.,1998; Nowinski & Belov, 2003; Ganser et al., 2004; Carballo-Barreda et al., 2007). However, some inaccuracies on the original atlases led to great 3D inconsistencies (Nieman et al., 1994; Nowinski et al., 2006a, 2006b).The orthogonal plates from the Talairach & Tournoux atlas are not consistent and as a result a given point in the stereotactic space may have up to three different labels. Another example is that 3D structures reconstructed from the Schaltenbrand and Wahren atlas from 1977 are often distorted and sometimes have unrealistic shapes (Nowinski et al., 1997). To overcome this, some techniques were developed. Nowinski in 1997 (Nowinski et al., 1997) opted to correct by manual correction of rotation and overlay-plate mis-registrations; however, the inherent inconsistencies from the original templates could not be corrected. St-Jean in 1998 (St-Jean et al., 1998) addressed the problem first by performing an interpolation of the 2D contours using Hermite polynomials to achieve a 3D representation of the structures. The second step was registering the atlas volume to an MRI reference volume, the Colin27 (average of 27 scans from the same subject). This was made by identifying 250 homologous landmarks at the atlas and at the MRI and then applying the Brookstein thin-plate spline approach to warp them. As a result, the Colin27 was a labeled 3D volume based on the Schaltenbrand & Wahren atlas and could be warped to a given patient MRI with better accuracy. In 2003, Nowinski (Nowinski & Belov, 2003) added structures to the original templates to improve 3D consistency, and developed algorithms to reformat the atlas to the intercommissural plane. In 2004, Ganser presented an algorithm to align and reconstruct three-dimensionally the Talairach and Tournoux atlas (Ganser et al., 2004). The authors therefore used the coronal plates and improved the spatial resolution by interpolating additional cross-sections between each pair of adjacent original plates. After processing the images with Delauney tetrahedrization of the object using the Nuages algorithm, smoothing the shapes by applying a spatial low pass convolution filter, extracting the surface representation of the object with the marching cubes algorithm (Lorensen and Cline, 1987 as cited in Ganser et al., 2004), and reducing the number of vertices by applying the polygon reduction algorithm proposed by Melax (Melax, 1998 as cited in Ganser et al., 2004), they obtained a better 3D surface from the Talairach and Tournoux atlas. The lateral symmetry of the brain gives rise to a high redundancy in brain cross-sections, for which reason Talairach and Tournoux drew only one hemisphere in detail. They exploited this symmetry for further reduction of data as well: They have only processed the right hemisphere of the atlas and mirrored it at the midsagittal plane to the left side.

Even with all the mathematical treatment and computation of the images, the 3D atlases based on the classical 2D atlases did not fully satisfy the functional neurosurgeon's needs. Therefore, three groups started building three-dimensional atlases based on own histological preparations, so they could cut and prepare the slices using modern technique.

Even with new methods, the slices continue to suffer linear and nonlinear transformations by the fixation and processing techniques. The Canadian group (Chakravarty et al., 2006) used a previously presented nonlinear transforming algorithm (ANIMAL-Automated Nonlinear Image Matching and Anatomical Labeling) to register and align slice-to-slice together to build a contiguous 3D histological volume. The French group (Yelnik et al., 2007) used MRI scans from the same subject and slice-to-slice alignment (crioblock corregistered to cryosections, Nissl, immunostained, T1 and T2 MRI images) to build the coherent volume. The corresgistration was made with software tools (TTS, YAv++ and BALADIN) through an intensity-based block-matching approach. The Swiss group (Krauth et al., 2010) calculated the distortion index of the tissue by measuring the ICL distance in MRI *in vivo* and *in vitro,* and comparing it with the ICL distance from the processed tissue. They extrapolated the results to the stacks in which no MRI was performed.

In fact, the use of MRI scans as parameter to align and correct tissue processing linear and nonlinear transformations is the gold standard at the moment; however, the methods so far used to readapt the histological slices into their original volume and form can be further developed to allow exact correlations between histology, immunostaining, and image.

The next challenging part of the process is how to adapt this histological 3D coherent volume obtained to a given patient.

### 6.2 Warping the atlas to the patient

As soon as we have consistent, validated, three-dimensional surfaces, we have to fit them into the patient's brain. Therefore, reliable (and visible in both atlas and patient image) reference points are needed to transform the atlas into the living brain ($\mathbb{R}^3 \rightarrow \mathbb{R}'^3$ transform). In the early 1950s, pneumoencephalography and ventriculography permitted the visualization of some intraventricular landmarks as the pineal gland calcification, habenular calcification, and ventricular landmarks (AC and PC). Based on this, Spiegel and Wyics developed the first intracerebral coordinate system used in their atlas. An imaginary line connecting the center of the PC with the pontomedullary sulcus at the posterior border of the pons (PO) defined the CP-PO line.

This system was not really easy to employ, so they and others have developed simpler and more useful ones. Talairach could prove a good and consistent relationship between the AC-PC line (and its derivative planes) with the deep brain nuclei (Talairach et al., 1957). This would change the standard for intracerebral localization. In their 1988 work Talairach & Tournoux present the proportional grid system, which permits the transformation of the models to fit individual variability.

These deformations can be performed using different strategies, as landmark-based deformation methods or automatic deformations based on registration algorithms.

The most widely used system to adapt a brain atlas to the individual anatomy of a living subject is the proportional system of Talairach. It relies primarily on the AC-PC distance, i.e., the length between the anterior and posterior commissural points, well-identifiable on a ventriculography or a mid-sagittal section of a MRI acquisition. The user has just to measure the AC-PC distance in the living brain and to adapt the antero-posterior length of the atlas to that of the brain. The proportional system of Talairach is a reliable system, although it is inhomogeneous since the adaptation along the antero-posterior dimension is based upon two deep brain ventricular landmarks, whereas adaptation along the medio-lateral and infero superior dimensions depends on the overall size of the cerebral cortex. This is due to the fact that with ventriculography, internal landmarks are less clear along these dimensions the height of the thalamus and width of the third ventricle are the best possible landmarks (Yelnik, 2009).

An automatic registration algorithm is based on the comparison of features (grey-level values, points, lines, graphs, etc.) present in the two images to be registered. The algorithm is defined by three main characteristics: the similarity measure, the space of allowed deformations (the number of degrees-of-freedom (DoF) of the deformation, e.g., 6 DoF for a 3D rigid transform), and the optimization method that is used. Deformations can be very constrained (limited number of DoF), e.g., linear scaling (7 DoF) or not, like elastic, fluid, or even free-form deformations. These last types of deformations are often referred to as morphing or warping transforms. The choice of the most adequate deformation type is important, as it directly influences the quality of the atlas-to-patient result.

Chakravarty, in 2009, has studied and compared the "atlas to patient warping techniques"(Chakravarty et al., 2009) describing and comparing the linear, piece-wise linear and nonlinear techniques. These are automatic developed algorithms, although in the piece-wise technique, twelve different landmarks must be identified on both atlas and patient data, performing a Talairach transformation.

Chakravarty resumes the most typically used methods to warp the atlas to patient MRI data in two. The first is matching the anatomical structures directly from the atlas to the same structures seen in pre-operative scans (Ganser et al., 2004; Nowinski et al., 2000; Xu & Nowinski, 2001 as cited in Chakravarty et al., 2009). The second method starts with a set of anatomical atlas contours, pre-aligned to an MRI template. A transformation is then estimated between the template MRI and patient's MRI. Once this template-to patient transformation is estimated, the transformation is then applied to the anatomical atlas contours, thus customizing it to patient's anatomy (Bardinet et al., 2005; Chakravarty et al., 2005; D'Haese et al., 2005; Sanchez Castro et al., 2006; Yelnik et al., 2007as cited in Chakravarty et al., 2009).

### 6.3 Do we need new atlases?

Currently, magnetic resonance imaging is the method of choice for anatomic delineation of the brain. Its noninvasive nature allied to the possibility of unlimited repetition provides the

option of *in vivo* applications for clinical purposes and basic science research with quite comfortable accessibility. Volumetric and multi-sequence acquisitions of MRI images supply different sets of data, for instance, macroscopic anatomy, differentiation of gray and white matter, detection of iron deposits, fiber tracking, spectroscopy, BOLD effect in addition to the possibility of re-slicing and generating 3D reconstructions of the brain. It is even possible to differentiate the cortical layers in MRI (Fatterpekar et al., 2002). However, the protocol used to achieve this definition was a 9.4 T machine and each specimen was submitted to an overnight acquisition time of 14 hours and 17 minutes. This is not possible in living patients, not only because of the long acquisition time, but also due to movement artifacts including breathing.
The subthalamic nucleus is a good example for this discussion, because it is an important target to place electrodes in Deep Brain Stimulation (DBS) for treatment of Parkinson's disease, (Limousin et al., 1995; Benabid et al., 2001; Hamani et al., 2004) dystonia and epilepsy, and obsessive-compulsive disorders (Mallet et al., 2002).The real limits of STh within the hypointense image in the region lateral to the red nucleus is still matter of debate (Littlechild et al., 2003; Pollo et al., 2003; Dormont et al., 2004 ;Andrade-Souza et al., 2005 ; Sather & Patil, 2007; Stancanello et al., 2008; Kitajima et al., 2008;Caire et al., 2009; Vertinsky et al., 2009).The problem seems bigger if we consider that most neurosurgery services use 1.5 to 3.0 T magnetic fields in MRI acquisition. Although MRI images have improved in recent years, no sharp limits are really observed. Additionally, the iron content of the nucleus is unevenly distributed, predominating in its anterior aspects. We cannot forget as well the artifacts such as partial volume effect that distort the images and blur the nuclear outlines when we target small volumes (Ballester et al., 2002). On the other hand, the pioneer experiences of the first atlases based in brain histology have recently obtained substantial improvement with the addition of new staining techniques, imunohistochemestry specific to different subcellular and membrane structures of neurons and glial cells, and the development of softwares and algorithms to warp and correct the errors induced by tissue processing, all of which have made it more reliable and precise. Functional neurosurgery is aimed at functional targets, but these functional units are linked to an anatomical substrate. If we can in the future overlap the cytoarchitecture, intraoperative electrophysiology, and high-resolution functional images, we will surely be able to better understand the function and structure relationship and propose new treatments for diseases that have seemed hopeless until now .

## 7. Future perspectives

The future directions of image-guided neurosurgery include coherent 3D histological and histochemical volumes which can be interactively visualized and precisely warped to a given MRI scan. Templates and 3D reconstructions should be in electronic format and available over the internet , with a user-friendly interface that allows neurosurgical planning and better understanding of complex brain structures and spatial and functional relationships.

## 8. Conclusion

The field of neurosurgery-driven brain localization is still open and growing. Technological progress will greatly improve the precision of brain targeting. Atlases are an important part of this process, and together with the developing brain imaging methods and electrophysiology, future works will open new frontiers to the knowledge of the human brain as a whole.

## 9. Acknowledgment

The authors would like to thank all the members of the team participating on the São Paulo-Würzburg collaborative project and their representatives: Dr. Lea T. Grinberg, Dr.Wilson Jacob Filho, Prof. Dr. Manoel Jacobsen Teixeira, Prof. Dr. Edson Amaro Jr, and Prof. Dr. Carlos Augusto Pascualucci.
The author, Eduardo Joaquim Lopes Alho, has a scholarship for doctoral studies in the Julius-Maximilian Universität Würzburg, supported by the Brazilian agency CAPES in cooperation with the German agency DAAD .
Special thanks also to Bruna Barbosa Teodoro Felix, and to David Rochester for reviewing the chapter.

## 10. References

Afshar, F.; Watkins, E. S. & Yap, J. C. (1978). *Stereotaxic atlas of the human brainstem and cerebellar nuclei,* Raven Press, New York

Andrade-Souza, Y. M.; Schwalb, J. M.; Hamani, C.; Hoque, T.; Saint-Cyr, J. & Lozano, A. M. (2005). Comparison of 2-dimensional magnetic resonance imaging and 3-planar reconstruction methods for targeting the subthalamic nucleus in Parkinson disease. *SurgNeurol,* 63, 357, pp. 363

Andrew, J. & Watkins, E. S. (1969). *A stereotaxic atlas of the human thalamus and adjacent structures,*Williams and Wilkins, Baltimore

Ballester, M. A. G.; Zisserman, A. P. & Brady, M. (2002). Estimation of the partial volume effect in MRI. *Medical Image Analysis,* 6, 389-405

Benabid, A. L.; Pollak, P.; Koudsie, A.; Benazzouz, A.; Piallat, B.; Krack, P.; Limousin, P. & Le Bas, J. F. (2001). Deep Brain stimulation for Parkinson's disease. *AdvNeurol,* 86, 405-412

Bauchot, R. (1967). Les modifications du poidencephalique au cours de la fixation. *J Hirnforsch,* 253-283

Caire, F.; Ouchchane, L.; Coste, J.; Gabrillargues, J.; Derost, P.; Ulla, M.; Durif, F. &Lemaire, J. J. (2009). Subthalamic Nucleus Location: Relationships between Stereotactic AC-PC-Based Diagrams and MRI Anatomy-Based Contours. *Stereotact Funct Neurosurg,* 87, 337-347

Carballo-Barreda, M.; Rodríguez-Rojas, R.; Torres-Montoya, A. & López-Flores, G. (2007). Atlas computarizado para la planificación de neurocirugías estereotácticas funcionales guiadas por imágenes. *Neurocirugía,* 18, 478-484

Chakravarty, M. M.; Bertrand, G.; Hodge, C. P.; Sadikot, A. F. & Collins, D. L. (2006). The creation of a brain atlas for image guided neurosurgery using serial histological data. *NeuroImage,* 30, 359-376

Chakravarty, M. M.; Sadikot, A. F.; Germann, J.; Hellier, P.; Bertrand, G. & Collins, D. L. (2009). Comparison of Piece-Wise Linear, Linear, and Nonlinear Atlas-to-Patient Warping Techniques: Analysis of the Labeling of Subcortical Nuclei for Functional Neurosurgical Applications. *Human Brain Mapping,* 30, 3574-3595

Coffey, R. J. (2009).Printed Stereotactic Atlases, Review, In:*Textbook of Stereotactic and Functional Neurosurgery,* Lozano, AM, Gildenberg, PL, and Tasker, RR, pp. 347-372, Springer, Berlin/Heidelberg

Dormont, D.; Ricciardi, K. G.; Tandé, D.; Parain, K.; Menuel, C.; Galanaud, D.; Navarro, S.; Cornu, P.; Agid, Y. & Yelnik, J. (2004). Is the Subthalamic Nucleus Hypointense on T2-Weighted Images? A Correlation Study Using MR Imaging and Stereotactic Atlas Data. *AJNR Am J Neuroradiol,* 25, 1516-1523

Emmers, R. &Tasker, R. R. (1975).*The human somesthetic thalamus, with maps for physiological target localization during stereotactic neurosurgery.*Raven Press, New York

Fatterpekar, G. M.; Naidich, T. P.; Delman, B. N.; Aguinaldo, J. G.; Gultekin, S. H.; Sherwood, C.; Hof, P. R. &Drayer, B. P. (2002). Cytoarchitecture of the Human Cerebral Cortex: MR Microscopy of Excised Specimens at 9.4 Tesla. *Am J Neuroradiol,* 23, 1313-1321

Ganser, K. A.; Dickhaus, H.; Metzner, R. & Wirtz, C. R. (2004). A deformable digital brain atlas system according to Talairach and Tournoux.*Med Image Anal,* 8, 1, pp. 3-22

Grinberg,L.T., Ferretti, R.E.L., Farfel, J.M., Leite,R., Pasqualucci, C.A., Rosemberg, S., Saldiva, P.H.N., Nitrini,R., and Jacob Filho, W. (2006)Brain bank of the Brazilian aging brain study group—a milestone reached and more than 1,600 collected brains. *Cell Tissue Banking*

Grinberg, L.T.; Amaro Jr.E; Teipel S; dos Santos DD; Pasqualucci CA; Leite REP; Camargo CR; Goncalves JA; Sanches AG; Santana M; Ferretti REL; Jacob-Filho W; Nitrini R & Heinsen H. (2008). Assessment of factors that confound MRI and neuropathological correlation of human postmortem brain tissue. *Cell Tissue Banking,* 9, 195-203

Grinberg, L. T.; Amaro, E. Jr.; Santos, D. D.; Pacheco, S.; Ferretti, R. E. L.; Leite, R. E. P.; Pasqualucci, C. A.; Teipel, S.; Flatz , W. & Heinsen , H. (2009). Improved detection of incipient vascular changes by a biotechnical platform combining post-mortem MRI in situ with neuropathology. *Brazilian Aging Brain Study Group*

Hamani, C.; Saint-Cyr, J. A.; Fraser, J.; Kaplitt, M. & Lozano, A. M. (2004).The subthalamic nucleus in the context of movement disorders. *Brain,* 127, 4-20

Heinsen, H. &Heinsen, Y. L. (1991). Serial Thick, Frozen, Gallocyanin Stained Sections of Human Central Nervous System. *The Journal of Hlstotechnology,* 14, 167-173

Heinsen, H. ; Arzberger, T.& Schmitz, C. (2000). Celloidin mounting (embedding without infiltration) - a new, simple and reliable method for producing serial sections of high thickness through complete human brains and its application to stereological and immunohistochemicalinvestigations.*Journal of Chemical Neuroanatomy,* 20, 49-59

Horsley, V. & Clarke, R. H. (1908).The structure and function of the cerebellum examined by a new method. *Brain,* 31, 54-124

Kitajima, M.; Hirai, T.; Korogi, Y.; Kakeda, S.; Moriya, J.; Ohnari, N.; Sato, T.; Hayashida, Y.; Okuda, T. & Yamashita, Y. (2008). Human subthalamic nucleus: evaluation with high-resolution MR imaging at 3.0 T. *Neuroradiology,* 50, 675-681

Krauth, A.; Blanc, R.; Poveda, A.; Jeanmonod, D.; Morel, A. &Székely, G. (2010). A mean three-dimensional atlas of the human thalamus: Generation from multiple histological data. *NeuroImage,* 49, 2053-2062

Kretschmann, H. J.; Tafesse, U. & Herrmann, A. (1982).Different volume changes of cerebral cortex and white matter during histological preparation. *Microscopicaacta,* 86, 1, pp. 13-24

Limousin, P.; Pollak, P.; Benazzouz, A.; Hoffmann, D.; Le Bas, J. F. &Broussolle, E. (1995). Effect of parkinsonian signs and symptoms of bilateral subthalamic nucleus stimulation. *Lancet,* 345, 91, pp. 95-

Littlechild, P.; Varma, T. R.; Eldridge, P. R.; Fox, S.; Forster, A.; Fletcher, N.; Steiger, M.; Byrne, P.; Tyler, K. &Flintham, S. (2003). Variability in position of the subthalamic nucleus targeted by magnetic resonance imaging and microelectrode recordings as compared to atlas coordinates. *Stereotact Funct Neurosurg,* 80, 82, pp. 87-

Mai, J. K.; Assheuer, J. &Paxinos, G. (1997). *Atlas of the human brain.* ,Academic Press, San Diego

Mallet, L.; Mesnage, V.; Houeto, J. L.; Pelissolo, A.; Yelnik, J.; Behar, C.; Welter, M. L.; Bonnet, A. M.; Pillon, B.; Cornu, P.; Dormont, D.; Pidoux, B.; Allilaire, J. F. &Agid, Y. (2002). Compulsions, Parkinson's disease, and stimulation. *Lancet,* 360, 9342, pp. 1302-1304

Morel, A.; Magnin, M. &Jeanmonod, D. (1997).Multiarchitectonic and stereotactic atlas of the human thalamus. *J Comp Neuro,* 387, 4, pp. 588-630

Morel A. (2007). *Stereotactic atlas of the human thalamus and basal ganglia,*Informa Healthcare, New York:

Mazziotta, J. C.; Toga, A. W.; Evans, A. C.; Fox, P. & Lancaster, J. (1995). A Probabilistic Atlas of the Human Brain: Theory and Rationale for its Development. *NeuroImage,* 2, 89-101

Mazziotta, J. C.; Toga, A. W.; Evans, A. C.; Fox, P.; Lancaster, J.; Zilles, K.; Woods, R.; Paus, T.; Simpson, G.; Pike, B.; Holmes, C.; Collins, L.; Thompson, P.; MacDonald, D.; Iacoboni, M.; Schormann, T.; Amunts, K.; Palomero-Gallagher, N.; Geyer, S.; Parsons, L.; Narr, K.; Kabani, N.; Le Goualher, G.; Boomsma, D.; Cannon, T.; Kawashima, R. &Mazoyer, B. (2001). A probabilistic atlas and reference system for the human brain: International Consortium for Brain Mapping (ICBM). *Philos Trans R SocLondSer B-BiolSci,* 356, 1412, pp. 1293-1322

Niemann, K.; Naujokat, C.; Pohl, G.; Wollner, C. &Keyserlingk, D. v. (1994). Verification of the Schaltenbrand and Wahren Stereotactic Atlas. *ActaNeurochir,* 129, 72-81

Nowinski, W. L.; Fang, A. & Nguyen, B. T. (1997).Multiple brain atlas database and atlas-based neuroimaging system. *Comput Aided Surg,* 12, 1, pp. 42-66

Nowinski WL &Belov D. (2003).The Cerefy Neuroradiology Atlas: a Talairach–Tournoux atlas-based tool for analysis of neuroimages available over the Internet. *NeuroImage,* 20, 50-57

Nowinski WL; Belov D; Pollak P &Benabid AL. (2004).A probabilistic functional atlas of the human subthalamicnucleus. *Neuroinformatics,* 12, 4, pp. 381-398

Nowinski WL; Belov D; Thirunavuukarasuu A &Benabid AL. (2006a). A probabilistic functional atlas of the VIM nucleus constructed from pre-, intra- and post-operative electrophysiological and neuroimaging data acquired during the surgical treatment of Parkinson's disease patients. *Stereotact Funct Neurosurg 2006,* 83, 5-6, pp. 190-196

Nowinski WL; Liu J &Thirunavuukarasuu A. (2006b).Quantification and Visualization of the Three- Dimensional Inconsistency of the Subthalamic Nucleus in the Schaltenbrand-Wahren Brain Atlas. *Stereotact Funct Neurosurg,* 84, 46-55

Ono, M.; Kubik, S. &Abernathey, C. D. (1990). *Atlas of the Cerebral Sulci,* Georg Thieme Verlag/Thieme Medical Publishers, Stuttgart

Pfefferbaum, A.; Sullivan, E. V.; Adalsteinsson, E.; Garrick, T. & Harper, C. (2004). Postmortem MR imaging of formalin-fixed human brain. *NeuroImage,* 21, 4, pp. 1585-1595

Pollo, C.; Meuli, R.; Maeder, P.; Vingerhoets, F.; Ghika, J. &Villemure, J. G. (2003).Subthalamic nucleus deep brain stimulation for Parkinson's disease: magnetic resonance imaging targeting using visible anatomical landmarks. *Stereotact Funct Neurosurg,* 80, 76-81

Quester, R. &Schröder, R. (1997).The shrinkage of the human brain stem during formalin fixation and embedding in paraffin.*J NeurosciMethods,* 75, 81-89

Sather, M. D. &Patil, A. A. (2007).Direct Anatomical Localization of the Subthalamic Nucleus on CT with Comparison to Schaltenbrand Wahren Atlas. *StereotactFunctNeurosurg,* 85, 1-5

Schaltenbrand, G. & Bailey, P. (1959). *Introduction to Stereotaxis with an atlas of the human brain,*Thieme, Stuttgart

Schaltenbrand, G. &Wahren, W. (1977).*Atlas for Stereotaxy of the Human Brain with an accompanying guide,*Thieme, Stuttgart

Small, C. S. & Peterson, D. I. (1982).The reliability of dimensions of formalin-fixed brains. *Neurology,* 32, 413, pp. 415

Simmons, D. M. & Swanson, L. W. (2009).Comparing histological data from different brains: Sources of error and strategies for minimizing them. *Brain Research Reviews,* 60, 349-367

Spiegel, E. A.; Wycis, H. T. & Marks, M. (1947). Stereotaxic apparatus for operations on the human brain. *Science,* 106, 349-350

Spiegel, E. A. &Wycis, H. T. (1952). *Stereoencephalotomy (thalamotomy and related procedures),* Grune and Stratton, New York:

Spiegel, E. A. &Wycis, H. T. (1962). *Stereoencephalotomy. II. Clinical and physiological applications.,* New York

St-Jean, P.; Sadikot, A. F.; Collins, L.; Clonda, D.; Kasrai, R.; Evans, A. C. & Peters, T. M. (1998). Automated atlas integration and interactive three-dimensional visualization tools for planning and guidance in functional neurosurgery. *IEEE Trans Med Imaging,* 17, 5, pp. 672-680

Stancanello, J.; Muacevic, A.; Sebastiano, F.; Modugno, N.; Cerveri, P.; Ferrigno, G.; Uggeri, F. &Romanelli, P. (2008). 3T MRI evaluation of the accuracy of atlas-based subthalamic nucleus identification. *Medical Physics,* 35, 7, pp. 3069-3077

Talairach, J.; David, M.; Tournoux, P. &Kvasina, T. (1957).*Atlas D'AnatomieStereotaxique :RéperageRadiologique Indirect des Noyaux Gris Centraux des RègionsMesencephalo-sous-optique et Hypothalamique de L'Homme,*Masson &Cie, Paris

Talairach, J. &Tournoux.P. (1988). *Co-planar stereotaxic atlas of the human brain: Three-dimensional proportional system : An approach to cerebral imaging,*Thieme, New York

Teipel, S. J.; Meindl, T.; Grinberg, L.; Heinsen, H. & Hampel, H. (2008). Novel MRI techniques in the assessment of dementia. *Eur J Nucl Med MolImaging,* 35, supp 1, pp. 58-69

Toga, A. W.; Thompson, P. M.; Mori, S.; Amunts, K. &Zilles, K. (2006).Towards multimodal atlases of the human brain.*Nat Rev Neurosci,* 7, 12, pp. 952-966

Van Buren, J. M. &Borke.R.C. (1972). *Variations and connections of the human thalamus,* Springer, Berlin

Uylings, H. B.; SanzArigita, E.; de Vos, K.; Smeets, W. J.; Pool, C. W.; Amunts, K.; Rajkowska, G. &Zilles, K. (2000). The importance of a human 3D database and atlas for studies of prefrontal and thalamic functions. *Prog Brain Res,* 126, 357-368

Vertinsky, A. T.; Coenen.V.A.; Lang.D.J.; Kolind, S.; Honey, C. R.; Li, D. & Rauscher, A. (2009). Localization of the Subthalamic Nucleus: Optimization with Susceptibility-Weighted Phase MR Imaging. *AJNR Am J Neuroradiol,* 30, 1717-1724

Yelnik, J. (2002). Functional Anatomy of the Basal Ganglia. *Movement Disorders,* 17, Suppl 3, pp. S15-S21

Yelnik, J.; Bardinet, E.; Dormont, D.; Malandain, G.; Ourselin, S.; Tandé, D.; Karachi, C.; Ayache, N.; Cornu, P. &Agida, Y. (2007). A three-dimensional, histological and deformable atlas of the human basal ganglia. I. Atlas construction based on immunohistochemical and MRI data. *NeuroImage,* 34, 618-638

Yelnik, J.; Bardinet, E. &Dormont, D. (2009).Electronic Stereotactic Atlases, In:*Textbook of Stereotactic and Functional Neurosurgery,* Lozano AM, Gildenberg PL, and Tasker RR, pp. 373-393, Springer, Berlin/Heidelberg

Yoshida, M. (1987).Creation of a three-dimensional atlas by interpolation from Schaltenbrand-Bailey's atlas. *Appl Neurophysiol,* 50, 1-6, pp. 45-48

Zaborszky, L.; Hoemke, L.; Mohlberg, H.; Schleicher, A.; Amunts, K. & Zilles, K. (2008). Stereotaxic probabilistic maps of the magnocellular cell groups in human basal forebrain. *NeuroImage,* 42, 3, pp. 1127-1141

# Part 4

## Procedures & Neuroscience

# 10

# Intracranial Arterial Collateralization: Relevance in Neuro-Endovascular Procedures

Peng R. Chen[1], Adnan H. Siddiqui[2] and Peng Roc Chen[3]
[1]*Department of Neurosurgery, University of Texas Medical School at Houston, Houston, Texas;*
[2]*Department of Neurosurgery, School of Medicine and Biomedical Sciences, State University of New York, University at Buffalo, Buffalo, New York,*
[3]*Department of Neurosurgery University of Texas Medical School at Houston, USA*

## 1. Introduction

Endovascular strategies for addressing intracranial and extracranial diseases continue to gain momentum. These techniques are limited principally by technology and imagination. As newer devices and implements are introduced to the endovascular surgeon, more diseases previously construed to be the realm of open surgery or untreatable are becoming amenable to endovascular interventions. Because of the nature of endovascular procedures, with liquid agents, flow-directed therapies, and embolic materials, it is critical for a neuro-interventionalist to be aware of the collaterals that exist between the vessels being embolized and other critical collaterally connected vessels, occlusion of which may result in undesirable outcomes. Similarly, for other occasions, such collaterals may provide unique conduits that may afford access in novel ways to the intracranial or extracranial circulation. The understanding of these collaterals is best undertaken with an initial understanding of the development of the cranial vasculature. The rich anastomotic connections and interlinked development shed great light and provide a firm basis for understanding the cranial collaterals. Secondly, the collateral circulation may be divided by collaterals between extracranial and intracranial systems on one hand and collaterals between the internal carotid and vertebrobasilar (VB) systems on the other. In this chapter, we endeavor to provide a brief overview of cranial vascular development, followed by specific clinically relevant examples of extracranial and intracranial anastomoses and the internal carotid artery (ICA) and vertebrobasilar (VB) anastomoses, intracranial and intracranial anastomoses.

## 2. Cranial vascular embryology

The cranial vasculature begins with the development of a vascular supply to the paired pharyngeal arches. This supply develops as vascular arches that emanate from the ventral aortic sac connect with the paired dorsal aortae. Each pharyngeal arch gets its own vascular arch. These vascular arches then develop and regress in rostrocaudal fashion. The pharyngeal arches become apparent at approximately 3 to 4 weeks' gestation. The pharyngeal arches develop plexiform vascular channels that ultimately connect the ventral aortic sac with the paired dorsal aortae, forming the vascular arch. The first arch gives rise to the primitive stapedial artery, whereas the second gives rise to the hyoid artery. These arches then regress and coalesce to form the primitive hyoidostapedial artery. These vessels are critical to the vascular development of the skull base. This primitive branch follows the three divisions of the trigeminal nerve such that one trunk that develops along the mandibular division becomes the adult internal maxillary artery; the superior trunk becomes the middle meningeal artery and contributes to the ophthalmic artery. The primitive maxillary artery develops as the meningohypophyseal trunk, whereas the third division becomes the corticotympanic branch, which communicates with the ICA in the petrous canal (Figure 1). An embryologic dorsal ophthalmic artery regresses to become the inferolateral trunk, rarely staying on as a cavernous origin to the adult ophthalmic artery.[9] The third vascular arch on either side becomes the cervical ICA, eventually incorporating parts of the dorsal aortae bilaterally to form more cranial sections up the posterior communicating artery (PCoA) segment. From the third arch sprouts the external carotid artery (ECA) trunk, which anastomoses with the primitive hyoidostapedial artery branches to complete the ECA circuitry. Additionally, a pair of plexiform networks, called the ventral pharyngeal arteries, develop early on and connect to the hyoidostapedial trunk. These ventral-pharyngeal networks form prior to the development of the ECA trunk, eventually mostly regressing, but retaining parts that allow for anastomoses between the ascending pharyngeal and caroticotympanic arteries.

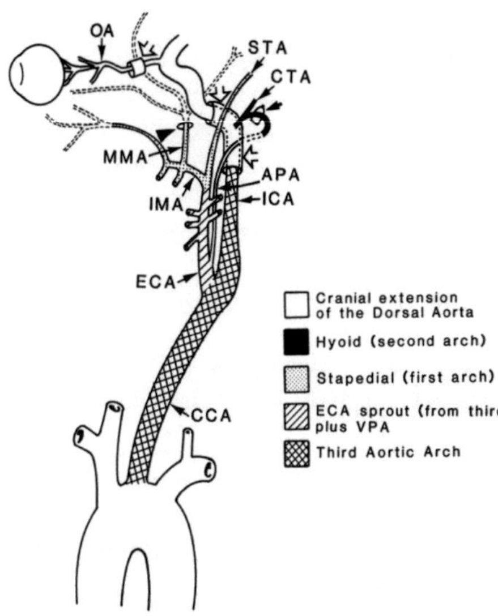


Fig. 1. Anatomic diagram turned from anteroposterior to a left anterior oblique (LAO) position depicts the definitive left common carotid artery (CCA) as well as the external carotid artery (ECA) and internal carotid artery (ICA). The embryonic origin of these vessels is also shown. CTA, caroticotympanic artery; small single arrow, stapes; (*arrowhead*), foramen spinosum; (*double arrows*), optic canal; (*open arrows*), carotid canal. Distal ramifications from the internal maxillary artery (IMA), middle meningeal artery (MMA), and orbital branches of the ophthalmic artery (OA) are indicated by the dotted lines. Stapedial artery (STA). *Permission requested from Osborn AG: Diagnostic Cerebral Angiography (2nd ed). Philadelphia: Lippincott Williams & Wilkins, Wolters Kluwer, 1999, figure 2-5, page 35.*

The posterior circulation develops in parallel, first appearing towards the beginning of the fifth gestational week as paired dorsal longitudinal neural arteries. These eventually form the intracranial VA and BA. Further caudally, a plexiform network of the cervical intersegmental arteries anastomoses to form the paired vertebral arteries (VAs). As these channels continue to develop, they reliably develop anastomotic connections with the ICAs, forming the trigeminal, otic, hypoglossal, and proatlantal intersegmental connections (Figure 2). The seventh cervical intersegmental artery coalesces with the right fourth

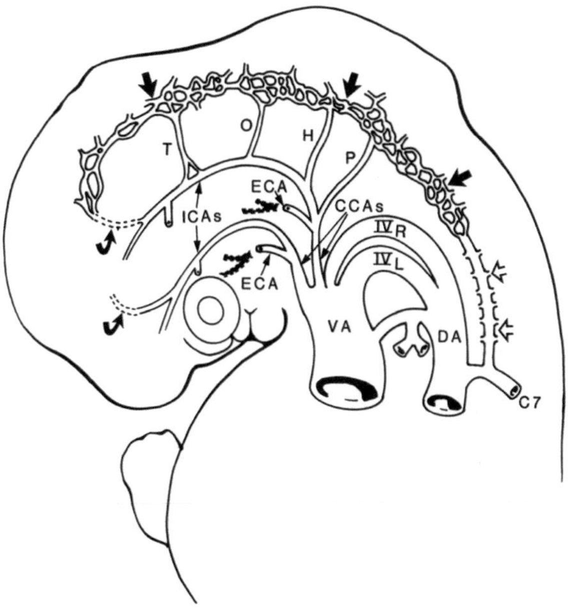


Fig. 2. Three-dimensional sketch at approximately 5 gestational weeks. Development of the paired plexiform longitudinal neural arteries (*solid black arrows*). The VAs (*open arrows*) form as longitudinal anastomoses between the seven cervical intersegmental arteries. The proximal connections between the C1-6 arteries and the dorsal aorta (DA) are regressing. For simplification, only one set of longitudinal neural and cervical intersegmental arteries is shown. These vessels are the precursors of the VB circulation. Initially, the longitudinal neural arteries are supplied from below via the intersegmental arteries. At this stage, several temporary connections between the developing VB circulation and the carotid arteries also form. From cephalad to caudad, these arteries are the trigeminal (T), otic (O), hypoglossal (H), and proatlantal intersegmental arteries (P) (this vessel forms slightly later). These transient anastomoses regress as the caudal divisions of the primitive internal carotid arteries (ICAs) anastomose with the cranial ends of the longitudinal neural arteries and form the future posterior communicating arteries (*dotted lines with curved arrows*). Persistence of the transient embryonic interconnections is abnormal and results in a so-called primitive carotid-basilar anastomosis. Sprouting of the external carotid arteries (ECAs) from the proximal common carotid arteries (CCAs) is also depicted. These vessels will annex first and second arch remnants (*solid black areas*). VA, ventral aorta. *Permission requested from Osborn AG: Diagnostic Cerebral Angiography (2nd ed). Philadelphia: Lippincott Williams & Wilkins, Wolters Kluwer, 1999, figure 1-2A, page 8.*

vascular arch (the right aortic arch) to form the proximal part of the subclavian artery and from it originates the VA. On the left side, the seventh cervical intersegmental artery coalesces with the left aortic arch (distal fourth arch–true adult aortic arch) to form the proximal left subclavian artery and from it originates the left VA (Figure 3). By 6 weeks' gestation, the cranial-most end of the ICAs have divided into rostral and caudal divisions. Although the rostral division will form the anterior, middle and anterior choroidal arteries, the caudal division fuses with the dorsal longitudinal neural arteries to form the PCoA. This results in eventual disappearance of the primitive carotid-basilar anastomoses.

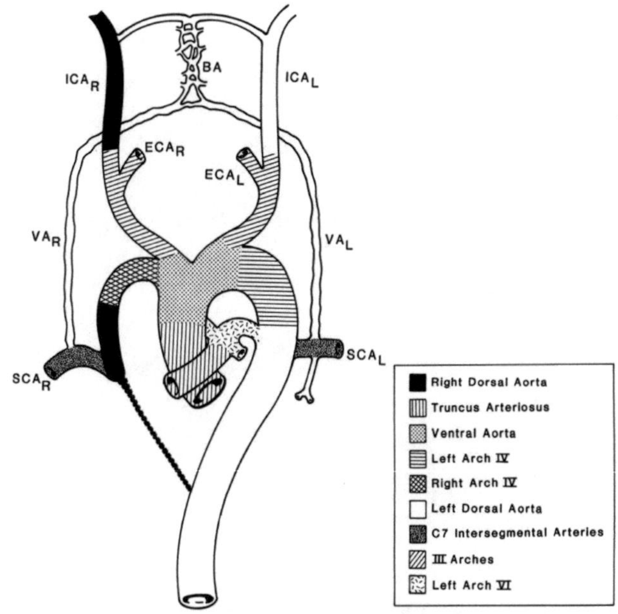


Fig. 3. Diagrammatic sketch of the craniocerebral vasculature at 7 weeks of development. The arch and great vessels are approaching their definitive form. Origins of these vessels from their embryonic precursors are depicted schematically. The fourth and sixth aortic arches are undergoing asymmetric remodeling to supply blood to the upper extremities, dorsal aorta, and lungs. The right sixth arch has involuted (leaving only part of the right pulmonary artery). The right dorsal aorta distal to the origin of the subclavian artery (SCA) is regressing (*dotted lines*) but remains connected to the right fourth arch. The right third and fourth arches are forming the brachiocephalic trunk; the left fourth arch becomes the definitive aortic arch. The left dorsal aorta becomes the proximal descending aorta. The first six cervical intersegmental arteries have become the definitive vertebral arteries (VAs); the C7 arteries have enlarged to become part of the developing subclavian arteries (SCAs). The longitudinal neural arteries are fusing across the midline to form the definitive basilar artery (BA). *Permission requested from Osborn AG: Diagnostic Cerebral Angiography (2nd ed). Philadelphia: Lippincott Williams & Wilkins, Wolters Kluwer, 1999, figure 1-4, page 11.*

Most of these changes are complete in the adult configuration by 8 weeks of gestation. For a review and further details, please see Osborn's detailed descriptions.[22] Further details have been described by Larsen[14] and Lasjaunias et al.[15]

## 3. Extracranial-to-intracranial anastomoses

For the purpose of grouping these anastomoses, Lasjaunias et al.[15,16] and Berenstein et al.[3] described regions within the cranial circulation that could be divided on the basis of primitive vascular connections. They divided the regions as follows:

1. Anterior or ophthalmic artery connections with facial and internal maxillary arteries
2. Middle or petrocavernous ICA branches with internal maxillary and ascending pharyngeal branches
3. Posterior or VB connections with ascending pharyngeal, occipital, and subclavian artery branches, especially the ascending and deep cervical arteries.

This division, although overlapping, serves to identify vascular territories of concern; that is, functional areas in which anastomotic dysfunction may become most apparent, thereby tailoring angiographic and neurologic examination during intraprocedural monitoring. Even when not apparent on routine angiography, these connections exist as byproducts of a unified vascular development for the entire head and neck region.[8] Under situations of increased flow, such as with arteriovenous fistulas (AVFs) or arteriovenous malformations (AVMs), there may be arterio-arterial embolization, resulting in deficits. In other cases, shared venous outflow may complicate options or results. Similarly, simply injecting materials, whether contrast or embolic materials, particularly liquid agents, may result in their crossing the anastomosis to occlude functional vessels supplying neural tissues, thereby creating unintended deficits. In addition, as embolization proceeds and the desired target vessel occludes, putative collateral anastomoses may be at increased risk. This may occur because of their presence as a relative lower-pressure sump (in the face of an occluded principal target vessel), resulting in the preferential shunting of embolic materials into these collaterals.[5] Although these collaterals may increase the risk of embolization procedures in the skull base, they serve to provide critical collaterals in the face of acute or subacute carotid or VB occlusion. They provide an innate bypass that grows under an increased demand from a hypoperfused intracranial territory. A recent review by Geibprasert et al.[9] describes these extracranial–intracranial anastomoses in considerable detail. These anastomotic connections are summarized in **Table 1**.

| Location | External Carotid Artery Branch | Internal Carotid Artery Branch |
|---|---|---|
| Orbit, Superior Orbital Fissure | Internal maxillary artery-Middle meningeal artery | Ophthalmic artery-Orbital branches |
| Falx | Internal maxillary artery-Middle meningeal artery | Ophthalmic artery-Anterior falcine artery |
| Orbit | Internal maxillary artery-Deep temporal artery, Inferior orbital artery | Ophthalmic artery-Orbital branches (Lacrimal branches) |
| Ethmoidal Sinus | Internal maxillary artery-Septal, Sphenopalatine, Greater palatine arteries | Ophthalmic artery-Anterior and Posterior ethmoidal arteries |
| Scalp | Superficial temporal artery | Ophthalmic artery-Superior orbital artery |
| Nose | Facial artery-nasal branches, Internal maxillary artery-Inferior orbital artery | Ophthalmic artery-Dorsal nasal artery |
| Cavernous Sinus | Internal maxillary artery-Middle meningeal artery, Accessory meningeal artery, deep temporal artery, Artery of the foramen rotundum | Internal carotid artery-Inferolateral trunk |
| Sphenopalatine Fossa | Internal maxillary artery-Artery of the vidian canal | Internal Carotid artery-Branch of the foramen lacerum (Primitive stapedial artery) |
| Inferotemporal Fossa | Internal maxillary artery-Accessory meningeal artery | Internal carotid artery-Inferolateral trunk (Artery of the foramen ovale) |
| Superior Nasopharynx | Ascending pharyngeal artery-Pharyngeal branches | Internal carotid artery-Artery of the foramen lacerum |
| Petrous Bone-Middle Ear | Ascending pharyngeal branches-Neuromeningeal branches | Internal carotid artery-Caroticotympanic branch |
| Hypoglossal Canal and Jugular Foramen | Ascending pharyngeal branches-Neuromeningeal branches (Hypoglossal canal and Jugular foramen branches) | Internal carotid artery-Meningohypophyseal trunk |
| Odontoid Process | Ascending pharyngeal artery-Neuromeningeal branches | Vertebral artery-Odontoid arch |
| Stylomastoid foramen | Posterior Auricular, Occipital artery-Stylomastoid branch | Internal carotid artery-Caroticotympanic branch (Facial nerve supply) |
| Transverse process of C1 | Occipital artery-Muscular branches | Vertebral artery-Muscular branches |
| Posterior cervical muscles/fascia | Deep and Ascending Cervical arteries-Muscular branches | Vertebral artery-Muscular branches |

Table 1. Extracranial-to-Intracranial Anastomoses

### 3.1 Ophthalmic artery anastomoses

The ophthalmic artery is the principal vascular supply for contents in the orbit.[13] It is the principal supply to the central retinal artery, which in turn, supplies the retina and choroid. Occlusion of this vessel will result in monocular blindness. Therefore, visualization of a choroid blush with an ECA injection should raise alarms about potential anatomic variations and dangerous collaterals.[25] The ophthalmic artery originates from the ICA; however, during its development, it necessarily develops connections with other sources of supply to the contents of the orbit. The primitive stapedial artery contributes to the middle meningeal artery, and this develops some connections to the ophthalmic artery through the superior orbital fissure.[26] The magnitude of this connection may vary; rarely, the middle meningeal and internal maxillary arteries completely assume the principal source of supply to the ophthalmic artery. In cases in which the ophthalmic artery is not visualized, such variation should be suspected.

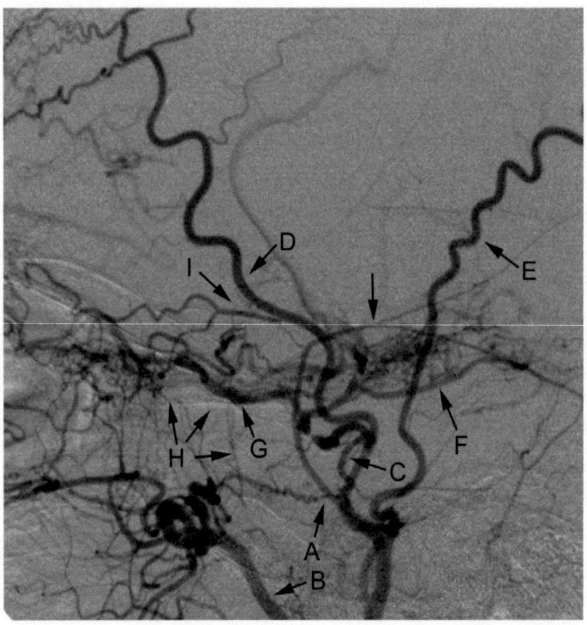


Fig. 4. An ECA angiogram in a patient with ICA occlusion, with reconstitution of the ICA through collaterals via the ophthalmic artery and the cavernous ICA. The vidian artery (A) is supplying collateral flow from the internal maxillary artery (B) to the petrous ICA (C). The frontal branch of the superficial temporal artery (D) is providing transosseous collaterals to the frontal meningo-pial collaterals, whereas the parietal branch (E) is not involved. The PCoA (F) is involved in the extensive neovascularization through its perforators, typical of Moya Moya disease. The ophthalmic artery (G) is the largest source of retrograde collateral flow to the ICA. It is receiving its supply principally through its ethmoidal arteries (H) via connections with the internal maxillary artery. Another source of supply to the ophthalmic artery is the recurrent meningeal branch (I) of the middle meningeal artery.

The anastomotic connections of the ECA branches with the ophthalmic artery may be divided according to the segments of the ophthalmic artery.[13] The first segment of the ophthalmic artery arises as the first supraclinoidal branch of the ICA and travels on the underside of the optic nerve in the optic canal. Upon entering the orbit, it maintains its close relationship with the optic nerve traveling towards the posterior globe. The recurrent meningeal artery is a reliable branch often noted by microvascular surgeons along the lateral aspect of the superior orbital fissure and is a branch of the middle meningeal artery. This supplies the contents of the superior orbital fissure and then anastomoses with the second segment of the ophthalmic artery in the orbit. This anastomosis is of particular importance when embolizing the middle meningeal artery branches, particularly for convexity meningiomas. The recurrent meningeal artery can often be visualized as the middle meningeal artery crosses the sphenoid wing. In cases in which embolization is desirable, it is best to obtain distal access close to or in the tumor proper and be vigilant to reflux to this more proximal branch point. In other cases where a branch is not noted, an intraarterial injection of sodium amytal and lidocaine may allow Wada testing[32] of the anastomosis, which may not be apparent (Figures 4 and 5).

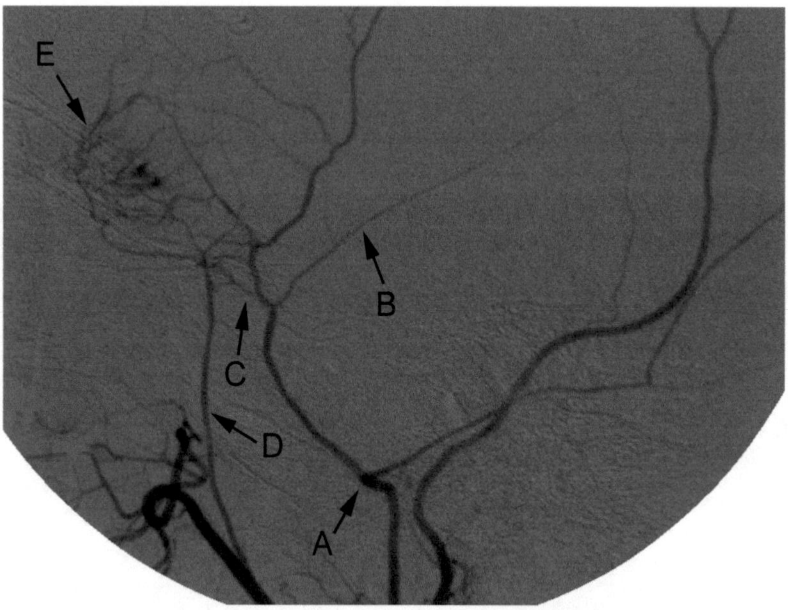


Fig. 5. Selective ECA angiogram reveals a tumor blush of an anterior cranial fossa meningioma. The principal supply is the middle meningeal artery (A), which divides into the parietal branch (B) and an enlarged recurrent meningeal branch (C) that, along with the accessory meningeal artery (D), is the principal supply for this tumor (E, tumor blush).

The second group of anastomoses is a product of the shared supply to the ethmoidal sinuses from the anterior and posterior branches of the ophthalmic artery as well as branches from septal, sphenopalatine, and greater palatine branches of the internal maxillary artery.[1] These occur along the second and third segments of the ophthalmic artery. In addition, anastomoses may also exist between the ophthalmic artery and deep temporal and infraorbital branches of the internal maxillary artery. These arise particularly because of shared ophthalmic and internal maxillary supply to the lacrimal apparatus (Figure 4). These anastomotic connections carry great significance during embolization for epistaxis. Most of the anastomotic connections through the lacrimal and ethmoidal arteries tend to be very small-caliber vessels (less than 80 microns). If embolization is desired, particles chosen should be greater than 150 microns. This prevents inadvertent passage of these particles into the ICA or ophthalmic artery through these collaterals. As noted above, one needs to identify an aberrant ophthalmic artery origin by always performing a cerebral angiogram to identify the origin of the ophthalmic artery from the ICA. Embolization of anterior fossa-based tumors, such as olfactory groove meningiomas, is considered high risk because the principal supply to these tumors is from the ethmoidal arteries, and transinternal maxillary or transophthalmic embolization of these branches may have an inordinate increased risk for some of the material refluxing into the central retinal artery or retrograde into the ICA (Figure 5).[1] Another consideration is with falcine meningiomas in which the anterior falcine artery, a branch of the ophthalmic artery, may anastomose with frontal branches of the middle meningeal artery, with retrograde flux of embolization materials into the ophthalmic artery from a middle meningeal artery branch embolization. Other situations in which these anastomoses need to be considered are during embolization for tumors in the head and neck region, particularly juvenile angiofibromas. Cavernous sinus DAVFs are particularly challenging because their inherent incorporation of these varied collateral channels may create significant risk for transarterial embolization (Figure 6).

The third group of anastomoses occurs along the third or terminal segments of the ophthalmic artery and its terminal branches, the dorsal nasal artery and superior orbital

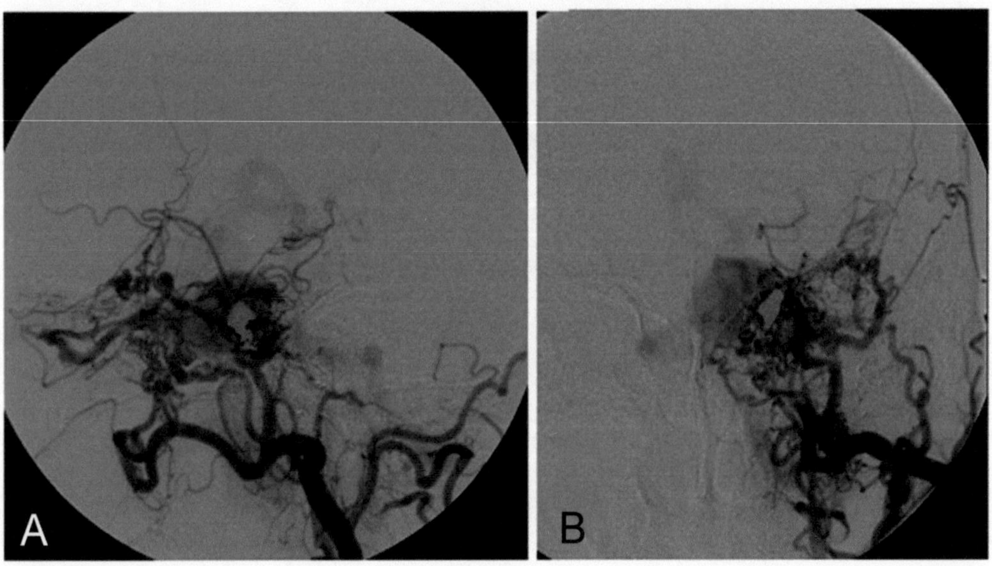


Fig. 6. An ECA angiogram in a patient with a surgical ICA occlusion and cavernous DAVF due to a gun shot (A). The hypertrophied ECA trunk (B) is supplying an enlarged internal maxillary artery (C) and its principal branches: middle meningeal artery (D), accessory meningeal artery (E), deep temporal artery (F), and sphenopalatine artery (G). The sphenoparietal artery branches to supply the small infraorbital artery (H), and the numerous septal arteries communicate with the ethmoidal arteries (I) to supply the enlarged ophthalmic artery (J). The enlarged recurrent meningeal branch (K) is noted off the middle meningeal artery. The accessory meningeal artery is seen communicating with the inferolateral trunk and artery of the foramen rotundum (L), with its typical corkscrew shape.

artery (Figure 7). The superior orbital artery anastomoses with the frontal branches of the superficial temporal artery. This anastomosis may gain relevance in situations in which the ICA is occluded with connections via the superior orbital artery supplying the ophthalmic artery and, in some cases, direct transosseous collaterals to frontal cortical meningo-pial anastomoses (Figure 4). The dorsal nasal artery anastomoses with terminal nasal branches of the facial artery as well as the inferior orbital artery (a terminal branch of the internal maxillary artery) (Figure 7). These anastomoses, particularly the latter, are of great significance during embolization procedures for epistaxis. A high-pressure angiogram through the microcatheter (micro-angiogram) prior to embolization may allow better identification of such dangerous collaterals as compared to an ECA angiogram from a more proximal location.

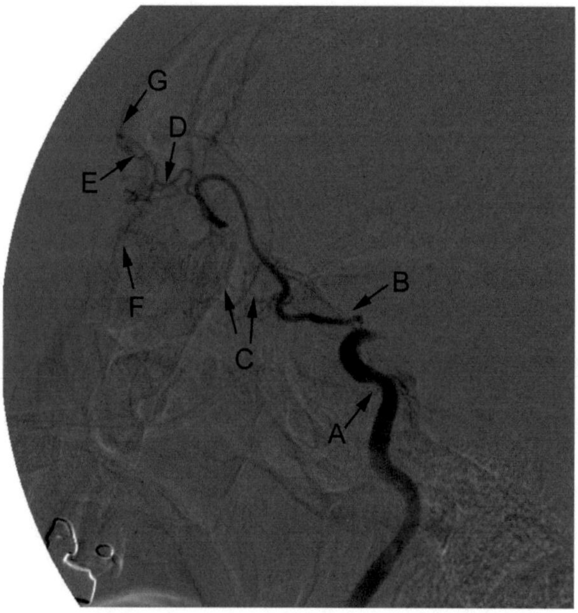


Fig. 7. Selective ICA injection demonstrates an occlusion beyond the origin of the ophthalmic artery. The ICA (A) gives rise to the ophthalmic artery (B), which is its first supraclinoidal branch. The ophthalmic artery then gives rise to multiple ethmoidal arteries (C), terminating as the dorsal nasal artery (D) and the supraorbital artery (E), which passes through the supraorbital notch (G) to anastomose with branches from the frontal branch of the superficial temporal artery. Inferiorly, the dorsal nasal artery anastomoses with the terminal angular branch of the facial artery (F).

### 3.2 Petrocavernous internal carotid artery collaterals

The anastomoses that fall within this region are complex and prone to multiple variations. Only the principal trunks are seen in good-quality angiograms. Although always there, these collateral pathways only become apparent in cases of increased flow across these connections, such as during petrocavernous AVF embolization or after cervical ICA occlusion (Figures 4, 6, and 8). A systematic discussion has recently been provided in detail by Geibprasert et al.[9] To understand the organization of these collaterals, one can attempt to look at these putative connections in terms of branches of the ICA, which are involved in the anastomosis. The first branch traveling rostrocaudal or distal to proximal along the ICA is the inferolateral trunk off the ICA in the cavernous sinus.

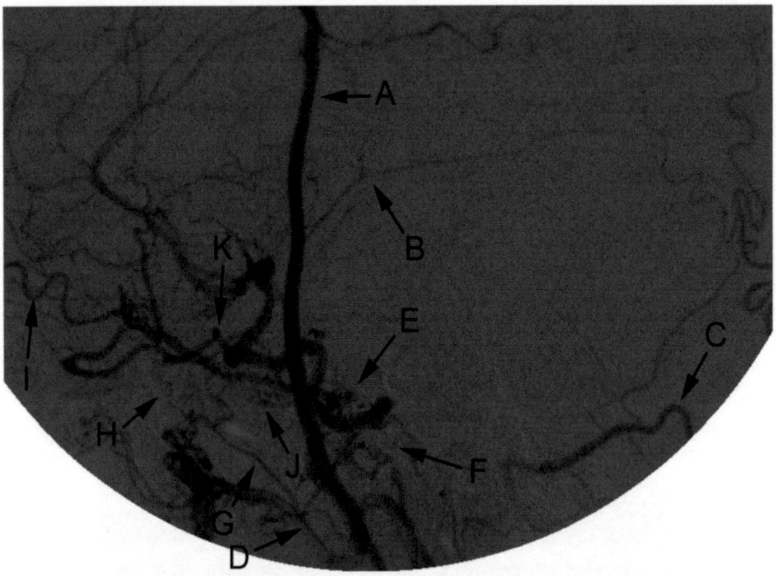


Fig. 8. An ECA angiogram following successful bypass with a radial artery graft from the ECA to the MCA. The radial artery graft (A) can be seen overlaid on the cavernous sinus anastomosis. Parietal branch of the middle meningeal artery (B). Occipital artery (C). Internal maxillary artery trunk (D). The caroticotympanic artery (E) anastomoses with branches from the ascending pharyngeal branches (F) to reconstitute the ICA. The accessory meningeal artery (G) is anastomosing with the inferolateral trunk branches. Additionally, the ethmoidal vessels (H) are supplying the ophthalmic artery (K). The inferolateral trunk is anastomosing with branches from the middle meningeal branches at the foramen spinosum (J) and through the artery of the foramen rotundum more anteriorly.

The inferolateral trunk has multiple branches, which supply the anterior and middle parts of the cavernous sinus structures.[4,15,17,30] It is a remnant of an embryologic dorsal ophthalmic artery and connects to its ECA counterparts principally along the foramina of cranial nerves or in the meningeal walls of the cavernous sinus. Anteriorly, it communicates with the internal maxillary artery through the artery of the foramen rotundum; laterally, it collateralizes with the cavernous branches of the middle meningeal artery, which arise soon after the artery exits the foramen spinosum; and, posteriorly, it communicates with the accessory meningeal artery through the artery of foramen ovale (Figure 8).

The second branch in this order is a remnant of the primitive stapedial artery and the subsequent mandibular trunk off the stapediohyoid artery, a small branch that pierces the foramen lacerum arising either directly off the carotid artery or as a branch off the meningohypophyseal trunk, which enters the vidian canal to anastomose with the sphenopalatine artery (a branch of the internal maxillary artery in the sphenopalatine fossa).[29] It also anastomoses with the superior pharyngeal artery (a branch of the pharyngeal trunk of the ascending pharyngeal artery) and the accessory meningeal artery to provide a branch to the pterygovaginal canal, which ends by anastomosing with internal maxillary artery branches (Figure 9).

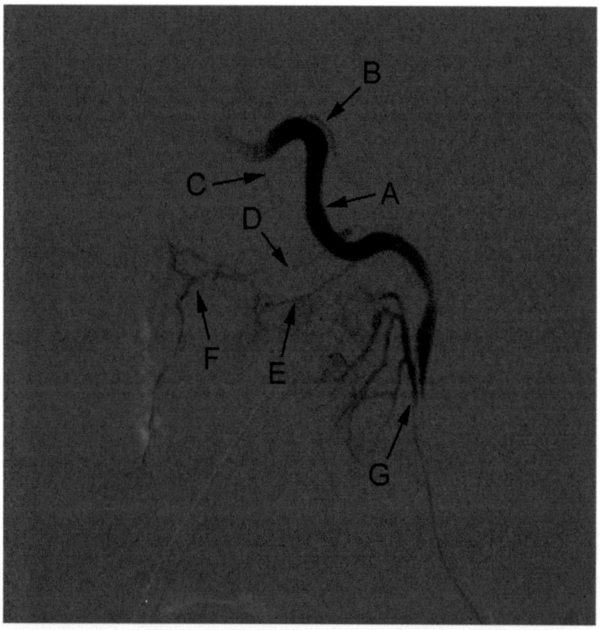


Fig. 9. Selective microinjection in an occluded ICA demonstrating connections with extracranial vessels. The ICA (A) is occluded at the distal cavernous segment. Its cavernous branches, the meningohypophyseal trunk (B) and inferolateral trunk (C) are noted. The inferolateral trunk is anastomosing with branches of the internal maxillary artery, particularly the sphenopalatine artery (F), through the artery of the foramen rotundum. More inferiorly, the primitive mandibular (petrous) branch anastomoses with the vidian artery (D), which originates from the sphenopalatine artery. Further inferiorly, the caroticotympanic artery is seen anastomosing with the ascending pharyngeal artery (G); and, together, these vessels are supplying the artery of the pterygovaginal canal (E).

The third branch of note is the primitive maxillary artery remnant, the meningohypophyseal trunk. This branch has widespread connections along the posterior cavernous sinus and clivus. Anteriorly, it anastomoses through its tentorial branch (of Bernasconi and Cassinari) with petrous branches from the middle meningeal artery. These branches are particularly noted during angiography for superior petrosal sinus or transverse-sigmoid junction DAVFs (Figure 10). More posteriorly, its major branch, the lateral clival artery, anastomoses extensively with neuromeningeal branches of the ascending pharyngeal artery, including branches that supply the hypoglossal and jugular foramina.

The most proximal branch of the ICA is the caroticotympanic artery in the petrous canal.[10,21,23,30] This embryologic remnant of the hyoid artery anastomoses with the tympanic plexus, which is supplied by the tympanic branches of the ascending pharyngeal artery, stylomastoid artery from the posterior auricular artery, and petrotympanic branches of the middle meningeal artery (Figure 9).

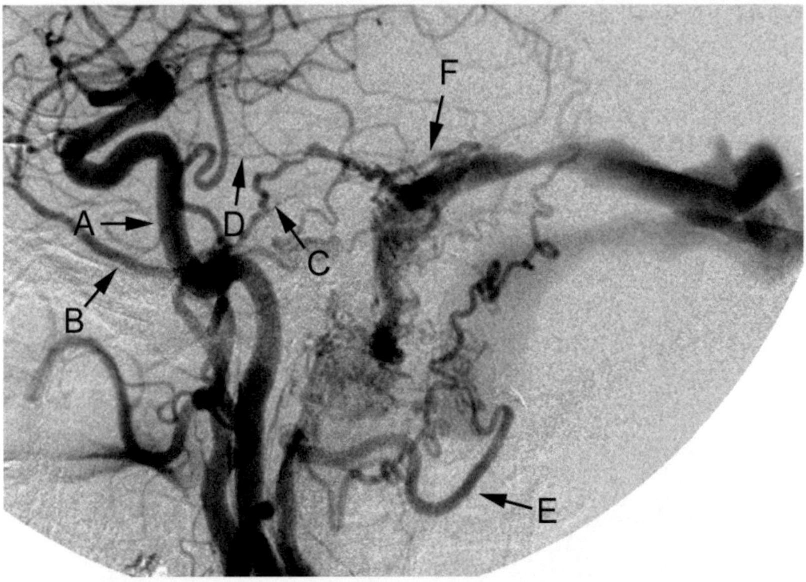


Fig. 10. A CCA angiogram revealing a transverse-sigmoid junction DAVF. ICA (A). The middle meningeal artery's (B) petrous branch (C) is supplying the DAVF, as is the tentorial branch (D) of the meningohypophyseal trunk of the ICA. The transosseous branches from the occipital artery (E) are a major supply to the DAVF (F).

These branches become most apparent as vascular sources for cavernous and petroclival meningiomas or for tympanic or jugular foramen glomus tumors. Because of the critical supply to cranial nerves and their ganglia in these foramina, embolization of these vessels carries potential for lower cranial nerve dysfunction.

### 3.3 Vertebrobasilar anastomoses

As noted above, the VB system develops through posterior paired longitudinal arteries that coalesce rostrally to form the basilar artery (BA), while inferiorly they remain separate as VAs. Rostrally, this system is supplied through collaterals of which only the PCoA remains in most adults. Primitive anastomoses include the trigeminal artery, which remains as a branch to Meckel's cave; the otic artery, as the labyrinthine artery; the hypoglossal artery, as an artery to the hypoglossal canal; and the proatlantal artery, as the occipital artery and its connections to the VA over the first cervical vertebra and separately at the second cervical vertebra, through segmental vertebral branches. Although regressed, these connections may remain viable and become prominent under conditions of increased flow. Rarely, they remain as principal supply to the posterior circulation with regression of the more proximal VB system.[18,24,27]

The occipital artery routinely has a prominent connection to the VA as it emerges from the C1 transverse foramen. Embolization of dural arteriovenous fistulas (DAVFs), particularly those involving the transverse sinuses at the transverse sigmoid junction or torcula, can have enlarged occipital feeders; and care must be exercised to ensure that no inadvertent posterior circulation embolization occurs. In other situations, this route may be used to treat intracranial lesions, such as acute occlusions,[33] or other pathologic conditions.

The neuromeningeal trunk of the ascending pharyngeal artery anastomoses with the VA, through connections at C3 through muscular collaterals, and more rostrally, as the remnant of the primitive hypoglossal artery with the odontoid arch vascular system.[11,19]
More caudally, the cervical branches of the subclavian artery anastomose with proximal sections of the VAs (C3-7). The ascending cervical artery arises from the thyrocervical trunk, while the deep cervical artery arises from the costocervical trunk. Both these branches form connections with the segmental vertebral branches through muscular collaterals. They are commonly noted to reconstitute the distal VA after proximal occlusion.

### 3.4 Extracranial to intracranial collateralization and complication avoidance in neurointervention procedures

First and foremost, one needs to be aware of the potential for collateral anastomotic channels. Such knowledge facilitates angiographic visualization. Even if the initial proximal external carotid or subclavian angiograms do not result in the visualization of these collaterals, we recommend that selective microcatheter angiograms be performed in as distal a position as is reasonably attainable immediately prior to embolization. These higher pressure selective injections are more likely to reveal these putative connections. If there is no visualization, a second element to further bolster confidence is to perform a Wada test with sodium amytal (75 mg) and lidocaine (30 mg) intraarterially through the microcatheter from the position planned for embolization and then immediately after injection to test for loss of appropriate neural function including that of the cranial nerves. Thirdly, if embolization is desired, polyvinyl alcohol particles, which considerably exceed the size (150 microns or greater) of most of these non-angiographically visualized collaterals (50-80 microns), should be used. Liquid embolics, such as glue (N-butyl cyanoacrylate; Trufill, Codman Neurovascular, Raynham, MA) and Onyx (EV3™, Irvine, California), provide superior visualization; however, they are not discriminatory with respect to vessel size and, therefore, their use may be associated with a higher likelihood of collateral vessel occlusion.
Angiographic visualization does not preclude embolization. One may attempt to attain distal purchase beyond the collateral communication and pay great attention to reflux during the embolization procedure. If such positioning is not attainable, pre-embolization occlusion of the collateral channel is another strategy. Typically, coil embolization of the collateral channel will not result in ischemic injury because of the multiple sources of vascular supply at the skull base; however, subsequent embolization of the intended vessel will prevent inadvertent passage of embolic materials through the occluded vessel to critical neural structures.

## 4. Intracranial anastomoses

In contrast to the extracranial-to-intracranial collateral anastomoses described above, which may be less obvious on non-superselective angiography, many of the ICA-to-ICA or ICA-to-VB anastomoses are rather easily identified and commonly seen. These common known collateral anastomoses as parts of the circle of Willis include the following: 1) anterior communicating artery (ACoA) connecting bilateral anterior cerebral arteries (ACAs); and 2) PCoA connecting the ipsilateral ICA to the posterior cerebral artery (PCA). Less obvious anastomoses occur among the various terminal cortical branches from each of the major vascular territories. The middle cerebral artery (MCA) branches anastomose with branches of the PCA and ACA. The pericallosal branches of the ACA connect to splenial branches of PCA. Distal branches of the superior cerebellar artery (SCA) connect to branches from posterior inferior cerebellar artery (PICA), or to branches from anterior inferior cerebellar artery (AICA). Branches of AICA could also have connection with PICA. These anastomoses not only provide collaterals to preserve potentially affected brain tissue in the case of an occlusion event but also provide crucial collateral supply in the situation if carotid artery or VA sacrifice becomes necessary; also, potentially, the collaterals may be utilized as alternative access routes to the target during interventional procedures. Typically, these distal branch anastomoses are not visible with standard angiogram runs. In order to delineate the present of the anastomoses, a superselective balloon test occlusion is often required.

### 4.1 Intracranial collateralization in neurointerventional procedures

#### 4.1.1 Flow replacement by collateral vessels

*Intracranial large artery sacrifice*

In patients with fusiform or giant aneurysms of the cavernous or supraclinoidal segment of the carotid artery or supraclinoidal carotid artery dissection with hemorrhage, sacrifice of the ipsilateral ICA can be a simple therapeutic solution with low risk if the ACoA and PCoA provide sufficient cross filling to the affected side. This is especially true if both angiographic and neurophysiologic tests are completed during a temporary balloon occlusion (TBO) test[6,28,31] (Figure 11). It should be noted that endovascular strategies for vessel preservation during treatment continue to gradually erode options for vessel sacrifice, e.g., flow diversion technique, (Pipeline stent by EV3™) in treating carotid artery giant aneurysms, which previously required carotid sacrifice.

Sacrifice of the VA is an effective strategy for the management of pathologic conditions of the VA, such as dissection with hemorrhage or endovascularly unmanageable aneurysms, simply because most patients are endowed with two vessels; and, after the sacrifice of one, unabated flow typically continues through the other. It is, however, important that the TBO test be performed before a vessel deconstruction procedure is carried out (Figure 12). There are other more complex situations involving the distal VAs, their junction, or the BA in which neither VA can be preserved, so flow reversal is desired. These situations include dissections with hemorrhage and complex, enlarging, symptomatic, or ruptured fusiform aneurysms.[2,20] The presence of a robust PCoA and a large-caliber ipsilateral PCA P1 segment may allow sacrifice of both VAs, thereby creating flow reversal with a diminution of flow, enough to reduce hemodynamic stresses on the diseased vessel and allowing it to heal. It should be borne in mind that, before such deconstruction, which is undoubtedly high risk, a comprehensive angiographic evaluation, including a VA angiogram with transient bilateral manual carotid artery compression, could be very useful to identify bilateral PCoA. Further hemodynamic and neurophysiologic testing should be completed prior to vessel deconstruction.

*Intracranial distal end artery sacrifice*

Occasionally, one may encounter dissecting, mycotic, or ruptured broad-based aneurysms involving the distal ACA, MCA or PCA and considered higher risk for surgical or endovascular reconstruction. Because of well-developed cortical collaterals from ipsilateral ACA to PCA or MCA to PCA or ACA to MCA territories, these collaterals typically are

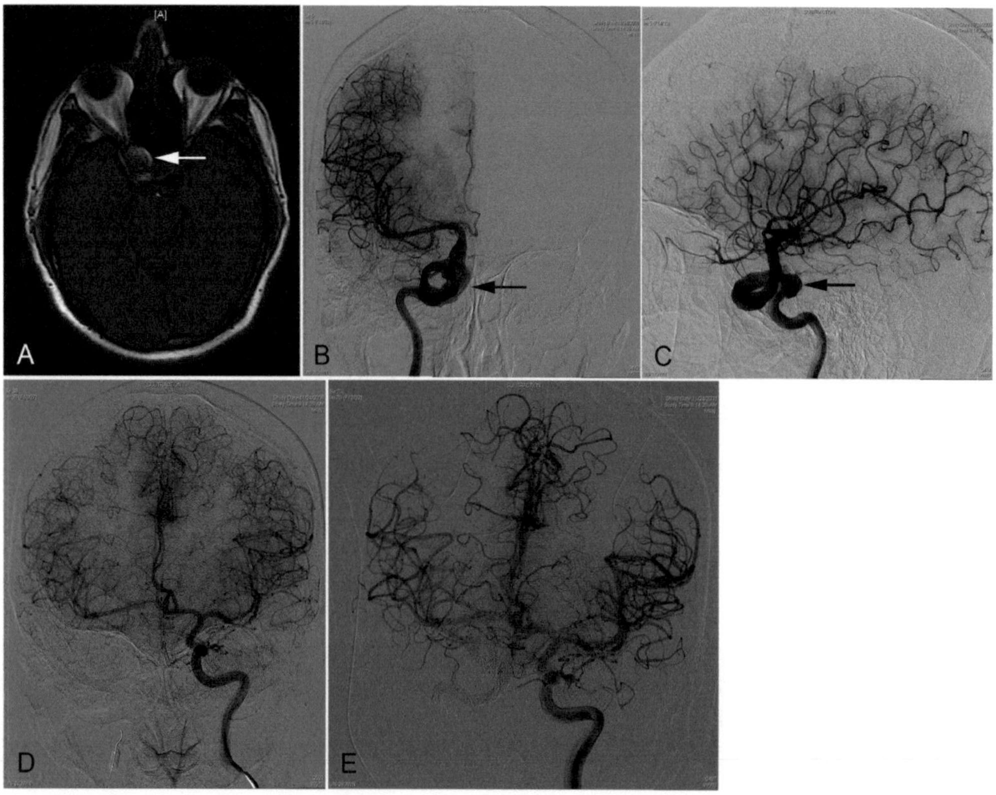


Fig. 11. A 40-year-old man presented with amaurosis fugax in the right eye. An imaging study confirmed a partially thrombosed giant aneurysm of the right ICA cavernous segment that likely had caused the embolic event. (A) T1-weighted magnetic resonance image reveals a partially thrombosed cavernous aneurysm (*arrow*). (B and C) Angiography shows the fusiform aneurysm with serpentine channel (*arrow*). (D) Right ICA TBO test with angiogram from left ICA reveals robust cross-filling of the contralateral circulation. The ACoA serves to opacify the right ACA and MCA without delay. (E) The patient tolerated TBO and was successfully treated with right ICA sacrifice.

revealed or opacified during angiography only after proximal vessel test occlusion. We typically perform a superselective micro-balloon test occlusion of the proximal vessel (as distal as possible remaining proximal to the aneurysm). Under micro-vessel occlusion we perform proximal angiograms as well as concurrent neurophysiologic testing to demonstrate angiographic and functional collateralization. If the patient tolerates the test occlusion, we then proceed immediately with endovascular embolization permanent occlusion of the tested vessel distal to the test site (Figure 13). If the patient does not tolerate test occlusion, one then has to weigh the risks of vessel-preserving strategies through microsurgical or endovascular means versus the expected neurologic deficit of vessel deconstruction. Obviously, microsurgical bypass anastomosis prior to artery sacrifice is one well-established treatment strategy. It should be noted that Hallacq et al.[12] reported a series of 10 cases of P2 PCA aneurysms treated with occlusion of the aneurysm and parent vessel without balloon test occlusion in which no postocclusion occipital lobe ischemia occurred.

Similar patterns of distal arterial collateralization can often be expected in PICA, AICA and SCA circulations. In cases of PICA ruptured dissections or dissecting aneurysms, proximal PICA can be occluded without needs of microsurgical bypass anastomosis. (Figure 21).

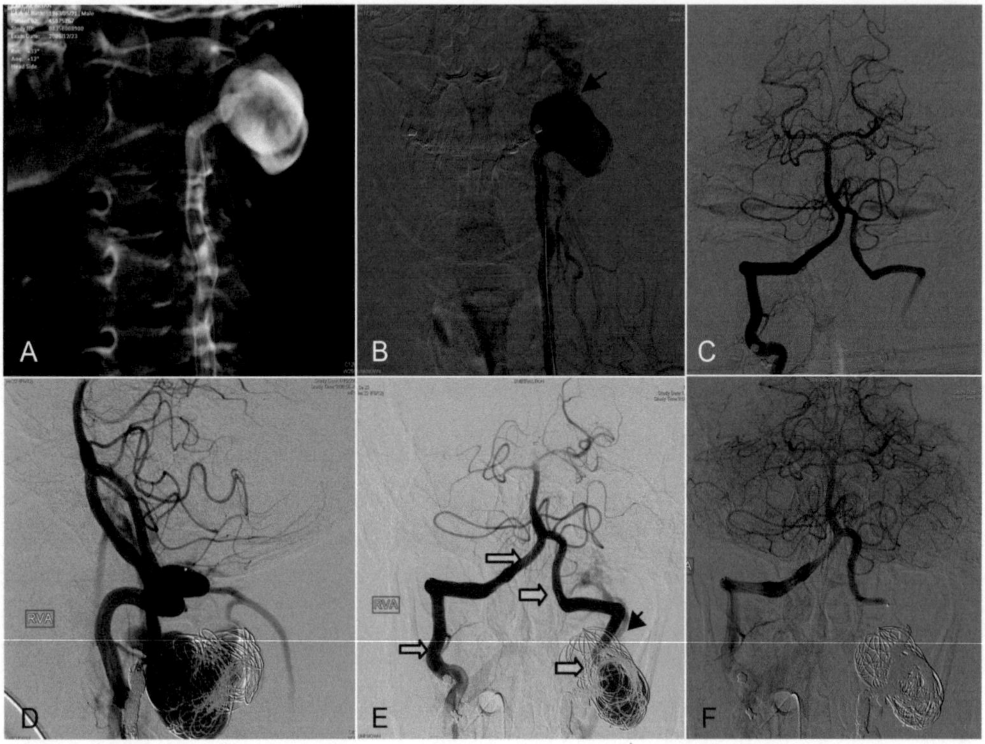


Fig. 12. A 38-year-old man with a left PCA territory embolic infarct was found to have a traumatic giant left VA dissecting aneurysm and DAVF from a fall 2 years prior to treatment. (A and B) Three-dimensional and two-dimensional angiograms show a giant left VA dissecting aneurysm and a DAVF. (C) The right VA angiogram demonstrates competent flow in the right VA. (D and E) Due to extremely high flow in the giant aneurysm, the DAVF was unable to be catheterized until occlusion of the left VA at the origin of the aneurysm. The left traumatic vertebral DAVF was catheterized from the right VA through the VB junction to the left VA. The *black arrow* indicates the fistula. *Open arrows* indicate the microcatheter route. (F) The fistula and residual filling of the giant aneurysm were treated successfully with coil occlusion through the contralateral VA to the left vertebral DAVF and giant aneurysm.

## 5. Alternative microcatheterization of target vessel via a collateral route

The circle of Willis provides a natural conduit to access contralateral or carotid to basilar (or vice-versa) circulations. In the vast majority of cases, adequate access may be obtained through direct ipsilateral routes; however, due either to proximal vessel occlusion or distal vessel entry angles, these alternate routes through the circle of Willis provide easier microcatheter entry angles.

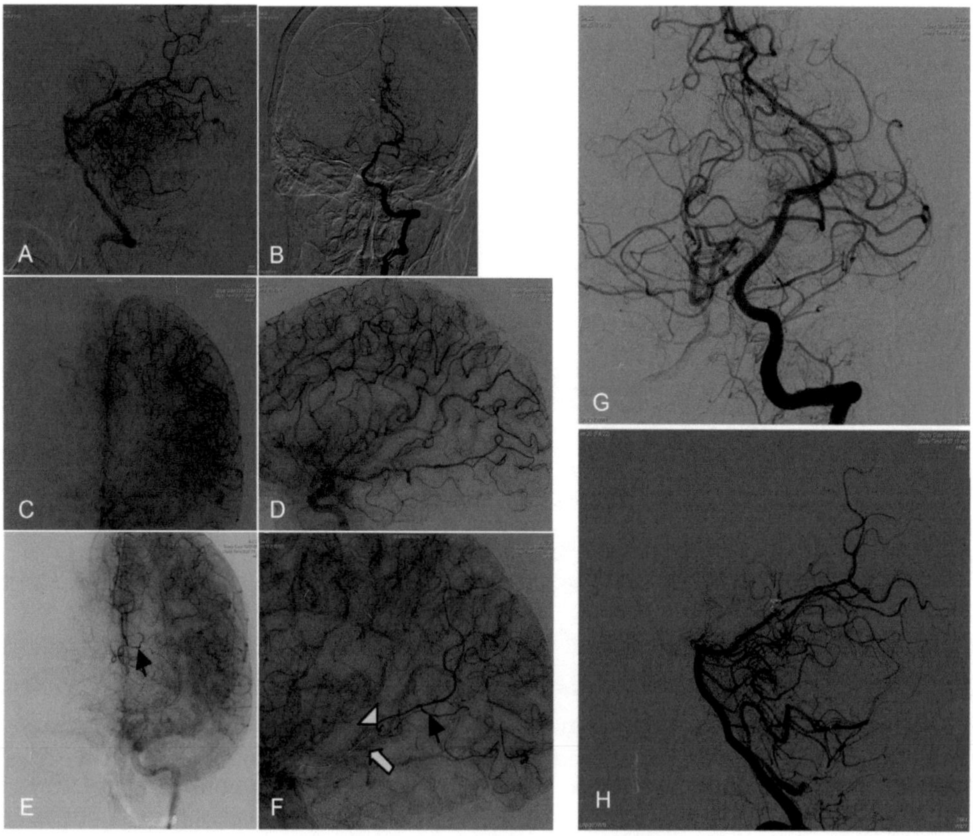


Fig. 13. A 48-year-old woman with a subarachnoid hemorrhage due to a left P2–P3 junction ruptured aneurysm. (A and B) Lateral view and anteroposterior (AP) view of original VA angiogram (*arrow in B*). (C and D) Left ICA AP and lateral angiography. (E and F) Left PCA P2 TBO. The left ICA angiogram, while the left P2 was occluded with a balloon, revealed left ACA to PCA cortical collateralization (*black arrow*) with retrograde opacification during the late arterial phase. In F, *open arrow* indicates the balloon; *arrowhead* indicates the retrograde partially opacified P2-P3 aneurysm. (G and H) Ultimately, this aneurysm was coil embolized completely with balloon-remodeling technique; and the distal PCA branches were preserved anterogradely.

A sharp reversely angulated origin of a vessel makes superselective ipsilateral catheterization difficult. For instance, access to the PICA or anterior inferior cerebellar artery (AICA) from the VA can be occasionally difficult, or in cases in which the carotid or bilateral VAs are occluded, the PCoA offers a distinct advantage. In these situations, if the caliber of the PCoA is adequate, effective catheterization of the desired vessel can be achieved (Figures 14 and 15). Naturally, a microcatheter can also go from one VA to the other through the VB junction (Figure 12, 16).[7] Similarly, during treatment of broad-based aneurysms at the basilar or ICA terminus, ipsilateral placement of a stent may be inadequate for complete coverage of the aneurysm neck, necessitating a Y-configuration with increased risk of thromboembolic complications. In these cases, the following strategies offer distinct advantages: access from the contralateral carotid artery to pass a stent across the AcoA so

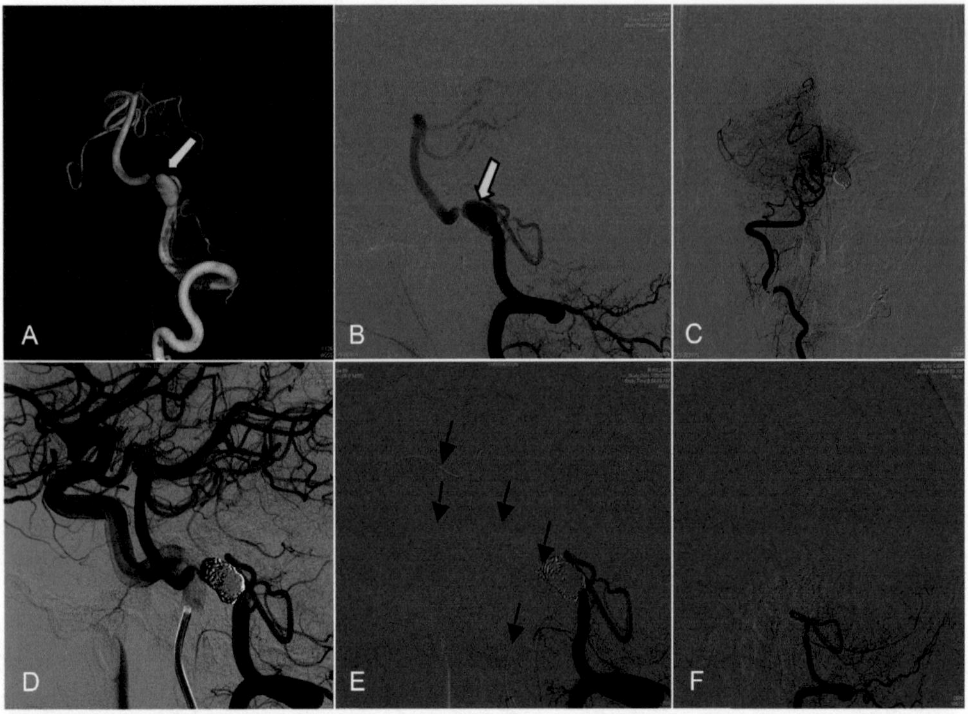


Fig. 14. A 40-year-old man with a left intracranial VA dissection with a pseudoaneurysm just distal to the left PICA origin. (A and B) three-dimensional angiogram and lateral view of left VA two-dimensional angiogram. *Arrows* indicate the pseudoaneurysm at the dissection site. (C) Left ICA angiogram revealed robust PCoA connecting the left ICA system to the VB system. (D) Due to limited distal flow from the dissecting aneurysm to the normal PICA origin, complete occlusion of the left VA was not achieved by balloon-remodeling coiling through left VA catheterization. Therefore, superselective catheterization through a left ICA-PCoA-BA-left VA route allowed us to successfully occlude the diseased segment of the VA. *Arrows* in E indicate the microcatheter route. By comparison with the angiogram in C, the 3-month follow-up angiogram with right VA (E) and left VA (F, lateral view) runs shows the left VA supplying the left PICA without evidence of recurrent aneurysm.

that it ultimately sits across the entire neck of the aneurysm in the ICA terminus (from the ipsilateral ACA to the MCA) or from the carotid artery across the PCoA so that it sits from the ipsilateral PCA to contralateral PCA (Figure 17). In cases in which there is occlusion of one or more vessels to the circle of Willis, the circle provides an optimal opportunity to access diseased segments of vessels that are proximally occluded. These routes can be used to treat a variety of conditions, such as aneurysms (Figure 18), AVMs, or AVFs. Similarly, in cases of acute occlusion, even if the proximal vessel cannot be adequately revascularized, reestablishing flow across the circle may alleviate acute cerebral ischemia (Figure 19). In other situations, the circle may allow passage of endovascular implements that, despite patency, cannot be brought up through ipsilateral routes (Figure 22 -24). This is particularly relevant to situations in which the ipsilateral vessel may have spasm after subarachnoid hemorrhage (Figure 20) or be congenitally hypoplastic.

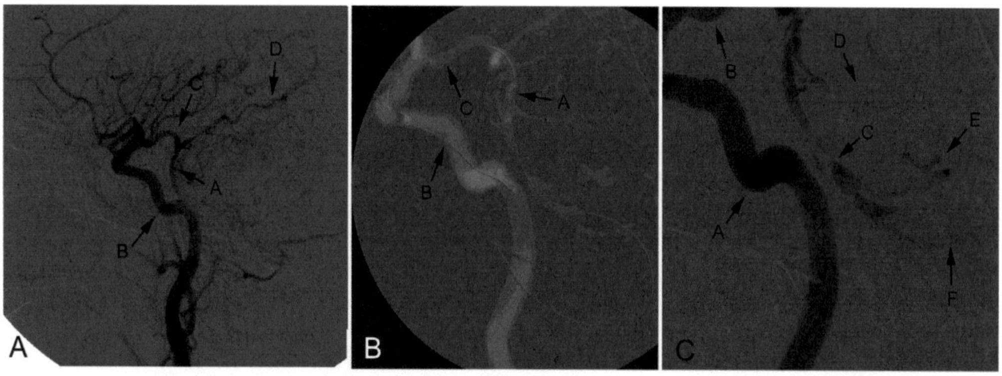


Fig. 15. A 70-year-old woman presented with multiple events of VB insufficiency. Evaluation revealed bilateral VA occlusions. A) Injection of the left ICA (C) revealed the PCoA (B) as the principal supply to the BA (A) and the PCA (D). (B) A road-map angiogram reveals a guide catheter in the left ICA (B) with a microwire through the PCoA (C) and through the proximal BA (A) across an obvious stenosis into the distal VA. (C) After retrograde BA angioplasty, an ICA (A) angiogram reveals robust filling through the PCoA (B) into the basilar artery with markedly improved flow across the stenotic lesion into the BA junction (C), bilateral PICA, and VA (E, F). *With permission from Chiam PT, Mocco J, Samuelson RM, Siddiqui AH, Hopkins LN, Levy EI: Retrograde angioplasty for basilar artery stenosis: bypassing bilateral vertebral artery occlusions.* ***J Neurosurg* 110:***427-430, 2009*

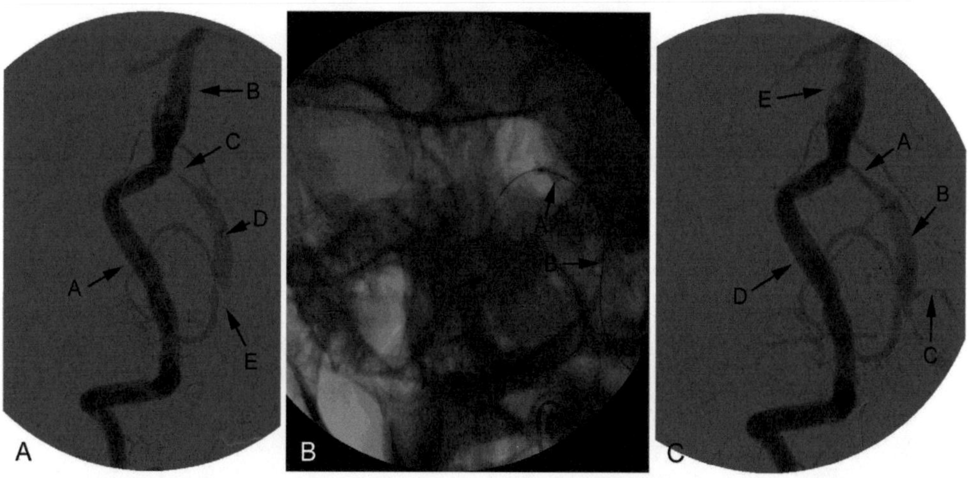


Fig. 16. A 65-year old man presented with neck-movement-related VB insufficiency. The left VA was noted to be occluded extracranially. (A) Right VA (A) angiogram revealed excellent flow into the BA with fenestration (B), a tight stenosis at the junction (C) of the left VA (D) with the BA, and a peak systolic angiographic jet opacifying the PICA (E). (B) A microballoon (A) was brought from the right VA (C) over a wire, which was placed into the left proximal VA (B). (C) Final angiogram revealing significant improvement (despite persistent stenosis) in distal left VA (A) flow noted into the proximal left VA (B) and left PICA (C) following a right VA (D) injection. (E) Basilar artery.

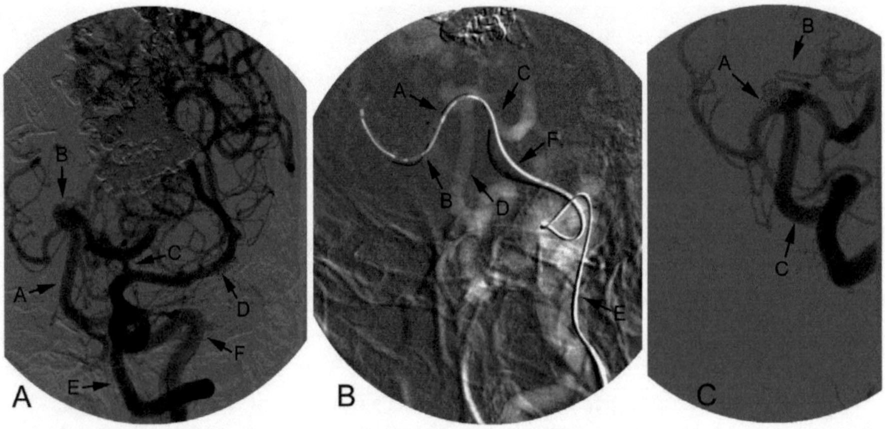

Fig. 17. A 44-year-old man with a Spetzler-Martin Grade IV AVM post-staged embolization and Gamma Knife radiosurgery presented with a residual, broad-based basilar terminus aneurysm. (A) Combined left carotid (E) and left VA (F) angiogram reveals a robust PCoA (C). BA (A), aneurysm (B), MCA (D). (B) Road-map image of an Enterprise stent (Codman Neurovascular) being deployed via the left ICA (E) through the left PCoA (F) from the ipsilateral P1 segment of the PCA (C) across the neck of the aneurysm into the contralateral PCA (B). Deployed stent markers (A). BA (D). (C) The patient was subsequently brought for a second coil embolization session with access to the BA aneurysm achieved from the left VA (C). Angiographically, complete aneurysm obliteration (A) was obtained. The left PCoA (B) is noted.

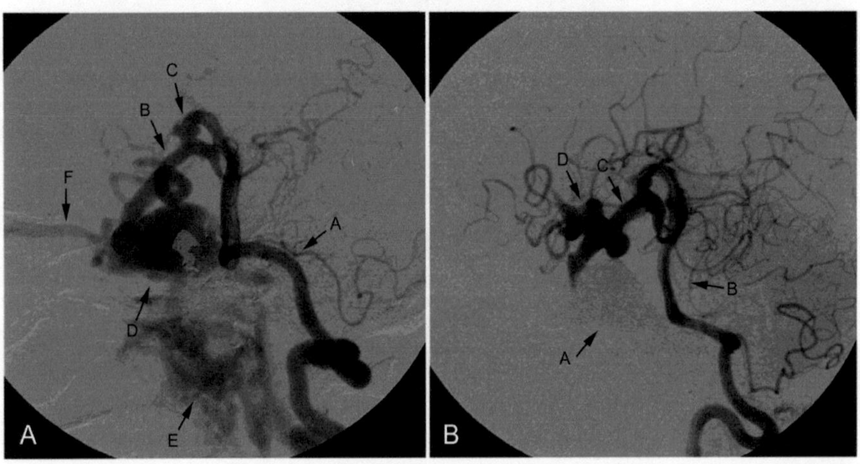

Fig. 18. A 40-year-old man presented with a history of a bullet injury to the head and neck and surgical ligation of the left ICA and now with acute development of a carotid-cavernous fistula. He was noted to have a ruptured, giant cavernous ICA pseudoaneurysm. (A) A left VA (A) angiogram reveals filling of the aneurysm (D) across the PCoA (C) to the supraclinoidal carotid artery (B) with early venous filling of the ophthalmic vein (F) and pterygoid venous plexus (E). (B) The aneurysm was accessed through the same route from the left VA (B) across the PCoA (C) to achieve complete obliteration of the aneurysm and carotid-cavernous fistula (A). MCA (D).

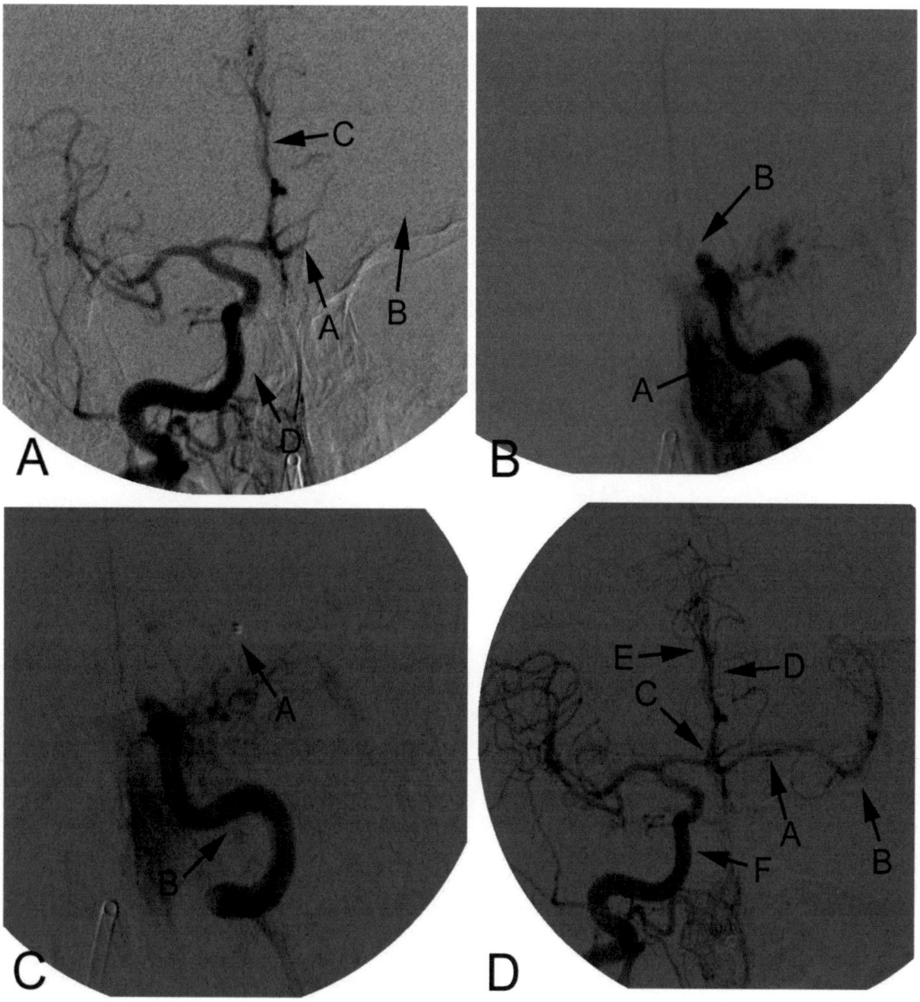


Fig. 19. A 65-year-old man presented with an acute stroke with occlusion of his left ICA. He was beyond the window for intravenous thrombolysis. His ancillary studies suggested potentially viable brain in the MCA territory. However, computed tomographic angiography suggested occlusion of the left MCA territory in addition to more proximal carotid occlusion. An emergent angiogram was planned. (A) A right carotid (D) angiogram performed to assess cross-flow reveals a left ICA terminus occlusion (A) with flow to the bilateral distal ACA circulation across the ACoA (C) but no flow to the left MCA (B). (B) Selective left ICA angiogram reveals complete cavernous occlusion (B) of the left ICA (A). (C) The occlusion (B) was carefully crossed, and a thrombectomy suction catheter (A) was advanced into the occluded left MCA. (D) Following suction aspiration, the clot was retrieved from the MCA (B), resulting in revascularization of the ICA terminus (A) and reestablishment of flow across the ACoA (C) from the right ICA (F). Both ACAs remained patent (E, D). Despite these efforts, the proximal occlusion remained recalcitrant to revascularization efforts and was therefore left occluded. The patient recovered from all deficits.

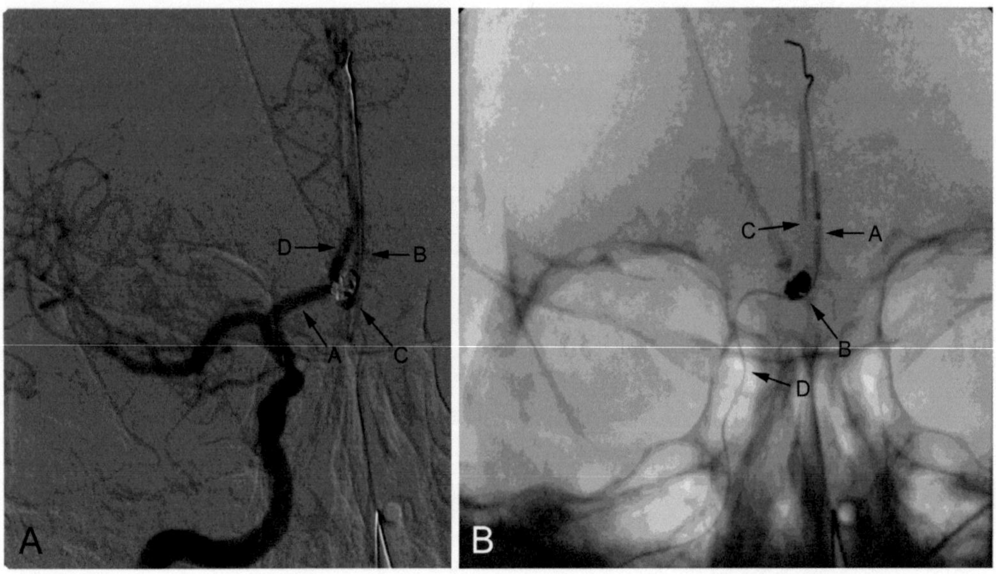


Fig. 20. A 42-year-old man presented with a ruptured ACoA aneurysm, which was treated via coil embolization. On Day 6, he developed severe symptomatic spasm, which remained refractory to maximal medical therapy. He had severe spasm of his left ACA, which resulted in the use of the ACoA artery as a conduit to angioplasty the left distal ACA. (A) Right carotid angiogram reveals a microcatheter and wire across the right ACA (A), AcoA, and aneurysm (C) into the left distal ACA (B). Right distal ACA (D). (B) Non-subtracted angiogram revealing the relationship of the aneurysm and the inflated balloon in the left distal ACA (A). AcoA (B), right distal ACA (C). Access microcatheter in the right ICA (D).

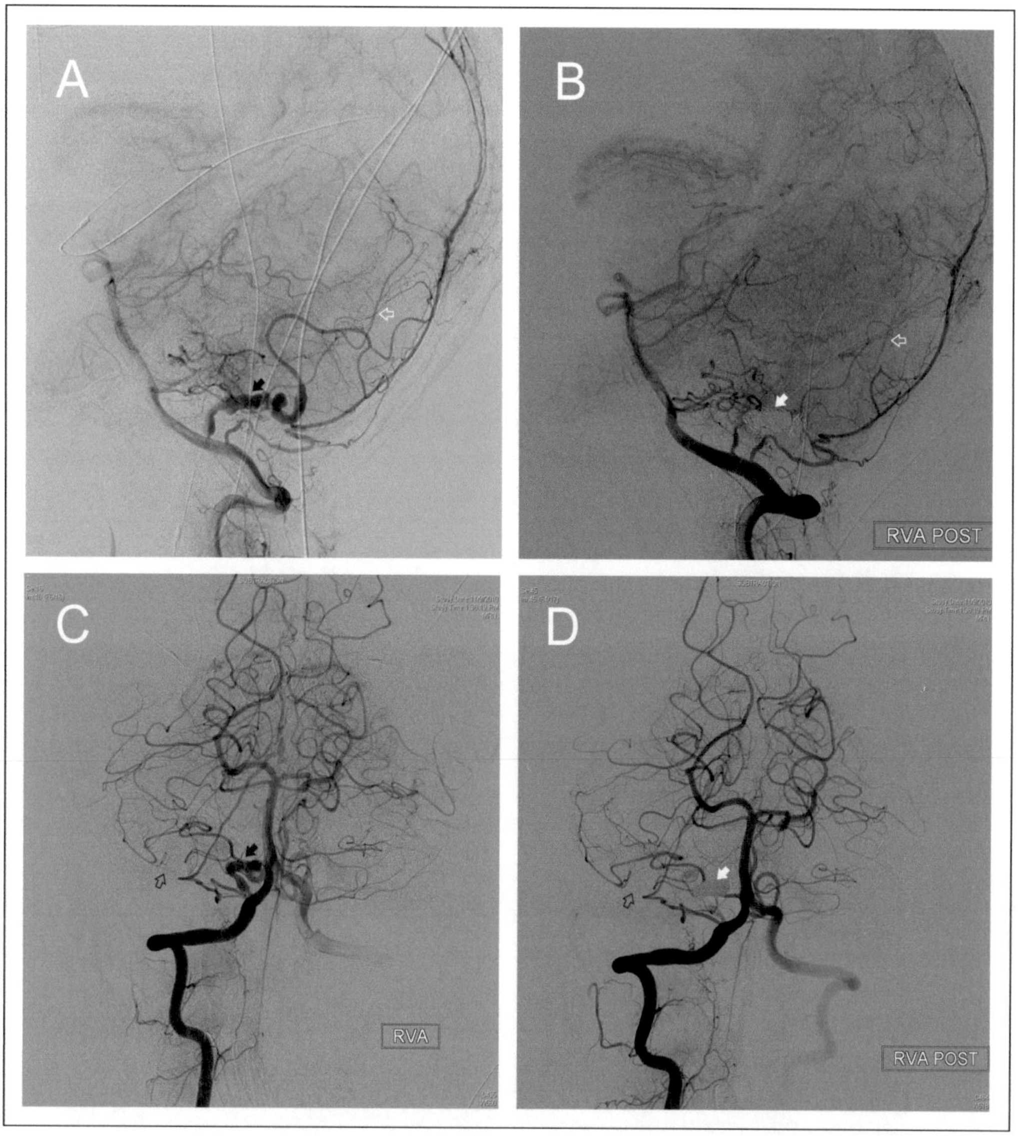


Fig. 21. A 24-year-old man presented with subarachnoid hemorrhage due to proximal right PICA dissection. After superselective micro-balloon test occlusion, it was clear that there are anastomoses from right SCA and AICA to right PICA distal branches. Therefore, the dissecting segment right PICA was successfully occluded with coils without the need of microsurgical bypass procedure, and the patient revealed no deficits following the procedure. The distal branches remains filling after the proximal PICA occlusion. (A) Right vertebral artery angiogram lateral view and (C) anterior-posterior view prior to the treatment. The *black arrows* point to the dissected proximal PICA. (B) Right vertebral artery angiogram lateral view and (D) anterior-posterior view after occlusion of proximal right PICA with coils. The *solid white arrows* indicate coil occlusion of the dissected proximal PICA. *Open white arrows* indicate the distal right PICA filling from collaterals.

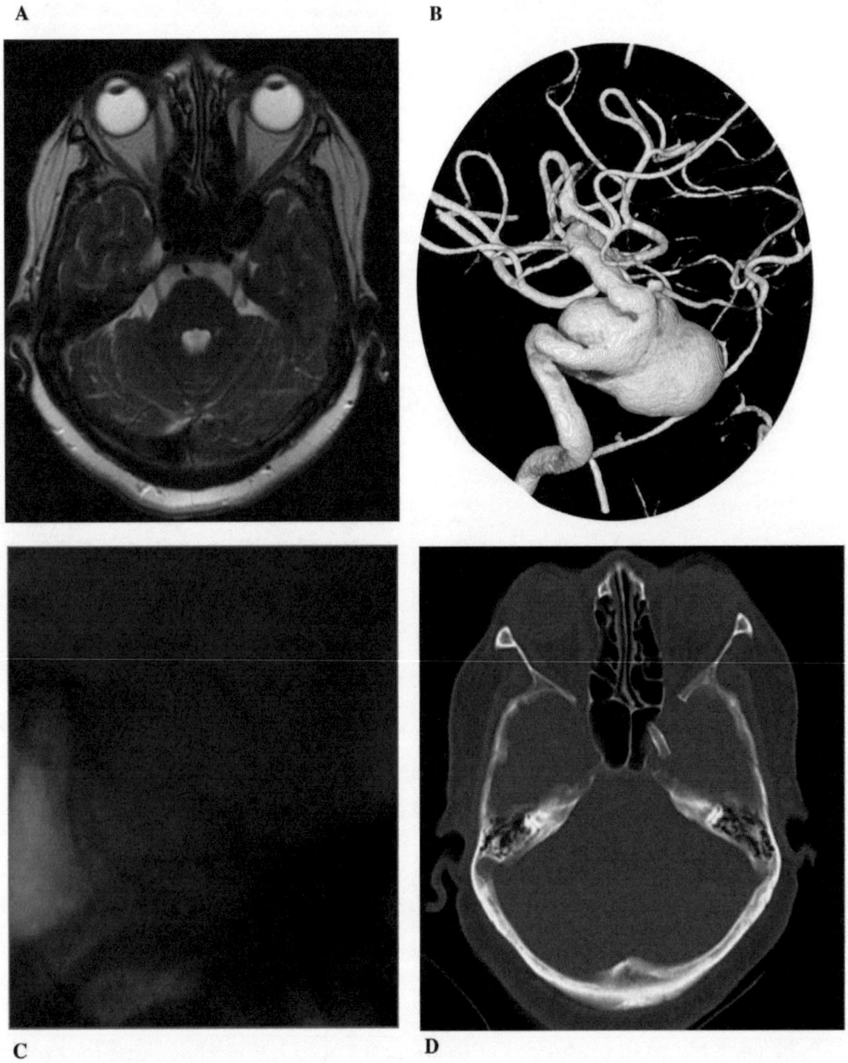


Fig. 22. 64-year old woman presented with increasing headaches after a motor vehicle accident. She was neurologically intact upon presentation. Diagnostic workup revealed a giant cavernous aneurysm (Figure 22 A, B). She was enrolled in the PUFFs trial for utilization of a flow diversion Pipeline Device™ for treatment of large proximal carotid aneurysms. After deployment of the first device the distal access through the aneurysm was lost and despite multiple attempts to regain access through the proximal end of the stent, which had migrated laterally into the aneurysm, distal anterograde access could not be established (Figure 22 C, D).

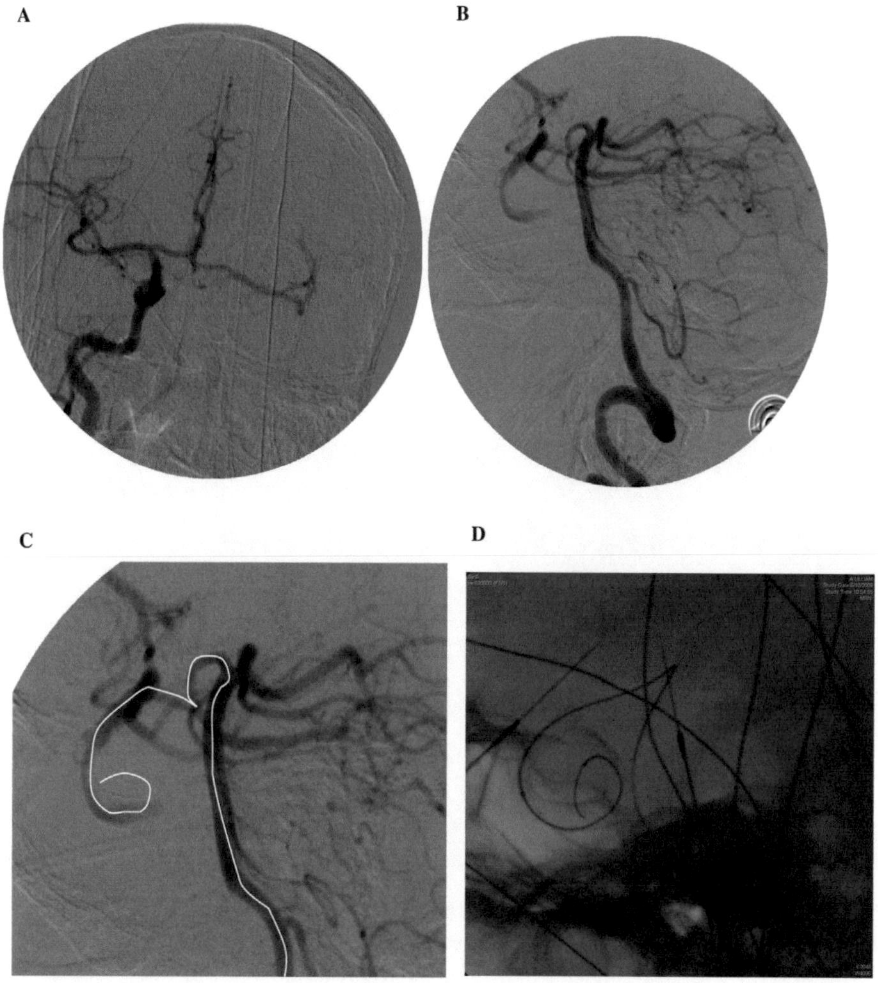

Fig. 23. Review of the circle of Willis appeared to demonstrate both a sizeable ACoA and PCoA arteries therefore a second groin access was established with the guide catheter in the vertebral artery (Figure 23 A, B). A microcatheter was used to catheterize the PCoA artery from the vertebral artery and thereby gain access into the aneurysm using retrograde catheterization of the proximally dislocated but distally tethered Pipeline Device™ (Figure 23 C, D).

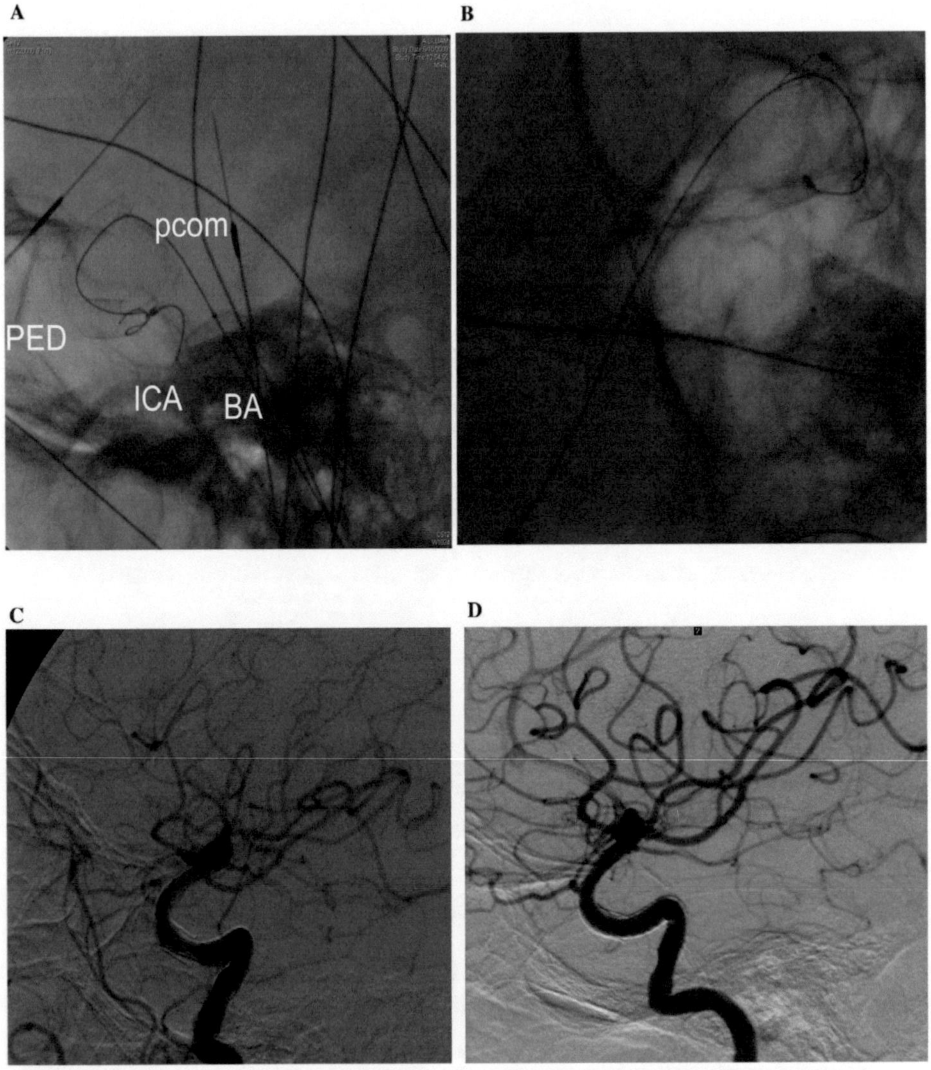


Fig. 24. Once the microwire was in the aneurysm a Snare was deployed to grab the microwire and the Marksman microcatheter was advanced using the snare over the microwire into the Pipeline device by pulling the microwire back out through the PCoA (Figure 24 A, B). Once distal access was reestablished additional Pipeline Devices were used to complete the endovascular reconstruction of the aneurysm. The aneurysm appeared almost completely obliterated at the end of the procedure (Figure 24 C) and remained obliterated at the 6-month follow-up (Figure 24 D).

## 6. Conclusion

An in-depth knowledge of intracranial and extracranial collateral anastomoses, overt or hidden, is crucial for a neurointerventionist to devise optimal endovascular strategies to manage a host of pathological conditions; to ascertain potential pitfalls; and ultimately, to avoid complications that could have been prevented by a better understanding of underlying vascular anatomy. As the scope and extent of endovascular interventions for cerebrovascular and cranial disease continues to expand, the recognition of these putative anastomoses will continue to become a larger part of diagnostic evaluation and interventional design.

## 7. References


[1] Agid R, Terbrugge K, Rodesch G, Andersson T, Soderman M: Management strategies for anterior cranial fossa (ethmoidal) dural arteriovenous fistulas with an emphasis on endovascular treatment. J Neurosurg 110:79-84, 2009

[2] Albuquerque FC, Fiorella DJ, Han PP, Deshmukh VR, Kim LJ, McDougall CG: Endovascular management of intracranial vertebral artery dissecting aneurysms. Neurosurg Focus 18:E3, 2005

[3] Berenstein A, Lasjaunias P, Kricheff, II: Functional anatomy of the facial vasculature in pathologic conditions and its therapeutic application. AJNR Am J Neuroradiol 4:149-153, 1983

[4] Capo H, Kupersmith MJ, Berenstein A, Choi IS, Diamond GA: The clinical importance of the inferolateral trunk of the internal carotid artery. Neurosurgery 28:733-738, 1991

[5] Casasco A, Houdart E, Biondi A, Jhaveri HS, Herbreteau D, Aymard A, et al: Major complications of percutaneous embolization of skull-base tumors. AJNR Am J Neuroradiol 20:179-181, 1999

[6] Chen PR, Ortiz R, Page JH, Siddiqui AH, Veznedaroglu E, Rosenwasser RH: Spontaneous systolic blood pressure elevation during temporary balloon occlusion increases the risk of ischemic events after carotid artery occlusion. Neurosurgery 63:256-265, 2008

[7] Chiam PT, Mocco J, Samuelson RM, Siddiqui AH, Hopkins LN, Levy EI: Retrograde angioplasty for basilar artery stenosis: bypassing bilateral vertebral artery occlusions. J Neurosurg 110:427-430, 2009

[8] Countee RW, Vijayanathan T: External carotid artery in internal carotid artery occlusion. Angiographic, therapeutic, and prognostic considerations. Stroke 10:450-460, 1979

[9] Geibprasert S, Pongpech S, Armstrong D, Krings T: Dangerous extracranial-intracranial anastomoses and supply to the cranial nerves: vessels the neurointerventionalist needs to nnow. AJNR Am J Neuroradiol doi 10.3174/ajnr.A1500; epub March 11, 2009

[10] Hacein-Bey L, Daniels DL, Ulmer JL, Mark LP, Smith MM, Strottmann JM, et al: The ascending pharyngeal artery: branches, anastomoses, and clinical significance. AJNR Am J Neuroradiol 23:1246-1256, 2002

[11] Haffajee MR: A contribution by the ascending pharyngeal artery to the arterial supply of the odontoid process of the axis vertebra. Clin Anat 10:14-18, 1997

[12] Hallacq P, Piotin M, Moret J: Endovascular occlusion of the posterior cerebral artery for the treatment of p2 segment aneurysms: retrospective review of a 10-year series. AJNR Am J Neuroradiol 23:1128-1136, 2002

[13] Hayreh SS: Orbital vascular anatomy. Eye 20:1130-1144, 2006

[14] Larsen WJ: Development of Vasculature. New York (NY): Churchill Livingstone, 1997

[15] Lasjaunias P, Berenstein A, ter Brugge K: Surgical Neuroangiography: 1 Clinical Vascular Anatomy and Variations. Berlin: Springer-Verlag, 2001

[16] Lasjaunias P, Berenstein A, ter Brugge K: Surgical Neuroangiography: 2 Clinical and Endovascular Treatment Aspects in Adults. Berlin: Springer-Verlag, 2004
[17] Lasjaunias P, Moret J, Mink J: The anatomy of the inferolateral trunk (ILT) of the internal carotid artery. Neuroradiology 13:215-220, 1977
[18] Miyachi S, Negoro M, Sugita K: The occipital-vertebral anastomosis as a collateral pathway: hemodynamic patterns--case report. Surg Neurol 32:350-355, 1989
[19] Nakamura M, Kobayashi S, Yoshida T, Kamagata M, Sasaki T: Persistent external carotid-vertebrobasilar anastomosis via the hypoglossal canal. Neuroradiology 42:821-823, 2000
[20] O'Shaughnessy BA, Getch CC, Bendok BR, Batjer HH: Late morphological progression of a dissecting basilar artery aneurysm after staged bilateral vertebral artery occlusion: case report. Surg Neurol 63:236-243, 2005
[21] Osawa S, Rhoton AL, Jr., Tanriover N, Shimizu S, Fujii K: Microsurgical anatomy and surgical exposure of the petrous segment of the internal carotid artery. Neurosurgery 63:210-239, 2008
[22] Osborn AG: Diagnostic Cerebral Angiography (2nd ed). Philadelphia: Lippincott Williams & Wilkins, Wolters Kluwer, 1999
[23] Osborn AG: The vidian artery: normal and pathologic anatomy. Radiology 136:373-378, 1980
[24] Papon X, Pasco A, Fournier HD, Mercier P, Cronier P, Pillet J: Anastomosis between the internal carotid and vertebral artery in the neck. Surg Radiol Anat 17:335-337, 1995
[25] Perrini P, Cardia A, Fraser K, Lanzino G: A microsurgical study of the anatomy and course of the ophthalmic artery and its possibly dangerous anastomoses. J Neurosurg 106:142-150, 2007
[26] Silbergleit R, Quint DJ, Mehta BA, Patel SC, Metes JJ, Noujaim SE: The persistent stapedial artery. AJNR Am J Neuroradiol 21:572-577, 2000
[27] Spetzler RF, Modic M, Bonstelle C: Spontaneous opening of large occipital-vertebral artery anastomosis during embolization. Case report. J Neurosurg 53:849-850, 1980
[28] Standard SC, Ahuja A, Guterman LR, Chavis TD, Gibbons KJ, Barth AP, et al: Balloon test occlusion of the internal carotid artery with hypotensive challenge. AJNR Am J Neuroradiol 16:1453-1458, 1995
[29] Takeuchi M, Kuwayama N, Kubo M, Umemura K, Hirashima Y, Endo S: Vidian artery as a collateral channel between the external and occluded internal carotid arteries--case report. Neurol Med Chir (Tokyo) 45:470-471, 2005
[30] Tubbs RS, Hansasuta A, Loukas M, Louis RG, Jr., Shoja MM, Salter EG, et al: Branches of the petrous and cavernous segments of the internal carotid artery. Clin Anat 20:596-601, 2007
[31] van Rooij WJ, Sluzewski M, Slob MJ, Rinkel GJ: Predictive value of angiographic testing for tolerance to therapeutic occlusion of the carotid artery. AJNR Am J Neuroradiol 26:175-178, 2005
[32] Wada J: A new method for determination of the side of cerebral speech dominance. A preliminary report of the intra-carotid injection of sodium amytal in man. Igaku Seibutsugaki 14:221-222, 1949
[33] Wang H, Fraser K, Wang D, Alvernia J, Lanzino G: Successful intra-arterial basilar artery thrombolysis in a patient with bilateral vertebral artery occlusion: technical case report. Neurosurgery 57:E398, 2005

# 11

# Haemolytic-Uraemic Syndrome: Neurologic Symptoms, Neuroimaging and Neurocognitive Outcome

Ana Roche Martínez[1], Pilar Póo Argüelles[1], Marta Maristany Cucurella[1], Antonio Jiménez Llort[2], Juan A Camacho[2] and Jaume Campistol Plana[1]
*Neurology (1) and Nephrology (2) Departments of Sant Joan de Déu Children's Hospital of Barcelona, Barcelona University (U.B.) Spain*

## 1. Introduction

Haemolytic-Uraemic Syndrome (HUS) was first described in 1955 by Gasser (Pérez del Campo et al., 2000) and defined as a multi-systemic syndrome, due to the association of microangyopathic haemolytic anemia, thrombopenia and multiorganic aggression. HUS affects mainly kidneys and leads to acute renal failure with high levels of urea and creatinin; it often involves digestive and central nervous systems. Central nervous system (CNS) lesions, typically at the basal ganglia, may also affect cortico-subcortical areas and in so doing determines motor and neurocognitive outcome, and modify the patients' quality of life.

Incidence of HUS varies among continents, highly influenced by migration movements, and it is estimated to be around 18/100,000 in children younger than 5 years old. Some countries, like Argentina and South Africa, are considered "endemic", with a steady and relatively high incidence of HUS during all the seasons of the year; other areas, such as Canada, most of the European countries, and the west coast of the USA, are said to be "epidemic", with sporadic cases and a lower incidence of HUS compared to Latin America and Africa during most of the year, but with self-limited relapses during summertime (Exeni, 2001).

HUS etiology is diverse and physiopathologic mechanisms are not yet well known, but infective microorganisms are frequently involved, especially *Escherichia coli,* serotype O15:H7; this bacteria is able to produce a toxic protein (vero-toxin -VT- or Shiga-toxin -Stx), which "recognizes" the endothelial cells and provokes an endothelial lesion (Scheiring, 2010). Other bacteria seem to be involved in different cases of HUS, like *Salmonella enteritidis* and *Streptococcus pneumoniae* (De Loos et al., 2002; Prestidge & Wong, 2009). Mutations in genes coding for different components of the complement system seem to be a risk factor for HUS (Skerka et al., 2009). However, the etiologic agent remains unidentified in most patients.

Clinical presentation in the acute phase includes acute renal failure (100% of patients), often high blood pressure (HBP) due to a volume surcharge (35-40% of patients), and neurological symptoms such as irritability, drowsiness, seizures, cortical blindness, hemiparesis or coma, in up to 35-50% of patients (Montoliu, 1989). These symptoms may be a consequence of different disturbances: metabolic distress (hyponatremia, hyperglycemia, acidosis, fluid imbalance), HBP itself, or CNS microangyopathy. Pancreatic failure and heart involvement are less frequent during the acute phase of HUS (2% of patients).

HUS treatment is based on hydro-electrolytic management: peripheral and central venous pressure must be monitored and cardiac function must be closely controlled; renal function control is especially important, as well as caloric intake adjustment. Neurologic evaluation at the acute phase and during follow-up is crucial to diagnose CNS damage and prevent medium- and long-term sequelae.

No complementary tests have yet been developed to help the clinician in establishing a medium- or long-term prognosis in patients with HUS presenting with neurologic symptoms. Although during the 1980s some authors observed a good clinical outcome in patients with microangyopathic lesions (Steinborn et al., 2004), few references have reported long-term follow-up in these patients. Over the last 20 years, some cases of posterior reversible leuko-encephalopathy syndrome of subacute onset (presenting with drowsiness, lethargy, visual disturbance or seizures) have been described in the context of HUS, sometimes not even associated with HBP (Bennett et al., 2003; Gómez-Lado et al., 2007; Kitamura et al., 2010).

Prognosis factors previously described in different series of patients (Cimolai et al., 1992; Roche et al. 2008), including patient age, acute gastroenteritis symptoms, etiologic agent, seizures at onset, CNS images at the acute phase and neurofunctional tests performance, are reviewed below; clinical course during follow-up and long-term outcome of HUS patients with neurological symptoms are also analyzed.

## 2. Material and methods

Over the last 30 years (1981-2011), a series of 64 patients (29 boys and 35 girls) have presented with HUS in our hospital. Clinical charts of children with neurological symptoms during the acute phase were reviewed, including:

- Clinical data: age at onset, male/female gender, clinical presentation as infectious disease (acute gastroenteritis); "D+" nomenclature is internationally accepted to define acute gastroenteritis history, not regarding infectious agent identification. "D-" is used if acute gastrointestinal infection history was not present.
- Laboratory tests (data not shown but available upon request).
- Infectious agent: *Escherichia coli, Salmonella enteritidis, Streptococcus pneumoniae,* etc.
- Neurological symptoms: seizures, drowsiness, irritability, visual disturbances and paresia.
- Electrophysiological findings in video-electroencephalogram (video-EEG), visual evoked potentials (VEP) and brainstem evoked auditory response (BEAR), during the acute phase and along follow-up.
- Brain perfusion: Medium brain artery (MBA) Doppler ultrasound (US).
- Eye funduscopy at the acute phase and during follow-up.
- Neuroimaging: transfontanelar US, brain computerized tomography (CT), brain magnetic resonance imaging (MRI) at the acute phase and during follow-up.
- Non-neurological complications: pancreatitis, heart dysfunction….

- Medium- and long-term outcome (2-18 years).

Neurologic evaluation was performed by a pediatric neurologist when abnormalities at the initial neurological examination or complementary tests were identified.

Neurological sequelae were considered "medium-term" when they were present between 4 weeks and 12 months after clinical onset; complications were considered "long-term" when they persisted for more than 1 year after admission.

Neurocognitive evaluation was performed when medium or long term sequelae were identified. In these patients, physiotherapy and neurocognitive intervention were started as soon as possible after hospital discharge and continued during the school years.

- Pathology data of the exitus are also summarized.

Follow-up was maintained until clinical normalization or at least 2 years after admission.

## 3. Results

The following tables summarize the patients' characteristics (sex, age at onset), causative agent, clinical presentation, diagnostic tests and clinical course of the 25 patients with HUS and neurological symptoms at onset.

Median age at presentation was 2 years 8 months (range 7 months-7 years old).

As shown in Table 1, sex distribution in HUS patients with neurologic symptoms reveals a higher proportion of girls (64%), with a boy/girl rate of 1:1.7; the rate among patients without neurologic symptoms was 1:1.2, slightly more frequent in girls.

Recent history of acute gastroenteritis (D+) was present in 24/25 patients with HUS and neurological symptoms at onset, although etiologic agent was only found in blood in 4/25 (two *Salmonella enteritidis* and two *E. coli*). One of these patients presented *E coli* both in blood and urine, and another had *Salmonella* in blood and *E. coli* in urine; *E. coli* was also present in urine in another patient.

The most frequent neurologic sign at onset was drowsiness alone (40%) or together with irritability (16%), while irritability alone was present in 10%.

| Patient | Age at onset | Sex M / F[#] | Acute Gastro enteritis[1] | Agent | Dialysis | Acute neurologic presentation |
|---|---|---|---|---|---|---|
| 1 | 1yr 3mo | M | D+ | Unknown | no | Accidental traumatic epidural hematoma |
| 2 | 2yr 3mo | F | D+ | Unknown | yes | Drowsiness |
| 3 | 8mo | F | D+ | Salmonella | yes | Drowsiness. GTCS. Hyponatremia |
| 4 | 7mo | F | D+ | Unknown | yes | Drowsiness → cardiac arrest → myoclonias. Plain EEG within 15 hours |
| 5 | 4yr 6mo | F | D+ | Unknown | yes | GTCS. HBP. Hypoglycemia |
| 6 | 1yr 2mo | M | D- | Unknown | yes | GTCS |
| 7 | 3yr 4mo | M | D+ | Unknown | no | Drowsiness |
| 8 | 3yr | F | D+ | Unknown | yes | HBP. Brain edema. Irritability and drowsiness |
| 9 | 2yr 2mo | M | D+ | Unknown | yes | Neurologic depression. Myoclonic seizures |

| | | | | | | |
|---|---|---|---|---|---|---|
| 10 | 4yr 6mo | M | D+ | Salmonella *E.coli* (urine) | yes | Consciousness decrease. Irritability |
| 11 | 1yr 10mo | F | D+ | Unknown | yes | Consciousness decrease. Myosis. Pyramidal signs |
| 12 | 1yr 6mo | F | D+ | Unknown | yes | Drowsiness, pyramidal signs |
| 13 | 2yr 2mo | M | D+ | Unknown | no | Irritability-drowsiness |
| 14 | 6yr | F | D+ | *E.Coli* (urine and blood) | yes | Drowsiness |
| 15 | 1yr 2mo | M | D+ | Unknown | yes | GTCS |
| 16 | 3yr 8mo | F | D+ | Unknown | yes | Drowsiness, irritability |
| 17 | 1yr 8mo | F | D+ | Unknown | yes | Drowsiness. Loss of consciousness |
| 18 | 2yr 2mo | F | D+ | Unknown | yes | GTCS. Anisocoria |
| 19 | 3yr 1mo | F | D+ | *E.Coli* (urine) | yes | Drowsiness |
| 20 | 7yr 4mo | F | D+ | Unknown | yes | Drowsiness |
| 21* | 3yr | F | D+ | E.Coli | yes | Stupor. Consciousness decrease. Slow ocular movements |
| 22 | 3yr 11mo | M | D+ | Unknown | yes | Irritability, agitation, drowsiness, orolingual dystonia. |
| 23 | 4 yr | F | D+ | Unknown | yes | Drowsiness |
| 24 | 12 mo | F | D+ | Unknown | yes | GTCS |
| 25 | 12 mo | M | D+ | Unknown | yes | GTCS |

GTCS: generalized tonic-clonic seizure; HBP: high blood pressure;#M:male / F:female;*Trip to Argentina a few days before acute gastroenteritis

Table 1. Acute neurologic presentation on HUS context.

Nine patients suffered seizures at onset (generalized tonic-clonic, tonic or myoclonic seizures), which stands for 14% of all HUS patients and 36% of neurologic HUS patients. All nine patients survived without important long term sequelae. However, patients presenting seizure recurrence (patient 6) or myoclonic seizures during the acute phase (patient 9) developed medium term sequelae.

One patient presented orolingual dystonia shortly after clinical onset with irritability and drowsiness; no other patients showed abnormal movements at the acute phase or during follow up.

Eleven children had some neurological complementary test performed: eye funduscopy showed fovea erythrosis in patient 4 (exitus), and patient 21 presented delayed and disorganized VEP with normal BEAR. Video EEG was abnormal for all the patients who underwent it (5/9), with slow background activity; transfontanellar US, BMA Doppler US brain CT and MRI (both in the acute phase and during follow-up) findings are summarized in Table 2.

Brain MRI findings of patients 6 (Figures 1 and 2) and 21 (Figures 3 and 4) are consistent with vasculitic lesions due to diffuse hypoxic-ischemic aggression, with cortico-subcortical and basal ganglia distribution. Despite these findings, which were persistent along follow-up, both patients presented a favorable course without important long-term sequelae.

| Patient | EEG | Brain ultrasound | Brain CT | Brain MRI acute phase | Brain MRI control |
|---|---|---|---|---|---|
| 4 | Plain EEG 15 hours after onset | Normal at the acute phase. Absence of supra-tentorial pulse 15h after onset | Not performed | Not performed | Not performed |
| 6 | Bilateral hemispheric abnormalities | Not performed | Not performed | Cortico-subcortical atrophy. Putamen necrosis | Putamen necrosis |
| 11 | Combination $\theta$,$\alpha$ and $\beta$ waves, without paroxysmal activity | Normal | Normal | Not performed | Not performed |
| 15 | Diffuse slow background. Left temporal paroxysms | Prominent sulci | Not performed | Not performed | Not performed |
| 17 | Paradoxal reactivity with slow background and slow high voltage waves in both hemispheres, no paroxysms | Not performed | Not performed | Not performed | Not performed |
| 21 | Not performed | Bilateral hemispheric abnormalities, of left predominance | Multiple cortico-subcortical hypointense images, consistent with brain edema | Basal ganglia necrosis and cortico-subcortical atrophy, consistent with vasculitis | Basal ganglia necrosis and cortico-subcortical atrophy also affecting cerebellum |
| 22 | Not performed | Normal brain medium artery Doppler ultrasound | Not performed | Normal diffusion brain MRI | Not performed |
| 24 | Not performed | Not performed | Not performed | Normal | Not performed |
| 25 | Not performed | Not performed | Normal | Not performed | Not performed |

Table 2. Results of the pathologic tests in patients with HUS and neurologic symptoms at the acute phase and MRI control.

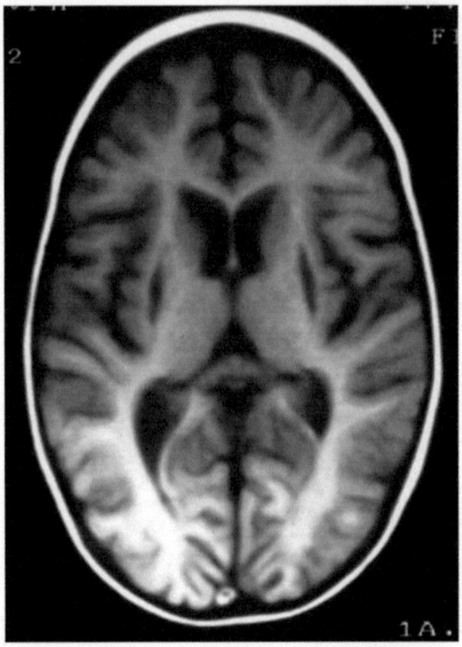

A

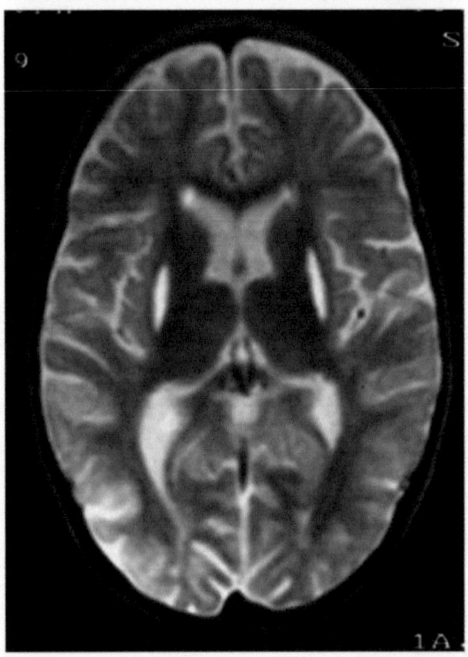

B

Fig. 1. Brain MRI of patient n. 6, six days after clinical onset.

T1 (A) and T2 (B) axial sequences, consistent with cortico-subcortical atrophy. Symmetrical areas of putamen necrosis.

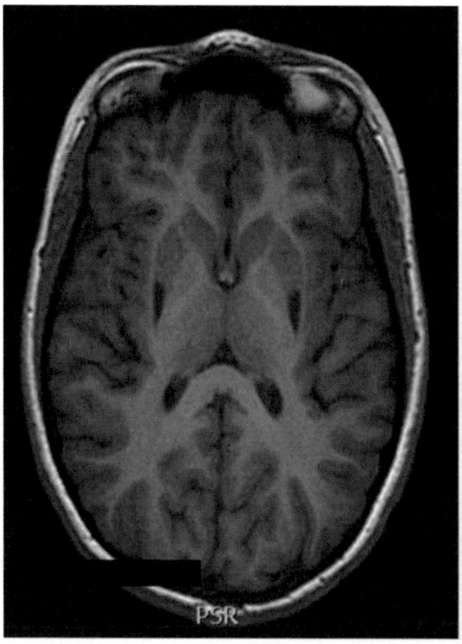


Figure 2.A

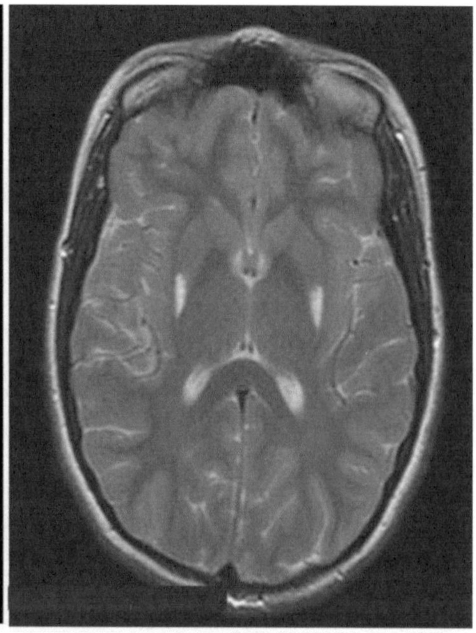

Figure 2.B

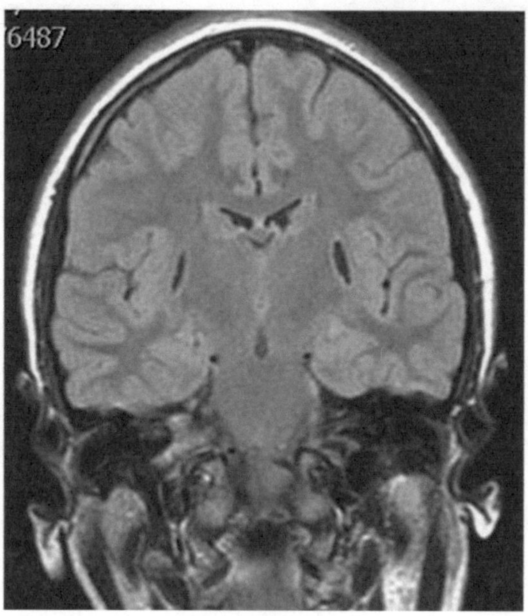


Figure 2.C

Fig. 2. Brain MRI of patient n. 6, fifteen years after clinical presentation. Axial T1 (A) and FLAIR (B), and coronal T2 (C) sequences. The bilateral putamen necrotic areas remain unchanged compared to the previous study.

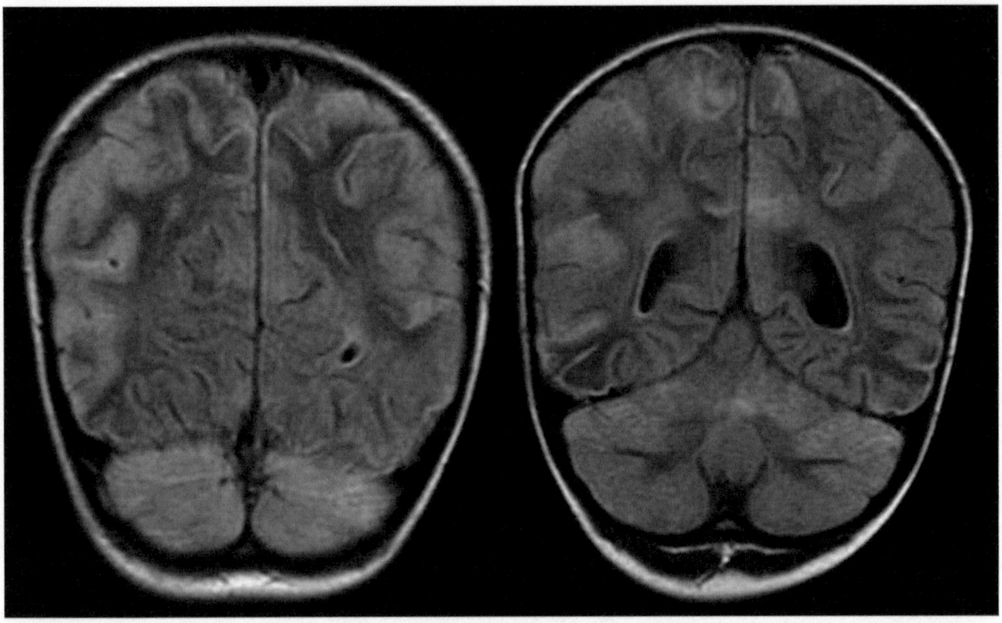

Figure 3.A Figure 3.B

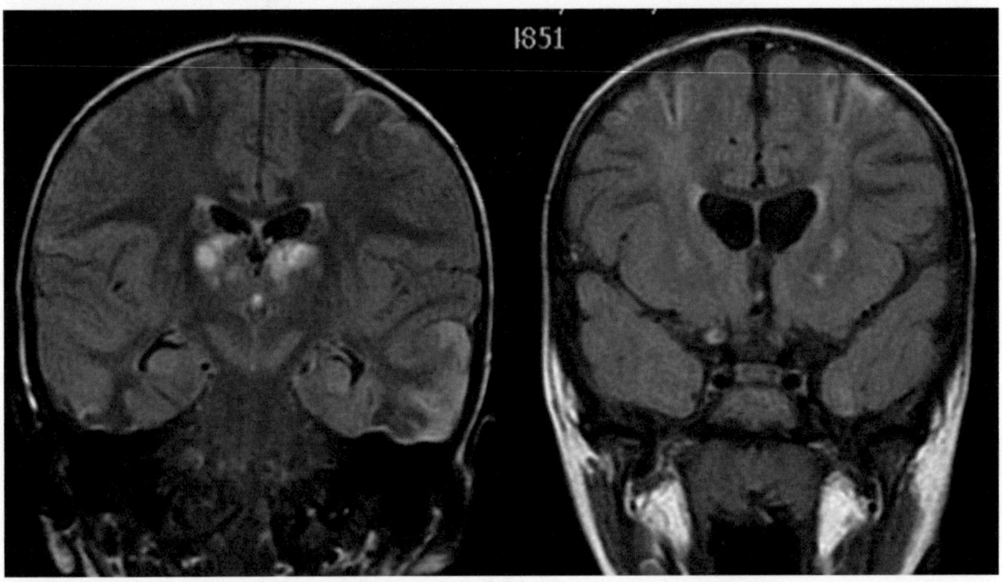


Figure 3.C Figure 3.D

Fig. 3. Brain MRI of patient n. 21, six days after clinical onset. Coronal FLAIR (A, B, C and D) sequences. Prominence of the convexity sulci and increased ventricular size, consistent with cortico-subcortical atrophy. Bilateral hyperintense areas at the basal ganglia. Multiple cortico-subcortical supratentorial hyperintensities, more subtle at the cerebellar lobes, suggestive of ischemic lesions.

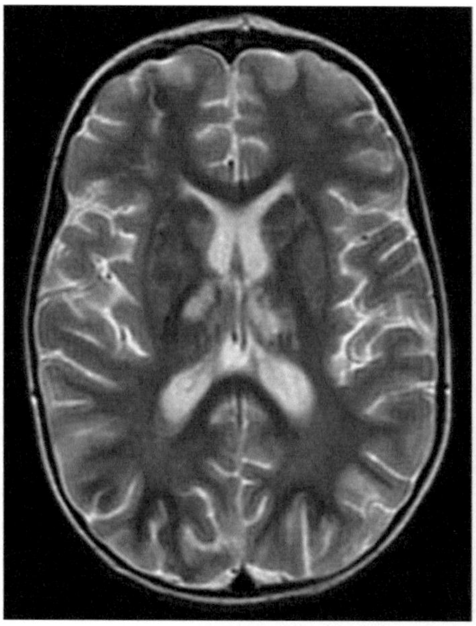

Figure 3.E

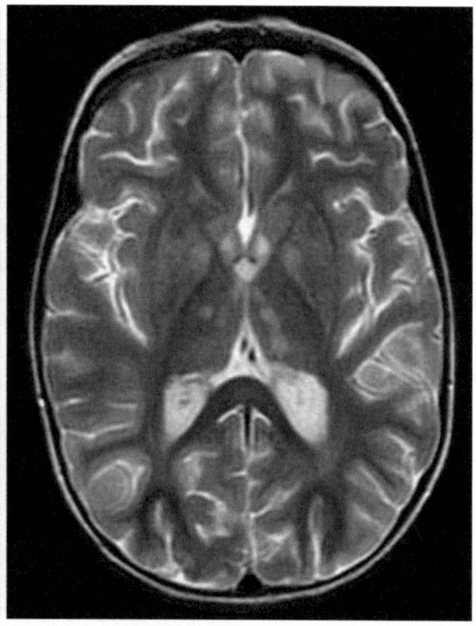

Figure 3.F

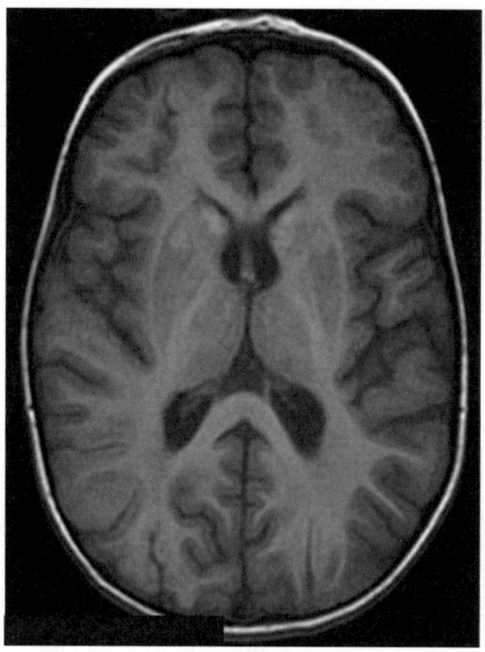

Figure 3.G

Fig. 3. Brain MRI of patient n. 21, six days after clinical onset. Axial T2 FS (E, F) and T1 (G) sequences. Prominence of the convexity sulci and increased ventricular size, consistent with cortico-subcortical atrophy. Bilateral hyperintense areas at the basal ganglia. Multiple cortico-subcortical supratentorial hyperintensities, milder at the cerebellar lobes, suggestive of ischemic lesions.

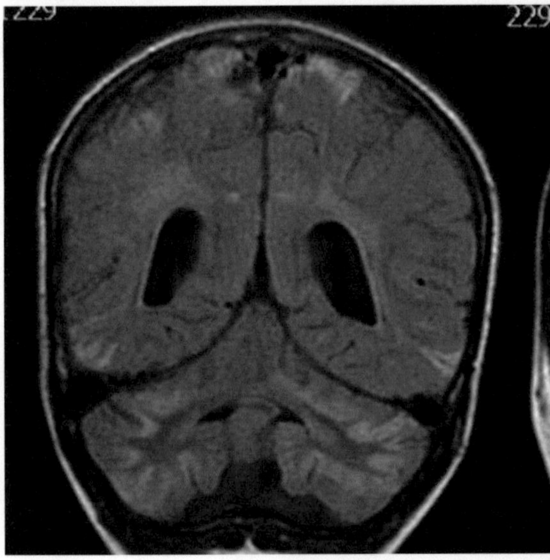

Figure 4.A

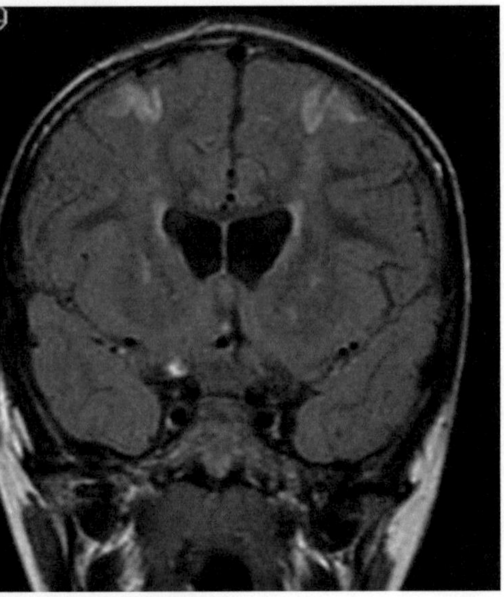


Figure 4.B

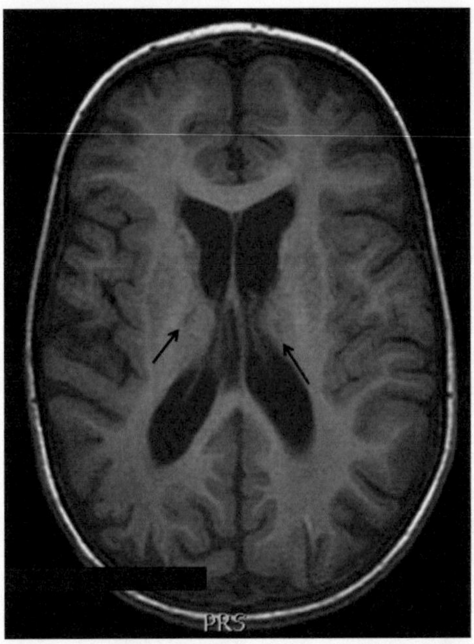


Figure 4.C

Fig. 4. Brain MRI of patient n. 21, 6 months after clinical onset. Coronal FLAIR sequences (Figures A and B). Increased ventricular size, bilateral hyperintense areas at the basal ganglia and multiple cortico-subcortical supratentorial hyperintense images, milder at cerebellar lobes, suggestive of subacute ischemic lesions, with laminar cortical necrosis. Axial T1 sequence (C) showing basal ganglia necrosis (arrows) and cortico-subcortical atrophy.

| Patient | Diagnostic Test | Medium-term outcome | Long-term outcome |
|---|---|---|---|
| 1 | No | Normal | Normal |
| 2 | No | Normal | Normal |
| 3 | No | Normal | Normal |
| 4 | Transfontanellar ultrasound* Pathology | Exitus in the acute phase | Exitus in the acute phase |
| 5 | No | Normal | Normal |
| 6 | EEG* Brain MRI* Renal biopsy. Heart Doppler and EKG | Left hemiplegia Hypertensive retinopathy Renal function worsening Hypertrophic myocardiopathy | Asymptomatic |
| 7 | No | Normal | Normal |
| 8 | Eye funduscopy | Normal | Normal |
| 9 | VEP. ERG. EEG* Brain MRI*. SPECT* | Cognitive and language delay and epilepsy due to cortical dysplasia. | Consistent with his base line neurodevelopment |
| 10 | No | Normal | Normal |
| 11 | EEG* Brain CT | Slight cognitive delay | Outside follow-up, described as normal |
| 12 | No | Normal | Normal |
| 13 | No | Normal | Normal |
| 14 | No | Normal | Normal |
| 15 | Transfontanellar ultrasound EEG* | Learning disability | Normal |
| 16 | No | Normal | Normal |
| 17 | EEG* | Normal | Normal |
| 18 | No | Normal | Normal |
| 19 | No | Acute pancreatitis | Normal |
| 20 | No | Normal | Normal |
| 21 | Brain CT*. Brain MRI* EEG*. VEP*. PEAT | Visual impairment | Slight visual impairment Slightly unstructured EEG |
| 22 | Diffusion MRI*. EEG Lumbar puncture Brain medium artery Doppler ultrasound | Visual impairment Cognitive impairment | Normal |
| 23 | No | normal | normal |
| 24 | Brain MRI | normal | normal |
| 25 | Brain CT | normal | normal |

Table 3. Diagnostic tests, medium- and long-term outcome of patients with neurologic symptoms at the acute phase; (*) abnormal test.

Five of the 25 patients with neurologic symptoms at the acute phase showed one or more medium-term neurological deficits (Table 3): 1/5 hemiparesia, 4/5 mild cognitive dysfunction and 2/5 visuo-perception and construction deficits, which almost normalized during long-term follow up. Nineteen of the 25 presented normal neurological examination at hospital discharge, and one year later.

Patient 4 died within the first 15 hours after admission, after a rapidly progressive neurologic deterioration and respiratory arrest. He presented lower limb myoclonias after life rescue. Thorax x-ray revealed right inferior lobe (RIL) pneumonia. Abdomen and transfontanellar US were normal. Pathology studies confirmed RIL pneumonia, severe segmentary glomerular and tubular nephropathy, acute pancreatitis, lung and heart interstitial inflammation, diffuse alveolar damage, intracapillary thrombi in lungs and kidneys, brain cortical necrosis with edema and cerebellar granular necrosis. *Steptococcus pneumoniae* was not identified. This represents a mortality of 1.5% of the HUS patients and 4% of the patients with HUS and neurologic symptoms at onset.

## 4. Comments

HUS is a multisystemic entity; its incidence in Europe has been sporadic in the past, although recent migration movements have facilitated a relapse of cases in several countries. In general, older patients tend to show milder neurologic symptoms at onset, like drowsiness or irritability, while younger patients, especially under 18 months, tend to present seizures during the acute phase.

Physiopathology is not yet well understood, but experimental and in vivo studies (Ren et al., 1999; Carter, 1986; Cimolai, 1896) have proved that *Escherichia coli* VT induces thrombopenia through consuming, kidnapping, aggregation and platelet dysfunction mechanisms; plasminogen inhibitor activity is also enhanced, and therefore fibrinolysis is inhibited. Released factors such as TNF, IL, FvW monomers, free radicals, thromboxane, etc., provoke endothelial lesions and vasculitic events in several organs, especially kidneys, digestive system and brain (Seth et al., 1896; Miller & Kin, 1987; Montoliu, 1989; Hahn et al., 1989; Erikson et al., 2001; Steinborn et al., 2004; Rivero et al., 2004). VT receptors are present in various troncoencephalic nuclei, the amygdala and the hippocampus, and in the posterior root neurons of the ganglia. This suggests VT may induce primary neuronal damage as well as a vasculitic lesion (Hahn et al., 1989; Hamano et al., 1993; Rivero et al., 2004). This probably happens also at the basal ganglia, especially at putamen nucleae, the most frequent localization of CNS lesions (Nakamura et al., 2003). The vasculitic damage (due to the diffuse hypoxic-ischemic aggression) observed in our patients was mainly localized at cortico-subcortical areas and the basal ganglia, as described in previous reports (Ren et al., 1999; Akasaka et al., 1999; Garel et al., 2004). Clinical course of patients with these lesions was favorable, and MRI lesions became smaller on follow-up controls. Brain MRI sequenced controls of patients 6 and 21 reinforce the hypothesis of vasculitic lesion as the main cause of tissue damage, although direct neuronal toxicity could not be disclosed (Hahn et al., 1989). In contrast with previous reports (Theobald et al., 2001), basal ganglia necrosis has not proved to be a bad prognosis factor in our series: our patients did not present extrapyramidal signs, as other authors have reported (Di Mario et al., 1987; Barnett et al., 1995).

Unfavorable neurologic outcome was formerly correlated with seizures at onset of symptoms and plasmapheresis (unnecessary for our patients) at diagnosis (Cimolai et al.,

1986). The nine patients who presented seizures at onset survived without long-term sequelae, whereas the only exitus presented initial drowsiness and rapidly progressive neurologic deterioration, without seizures (myoclonias happened after resuscitation maneuvers). This was the only patient with neurologic symptoms, acute pancreatitis, endocarditis and RIL pneumonia; *Streptococcus pneumoniae* was not detected (De Loos et al., 2002; Prestidge & Wong, 2009). Neurologic evaluation and follow-up of patients with CNS symptoms allowed early detection of subtle vision dysfunction, visual perception deficit, and mild cognitive disabilities.

Incidence of neurologic symptoms in acute phase of HUS in this group (39%) was similar to former descriptive studies (Sheth et al., 1986; Hahn et al., 1989; Garel et al., 2004; Steinborn et al., 2004); orolingual dystonia was previously observed, but cortical blindness, hallucinations (Cimolai et al., 1896) and cerebellar mutism/anarthria (Mewasingh et al., 2003) were not observed in our group. A slightly higher prevalence in girls was identified (boy/girl rate 1:1.2), as reported by other authors (Cimolai et al., 1986; Rivero et al., 2004; Zambrano et al., 2005); this rate is increased to 1:1,7 when regarding the neurologic patients, perhaps related to specific auto-immune characteristics.

It was previously reported that HUS patients with partial seizures tend to present epilepsy or abnormal movements after HUS recovery (Dhuna et al., 1992; Hue et al., 1992; Koehl et al., 2010). However, none of our patients developed abnormal movements during medium- and long-term follow-up, and seizures or EEG abnormalities at the acute phase did not determine a poor outcome (only the patient with previously diagnosed cortical dysplasia presented focal seizures).

SHU mortality has decreased in recent years, from 25% in the 1980s to 2% in more recent publications (Rivero et al., 2004). Despite this low mortality rate, a small percentage of patients with neurological symptoms at the acute stage subsequently present neurological sequelae. In our series of 25 children with neurological symptoms, one patient died and 5 had medium-term neurological complications (hemiparesia, cognitive delay or visual perception deficit). The rates of medium-term neurologic morbidity (20%) and mortality (4%) were similar to those of other authors (Hahn et al., 1989; Erikson et al., 2001). Only in one patient after 3 years of follow-up were there persistent minor neurological sequelae (slight cognitive, visual perception and visual construction impairments), with gradual improvement despite the absence of significant changes on MRI and visual evoked potentials monitoring. Although neurocognitive impairment is not frequently reported in HUS (Roche et al., 2008), neuropsychological evaluation and follow-up of these children, especially when basal ganglia (mainly putamen) and cortico-subcortical regions are damaged at the initial brain MRI, helps to identify neurocognitive disabilities. Even if they are not severe, a good neurofunctional diagnosis and rehabilitation can help patients with their school performance and day-to-day life.

## 5. Conclusions

In summary, HUS is not yet completely understood from a physiological point of view. The most common neurological manifestations in the acute phase are drowsiness, stupor, irritability and convulsions. Neurological morbidity is important: it affects 20% of children with acute neurological presentation (8% of all patients with HUS). Seizures at presentation were not a risk factor for poor outcome in our series. Electrophysiological abnormalities at the acute phase tend to normalize; when they persist, clinical expression is very subtle. Importantly, brain lesions may persist during follow-up despite clinical recovery. No clear correlation can be established between MRI findings and long-term clinical outcome. Neurocognitive evaluation of children with neurological impairment in the context of SHU should be part of the medium- and long-term follow-up in these patients.

## 6. References

Akasaka N, Hayakawa H, Okugawa T, Kasahara T, Ishikawa N, Tojo M et al. Serial cerebral computed tomography and magnetic resonance imaging in a case of hemolytic uremic syndrome with the complication of the central nervous system due to Escherichia coli O157:H7. *No To Hattatsu* 1999;31:565-70

Barnett ND, Kaplan AM, Bernes SM & Cohen ML. Hemolytic uremic syndrome with particular involvement of basal ganglia and favorable outcome. *Pediatr Neurol* 1995;12:155-58

Bennett B, Booth T & Quan A. Late onset seizures, hemiparesis and blindness in hemolytic uremic syndrome *Clin Nephrol* 2003;59:196-200

Cimolai N & Carter JE. Bacterial genotype and neurological complications of Escherichia coli O157:H7-associated haemolytic uraemic syndrome. *Acta Pediatr* 1986;87: 593-94

Cimolai N, Morrison BJ & Carter JE. Risk factors for the CNS manifestations of gastroenteritis associated HUS. *Pediatrics* 1992;90:616-21

De Loos F, Huijben K, van der Kar NCAJ, Monnens LAH, van den Heuvel LPWJ, Groener JEM et al. Hemolytic uremic syndrome attributable to *Streptococcus pneumoniae* infection: a novel cause for secondary protein n-glycan abnormalities. *Clinical Chemistry* 2002 48;781-84

Dhuna A, Pascual-Leone A, Talwar D & Torres F. EEG and seizures in children with hemolytic-uremic syndrome. *Epilepsia* 1992;33:482-86

DiMario FJ Jr, Brönte-Stewart H, Sherbotie J & Turner ME. Lacunar infarction of the basal ganglia as a complication of hemolytic-uremic syndrome. MRI and clinical correlations. *Clin Pediatr (Phila)* 1987;26:586-89

Exeni R. Aspectos Clínicos del Síndrome Hemolítico Urémico. http://www. medwave.cl /congresos/2nefro2001

Erikson KJ, Boyd SG & Tasker RC. Acute neurology and neurophysiology of haemolytic-uraemic syndrome. *Arch Dis Child* 2001;84:434-35

Garel L, Vázquez E & Lucaya J. Clinical quiz. Pediatr Radiol 2004;34:92-93

Gómez-Lado C, Martinón-Torres F, Álvarez-Moreno, Eiris-Puñal J, Carreira-Sande N, Rodríguez-Núñez A & Castro-Gago M. Leucoencefalopatía posterior reversible: una complicación infrecuente en el curso del síndrome hemolítico urémico. *Rev Neurol* 2007;44:475-78

Hahn JS, Havens PL, Higging JJ, O'Rourke PP, Estroff JA & Strand R. Neurologycal complications of hemolytic-uremic syndrome. *J Child Neurol* 1989;4:108-13

Hamano S, Nakanishi Y, Nara T, Seki T, Ohtani T, Oishi T et al. Neurological manifestations of hemorrhagic colitis in the outbreak of Escherichia coli O157:H7 infection in Japan. *Acta Paediatr* 1993;825:454-58

Hue V, Leclerc F, Martinot A, Vallee L & Saunier P. Striatal involvement with abnormal movements in hemolytic-uremic syndrome. *Arch Fr Pediatr* 1992;49:369-71

Kitamura M, Furusu A, Hirose M, Nishino T, Obata Y, Uramatsu T & Kohno S. A case of reversible posterior leukoencephalopathy syndrome in a patient on peritoneal dialysis. *Clin Exp Nephrol* 2010;14:633-36

Koehl B, Boyer O, Biebuyck-Gougé N, Kossorotoff M, Frémeaux-Bacchi V, Boddaert N & Niaudet P. Neurological involvement in a child with atypical hemolytic uremic syndrome. *Pediatr Nephrol* 2010;25:2539-42

Miller K, Kin Y. Hemolytic Uremic Syndrome. In: Holliday AA, Martin Barrat J & Vernier RK. Pediatric nephrology, 2nd ed. Baltimore, USA: Williams and Wilkins, 1987: 482-89

Mewasingh LD, Kadhim H, Christophe C, Christiaens FJ & Dan B. Nonsurgical cerebellar mutism (anarthria) in two children. *Pediatr Neurol* 2003;28:59-63

Montoliu J. Microangiopatía trombótica. Síndrome urémico-hemolítico y púrpura trombótica trombocitopénica. MTA *Medicina Interna* 1989;7:517-46

Nakamura H, Takaba H, Inoue T, Saku Y, Saito F, Ibayashi S & Fujishima M. MRI findings of hemolytic uremic syndrome with encephalopathy: widespread symmetrical distribution. *J Neuroimaging* 2003;13:75-78

Pérez del Campo Y, Espinosa López DM., Florín Yrabien J, Levy ON, Alvarez Arias CZ & Infante Velázquez E. Síndrome hemolítico urémico: Aspectos epidemiológicos y patogénicos. *Rev Cubana Pediatr* 2000;3:203-13

Prestidge C & Wong W. Ten years of pneumococcal-associated haemolytic uraemic syndrome in New Zealand children. *J Paediatr Child Health* 2009;45:731-5

Ren J, Utsunomiya I, Taguchi K, Ariga T, Tai T, Ihara Y & Miyatake T. Localization of verotoxin receptors in nervous system. *Brain Research* 1999;825:183-88

Rivero MA, Padola NL, Etcheverría AI & Parma AE. Escherichia coli enterohemorrágica y síndrome hemolítico urémico en Argentina. *Medicina (Buenos Aires)* 2004;64:352-56

Roche Martínez A, Póo P, Maristany-Cucurella M, Jiménez-Llort A, Camacho JA & Campistol J. Neurologic presentation in haemolytic-uraemic syndrome. *Rev Neurol* 2008 16-31;47:191-96

Scheiring J, Rosales A & Zimmerhackl LB. Clinical practice. Today's understanding of the haemolytic uraemic syndrome. *Eur J Pediatr 2010*;169:7-13

Skerka C, Jazsi M, Zipfel PF, Dragon-Durey MA & Fremeaux-Bacchi V. Autoantibodies in haemolytic uraemic syndrome (HUS). *Thromb Haemost* 2009;101:227-32

Sheth KJ, Swick HM & Haworth N. Neurological involvement in HSU. *Ann Neurol* 1986;19:90-93

Steinborn M, Leiz S, Rûdisser K, Griebel M, Harder T & Halm H. CT and MRI in haemolytic uraemic syndrome with central nervous system involvement: distribution of lesions and prognostic value of image findings. *Pediatr Radiol* 2004;34:805-10

Theobald I, Kuwertz-Bröking E, Schiborr M & Heindel. Central nervous system involvement in hemolytic uremic syndrome (HUS), a retrospective analysis of cerebral CT and MRI studies. *Clin Nephrol* 2001;56:S3-8

Zambrano O, Deluchi B & Hevia J. Síndrome hemolítico urémico en Santiago de Chile: Evolución de la función renal y factores pronósticos. *Rev Chil Pediatr* 2005;76: 48-56

# 12

# Clinical and Genetic Aspects in Patients with Idiopathic Parkinson Disease

Arben Taravari, Marija Milanovska, Igor Petrov, Vera Petrova, Merita Ismajli-Marku, Besim Memedi, Fadil Cana and Fatmir Mexhiti
*PHO University Clinic of Neurology Skopje,*
*R. Macedonia*

## 1. Introduction

Parkinson syndrome is one of the most often neurodegenerative diseases, which affects the Central Nervous system. James Parkinson was the first who described the clinical symptoms of factor complex, a complex which can be present as a combination of six cardinal signs: tremor, rigor, bradikinesia-hypokinesia, curve pose, lose of postural reflexes and freezing phenomena. To get to the final diagnose, the clinicians usually use the Brain Bank Criteria of UKPDS [9].

Generally, there are four categories of Parkinsonism: Idiopathic Parkinson Disease; Secondary Parkinsonism; Parkinson plus syndrome and other neurodegenerative diseases in which Parkinsonism is main clinical manifestation [7].

Idiopathic Parkinson disease is the most represented type of Parkinsonism and it is maintained in almost 80 percents of the patients with movement disorders. Mostly with unilateral presentation, well respons on Dopamine-agonists and Levodopa, characterized with general slowness and typical tremor, from 4 to 6 Herz.

The basic patho-anatomical findings in patients with Idiopathic Parkinson Disease, is loss of neurons which contain neuromelanin. These neurons are located in particular parts of the brain, such as substantia nigra and locus ceruleus. Dopamine level is reduced for almost 80 percents under normal level, especially in striatum [7].

Hystopatological findings direct to presence of intracellular inclusions called Lewy-body, primary in substantia nigra, and they contain alpha-synuclein.

Alpha-synuclein is present in many parts of the brain, but mostly in substantia nigra, and it is the only synuclein included in Parkinson disease. It was found that two non-sence mutations in gene of alpha-synuclein, A53T and A30P, are closely related with early appearance of Idiopathic Parkinson Disease between populations in Europe. Accumulation of this protein in dopaminergic neurons is responsible for the process of neurodegeneration [20].

## 2. Aims

1. To determinate age, sex and difficulty of clinical manifestations in patients with Idiopathic Parkinson Disease, using UPDRS scale.
2. To compare the findings of genetic researches, by age and sex in patients with Idiopathic Parkison's Disease, with those in control group.

## 3. Materials and methodes

This is a prospective study, clinical and genetic, approved by the Ethical Committee, at Medical Faculty of Skopje. The clinical part of the study was made at University Clinic of Neurology in Skopje. Laboratory and genetic part of the study was made at the laboratory of molecular biology at Faculty of Math and Natural sciences at University of "St. Cyril and Methodius" in Skopje.
In the study were included and were analyzed 30 patients. At each of them, Idiopathic Parkinson Disease was diagnosed, by using many diagnostic criteria such as: History of the patient's disease; Neurological examination; Neurophysiologic examinations such as EEG, ENMG, EP (VEP, SEP, BAEP); Neuroimaging methods, such as CT scan and MRI of brain; Neuropsychological tests.

## 4. Genetic analysis: Detection of mutations in gene of alpha-synuclein (SNCA)

*DNA Isolation:* under aseptic conditions, from each one of the patients, blood sample was taken, with the function of a vein. Each of those blood samples are kept invaccum pots (Vaccutainer), and anticoagulant EDTA Na2 is added in each of the pots.
*Amplification:* amplification of regions of SNCA gene was made with polymerase chain reaction.
*Detection of mutations:* to detect the mutations in selected regions of SNCA gene, polymerase chain reaction- Restriction Fragment Length Polymorphism, was used.
Amplification of the region of egzon 3 of SNCA gene was made, using the primers 5'- GTC TCA CAC TTT GGA GGG TTT C-3' and 5' CAC CTA CCT ACA CAT ACC TCT GAC and TC-3'.
PCR amplification of region of egzon 4 of SNCA gene was made by using the primers 5' GCT AAT CAG CAA TTT AAG GCT AG-3' and 5' GAT ATG TTC TTA GAT GCT and CAG-3'. All of these amplifications have length of 215 bp.
Amplificated products were digested with appropriate restrictive endonuclease under the optimal conditions.
G88C mutation in egzon 3 of SNCA gene was detected with restricted digestion with enzyme Mval.
G209A mutation in egzon 4 of SNCA gene was detected with enzyme Mael.

## 5. Results

In this part of the article, we have a presentation of the results gained with processing, in other words, a statistic data analysis, needed for fulfilling the research aims set.
As respondents in the research, we've included 32 patients with clinically confirmed Idiopathic Parkinson's disease (IPD), diagnosed to Brain Bank Criteria, treated in the University Clinic of Neurology in Skopje - ward for extra pyramidal diseases.
The gender structure of the respondents is presented with 18 (56.25%) males and 14 (43.75%) females, table 1 and picture 1.
The average age of the respondents is 52, 7+10.3 years. The youngest respondent is 30 years and the oldest is 78 years. The median value with value of 50 years shows that 16 of the respondents (50%) are in the age group of 50-59 years, and even 23 of the patients are older than 50 years, table 2 and picture 2.

| Gender | N | % |
|---|---|---|
| Males | 18 | 56.25 |
| Females | 14 | 43.75 |
| Total | 32 | 100 |

Table 1. Respondents distribution by gender

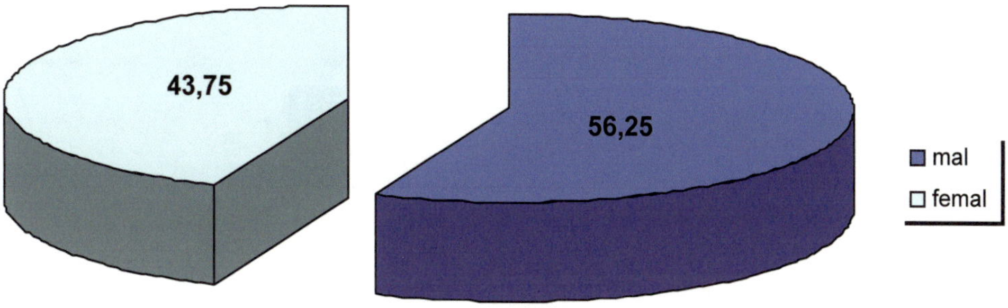


Fig. 1. Respondents distribution by gender

| Years | N | % |
|---|---|---|
| 30-39 | 4 | 12.5 |
| 40-49 | 5 | 15.62 |
| 50-59 | 16 | 50.0 |
| 60-69 | 5 | 15.62 |
| 70 > | 2 | 6.26 |
| Total | 32 | 100 |
| Mean = 52.75±10.3<br>Median = 50 | Min=30 | Max=78 |

Table 2. Respondents distribution by age

In table 3 and picture 3, the representation of neurological symptoms with extra pyramidal origin, typical for diagnosed with IPD, is presented.
The objective neurogical finding, confirmed the presence of rigidity and hypertonia with extrapyramidal origin, to all 32 respondents. This also happened with tremor, which is one of the key symptoms of IPD.
Dyskinesia, as a symptom of long-lasting usage of substitution therapy (levodopa), is found in 15 patients (46.9%) and lack of these symptoms is seen in 17 patients (53.1%).

| Symptoms | Rigidity | | Tremor | | Dyskinesia | |
|---|---|---|---|---|---|---|
| | Number | % | Number | % | Number | % |
| Present | 32 | 100 | 32 | 100 | 15 | 46.88 |
| Absent | / | / | / | / | 17 | 53.12 |
| Total | 32 | 100 | 32 | 100 | 32 | 100 |

Table 3. Rigidity, tremor and dyskinesia distribution

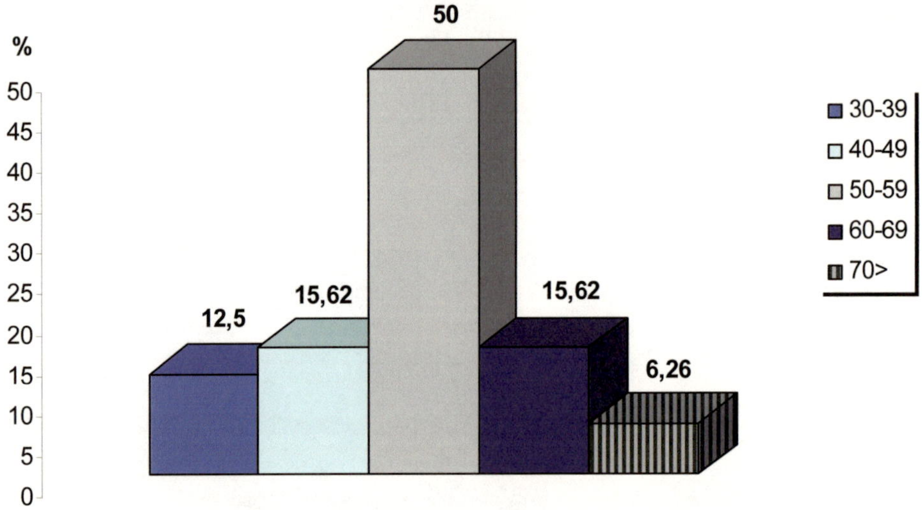


Fig. 2. Respondents distribution by age

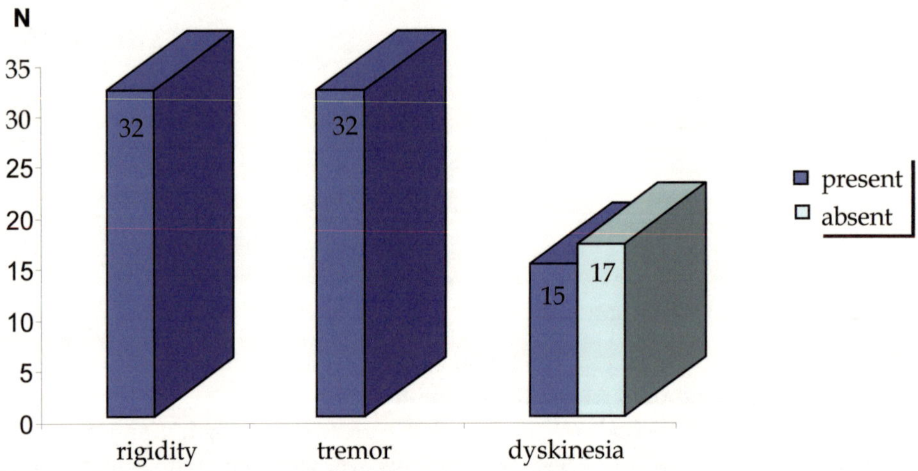


Fig. 3. Rigidity, tremor and dyskinesia distribution

Bradykinesia or stuntment in movements, as main of the list of cardinal symptoms, according to Brain Bank Criteria of UK Parkinson's Disease, was found present in all respondents.

Reduced postural reflexes are positive in dominant number of respondents, 31 (96.6%).

Bradydilalia or the changes in speech (stunt and monotonous speech), is found in 28 patients (87.5 %) and in 4 of our patients (12.5%) a fully normal speech is present, table 4 and picture 4.

Dominant patients with bradydilalia are those with minimal changes in speech, estimated by UPDRS scale, with 1 are 16 patients(50%), with 2,8 patients (25%), with 3 and 4, 2 patients(6.25%) and in 4 patients(12.5%) a fully normal speech is present and the speech itself is estimated with 0, according to UPDRS scale.

| Symptoms | Bradykinesia | | Reduced postural reflexes | | Bradylalia | |
|---|---|---|---|---|---|---|
| | Number | % | Number | % | Number | % |
| Present | 32 | 100 | 31 | 96.87 | 28 | 87.5 |
| Absent | / | / | 1 | 3.13 | 4 | 12.5 |
| Total | 32 | 100 | 32 | 100 | 32 | 100 |

Table 4. Bradykinesia, reduced postural reflexes and bradydilalia distribution

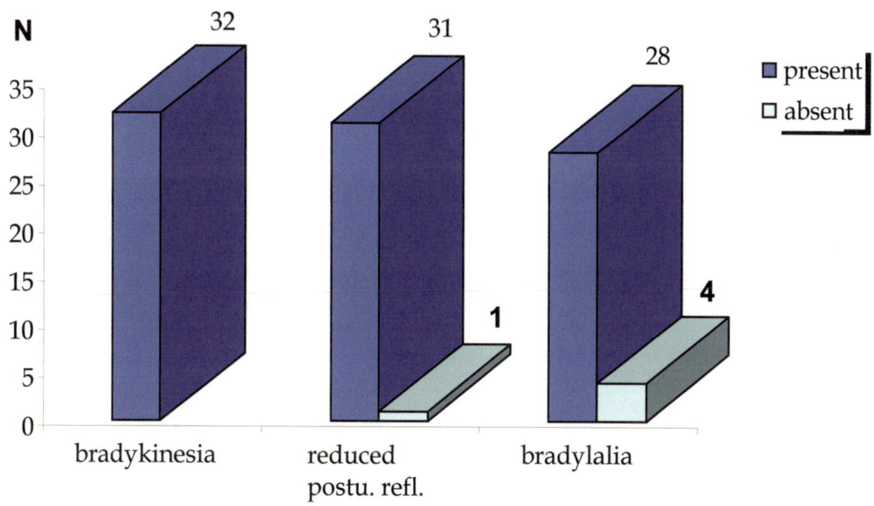


Fig. 4. Bradykinesia, reduced postural reflexes and bradydilalia distribution

The respondents gained the following neurophysiologic examinations: visual evoked potentials (VEP), somatosensory evoked potentials (SSEP), acoustic evoked potentials (BAEP) and electroencephalography (EEG).

The VEP is with proper finding in 29 respondents (90.6%), 2 of them (6.3%) have prolonged latency and the finding of one respondent shows low-volted response, table 5 and picture 5.

| VEP | N | % |
|---|---|---|
| Proper finding | 29 | 90.62 |
| Low-volted response | 1 | 3.12 |
| Prolonged latency | 2 | 6.26 |
| Total | 32 | 100 |

Table 5. Visual evoked potentials (VEP) in patients with IPD

30 of the respondents have proper finding of somatosensory potentials SSEP and in 2 of them (6.2%), those potentials show low-volted responses, table 6 and picture 6.

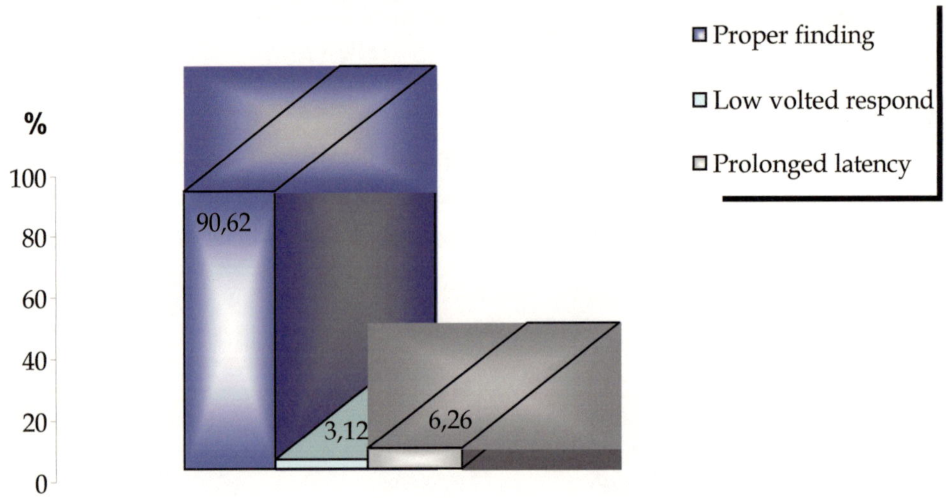


Fig. 5. Visual evoked potentials (VEP) in patients with IPD

| SSEP | N | % |
|---|---|---|
| Proper finding | 30 | 93.75 |
| Low-volted responses | 2 | 6.25 |
| Total | 32 | 100 |

Table 6. Somatosensor evoked potentials in patients with IPD

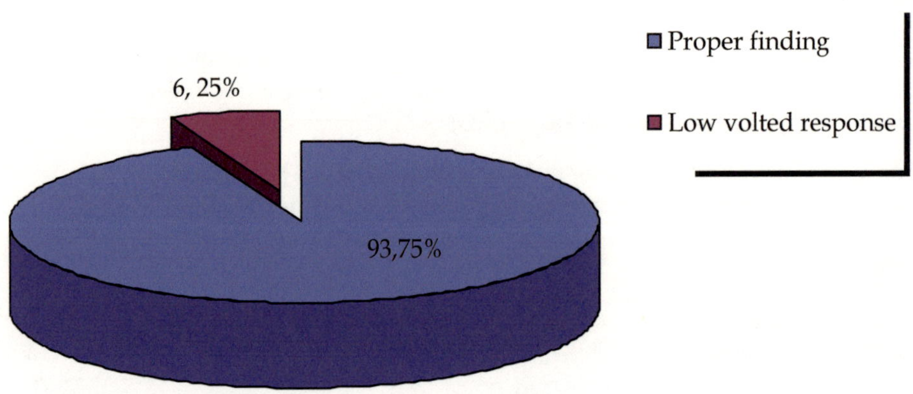


Fig. 6. Somatosensory evoked potentials in patients with IPD

22 of the respondents (68.7%) have proper finding of caustic evoked potentials BAEP and 10 of them (31.2%) are with low-volted responses, table 7 and picture 7.

| BAEP | N | % |
|---|---|---|
| Proper finding | 22 | 68.75 |
| Low-volted responses | 10 | 31.25 |
| Total | 32 | 100 |

Table 7. Caustic evoked potentials BAEP in patients with IPD

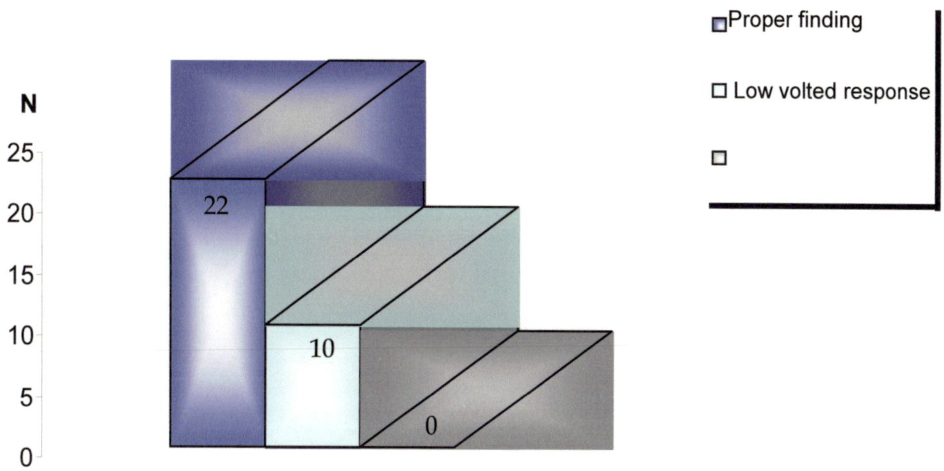


Fig. 7. Caustic evoked potentials BAEP in patients with IPD

19 of the responders (59.4%) have proper finding of electroencephalography; the finding of 12 of them (37.5%) shows unstable basic brain activity, without pathological graph elements and in only one patient, unstable brain activity with presence of different types of pathological graph elements is found, table 8 and picture 8.

| EEG findings | N | % |
|---|---|---|
| Proper finding | 19 | 59.37 |
| Unstable basic brain activity without pathological graph elements | 12 | 37.5 |
| Unstable basic brain activity, with presence of pathological graph elements | 1 | 3.13 |
| Total | 32 | 100 |

Table 8. EEG in patients with IPD

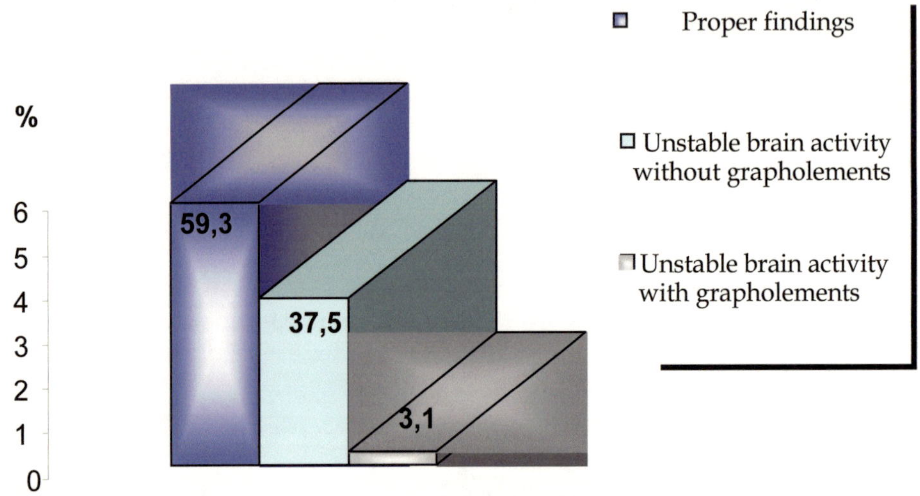


Fig. 8. EEG in patients with IPD

| CT and MRI of brain findings | N | % |
|---|---|---|
| Proper finding | 12 | 37.5 |
| Discrete cortical reductive changes | 11 | 34.37 |
| Global cortical reductive changes | 9 | 28.13 |
| Total | 32 | 100 |

Table 9. CT and MRI of brain in patients with IPD

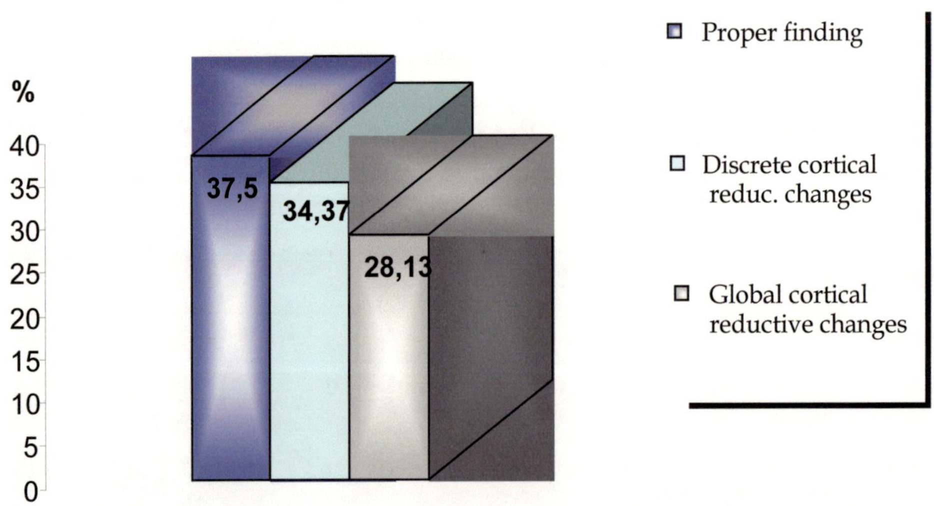


Fig. 9. CT and MRI of brain in patients with IPD

All patients gained neuroimaging examinations (CT and MRI of brain) and the examination results are presented in table 9 and picture 9.

In 12 patients (37.5%), the results of CT and MRI of brain are normal; 11 (34.4%) have discrete cortical reductive changes and 9 (28, 1 %) have global cortical changes.
Doppler color sonography of the extra cranial blood vessels is with proper finding in 20 respondents (62.5%), 7 (21.9%) are with lightly expressed intimacy and proper hemodynamic parameters; 5(15.6%) have expressed arteriosclerosical changes of carotidal blood vessels, table 10 and picture 10.

| Doppler color sonography of the carotid system | N | % |
|---|---|---|
| Normal finding | 20 | 62.5 |
| Lightly expressed intimacy with proper chemo dynamic parameters | 7 | 21.87 |
| Expressed arteriosclerotic changes of the blood vessels of the carotid system | 5 | 15.63 |
| Total | 32 | 100 |

Table 10. Doppler color sonography of the carotid system in patients with IPD

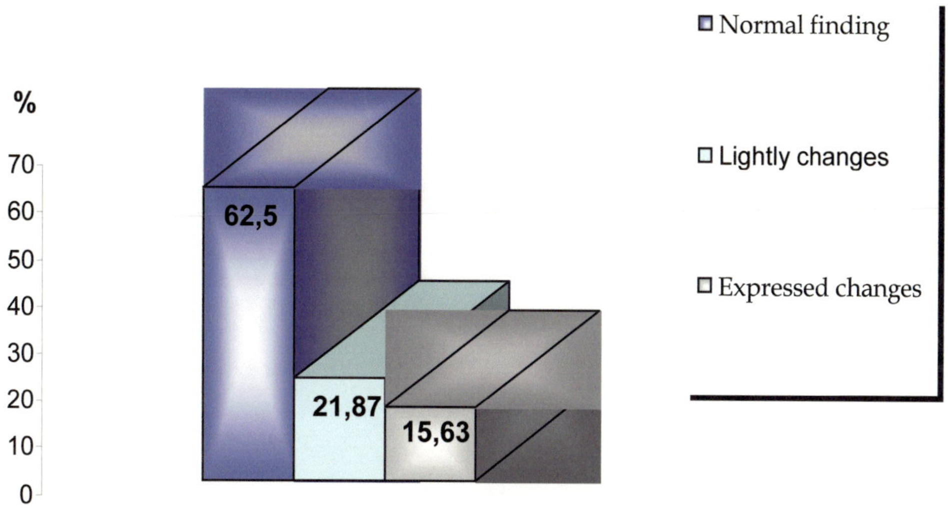


Fig. 10. Doppler color sonography of the carotid system in patients with IPD

In tables 11a and 11b, the results of the neuropsychological testing are shown. It's visible that only 3 patients (9.4%) have proper cognitive capacities. In table 11a all neuropsychological findings are examined individually, with percentage representation in our 32 respondents. Depression is found in 24 patients (84.4%); anxiety in 3 patients (9.4%); in 13 patients (40.6%), initial or global cognitive and mnestic reduced changes are found.
In table 11b, a statistic analysis of different combinations of findings from neuropsychological testing is presented, so between the patients dominant are those with depression and initial reduced cognitive capacities, as well as global reduced cognitive capacities. According to the frequency of occurrence, next is the finding of depression and global reduced cognitive and mnestical capacities, found in 3 respondents (9.4%).
The rest findings from the neuropsychological testing: depression, anxiety, initial reduced cognitive capacities, depression and anxiety together, as well as the mutual presence of

depression and anxiety, joined with initial reduced cognitive and mnestical capacities, are found only in one of the respondents.

| Neuropsychological testing | N | % |
|---|---|---|
| Proper finding | 3 | 9.37 |
| Depression | 27 | 84.37 |
| Anxiety | 3 | 9.37 |
| Initial reduced cognitive and mnestical capacities | 13 | 40.62 |
| Global reduced cognitive and mnestical capacities | 13 | 40.62 |

Table 11.a. Neuropsychological testing of respondents with IPD

| Neuropsychological testing | N | % |
|---|---|---|
| Proper finding | 3 | 9.37 |
| Depression | 1 | 3.12 |
| Anxiety | 1 | 3.12 |
| Global reduced cognitive and mnestic capacities | 10 | 31.25 |
| Initial reduced cognitive and mnestic capacities | 1 | 3.12 |
| Depression and anxiety | 1 | 3.12 |
| Depression and global reduced cognitive and mnestic capacities | 3 | 9.37 |
| Depression and initial reduced cognitive and mnestical capacities | 11 | 34.37 |
| Depression and anxiety and initial reduced cognitive and mnestical capacities | 1 | 3.12 |
| Total | 32 | 100 |

Table 11.b. Neuropsychological testing of respondents with IPD

| UPDRS | Gender | | Total |
|---|---|---|---|
| | Males | Females | |
| Minimal signs | 2<br>11.11% | 9<br>64.29% | 11 |
| Light signs | 9<br>50.00% | 4<br>28.57% | 13 |
| Expressed symptoms | 3<br>16.67% | 1<br>7.14% | 4 |
| Extremely expressed symptoms | 4<br>22.22% | 0 | 4 |
| Total<br>% of total number | 18<br>56.25% | 14<br>43.75% | 32 |

Table 12. The immensity of the clinical state, according to the respondents' gender Mann-Whitney U=47,5 Z=2,98 p=0,0029

The immensity of the clinical state of Parkinson's disease in our respondents, of different gender, is presented in table 12 and picture 11. The male respondents have significantly tougher clinical state comparing to female respondents. This statistic comment is a result of the distribution shown in the table. It is noticeable that half of the male respondents (9.50%), have light disease symptoms; 2 (11.1%) have minimal signs or symptoms according to UPDRS scale; 4 (22.2%) are with extremely visible symptoms. In the female respondents, the disease is often manifested with minimal symptoms; 9(64.3%) and 4(28.6%) have light symptoms and there aren't any female respondents with extremely visible symptoms.

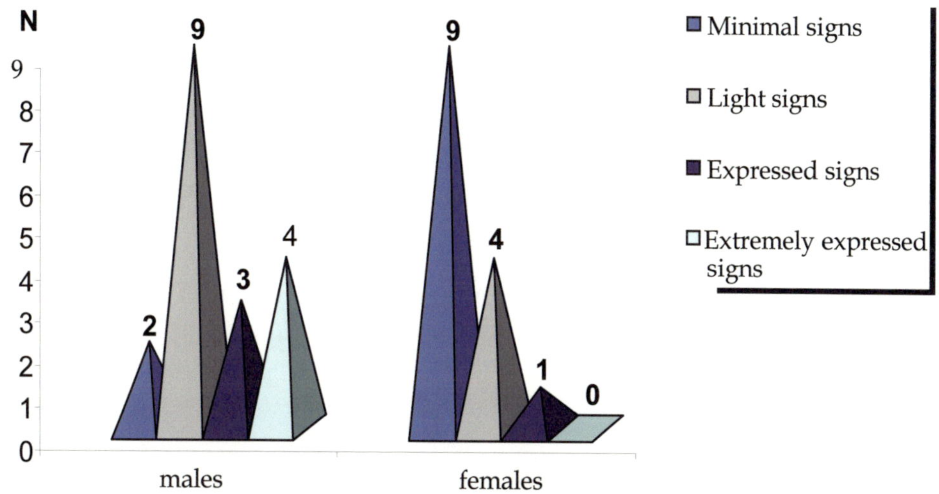


Fig. 11. The immensity of the clinical state, according to the respondents gender

The average age of the respondents, which according to UPDRS scale, have minimal symptoms of Parkinson's disease, is 53, 6+10.3 years.
The respondents with light signs have average age of 52.8+8.1 years; the respondents with extremely expressed symptoms have average age of 45+15.3 years, table 13 and picture 12.

| UPDRS | N | Age (Mean) | Age (SD) |
|---|---|---|---|
| Minimal signs | 11 | 53.63 | 10.28 |
| Light signs | 13 | 52.85 | 8.10 |
| Expressed signs | 4 | 57.75 | 11.73 |
| Extremely expressed symptom | 4 | 45.00 | 15.30 |

Table 13. The immensity of the clinical state (UPDRS), according to the patient's age

The connection between the age and the immensity of the clinical state of the respondents, estimated by UPDRS scale is presented in picture 13. That correlation has value for Spearmenov's correlation coefficient, R=0.039, which indicates indirect or negative correlation. Parkinson's disease has more difficult clinical state in younger patients and vice versa lighter symptoms in older patients. But, considering the value of the coefficient, we can conclude that the correlation between these two parameters is weak and statistically insignificant ($p>0.05$).

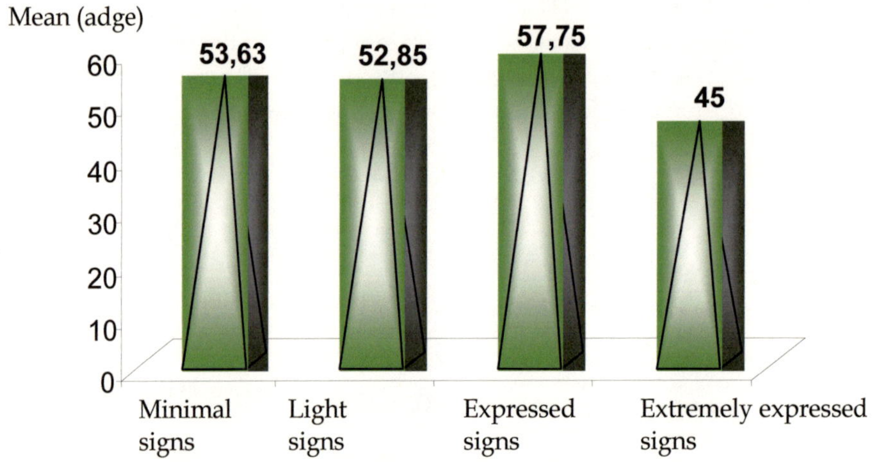


Fig. 12. The immensity of the clinical state (UPDRS), according to the patient's age

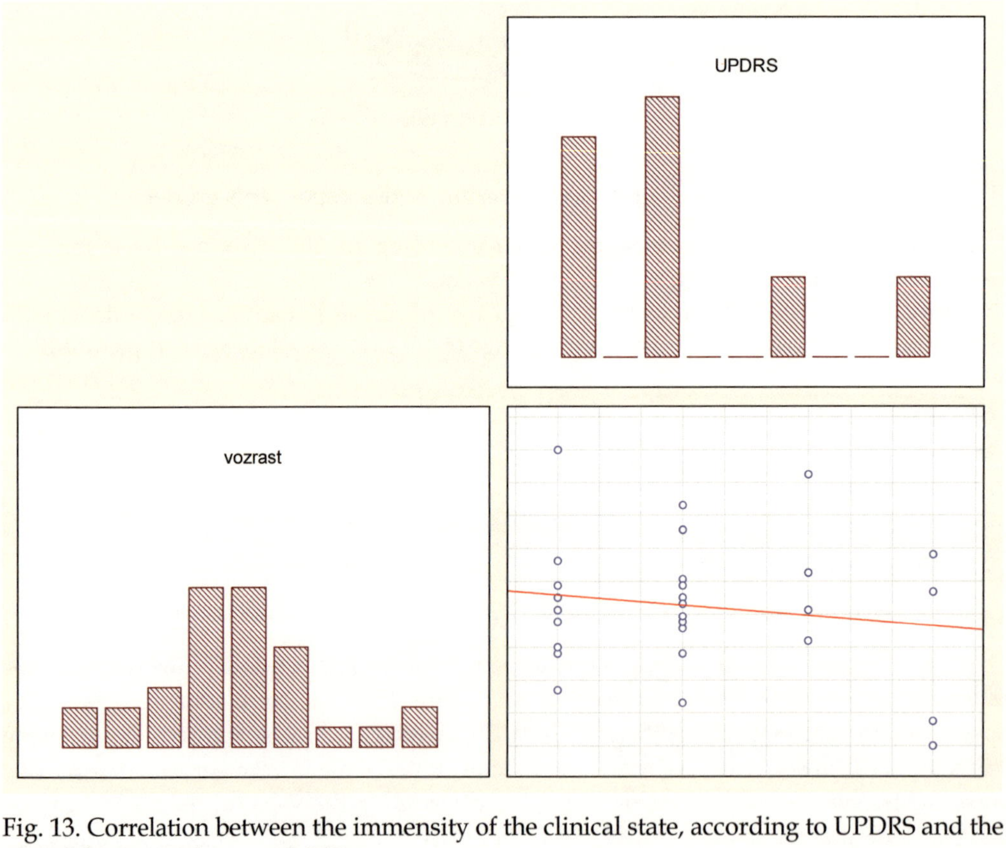


Fig. 13. Correlation between the immensity of the clinical state, according to UPDRS and the age of the respondents with IPD

## 6. Spearman rank order correlations R=-0.039 p>0.05

In our research, we've concluded that direct or positive statistic significant correlation between the number of hospitalizations and the immensity of the clinical state, according to UPDRS, indeed exists.

The value of the Spermen's coefficient (r=0.48), shows that these two parameters are proportionally connected, in other words, patients with IPD difficult manifestations of the disease, according to UPDRS scale, have more hospitalizations in the University clinic of Neurology in Skopje.

Table 14 and picture 14, show the results from the crostabulation between the CT finding and MRI of brain and the immensity of the clinical state, determined according UPDRS scale. In the respondents group with light disease symptoms, according to UPDRS scale, dominant are the findings with normal level, previously determined with CT and MRI of brain, present in 5 patients (45.4%), from this group. Between the respondents with light disease symptoms, the finding from CT and MRI of the brain shows discrete cortical reduced changes in 6 patients (46.1%). In half of the respondents, the finding from CT and MRI of brain, shows presence of discrete cortical reduced changes.75% of the respondents with highly expressed disease symptoms, have global cortical reduced changes, proved on CT and MRI of brain.

| CT and MRI of brain | Immensity of the clinical state (UPDRS) | | | | Total |
|---|---|---|---|---|---|
| | Minimal signs | Light signs | Expressed signs | Extremely expressed signs | |
| Normal finding | 5<br>45.45% | 5<br>38.46% | 1<br>25.00% | 1<br>25.00% | 12 |
| Discrete cortical reductive changes | 3<br>27.27% | 6<br>46.15% | 2<br>50.00% | 0 | 11 |
| Global cortical reductive changes | 3<br>27.27% | 2<br>15.38% | 1<br>25.00% | 3<br>75.00% | 9 |
| Total | 11 | 13 | 4 | 4 | 32 |

Table 14. Immensity of the clinical state (UPDRS) in relation to CT and MRI of brain

The connection or the correlation between the immensity of the clinical state, determined by UPDRS scale and brain CT/MRI finding, is also proved with the usage of Spearsmen's correlation coefficient. Its value (r=0.2) shows presence of direct, positive correlation between these two parameters, in other words, there is a match between the brain CT/MRI finding and the results from the UPDRS scale. In patients with difficult clinical forms of IPD, most often the brain CT/MRI finding shows global cortical reduced changes. But, the confirmed correlation is statistically insignificant, (p>0.05), picture 15.

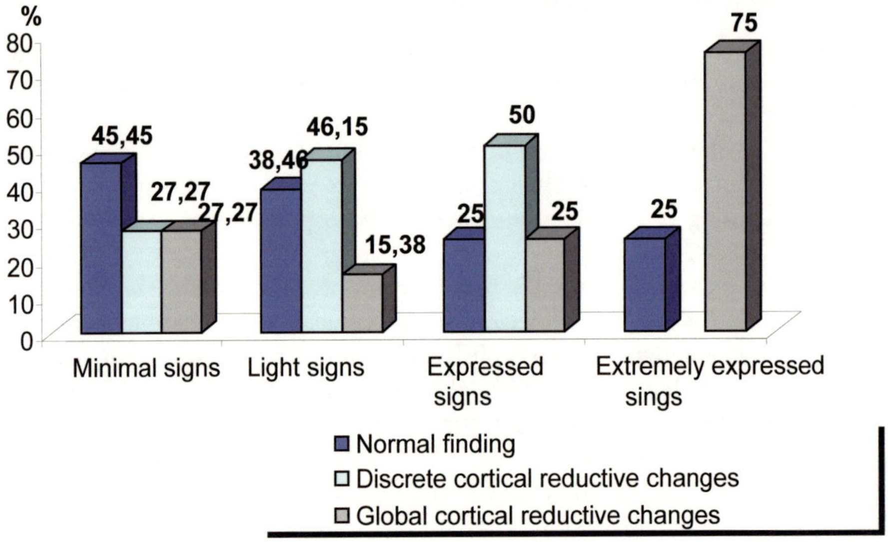


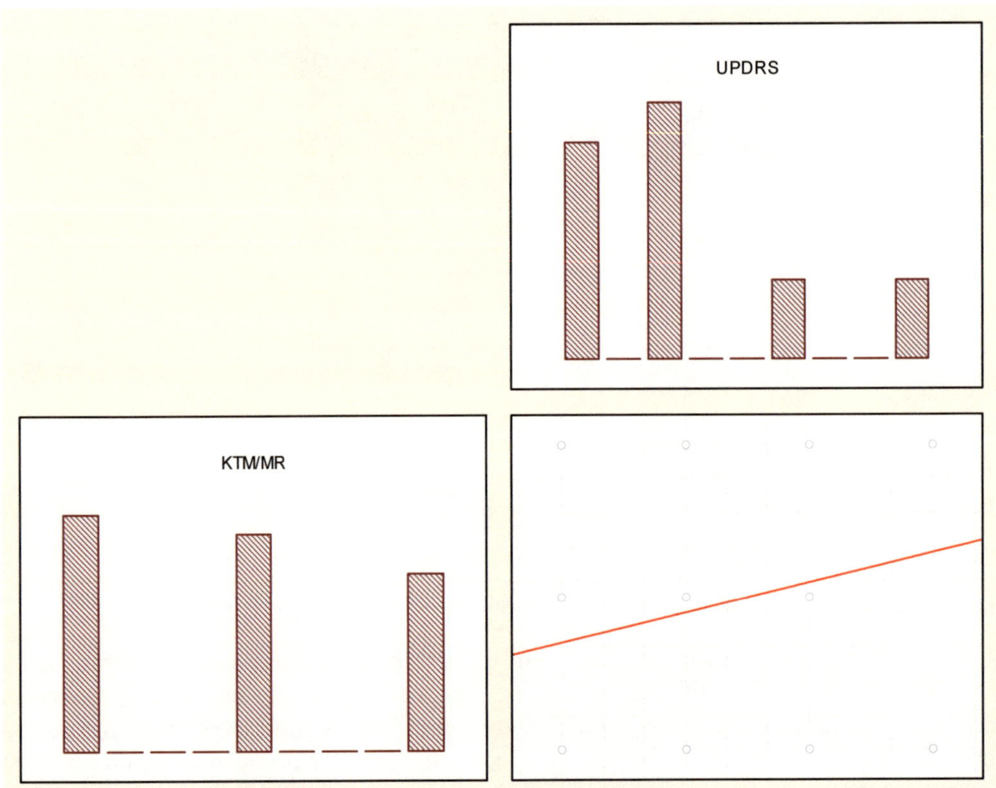


Fig. 15. Correlation between the immensity of the clinical state (UPDRS) and brain CT/MRI finding Spearman Rank Order Correlations R=0, 2 p>0.05

## 7. Mutation detection

After amplification of a region from egzon 3 of SNCA gene, with usage of the following primers: 5'GTC TCA CAC TTT GGA GGG TTT C-3 and 5'-CAC CTA CCT ACA CAT ACC TCT GAC TC-3', the result was an amplified product with length of 395 base pairs (bp). PCR amplification of a region from egzon 4 of SNCA gene, was performed with these primers 5'-GTC AAT CAG CAA TTT AAG GCT AG-3' and 5'-GAT ATG TTC TTA GAT GCT CAG-3', and the amplifications have length of 215 bp. The amplified products were digested with proper restrictive endonuclease under optimal conditions (puferian solutions suitable for each enzyme separately on temperature of 37 c). With that, no mutated sequence in the PCR product is found.

G88C mutation in egzon 3 of SNCA gene isn't detected in our 32 respondents with IPD. No mutations were found in the G209A in the enzon 4 from SNCA gene, also.

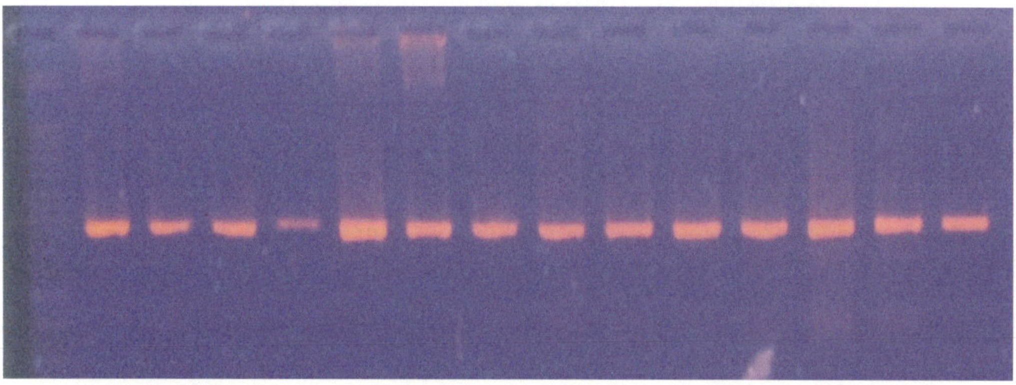

Fig. 16. Electroforetogram from PCR-RELP analysis (agaros gels colored with etidium bromide and photographed on ultraviolet light.

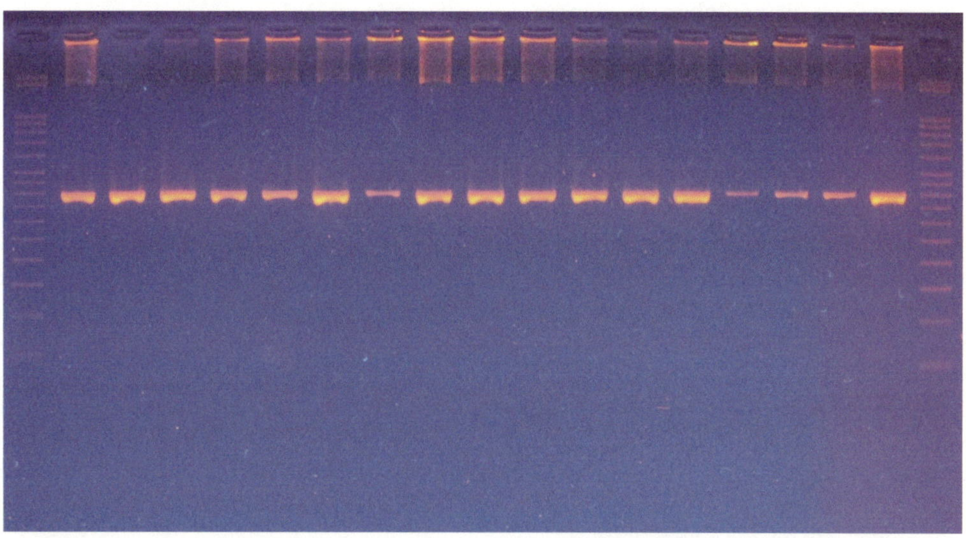

Fig. 17. Electroforetogram from PCR-RELP analysis (agaros gels colored with etidium bromide and photographed on ultraviolet light

## 8. Discussion

IPB is found in both genders, with discretely higher representation in males. Our study shows that the gender representation for 32 patients with clinically confirmed diagnosis of JPB, by Brain Bank Criteria, is 18 males (56.25%) and females (43.75%). In most studies, as those of Haksma and all. (2007), Lions and all (2009); Linder and all. (2010), conducted in different periods and different populations, the results have big similarity with ours (8, 17, and 12).

In our study the average age of the respondents is 52.7 years. The youngest is only 30 years and the oldest is 78 years. The median value (50 years) shows that 16 respondents (50%) are in the age group of 50-59 years, and even 23 patients (71.87%) are older than 50 years (table 2, picture 2 from the results).

From the analyzed articles about the average beginning of IPD, dominant are those where the average beginning is in the sixth decade from life [21, 16, and 1].

Alves and all. (2009) in their epidemiological study in Norway, conducted on 554 patients with IPD, noted that the average age for beginning of symptoms manifestation of IPD is 54.3 years (this fits perfectly with the average age of our 32 respondents) [1].

Bradykinesia or the of stuntment in movements, as main from the list of cardinal symptoms according to Brain Bank Criteria of UK Parkinson's Disease (BBC-UKPCD), was present in all respondents. According to BBC-UKPCD criteria, to set the JPD diagnosis, the patient should have bradykinesia plus one of the rest cardinal symptoms such as tremor, rigidity or reduced postural reflexes. With the presence of only 2 symptoms (from which one must be bradykinesia) IPD can be confirmed.

Bradykinesia as cardinal symptom according to UPRDS, was estimated in the following way: 15 patients (47.87%) with 1; 10 (31.25%) with 2; 5 (15.62%) with 3 and only 2 respondents (6.25%) with 4 according to UPRDS scale.

Stefanie Lui and all. (2009) in their study make analysis of the development of bradykinesia as symptom in different disease stadiums. According to them, the disease progression is influenced from the bradykinesia as main cardinal symptom [19].

When our respondents are in question, in only one of them (3.12%), the lack of symptom reduced postural reflexes was confirmed and its value was 0, according to UPDRS scale. In our respondents, 75% had reduced postural reflexes, estimated with 1; 5 (15.62 %) with 2 and 1 (3.12%) were with values of 3 and 4.

Spildoren I and all. (2010), in their article described the postural instability as common and very important symptoms in IPD. In their patients, this instability is seen through partial walking instability in the initial disease stadium and as freezing phenomena in the advanced disease stadiums. According to them, the freezing phenomena are often expressed in simultaneous double activities and in the act of turning after short walking [13].

Kerstin Ziegler and all. (2010), describe festination and freezing in all 33 patients with more advanced stadium of IPD. The way they estimated festination and freezing in walking, was with 12 episodes walking capturing, in which motor block was seemed in 4 situations with 3 levels of double activities. Practically, these phenomenas are reflected in parameters expressed by measuring the number of steps of those patients, walking on special stripe and analysis on walking on distance of 10 meters. This is how you make assessment on expression of the postural instability [14].

Besides bradykinesia, as main cardinal symptom, as symptoms od IPD, are also found tremor and rigidity. We've found their presence in all our respondents (100%).

Tremor is estimated with 2, according to UPDRS scale in 18 respondents (56.25%); 10 (31.25%) with 1; 3 (9.4%) with 3 and only one patient (3.1%) we've found tremor estimated with 4.

Petra Vingensuh and all (2010) conducted examination on 25 respondents in initial stadium of IPD. In all of them, unilateral tremor pointed with bradykinesia was found, and it was possible to make diagnosis. Additionally, all these patients gained SPECT testing and in only 10% a proper finding of SPEKT was found. Lately, a number of articles are published, which through examination of cardinal secondary symptoms in patients with IPD, make analysis on their life quality. In our article, the estimation of the immensity of the clinical state was made using the UPDRS scale, which is generally accepted and applied in most scientific articles for Parkinson's disease [6].

The correlation between respondents' age and the immensity of the clinical state, estimated according to UPDRS scale, is shown in picture 26 in our results. This relation points the existence or negative correlation. Parkinson's disease has fairly difficult clinical state in younger patients and vice verse; the disease is manifested with lighter symptoms in elder patients. But, considering the coefficient value, we can conclude the correlation between these two parameters is statistically insignificant ($p>0.05$).

Barone P and all. (2009), this multicentrical article shows the frequency of the nonmotor signs and symptoms such as hyposmia, mood, sleeping, tiredness, perception difficulties, attention, memory capacity, erectil disfunction [3].

All these signs are examined in patients on different disease stadiums, and than analyzed to present their influence on the life of these patients.

The authors monitor 524 patients with Parkinson's disease, and they register their nonmotor symptoms and their influence on patients' life in different disease stadiums. They stated, that in younger patients the clinical state is tougher according to UPDRS, comparing to elder patients. Also, the study witnessed that disease progression is much faster in younger patients comparing to elder patients [3].

Keush SH and all. (2009), conducted their clinical examination of motor and nonmotor symptoms of Parkinson's disease in Holland. The authors developed a specific scale through which, the possibilities and capabilities for daily activities were analyzed, and according to which the degree of disease progression can be determined.

According to them, in younger patients we have faster symptoms progression, comparing to patients where the clinical state is manifested later [15].

The immensity of the clinical state of Parkinson's disease in our respondents of different gender, show that male patients have significantly tougher clinical state comparing to female patients.

Ivi Miler and Golomb AC (2010) made interesting, clinical-epidemiological study, in which is clearly shown that the disease is nearly equally manifested in two genders, but specific symptoms are more frequent in females and others in males. Motor symptoms which appear as a consequence of reduced function of dopaminerigic system, those which we often examine, are dominant in males, and only rigidity as motor symtoms and nonmotor signs are dominant in females [11].

It is assumed that this difference in manifestation by gender, most likely, is influenced by unknown hormonal mechanisms.

From the list of the neuropsychological examinations, the respondents gained: visual evoked potentials (VEP); somatosesoral evoked potentials (SSEP); caustic evoked potentials (BAEP) and electroencephalography (EEG). Generally in our 32 respondents, the most

findings for evoked potentials (VEP, SSEP and BAEP) are proper. Proper VEP is found in 29 respondents (90.6%); prolonged latencies and low-volted responses are found in 2 (6.3%) and only in 1 respondent (3.1%), the finding is with low-volted response.
SSEP is with proper finding in 30 respondents (93.8%) and low-volted responses are found in 2 (6.2%). Proper BAEP finding is found in 22 (68.72%) and low-volted different components are found in 10 (31.25%).
In our patients, neuroimaging examination (CT and MRI of brain) are made; 37.5% have proper results; in 34.4% of them discrete cortical reduced changes are found and in 28.1% the pathological process is manifested with global cortical reduced changes.
Doppler color sonography on extra cranial blood vessels, shows proper finding in 62.5% of the respondents; in 21.9% lightly expressed intimacy and proper chemo dynamic parameters are found; in 15.6% of our patients have arteriosclerotical changes of the caroted blood vessels.
Lio CH and all. (2010) made a study on 84 patients with IPD, without dementia signs. They made several short capturing with MRI of brain, examining the regions which are most often damaged in these patients. Patients with medium developed clinical state were selected. They also had plenty symptoms and the exact regions which influenced the domination on specific motor and nonmotor symptoms, were determinated. Dementia as a symptom was excluded [4].
Table 11a and 11b from our results, presents the results from the neuropsychological testing. Proper cognitive capacities of testing were found only in 3 patients with IPD. Between the patients dominant are those with depression and initial reduced cognitive capacities (34.4%), as well as 31.2% with global reduced cognitive capacities.
According to the frequency of occurrence, next is the finding of depression and global reduced cognitive capacities, found in 9.4% of our respondents.
The rest findings of the neuropsychological testing: depression in behavior, anxiety in behavior, initial reduced cognitive capacities; depression and anxiety in behavior, as well as the mutual presence of depression and anxiety in behavior and initial reduced cognitive capacities are found only in 1 patient with IPD.
Lately, in different magazines and congresses, scientists try to prove the correlation between the IPD and depression as secondary symptom, as well as, dementia, found in high percent of patients with Parkinson's disease.
Ivi N Miler and Golumb AC (2010) made interesting clinical and epidemiological study, where they proved that the disease is nearly equally manifested in both genders. But, certain symptoms more often appear in females and other in males. Etiopathogenetical mechanisms for these symptoms division, is still unknown, but it is assumed that the hormonal status influences on manifestation of these symptoms. Consequently, the nonvoter symptoms (mood, hyposmia, sleeping, attention, memory, perception difficulties and depression) are dominant in females [11].
Huijuan Li and all. (2010), made a study on 82 Chinese patients, 46 males and 36 females with IPD, which lasted 18 months. Patients were on average age of 65 years. Generally, they examined the motor signs such as: mood, sleeping, depression, attention, memory capacity and perception disorder. To determinate the degree of disease, the authors used UPDRS scale. Then using a special scale for determination of nonmotoral symptoms development, they determined the degree of these symptoms. They concluded that there is a positive correlation between the development of the nonmotor and psychological symptoms in relation to the development of motor signs of the disease, according to UPDRS. Actually, all

these symptoms, nonmotor and motor, develop parallel, meaning that in the early disease stadiums, all symptoms are lightly developed, no matter what they are like, while in the more advanced stadiums, all symptoms are expressed and visible [10].

Ajlin Juxel and all. (2010) in their study of 28 patients with IPD, conducted in Turkey, made multiple capturing with nuclear magnetic resonance on brain (MRI), measuring the thickness of brain callus in different brain regions. A correlation between the immensity of the clinical state, determined by UPDRS scale and the finding from MRI (measurement of the brain callus thickness), was set. The authors concluded that the thinner brain callus is, the more developed the clinical state of patients with IPD is [2].

In our study, G88C mutation in egzon 3 form SNCA genes isn't detected in our 32 respondents with IPD. The same happens with G209A in egzon 4 form SNCA gene.

Suterland GT and all (2009) in their immense study conducted on Australian population, of 331 patients with scattered form and family form of Parkinson's disease and 296 healthy people. The authors examined 11 known genes and all kinds of combinations of these genes correlations with symptoms manifestations of Parkinson's disease. They concluded that only LRRK2 gene has hardly any influence only in the family form of Parkinson's disease, while the rest genes, between which SNCA, have no influence at all in scattered Parkinson's disease manifestation in Australians, a result which fits the findings of our research [20].

Sarah Kamargos and all. (2009) made a study to evaluate the frequency and the phonotypical and genotypical manifestation in family and scattered forms of Parkinson's disease in Brazilian population. The examination was conducted on 575 patients with Parkinsonism, where the ones with IPD are 428. Mutations and polymorphisms on many different genes, typical for Parkinson's disease, such as alpha synuclein and LRRK2 gene, were examined. In the end, they concluded that there wasn't any mutation on alpha synuclein in all respondents and in only one patient with initial symptoms of IPD, a slight mutation of LRRK2 gene, was found [18].

Kristian Vajder and all. (2009), made immense study on 1262 patients with IPD and control group of 1881 patient. They checked the correlations between the fibroblastic growing factor 20 and alpha synuclein in patients with Parkinson's disease. They examined their correlations on 9 brains on deceased patients, which were previously diagnosed with IPD. The authors concluded that the role of alpha synuclein in Parkinson's disease is undisputable, but the changes in sequences in this gene, were negative [5].

## 9. References


[1] Alves G, Muller B,Herlofson K. Incidence of Parkinson's disease in Norway. The Norwegian Park West study. J Neural Neurosurgery Psychiatry 2009; 80: 851–857

[2] Aylin Yucel, Ozge Yilmaz Kusbeci. Magnetic resonance imaging findings of shoulders in Parkinson's disease. Mov Disord 2010; 25 (15): 2524-2530.

[3] Barone P, Antonini A, Colosimo C, et al. The PRIAMO study: A multicenter assessment of nonmotor symptoms and their impact on quality of life in Parkinson's disease. Mov Disord 2009; 24: 1641–1649.

[4] Chul Hyoung Lyoo, Young Hoon Ryu, Myung Sik Lee. Topographical distribution of cerebral cortical thinning in patients with mild Parkinson's disease without dementia. Mov Disord 2010; 25 (4): 496-499.

[5] Christian Wider, Justus C. Dachsel, Alexandra I. Soto et al. FGF20 and Parkinson's disease: No evidence of association or pathogenicity via α-synuclein expression. Mov Disord 2009; 24 (3): 455-9.

[6] Christopher G. Goetz, Glenn T. Stebbins, Teresa A. Chmura, Stanley Fahn, Werner Poewe, Caroline M. Tanner. Teaching program for the movement disorder society-sponsored revision of the Unified Parkinson's disease Rating Scale: (MDS-UPDRS). Mov Disord 2008; Vol. 23 (9): 1190–1194.
[7] Galvan A, Wichmann T. Pathophysiology of Parkinsonism. Clin Neurophysiol 2008; 119: 1459–1474.
[8] Haaxma CA, Bloem BR, Borm GF et al. Gender differences in Parkinson's disease. J Neurol Neurosurg Psychiatry 2007; 78: 819–824.
[9] Hughes AJ, Daniel SE, Kilford L, Lees AJ. Accuracy of clinical diagnosis of idiopathic Parkinson's disease. A clinico-pathological study of 100 cases. JNNP 1992;55:181-184.
[10] Huijuan Li, Meifen Zhang, Ling Chen, June Zhang, Zhong Pei, Ailing Hu, Qing Wang. Nonmotor symptoms are independently associated with impaired health-related quality of life in Chinese patients with Parkinson's disease. Mov Disord 2010; 25 (16): 2740-2746.
[11] Ivy N. Miller, Alice Cronin-Golomb. Gender differences in Parkinson's disease: Clinical characteristics and cognition. Mov Disord 2010; 25 (16): 2695-2703.
[12] Jan Linder, Hans Stenlund, Lars Forsgren. Incidence of Parkinson's disease and Parkinsonism in northern Sweden: A population-based study. Mov Disord 2010; 25 (3): 341-348.
[13] Joke Spildooren, Sarah Vercruysse, Kaat Desloovere, Wim Vandenberghe, Eric Kerckhofs, Alice Nieuwboer. Freezing of gait in Parkinson's disease: The impact of dual-tasking and turning. Mov Disord 2010; 25 (15): 2563-2570.
[14] Kerstin Ziegler, Frauke Schroeteler, Andres O. Ceballos-Baumann, Urban M. Fietzek. A new rating instrument to assess festination and freezing gait in Parkinsonian patients. Mov Disord 2010; 25 (8): 1012-1018.
[15] Keus SH, Nieuwboer A, Bloem BR, Borm GF, Munneke M. Clinimetric analyses of the Modified Parkinson Activity Scale. Parkinsonism Relat Disord 2008; 15: 263–269.
[16] Levy G. The relationship of Parkinson disease with aging. Arch Neurol 2007; 64: 1242–1246.
[17] Lyons KS,Steward BJ,Archbold PG,Carter JH. Optimism, pessimism, mutuality and gender: predicting 10-year role strain in Parkinson's disease spouses. Gerontol 2009; 49: 378–387.
[18] Sarah Teixeira Camargos, Leonardo Oliveira Dornas, Parastoo Momeni, Andrew Lees, John Hardy, Andrew Singleton, Francisco Cardoso. Familial Parkinsonism and early onset Parkinson's disease in a Brazilian movement disorders clinic: Phenotypic characterization and frequency of SNCA, PRKN, PINK1, and LRRK2 mutations. Mov Disord 2009; 24 (5): 662-6.
[19] Stephanie Louie, Mandy Miller Koop, Anna Frenklach, Helen Bronte-Stewart. Quantitative lateralized measures of bradykinesia at different stages of Parkinson's disease: The role of the less affected side. Mov Disord 2009; 24 (13): 1991-97.
[20] Sutherland GT, Halliday GM, Silburn PA, Mastalgia FL, Rowe DB, Boyle RS, O'Sullivan JD, Ly T, Wilton SD, Mellick GD. Do polymorphisms in the familial Parkinsonism genes contribute to risk for sporadic Parkinson's disease? Mov Disord 2009; 24 (6):833-8.
[21] Wermuth L, Bech S, Petersen MS, Joensen P, Weihe P, Grandjean P. Prevalence and incidence of Parkinson's disease in The Faroe Islands. Acta Neurol Scand 2008; 118: 126–131.

# 13

# New Insights for a Better Understanding of the Pusher Behavior: From Clinical to Neuroimaging Features

Taiza E.G. Santos-Pontelli, Octavio M. Pontes-Neto and Joao P. Leite
*University of Sao Paulo School of Medicine at Ribeirao Preto*
*Brazil*

## 1. Introduction

Disorders of postural balance are common in patients with encephalic lesions. According Tyson et al. (Tyson et al., 2006), around 80% of patients experiencing their first cerebrovascular event have static or dynamic postural imbalance. Historically, the first description of postural balance dysfunction in stroke patients dates back to more than one hundred years ago. In 1909, Beevor described the occasional lack of lateral balance in stroke patients that cause them to fall towards their contralesional side due to their paresis (Beevor, 1909). Later, Brunnstrom reported the 'listing phenomenon' as a list toward the affected side that patients cope by climbing onto something with their nonparetic hand to prevent listing (Brunnstrom, 1970).

In 1968, a tendency to fall towards the lesion side and lateropulsion were described by Bjerver and coworkers in patients with Wallenberg's syndrome due to dorsolateral medullary infarction (Bjerver &Silfverskiold, 1968). These patients also presented with transient ocular tilt reaction and ipsiversive deviations of the subjective vertical, which indicate a pathological shift in the internal representation of the gravitational vector (Dieterich &Brandt, 1992; Brandt &Dieterich, 2000; Dieterich, 2007).

Another postural imbalance observed in patients with encephalic lesions is thalamic astasia. According to Masdeu and Gorelick, this disorder is characterized by the inability to maintain an unsupported upright posture even without paresis or sensory or cerebellar deficits.[8] When asked to sit up, patients with this disorder use the unaffected arm to pull themselves up (Masdeu & Gorelick, 1988). This behavior could be explained in part by a vestibular tone imbalance in the roll plane, especially since skew deviation was included as a feature of the syndrome (Brandt & Dieterich, 2000; Dieterich, 2007).

As opposed to all other syndromes and phenomena described above, the pusher behavior (PB) is characterized by actively pushing away from the nonparetic side (Davies, 1985). Moreover, patients with PB lean to the side opposite the lesion and strongly resist any attempt at passive correction of their tilted body while sitting or standing. In the most severe cases, this resistance occurs even in a supine position (Pedersen et al., 1996; Lafosse et al., 2005). Such patients report a fear of falling towards their ipsilesional side (Davies, 1985; Pedersen et al., 1996; Lafosse et al., 2005) and are not aware that their active pushing is counterproductive and makes it impossible for them to stand without assistance (D'Aquila et al., 2004). Thus, the listing phenomenon, thalamic astasia and Wallenberg's syndrome need to be considered in the differential diagnosis of PB. Although the PB was originally described in association with neglect and anosognosia as a syndrome that is related to right encephalic lesions by the physical therapist Davies (Davies, 1985), several studies have demonstrated that it can occur in patients with lesions in both hemispheres and is distinct from those neuropsychological deficits (Pedersen et al., 1996; Karnath et al., 2000b, 2000a; Premoselli et al., 2001; Pérrenou, 2002; Bohannon, 2004; Santos-Pontelli et al., 2004). Since the definition of 'syndrome' is "a set of qualities, events or behaviors that is typical of a particular kind of problem' (Longman dictionary of Contemporary English; 1995) and the diagnostic criteria for PB are presence of the 3 behaviors observed by the examiner described above, the term 'pusher syndrome' can be considered appropriate. Alternative labels of the PB are 'contraversive pushing' (Santos-Pontelli et al., 2004; Lafosse et al., 2005; Baccini et al., 2006; Karnath &Brotz, 2007), 'ipsilateral pushing' (Pedersen et al., 1996) and 'lateropulsion' (Babyar et al., 2009). D'Aquila et al (2004) (D'Aquila et al., 2004) referred to this behavior as being synonymous with the 'listing phenomenon', but Brunnstrum's first description mentions neither the behavior of active pushing away from the nonparetic side nor the resistance to posture correction (Brunnstrom, 1970).

Since it was first described in 1985 (Davies, 1985) , interest in PB has been increasing. The aim of this review is to summarize and critically discuss several aspects of this intriguing disorder that are described in the literature.

## 2. Assessment

The assessment of PB has been conducted either by clinical examination according the recommendations of the physiotherapist Davies (Pedersen et al., 1996; Lafosse et al., 2005; Baccini et al., 2006) or by ordinal scales (Babyar et al., 2009). According to the systematic review by Babyar and coworkers, there are three appropriate clinical examination scales for evaluation of PB (Babyar et al., 2009): the Scale for Contraversive Pushing (SCP), the Modified Scale for Contraversive Pushing (mSCP) and the Burke Lateropulsion Scale (BLS).

Based on the Davies' criteria, Karnath et al. (Karnath et al., 2001) created the SCP that assesses three distinct aspects of postural control: A) symmetry of spontaneous posture while sitting and standing, B) the use of the ipsilesional extremities to abduct and extend the area of physical contact with the surface (arm/hand on mattress; leg/foot on floor) while sitting and standing, and C) resistance to passive correction of posture while sitting and standing. The authors made the diagnosis of PB if all three criteria were present, reaching a total score of at least 1 in each criterion (sitting plus standing in the three situations).

By analyzing the clinimetric properties of the SCP, Baccini et al. (Baccini et al., 2006) found that a cutoff score of greater than 0 in each SCP section might be more appropriate for studies aimed at investigating the prevalence of the PB or its association with other features, such as presence of neglect because this cutoff enhanced the specificity without any decrease in sensitivity or the predictive value of a negative test. Nevertheless, this cutoff criterion requires further investigation in an unselected group of acute neurologically injured patients (Karnath &Brotz, 2007). Since the original cutoff score suggested by Karnath et al. has no false-positive diagnoses (Baccini et al., 2006), it should be better used for pathophysiological studies or investigations about the neural substrates involved with the PB.

Recently, more specific instructions of the SCP were published (Karnath &Brotz, 2007). The use of the nonparetic extremities to bring about the pathological lateral tilt of the body axis was called 'variable B', and its standing assessment was described as follows: 'The examiner first observes whether the ipsilesional leg is spontaneously (already when rising from the sitting position) abducted and extended. If so, variable B is given the value 1 for standing. If abduction and extension of the nonparetic leg are not spontaneously performed, the examiner asks the patient to start walking. The examiner observes whether the patient now abducts and extends the ipsilesional leg. If so, variable B is given the value 0.5 for standing'. Because the instructions above do not consider the reaction of the arm/hand in standing position and does not include any recommendation for the examiner's performance during the assessment, we suggest the following additional instructions that we found very helpful for the SCP assessment: (1) while the patient is in the standing position, his/her paretic/plegic leg should be supported by using a knee extension split or by the examiner's stabilization (see figure 1); (2) also in the standing position, the examiner should guarantee the presence of a surface next to the patient to observe the behavior of the ipsilesional arm/hand in searching for contact with the surface and achieving extension of the elbow. Another slight but noteworthy detail that should be remembered when assessing the SCP in the sitting position is that patients should be evaluated with plantar support. Nevertheless, an additional bedside tool to detect PB is the investigation of the pusher patients' leg-to-trunk orientation (Johannsen et al., 2006a). When seated upright without contact with the ground, an ipsiversive tilt of the non-paretic leg in relation to the trunk of about 9° is observed. The inclined leg position is maintained throughout the entire tilt cycle. This reaction was not observed in non-brain-damaged subjects, in patients with acute unilateral vestibular dysfunction, or in patients with stroke without PB and vestibular dysfunction (Johannsen et al., 2006a).

The Modified Scale for Contraversive Pushing (mSCP) consists of a composite score that quantifies the PB and includes four functional conditions: (1) static sitting at the bedside with the feet on the floor; (2) static standing with a fully erect posture; (3) transferring from the bed to a chair or wheelchair (with armrests) while maintaining hip flexion; (4) transferring from the bed to a chair or wheelchair by coming to a full standing position and stepping or pivoting 90 degrees (Lagerqvist &Skargren, 2006). Each part is scored separately and the degree of pushing is evaluated on a scale from 0 to 2 points, where 0 indicates no symptoms, and 2 indicates very severe symptoms. The highest possible score is 8 and the recommended diagnostic cutoff score is 3 (Lagerqvist &Skargren, 2006). As suggested by Baccini et al. (Baccini et al., 2006), this modified version is so different from the original SCP that it should be considered a different instrument. Adding transfers and using specific scoring criteria may help examiners of patients whose PB tends to manifest with dynamic balance activities. The concurrent validity of the mSCP with Berg Balance Scale and Swedish Physiotherapy Clinical Outcome was low to moderate, and the inter-rater reliability was moderate to good. Although the mSCP seems to be practical and more sensitive for small changes in the PB's status, further studies are needed because the sample size of its only clinimetric properties' study was small, and all patients exhibited signs of PB. Moreover, sensitivity/specificity data, internal consistency and responsiveness are not available for this scale (Lagerqvist &Skargren, 2006).

The Burke Lateropulsion Scale (BLS) was first developed in 1993 and revised several times by the physiotherapist team of the Burke Rehabilitation Hospital (D'Aquila et al., 2004). This scale is rated according to the severity of resistance to passive correction of the posture or the presence of PB sensed by the examiner during supine rolling, sitting, standing, transferring and walking (0, 1=mild, 2=moderate, 3=severe). According to the authors, to test sitting and standing, the patient is passively tilted 30° (15–20° for standing) towards his/her paretic side (contralesional tilt) and then brought back to vertical alignment. Scores are then based on any voluntary or reflex movements noted in trunks, arms or legs according to the angle from true vertical where the resistance starts. For example, the sitting scores are as follows: 0=no resistance; 1=resistance starts at 5° tilt before full vertical; 2=resistance starts at 10° tilt before full vertical; and 3 is scored if they sense true vertical between 30° and 10° (D'Aquila et al., 2004). Total scores range from 0 for those without resistance to a maximum score of 17. Patients scoring 2 or greater are considered to exhibit PB (lateropulsion).

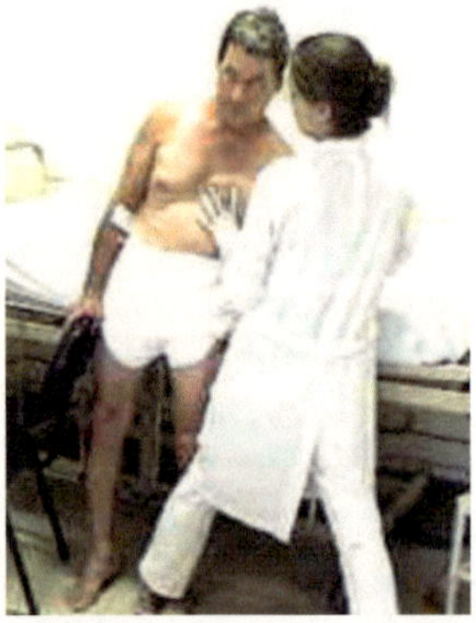

Fig. 1. A patient with left brain damage and severe pusher behavior. Examiner stabilizes the paretic leg of the patient in order to evaluate PB sings in standing position. The absence of this stabilization makes the observation of the characteristics of the disorder significantly difficult. Also, the examiner should guarantee the presence of a surface besides the patient in standing position, in order to observe the behavior of ipsilesional arm/hand activity to search for contact with the surface and of achieving extension of the elbow.

D`Aquila et al. (2004) analyzed the concurrent validity of the BLS with Fugl-Meyer Balance score, Functional Independence Measure and length of rehabilitation stay is moderate and the inter-rater reliability is very high. However, there are no available data about sensitivity, specificity, internal consistency and responsiveness for this scale. According to the authors, one of the weaknesses of the BLS is that the assessments are subjective and can be affected by both patient and therapist comfort and familiarity with the test protocol (D'Aquila et al., 2004). It could be difficult for untrained examiners to interpret the 5 or 10-degree increments from true vertical to determine the resistance to passive correction during functional activities. Nevertheless, this is the only scale that includes PB evaluation during supine rolling and walking.

Another assessment of PB was proposed by Lafosse et al.[11] based on Davies' criteria (Lafosse et al., 2005), including (a) the presence of an asymmetrical posture or the midline of the body towards the hemiplegic side, and (b) the presence of resistance against any attempt at passive correction of any of these postures across the midline of the body towards the 'non-affected' or ipsilesional side. A patient is classified as having PB if both criteria are present. No ordinal scale is specified in this analysis. Further differentiation is used with the help of a 4-point scale that is based on the number of postures (standing, sitting and/or lying) in which contraversive pushing is present as follows: a score of 0 indicated no PB, a score of 1 indicated PB when standing, a score of 2 indicated PB when standing and sitting and a score of 3 indicated PB when standing, sitting and lying. Measurement of inter-rater reliability revealed a percentage of agreement of 88.4% and a Kendall's coefficient of concordance of 0.83 (Lafosse et al., 2005). According to the authors, this assessment of PB is closely related to the SCP. However, it also has no available data about sensitivity, specificity, internal consistency and responsiveness.

## 3. Incidence

Among the studies that considered the PB according to Davies' description, the incidence of this disorder ranges from 1.5 % to 63 % of patients with acute encephalic lesions (Table 1) (Pedersen et al., 1996; Danells et al., 2004; Santos-Pontelli et al., 2004; Lafosse et al., 2005; Baccini et al., 2006). Pedersen et al. (Pedersen et al., 1996) found an incidence of 5.3 % of PB in all stroke patients who were admitted in study period and 10.4 % of patients without lower extremity paresis on admission, when early death or early recovery were excluded. Danells et al. (Danells et al., 2004) found a PB incidence of 23% and 63% among 65 stroke patients with moderate to severe hemiparesis depending on the assessment cutoff. We found 1.5 % of pusher patients among all neurological inpatients of an emergency hospital (Santos-Pontelli et al., 2004), and Lafosse et al. (Lafosse et al., 2005) found an incidence of 40 % of left-brain-damaged patients and 52% of right brain damaged patients at a rehabilitation center. More recently, Baccini and coworkers (Baccini et al., 2006) compared the incidence of the PB based on 4 different criteria: 3 different cutoffs of the SCP (SCP > 0; SCP≥ 1,75; SCP ≥ 3) and a clinical examination according to Davies' recommendations that focused on careful observation of patients while lying down, sitting, standing, weight transferring and walking (table 1).

The comparison of the reported frequencies of PB is very complicated due to the differences in the timing of the first post ictal evaluation, inclusion/exclusion criteria, characteristics of the institutions where patients were investigated, etiologies included in the screening and the assessments of PB and their cutoffs.

The post ictal timing of the first identification of PB is an important aspect for incidence analysis. PB may not be observed if the assessment is done in outpatients or after several weeks because of early resolution of the behavior. On the other hand, if the assessment is conducted too early, pusher behavior can appear as a fluctuated symptom. Therefore, the screening of this behavior should be conducted as soon as clinical conditions allow and repeated afterwards during several weeks after the ictus onset.

## 4. Demographic and clinical characteristics

The comparison of demographic and clinical characteristics between series of pusher patients is complicated not only because of the several selection criteria discussed above but also due to the differences among the designs of the studies. Nevertheless, we summarized some demographic and clinical characteristics that have been published so far (table 2).

Pusher behavior has been found more frequently in older patients (table 2). More recently, Barbieri et al. found a correlation between age and perception of posture in healthy subjects (Barbieri et al., 2009). If the internal model of verticality is less robust in elderly people, it would be possible that this population could be more vulnerable to present PB. Though, the incidence of strokes is much greater in old than in young adults. It remains unclear the influence of the deterioration of postural control related to aging on the development of PB. Moreover, there is no investigation about the occurrence of PB in children with an acute encephalic lesion.

| Author (year) | Institution characteristics | Etiologies included for screening | Time of PB evaluation (mean±SD) | Assessment | Cutoff | Incidence |
|---|---|---|---|---|---|---|
| Pedersen et al. (1996) | Stroke Unit (acute care, workup and rehabilitation stages) | Stroke | NA | - Lean towards the hemiplegic side in any position<br>- Resistance of any attempt of correction | PB presence considered if 'pushing were present in any posture'. | 5,3%*<br>10,4%** |
| Danells et al. (2004) | 5 different acute care hospitals | Stroke | 8±2 days | SCP | SCP > 0<br>SCP = 3 | 63%<br>23% |
| Santos-Pontelli et al. (2004) | Neurological Unit of an Emergency Hospital | All acute neurologic diseases | 31,7 days (range=8-57 days) | SCP | SCP ≥ 3¥ | 1,5% |
| Lafosse et al. (2005) | Rehabilitation Center | Stroke | 52,71±39,58 | - Lean towards the hemiplegic side<br>- Resistance of any attempt of correction (Plus a 4-point scale) | PB presence considered if both criteria were present. | 40-52% |
| Baccini et al. (2008) [26] | 2 Inpatient rehabilitation hospitals | Stroke | <=30 | - Clinical examination based on Davies recommendations<br>- SCP | - At least 2 of the authors mentioned singns were present, with one of them judge as severe<br>- SCP > 0<br>- SCP≥ 1,75+<br>- SCP ≥ 3 | - 16,2%<br>- 61,9%<br>- 18,1%<br>- 10,5% |

SCP= Scale for Contraversive Pushing. NA= not available. SD= Standard Deviation *All stroke patients admitted in study period. **Patients without lower extremity paresis on admission, with early death or early recovery were excluded. ¥ At least one point in each criterion. + More than 0 in each criterion.

Table 1. Dependent factors for the incidence of pusher behavior. PB= Pusher Behavior.

| Author (year) | Whole Sample (pusher patients) | Male % | Age (mean±SD) | Right encephalic lesion % | Paresis % | Sensory deficit % | Neglect / Anosognosia | Aphasia |
|---|---|---|---|---|---|---|---|---|
| Pedersen et al. (1996) | 327 (34) | 47,1% | 75±7,6 | 52,9%** | NA | NA | 40% / 27,3% | 47,1% |
| Karnath et al. (2000) | 10 (5) | 40%** | 73,6±4,56** | 100% | 100% | 100% | 100% | 0% |
| Karnath et al. (2000) | 46 (23) | 60,87%** | 71 (39-81)■<br>68 (38-89)#<br>Median (range) | 65,2% | 100% | 80%■<br>62%# | 80%■<br>0%# | 7%■<br>100%# |
| Pérennou et al. (2002) | 14 (3) | 66,67%** | 52,67±5,03** | 100%** | 100%** | 100%** | 100% | NA |
| Karnath et al. (2002) | 23 (12) | 66,6% | 68,5 (38-81)<br>Median (range) | 75%** | 100% | 58% | 67%■<br>0%# | 0%■<br>100%# |
| Broetz et al. (2004) | 8 (8) | 100% | 63 (51-79)<br>Median (range) | 75% | 100% | 71% | 83%■<br>0%# | 0%■<br>50%# |
| Danells et al. (2004) | 62 (39) | 59% | 69 (NA) | 59% | 82%▲ | 56% | 62% | NA |
| Santos-Pontelli et al. (2004) | 530 (8) | 62,5% | 65,4±12,32** | 75%* | 87,5%▲** | 50%** | 75%** | 25%* |
| Saj et al. (2005) | 17 (5) | 40%** | 69±6,6** | 100% | NA | NA | 80% | NA |
| Karnath et al. (2005) | 40 (14) | 57,14%** | 66,1±7,5■<br>63,9±9,7# | 64,28%** | 100% | 89%■<br>80%# | 67%■<br>0%# | 0%■<br>60%° |
| Pontelli et al. (2005) | 9 (9) | 55,50%** | 71,8±5,9 | 55,50%** | 100%** | 66,6%** | 33,30%** | NA |
| Johannsen et al. (2006) | 25 (15) | 80%** | 70 (41-88)<br>Median (range) | 86,6%** | 100% | NA | 73% | 7% |
| Johannsen et al. (2006) | 45 (21) | 80,95%** | 68±9,4■<br>67,8±8,3# | 52,3%** | 91%■<br>100%# | 73%■<br>90%# | 100%■<br>10%# | 0%■<br>80%# |
| Johannsen et al. (2006) | 25 (9) | 66,67%** | 69,7±13 | 88,88%** | 100% | NA | 88% | 0% |
| Pérrenou et al (2008) | 86 (6) | 66,67%** | 62,67±11,33** | 83,30%** | NA | NA | NA | NA |
| Babyar et al. (2008) | 72 (36) | 52,77%** | 74,6±9,1■<br>72,5±8,5# | 58,33%** | NA | NA | 0%■**<br>27,77%#** | 73,33%■**<br>0%** |
| Honoré et al (2009) | 18 (3) | 33,3%** | 66,3±6,7 | 100% | NA | NA | 100% | NA |
| Ticini et al. (2009) | 19 (9) | 66,66%** | 67,8±6,1 α<br>64,5±16,6 β | 66,6%** | 100% | NA | 100%■**<br>0%#** | 33,3%** |

NA= not available. *Data informed by the authors. **Calculated from the data available in the reference. ■Right brain damaged patients. #Left brain damaged patients. ▲Severe hemiparesis. αThalamic brain damaged patients. βExtra-thalamic brain damaged patients.

Table 2. Overview of demographic and clinical characteristics observed on the first evaluation of pusher patients in published literature.

A possible gender influence on the incidence of PB was initially suggested (Lafosse et al., 2005). Nevertheless, analysis of several studies performed in large samples of neurologic injured patients found no persistent gender predominance (Danells et al., 2004; Santos-Pontelli et al., 2004; Lafosse et al., 2005).

Paresis of the contralesional extremities seems to be more frequent and more severe in pusher patients than in control encephalic lesioned patients (Karnath et al., 2005). On the other hand, severe PB can occur despite mild degree of hemiparesis (Santos-Pontelli et al., 2007). This observation raises an interesting question: is hemiparesis necessary for the development of the pushing behavior? We reported a patient that the resolution of the contraversive pushing did not depend on the resolution of the hemiparesis (Santos-Pontelli et al., 2007). Therefore, it is possible that hemiparesis may be more properly considered a commonly associated symptom of PB rather than an essential component of the syndrome and its damaged graviceptive circuitry. Further studies involving patients with pusher syndrome controlled for the degree of hemiparesis may be necessary to clarify the impact of PB itself on long-term prognosis after neurologic conditions.

## 5. Postural control

The mechanisms underlying PB have been attributed to a dysfunction of sensory (vertical) perception that leads to a postural reactive behavior (Karnath et al., 2000b; Karnath &Broetz, 2003; Saj et al., 2005; Johannsen et al., 2006c; Perennou, D. A. et al., 2008). These perceptions represent the subjective spatial perceptions, which include the haptic vertical (SHV), visual vertical (SVV), postural vertical (SPV) and the subjective straight ahead (SSA). Figure 2 shows the methodology and sensorial systems involved with these perceptions, and table 3 summarizes the available data about the subjective spatial perceptions of pusher patients published so far.

Karnath et al. found 5 patients with severe PB (SCP=6) who experience their body as being oriented "upright" when it is actually tilted about 18° towards the side of the brain lesion and with no SVV bias (Karnath et al., 2000b). According to the authors, the possible explanation for the PB is that when patients try to move their body to a subjectively 'upright' position, they became laterally unstable because their center of mass was shifted too far to the ipsilesional side and they react to this imbalance by pushing themselves to the contralesional side (Karnath et al., 2000b; Karnath, 2007).

In contrast, Pérrenou et al. recently found a contralesional bias of SPV in 6 pusher patients with an SCP score ranging from 3 to 6. Moreover, all these patients also presented with contralesional tilts in SHV and SVV (Perennou, D. A. et al., 2008). Their hypothesis was that pushing is an implicit active body postural alignment with the perceived vertical. Interestingly, Johannsen et al. demonstrated that patients with PB align their nonparetic leg upright when their trunks are actually tilted to the side opposite to the encephalic lesion (Johannsen et al., 2006a). The authors pointed out that observing the spontaneous posture of the body segments in a seated subject may be a reasonable approach to predict the subject's SPV (Johannsen et al., 2006a). However, future research is needed to verify the correlation between SPV and non-paretic leg orientation in the same sample of pusher patients.

The contradictory findings described above may reflect a difference in the methodology and inclusion/exclusion criteria. Karnath et al. (Karnath et al., 2000b) evaluated the SPV with the patients' legs hanging freely, while Pérennou et al. used a plantar support (Perennou, D. A. et al., 2008). Additionally, Pérrenou et al. did not screen for neglect. The influence of the presence of plantar support or neglect on the measurement of the SPV is unknown.

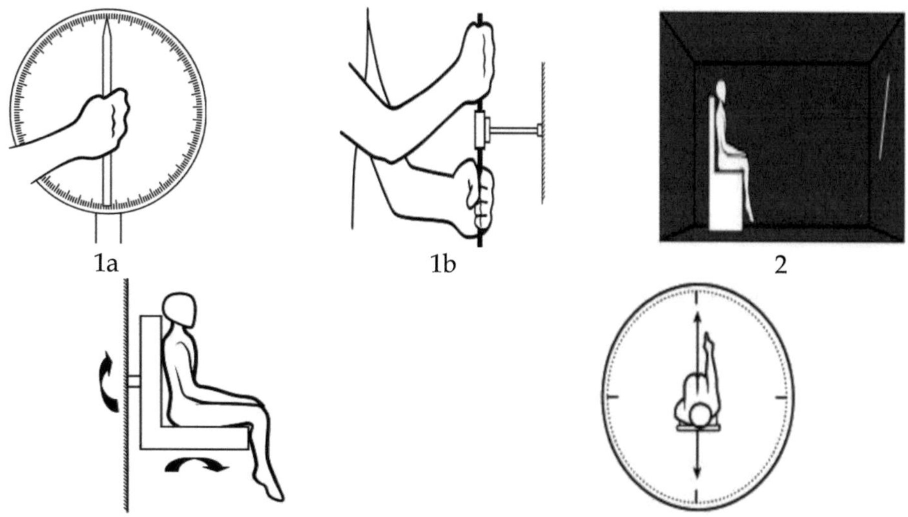


1. SHV: determined by manipulation of a wooden or metal rod to the earth-vertical position with the patients' eyes closed: this is essentially driven by proprioceptive afferences (Sharpe, 2003). 1a: with one hand.1b: with two hands.
2. SVV: assessed by the patients' verbal command to adjust a visible line in complete darkness. It depends only on vestibular information with the assistance of the visual cues, independent of the proprioceptors and truncal graviceptors when the subjects are positioned in alignment with Earth vertical (Anastasopoulos et al., 1997; Mittelstaedt, 1998; Trousselard et al., 2004; Lopez et al., 2011).
3. SPV: assessed with subjects seated on a tiltable chair that is capable of rotating in a particular plane and is immobilized by lateral stabilization to prevent postural reactions. The examiner asks the subjects to state, in absence of vision, when they feel their body as vertically oriented (Karnath et al., 2000b; Sharpe, 2003; Perennou, D. A. et al., 2008). The tilting velocity must be 1.5°/s to minimize semicircular canal stimulation (Sadeghi et al., 2007), and acoustic and vibration feedback should also be taken into account. This is determined essentially by interoceptive inputs (Mittelstaedt, 1998; Karnath et al., 2000b).
4. SSA: evaluated by asking the patient to point to the position they perceived as straight ahead and represents an egocentric reference framework (Richard et al., 2004; Saj et al., 2006).

Fig. 2. Methodology description and the sensorial systems involved with SHV, SVV, SPV and SSA.

The SVV (with a haptic component) and the SSA was found to be tilted to the side of the lesion in patients with neglect without PB and tilted to the contralesional side in patients with neglect and PB (Saj et al., 2005; Honore et al., 2009). Nevertheless, the SVV with no haptic influence conducted in a representative sample of pusher patients with and without neglect did not reveal a tilt of this perception[46]. Unfortunately, none of the above studies performed a systematic evaluation of the vestibular system for review see (Eggers & Zee, 2003). Although the dysfunction of the vestibular system is not assumed to be involved with PB (Perennou, D., 2005; Pontelli et al., 2005), its evaluation became imperative to dissociate vestibular dysfunction from the vertical misperceptions of pusher patients because SVV is essentially driven by this system (Anastasopoulos et al., 1997; Mittelstaedt, 1998; Trousselard et al., 2004). Other aspects to be considered for the evaluation of verticality perception are the learning effect and the number of trials performed. Therefore, in order to state which vertical perception is disturbed in pusher patients, the studies' designs require a meticulous methodology and a large sample of pusher patients. The underlying mechanisms of PB still remain unclear.

| Author (year) | Number of patients | Lesion side | Neglect | SVV Mean (SD) | SPV Mean (SD) | SHV Mean (SD) | SSA Mean (SD) |
|---|---|---|---|---|---|---|---|
| Karnath et al. (2000) | 5 | RBD | 100% | -0,4 ° (2,5°) | +17,9 ° (4,7°) | NA | NA |
| Saj et al (2005) | 4<br>1 | RBD | 100%<br>0% | +4,8 ° (5,1°)<br>+2,2° | NA | NA | NA |
| Johannsen et al. (2006) | 15 | 13 RBD<br>2 LBD | 73% | -3,2° (4,8°) | NA | NA | NA |
| Pérennou et al. (2008) | 6 | 5RBD<br>1LBD | NA | -6,53° (1,86)** | -10,6° (5,85°)** | -7,48° (1,71°)** | NA |
| Honnoré et al. (2009) | 3 | RBD | 100% | NA | NA | NA | -8,7° (2,4°) |

SD: Standard Deviation; RBD: Right Brain Damage; LBD: Left Brain Damage; *(with haptic component)
** Mean and standard deviation calculated from the data available in the reference (Perennou, D. A. et al., 2008).

Table 3. Summarized available data about the subjective perceptions of pusher patients.

## 6. Prognosis and rehabilitation

There are few studies that address the resolution of PB (Karnath et al., 2002; Broetz et al., 2004; Danells et al., 2004; Santos-Pontelli et al., 2004; Lafosse et al., 2005). Until now, the PB is described as having good prognosis with a maximum recovery time of 6 months (Karnath et al., 2002). Dannels and coworkers showed that the recovery of PB is neither strongly associated with age nor with the recovery of motor control evaluated by Fugl-Meyer motor scale (Danells et al., 2004). However, patients with neglect and those who presented higher initial SCP scores had longer PB recovery times (Danells et al., 2004; Lafosse et al., 2005). Recently, Babyar and coworkers demonstrated that pusher patients following stroke have a lower Functional Independence Measure efficiency and more dependency at discharge when compared with matched controls with equal functional limitations (Babyar et al., 2009). In addition, stroke patients seem to have worse PB prognosis than patients with brain trauma (Santos-Pontelli et al., 2004); this difference in recovery time may be related to etiology, extension, or inherent resolution mechanisms of the causative lesion.

Based on the Bobath concept, Davies described several activities using manual guidance (somesthetic information) to induce the midline body position in the pusher patients (Davies, 1985). Later, Broetz and Karnath suggested a visual feedback approach for PB based on their findings in 5 patients who presented with tilted SPV with unaffected SVV, as discussed above (Broetz et al., 2004; Broetz &Karnath, 2005). According to the authors, because the orientation perception of visual cues in pusher patients is not impaired, they can be trained to use conscious strategies to realign their body.

However, the contralesional tilts of SPV, SVV and SHV recently described in patients with PB raise the question about the utility of visual feedback treatment in all pusher patients (Pedersen et al., 1996). Some findings with healthy subjects have shown a difference in performance if the learner directs attention toward the effect of the movement (an external focus) instead of to the movement itself (an internal focus) (Wulf et al., 1998). It is possible that in pusher patients with multimodal misperception, we could induce the patient to perceive that their body position is tilted by showing the difference between the effect of the movement using their perceived (wrong) vertical reference and using the (somesthetic or verbal) reference given by the therapist. Broetz and Karnath recommended this demonstration of the ineffective result of the pathological pushing in patients with unimodal misperception (Broetz et al., 2004).

Recently, Shepherd and Carr suggested that the behavioral development may be a natural adaptive response to rehabilitation methods that have the potential to increase the fear of falling and provoke defensive pushing (Shepherd &Carr, 2005). The fact that PB has been identified early after the encephalic lesion argues against this possibility. Additionally, we performed a systematic screening of PB in an acute neurological unit (Santos-Pontelli et al., 2004), and we often identified the PB while the patients were positioned sitting on the edge of the bed for the first time after the onset. Nevertheless, as pointed out by the authors, it is imperative to take the fear of falling into account and to be careful to perform the exercises without evoking fear.

Other general evidence-based methods of intervention are naturally applied for pusher patients because other neurological deficits are present. So far, several studies suggest the following: task-oriented exercises, patients' focus on the actual activity, strength and skill training, specific strategies for spatial neglect (when present), patients' awareness of their deficits, attention to the intensity of skill practice and the extent of cardiovascular stress, proper rehabilitation environment, and the use of a treadmill with and without body weight support [for review see (Carr & Shepherd, 2006)].

A consensus on neurological rehabilitation is that intervention requires specificity and that the postural balance is essential in regaining independence in the activities of daily living. Thus, exercises must be individualized, and the best therapeutic strategy for PB should be chosen based on the vertical misperception of each pusher patient as soon as possible. The absence of controlled trials that investigate the treatment of PB supports the need for further research. Moreover, we should be careful about making statements about the PB based on few samples. Multicenter researches could help PB investigative groups to perform more representative studies in order to clarify all the underlying aspects of this still largely unknown neurological disorder.

## 7. Neuroimaging analysis

Several brain structures have been associated with PB. In this context, Pedersen et al.(Pedersen et al., 1996) and Santos-Pontelli et al. (Santos-Pontelli et al., 2011) have indicated a wide range of findings from no visible lesion to massive hemispheric lesions on neuroimaging scans in a large sample of PB patients. In these studies, radiologists and neurologists analyzed computed tomography or magnetic resonance imaging in order to determine the type and location of the encephalic lesions. Pedersen at al. determined the size of the stroke by the largest diameter of the lesion (Pedersen et al., 1996).

Nevertheless, the location of lesion more consistently described as related to PB occurrence is the posterior thalamus (Karnath et al., 2000a; Karnath et al., 2005). Besides the usual consideration as a relay structure of vestibular pathway (Deecke et al., 1974; Buttner &Henn, 1976), the posterior thalamus is also assumed to be essentially involved in the control of upright body posture. For the lesion analysis, Karnath et al. (Karnath et al., 2000a) compared patients with PB to patients without PB but comparable demographic and clinical data. Using the Talaraich space, the central area of overlap was defined as those voxels in the MRI template that were lesioned in at least 53% or more of their series (number of PB patients=15). The center of lesion overlap was located in the ventral posterior and lateral posterior of the posterolateral thalamus.

Among 40 patients with thalamic strokes (14 pusher patients and 26 control patients), Karnath et al. (Karnath et al., 2005) found that pusher patients had lesions that typically were caused by thalamic hemorrhage. This observation seems to resemble the fact that thalamic hemorrhages predominantly affect the posterolateral part of the thalamus (Hungerbuhler et al., 1984; Kawahara et al., 1986; Kumral et al., 1995; Chung et al., 1996) and that infarctions are less frequent in the posterior thalamus vs. the anterior and paramedian thalamus (Bogousslavsky et al., 1988; Van der Werf et al., 2000). Nevertheless, their control patients presented more ischemic than hemorrhagic thalamic strokes. Using two standard protocols, the authors carried out MRI or spiral CT imaging that were fit the canonical AC-PC orientation of the MRI scans (Karnath et al., 2005). The boundary of the lesion was delineated directly on the individual MRI for every single transversal slice using MRIcro software (Roden & Brett, 2000). Both the scan and lesion shape were then transferred into stereotaxic space using the spatial normalization algorithm provided by SPM2. The MRIcro software was also used to map the lesion from transversal slices of the T1-template MRI from Montreal Neurologic Institute (MNI) space. The authors used the Talairach Z-coordinates in Talairach space by using the identical or the closest matching transversal slices of each individual. Lesion location in the thalamic stroke patients with and without PB was compared using the subtraction technique (Karnath et al., 2005). The percentage of overlapping lesions of the PB patients after subtraction of controls ranged 20%.

The PB is also observed in patients with brain lesions that spare the thalamus as postcentral gyrus (Johannsen et al., 2006b), internal capsule (Pedersen et al., 1996; Saj et al., 2005), temporal lobe (Pedersen et al., 1996; Johannsen et al., 2006b), supplementary motor area (Reding et al., 1997), superior parietal lobule (Reding et al., 1997), inferior parietal lobule (Johannsen et al., 2006b), globus pallidus (Reding et al., 1997), striatum (Saj et al., 2005), centrum semi-ovalum (Saj et al., 2005), insula (Reding et al., 1997; Johannsen et al., 2006b), isolated cerebellum (Paci &Nannetti, 2005) and isolated anterior cerebral artery territory (Karnath et al., 2008).

By analyzing neuroimaging scans of patients with and without PB with the same methodology of Karnath et al. (Karnath et al., 2005), Johannsen et al. found very small regions for pusher patients when subtracted from matched controls (Johannsen et al., 2006b). In both hemispheres, the lesion of the pusher patients centered at the insular cortex and the postcentral gyrus. However, these areas were identified with the subtraction technique where the percentage of difference between the pusher and control patients neuroimaging scans was not exclusively 100% (ranged from 81 to 100%). Although both were meticulous studies (Karnath et al., 2005; Johannsen et al., 2006b), this analysis does not exclude the same lesion location in control patients.

Recently, Ticini et al. (Ticini et al., 2009), found that the posterior thalamus itself is integral to the occurrence of PB rather than additional malperfusion in distant cortical areas by using perfusion-weighted imaging (PWI), diffusion-weighted imaging (DWI) and T2-weighted fluid-attenuated inversion-recovery (FLAIR) imaging,. Moreover, they found no damage or malperfusion of the thalamus in patients with PB caused by extra-thalamic lesions. While DWI and FLAIR imaging reveal information about irreversibly damaged neural tissue, PWI allows the identification of structurally intact but not enough to function normally. These interesting findings indicate that the thalamic as well as the extra-thalamic brain structures previously related to the PB contribute to the network controlling upright body posture (Ticini et al., 2009).

Most recently, the relationship between neuroimaging data of stroke and non-stroke PB patients and the severity and prognosis of PB was analyzed (Santos-Pontelli et al., 2011). In order to measure the hemorrhage stroke volume (HSV) in patients with hemorrhagic stroke it was used the ABC/2 method (Zazulia et al., 1999) on CT scans of the acute stroke stage. A positive correlation of the National Institute of Health Stroke Scale (NIHSS) score with HSV in hemorrhagic stroke PB patients was found. In spite of this fact, neither the NIHSS score nor HSV were related with the severity or recovery time of PB. Conversely, previous studies showed that the hemorrhagic volume is highly associated with functional and neurologic deficits (NINDS ICH Workshop Participants, 2005). These data and the fact that the NIHSS score is a good neurologic outcome predictor (Wilde et al, 2010; Wityk et al., 1994; Aslanyan et al., 2004) indicate that the PB evolution and severity may be independent from other neurologic deficits such as those measured by the NIHSS. However, more research is needed to confirm this observation.

The fact that all the pusher patients described in literature had an acute event raises the question that the velocity of lesion´s onset may be essential for PB occurrence. In fact, PB also has been reported in patients with other acute brain lesions other than stroke, but not in patients with chronic neurodegenerative disorders (Santos-Pontelli et al., 2004). These observations may indicate that the related alteration of postural control observed in PB may be a consequence of any acute encephalic lesion that lead to a dysfunction in the neural network which processes the input for vertical perception. Figure 3 and 4 show examples of neuroimaging scans of stroke and non-stroke patients with PB.

## 8. Clinical implications of neuroimaging findings

The analysis of the clinical implications of neuroimaging findings requires an important discussion about some limitations of the neuroimaging methods in order to critically interpret the results of the several PB studies.

The localization of human brain functions by studying the correlation between a behavioral disorder and the region of brain lesion has an historical and huge contribution to the understanding of brain function. Nevertheless, as well as all the neuroimaging techniques, the 'lesion method' has some noteworthy limitations.

Roden and Karnath pointed out that the lesion method usually assumes that after a focal lesion, the intact regions of the brain continue to function in the same manner as before the lesion (Roden & Karnath, 2004). However, with tasks controlled by spread and changeable circuits, the brain start to adapt rapidly following the lesion. This rearrangement is helpful for recovery, but makes it difficult to infer the original function of the healthy brain. Also, the design of the brain, its blood supply and the surrounding skull mean that some areas of the brain are injured more often than others what implicate that the locations of brain damage are not randomly distributed in the brain. Roden and Karnath highlighted that this makes it difficult to interpret lesion overlay plots (Roden & Karnath, 2004). Moreover, if we test patients in the acute stage of their disease, we will not be able to accurately identify all of the brain regions that are damaged. However, if we wait for these initial issues to resolve, the issues associated with brain plasticity will become more evident.

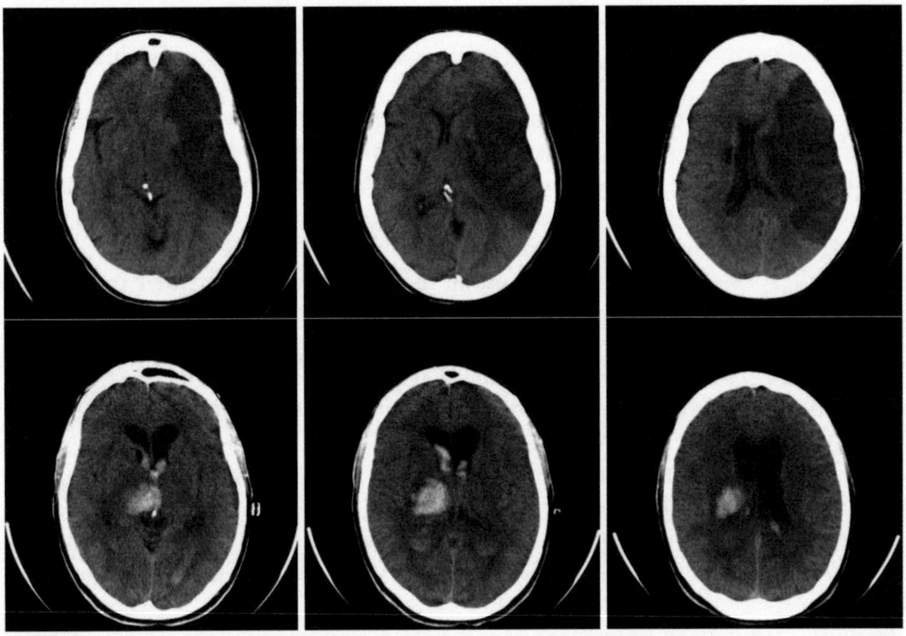

1: Ischemic stroke of the left M1 segment of the middle cerebral artery and significant midline shift (midline shift of the septum pellucidum = 8mm; interthalamic adhesion = 6mm; pineal = 7mm).
2: Right thalamic hemorrhagic stroke with intraventricular hemorrhage and midline shift (midline shift of the septum pellucidum = 2mm; interthalamic adhesion = 5mm; pineal = 9mm).

Fig. 3. CT scans of PB patients in the acute stage.

Although lesion data do not provide the precision of fMRI activation foci, they can tell us which areas are necessary for controlling a cognitive function (Roden & Karnath, 2004). According to Roden and Karnath, simple overlay plots for patients who have a disorder can be inaccurate due to the fact that the regions that they highlight might reflect increased vulnerability of certain regions to injury (as discussed above), rather than any direct involvement with the disorder of interest. A control group of neurological patients who do not exhibit the deficit of interest is, therefore, fundamental for valid anatomical conclusions (Roden & Karnath, 2004). Each technique on its own has only limited explanatory power. However, the strengths and weaknesses of these tools are complementary.
In neuroimaging studies, it is a common practice to spatially normalize subject brains to a standard coordinate system in order to reduce intersubject variability, enable intersubject image averaging, and facilitate the reporting of reduced results in the form of stereotactic coordinates. Numerous registration methods exist, and the two most established are based on the Talairach atlas (Talairach & Tournoux, 1988) and the Montreal Neurological Institute (MNI) templates (Evans et al., 1993; Collins et al., 1994; Laird et al, 2010). The Talairach cannot reflect an excellent representation of the neuroanatomy for the general population atlas because it was created based on the postmortem brain of single subject. In order to

allow better representation of average neuro-anatomy, the MNI created an average brain template based on the MRI scans from several hundred individuals (Evans et al., 1993;Collins et al., 1994). However, the Talairach coordinate system is still the standard reference system used by the neuroimaging community and it is a common practice to report the results in terms of Talairach coordinates even when different brain templates have been used to analyze imaging data. Nevertheless, there is no simple way to transform multiple subject data from the MNI space to the Talairach space. It is actually possible that the coordinate location in MNI space of two subjects would map to different points of Talairach space (Chau & MacIntosh, 2005). The discrepancy becomes a problem when the data are analyzed in the MNI space but the results are reported using the Talairach space (Brett et al., 2002; Chau & MacIntosh, 2005; Laird et al, 2010). Certainly, there is no perfect solution to the conversion problem. According to Laird et al. (Laird et al, 2010), authors should be encouraged to make a clearer distinction between the basic coordinate system as defined by Talairach and Tournoux (1998) and the reference template corresponding to a standard brain that was used during spatial normalization.

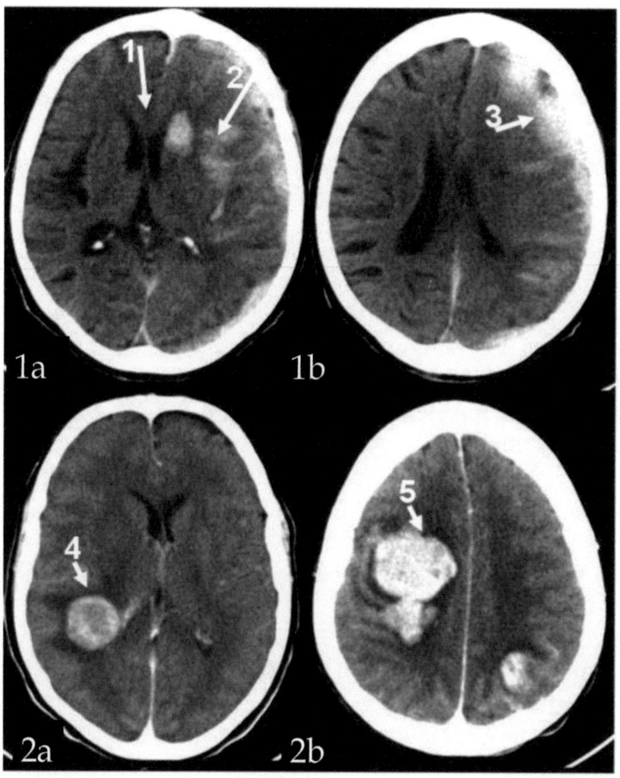


1: Scans from a PB patient with traumatic brain injury. Note the left subdural haematoma and mass effect with midline shift and multiple areas of contusion over the left hemisphere.
2: Scans from a PB patient with multiple hemorrhagic metastasis from a pelvis rabdomiosarcoma. The larger lesions were located in the right frontal and parietal lobes causing a mild falx displacement. (from Santos-Pontelli et al., 2005)

Fig. 4. CT scans of patients showing different etiologies for PB.

In this context, the PB neuroimaging studies greatly advanced our understanding of this interesting behavior. Although without a major precision, the qualitative analysis can be hepful to identify a patient that has a tendency to develop PB by the analysis of his/her neuroimage scan., specially in patients with thalamic lesions. In addition, the knowledge that several lesion locations can elicit PB reinforces the concept that this behavior can be accompanied by several neurologic deficits and all the neurologic condition can be critical for the functional prognosis of PB.

As discussed by Roden and Karnath (Roden & Karnath, 2004), the strength of cognitive neuroscience comes from using convergent tools to investigate the same theoretical question. Although there are neuroimaging studies regarding the PB, it remains an issue of future studies to investigate several aspects of PB using brain activation techniques (funcional magnetic resonance, single-photon emission computed tomography, positron emission tomography, magnetoencephalography, event related potential) and transcranial magnetic stimulation techniques in order to better understand this intriguing behavior.

## 9. Acknowledgement

The authors acknowledge the Coordenaçao de Aperfeiçoamento de Pessoal de Nível Superior (CAPES) and Fundaçao de Amparo à Pesquisa do Estado de Sao Paulo (FAPESP) for the financial support.

## 10. References

Anastasopoulos, D., Haslwanter, T., Bronstein, A., Fetter, M., & Dichgans, J. (1997). Dissociation between the perception of body verticality and the visual vertical in acute peripheral vestibular disorder in humans. Neurosci Lett, 233(2-3), 151-153.

Babyar, S. R., Peterson, M. G., Bohannon, R., Perennou, D., & Reding, M. (2009). Clinical examination tools for lateropulsion or pusher syndrome following stroke: a systematic review of the literature. Clin Rehabil, 23(7), 639-650.

Baccini, M., Paci, M., & Rinaldi, L. A. (2006). The scale for contraversive pushing: A reliability and validity study. Neurorehabil Neural Repair, 20(4), 468-472.

Barbieri, G., Gissot, A. S., & Perennou, D. (2009). Ageing of the postural vertical. Age (Dordr).

Beevor, C. E. (1909). Remarks on paralysis of the movements of the trunk in hemiplegia. Br Med J, 881-885.

Bjerver, K., & Silfverskiold, B. P. (1968). Lateropulsion and imbalance in Wallenberg's syndrome. Acta Neurol Scand, 44(1), 91-100.

Bogousslavsky, J., Regli, F., & Uske, A. (1988). Thalamic infarcts: clinical syndromes, etiology, and prognosis. Neurology, 38(6), 837-848.

Bohannon, R. W. (2004). Pusher syndrome. Phys Ther, 84(6), 580-581; author reply 582-583.

Brandt, T., & Dieterich, M. (2000). Perceived vertical and lateropulsion: clinical syndromes, localization, and prognosis. Neurorehabil Neural Repair, 14(1), 1-12.

Brett, M., Johnsrde, I.S., Owen, A.M. (2002). The problem of functional localization in the human brain. Nat Rev Neurosci, 3, 243–249.

Broetz, D., Johannsen, L., & Karnath, H. O. (2004). Time course of 'pusher syndrome' under visual feedback treatment. Physiother Res Int, 9(3), 138-143.

Broetz, D., & Karnath, H. O. (2005). New aspects for the physiotherapy of pushing behaviour. NeuroRehabilitation, 20(2), 133-138.

Brunnstrom, S. (1970). Movement therapy in hemiplegia. A neurophysiological approach. New York.

Buttner, U., & Henn, V. (1976). Thalamic unit activity in the alert monkey during natural vestibular stimulation. Brain Res, 103(1), 127-132.

Carr, J. H., & Shepherd, R. B. (2006). The changing face of neurological rehabilitation. Rev Bras Fisioter, 10, 147-156.

Chau, W., & McIntosh, A.R. (2005). The Talairach coordinate of a point in the MNI space: how to interpret it. Neuroimage, 25, 408–416.

Chung, C. S., Caplan, L. R., Han, W., Pessin, M. S., Lee, K. H., & Kim, J. M. (1996). Thalamic haemorrhage. Brain, 119 ( Pt 6), 1873-1886.

Collins, D.L., Neelin, P., Peters, T.M., Evans, A.C. (1994). Automatic 3D intersubject registration of MR columetric data in standardized Talairach space. J. Comput. Assist. Tomogr. 18, 192–205.

D'Aquila, M. A., Smith, T., Organ, D., Lichtman, S., & Reding, M. (2004). Validation of a lateropulsion scale for patients recovering from stroke. Clin Rehabil, 18(1), 102-109.

Danells, C. J., Black, S. E., Gladstone, D. J., & McIlroy, W. E. (2004). Poststroke "pushing": natural history and relationship to motor and functional recovery. Stroke, 35(12), 2873-2878.

Davies, P. M. (1985). Steps to follow: a guide to the treatment of adult hemiplegia. New York: Springer.

Deecke, L., Schwarz, D. W., & Fredrickson, J. M. (1974). Nucleus ventroposterior inferior (VPI) as the ventibular thalamic relay in the rhesus monkey. I. Field potential investigation. Exp Brain Res, 20(1), 88-100.

Dieterich, M. (2007). Central vestibular disorders. J Neurol, 254(5), 559-568.

Dieterich, M., & Brandt, T. (1992). Wallenberg's syndrome: lateropulsion, cyclorotation, and subjective visual vertical in thirty-six patients. Ann Neurol, 31(4), 399-408.

Eggers, S. D., & Zee, D. S. (2003). Evaluating the dizzy patient: bedside examination and laboratory assessment of the vestibular system. Semin Neurol, 23(1), 47-58.

Evans, A.C., Collins, D.L., Mills, S.R, Brown, E.D., Kelly, R.L., Peters, T.M. (1993). 3D statistical neuroanatomical models from 305 MRI volumes. Proc. IEEE Nucl. Sci. Symp. Med. Imaging Conf., 1813 - 1817.

Honore, J., Saj, A., Bernati, T., & Rousseaux, M. (2009). The pusher syndrome reverses the orienting bias caused by spatial neglect. Neuropsychologia, 47(3), 634-638.

Hungerbuhler, J. P., Assal, G., & Regli, F. (1984). Thalamic hematomas: neuropsychological aspects. Report of 11 cases and review of literature. Schweiz Arch Neurol Neurochir Psychiatr, 135(2), 199-215.

Johannsen, L., Broetz, D., & Karnath, H. O. (2006a). Leg orientation as a clinical sign for pusher syndrome. BMC Neurol, 6, 30.

Johannsen, L., Broetz, D., Naegele, T., & Karnath, H. O. (2006b). "Pusher syndrome" following cortical lesions that spare the thalamus. J Neurol, 253(4), 455-463.

Johannsen, L., Fruhmann Berger, M., & Karnath, H. O. (2006c). Subjective visual vertical (SVV) determined in a representative sample of 15 patients with pusher syndrome. J Neurol, 253(10), 1367-1369.

Karnath, H. O. (2007). Pusher syndrome-a frequent but little-known disturbance of body orientation perception. J Neurol, 254(4), 415-424.

Karnath, H. O., & Broetz, D. (2003). Understanding and treating "pusher syndrome". Phys Ther, 83(12), 1119-1125.

Karnath, H. O., & Brotz, D. (2007). Instructions for the Clinical Scale for Contraversive Pushing (SCP). Neurorehabil Neural Repair, 21(4), 370-371; author reply 371.

Karnath, H. O., Brotz, D., & Gotz, A. (2001). [Clinical symptoms, origin, and therapy of the "pusher syndrome"]. Nervenarzt, 72(2), 86-92.

Karnath, H. O., Ferber, S., & Dichgans, J. (2000a). The neural representation of postural control in humans. Proc Natl Acad Sci U S A, 97(25), 13931-13936.

Karnath, H. O., Ferber, S., & Dichgans, J. (2000b). The origin of contraversive pushing: evidence for a second graviceptive system in humans. Neurology, 55(9), 1298-1304.

Karnath, H. O., Johannsen, L., Broetz, D., Ferber, S., & Dichgans, J. (2002). Prognosis of contraversive pushing. J Neurol, 249(9), 1250-1253.

Karnath, H. O., Johannsen, L., Broetz, D., & Kuker, W. (2005). Posterior thalamic hemorrhage induces "pusher syndrome". Neurology, 64(6), 1014-1019.

Karnath, H. O., Suchan, J., & Johannsen, L. (2008). Pusher syndrome after ACA territory infarction. Eur J Neurol, 15(8), e84-85.

Kawahara, N., Sato, K., Muraki, M., Tanaka, K., Kaneko, M., & Uemura, K. (1986). CT classification of small thalamic hemorrhages and their clinical implications. Neurology, 36(2), 165-172.

Kumral, E., Kocaer, T., Ertubey, N. O., & Kumral, K. (1995). Thalamic hemorrhage. A prospective study of 100 patients. Stroke, 26(6), 964-970.

Lafosse, C., Kerckhofs, E., Troch, M., Vereeck, L., Van Hoydonck, G., Moeremans, M., et al. (2005). Contraversive pushing and inattention of the contralesional hemispace. J Clin Exp Neuropsychol, 27(4), 460-484.

Lagerqvist, J., & Skargren, E. (2006). Pusher syndrome: Reliability, validity and sensitivity to change of a classification instrument. Advances in Phisiotherapy, 8, 154-160.

Laird, A.R., Robinson, J.L., McMillan, K.M., Tordesillas-Gutiérrez, D., Moran, S.T., Gonzales, S.M., Ray, K.L., Franklin, C., Glahn, D.C., Fox, P.T., & Lancaster, J.L. (2010). Comparison of the disparity between Talairach and MNI coordinates in functional neuroimaging data: validation of the Lancaster transform. Neuroimage, 51(2), 677-83

Masdeu, J. C., & Gorelick, P. B. (1988). Longman dictionary of contemporary English. (1995). London: Longman. Thalamic astasia: inability to stand after unilateral thalamic lesions. Ann Neurol, 23(6), 596-603.

Lopez, C., Mercier, R., Halje, P. & Blanke, O. (2011). Spatiotemporal dynamics of visual vertical judgments: early and late brain mechanisms as revealed by high-density electrical neuroimaging. Neuroscience 181, 134-149.

Mittelstaedt, H. (1998). Origin and processing of postural information. Neurosci Biobehav Rev, 22(4), 473-478.

NINDS ICH Workshop Participants (2005). Priorities for clinical research in intracerebral hemorrhage: report from a National Institute of Neurological Disorders and Stroke workshop. Stroke 36(3), e23-41.

Paci, M., & Nannetti, L. (2005). The pusher syndrome in a patient with cerebellar infarction. Physiother Res Int, 10(3), 176-177.

Pedersen, P. M., Wandel, A., Jorgensen, H. S., Nakayama, H., Raaschou, H. O., & Olsen, T. S. (1996). Ipsilateral pushing in stroke: incidence, relation to neuropsychological symptoms, and impact on rehabilitation. The Copenhagen Stroke Study. Arch Phys Med Rehabil, 77(1), 25-28.

Perennou, D. (2005). [Towards a better understanding and quantitative assessment of pushing, a postural behaviour caused by some strokes]. Ann Readapt Med Phys, 48(4), 198-206.

Perennou, D. A., Mazibrada, G., Chauvineau, V., Greenwood, R., Rothwell, J., Gresty, M. A., et al. (2008). Lateropulsion, pushing and verticality perception in hemisphere stroke: a causal relationship? Brain, 131(Pt 9), 2401-2413.

Pérrenou, D. A., B; Laassel, EM; Benaim, C; Herisson, C; Pelissier, J. (2002). Understanding the pusher behavior of some stroke patients with spatial deficit: A pilot study. Phys Med Rehabil, 83, 570-575.

Pontelli, T. E., Pontes-Neto, O. M., Colafemina, J. F., Araujo, D. B., Santos, A. C., & Leite, J. P. (2005). Posture control in Pusher syndrome: influence of lateral semicircular canals. Rev Bras Otorrinolaringol (Engl Ed), 71(4), 448-452.

Premoselli, S., Cesana, L., & Cerri, C. (2001). Pusher syndrome in stroke: clinical, neuropsychological, and neurophysiological investigation. Eur Med Phys, 37, 143-151.

Reding, M., David, A., & Volpe, B. (1997). Neuroimaging study of the pusher syndrome post stroke. XVI World Congress of Neurology, Buenos Aires, Argentina, September 14-19. J Neurol Sci, 150, S129.

Richard, C., Rousseaux, M., Saj, A., & Honore, J. (2004). Straight ahead in spatial neglect: evidence that space is shifted, not rotated. Neurology, 63(11), 2136-2138.

Rorden, C., & Brett, M. (2000). Stereotaxic display of brain lesions. Behav Neurol, 12, 191-200.

Roden, C., & Karnath, H-O. (2004). Using brain lesions to infer function: a relic from a past era in the fMRI age? Nat Rev Neurosci, , 813-819.

Sadeghi, S. G., Chacron, M. J., Taylor, M. C., & Cullen, K. E. (2007). Neural variability, detection thresholds, and information transmission in the vestibular system. J Neurosci, 27(4), 771-781.

Saj, A., Honore, J., Coello, Y., & Rousseaux, M. (2005). The visual vertical in the pusher syndrome: influence of hemispace and body position. J Neurol, 252(8), 885-891.

Saj, A., Honore, J., Richard, C., Coello, Y., Bernati, T., & Rousseaux, M. (2006). Where is the "straight ahead" in spatial neglect? Neurology, 67(8), 1500-1503.

Santos-Pontelli, T. E., Pontes-Neto, O. M., Colafemina, J. F., Araujo, D. B., Santos, A. C., & Leite, J. P. (2007). Pushing behavior and hemiparesis: which is critical for functional recovery in pusher patients ? Case report. Arq Neuropsiquiatr, 65(2B), 536-539.

Santos-Pontelli, T. E., Pontes-Neto, O. M., Colafemina, J. F., de Araujo, D. B., Santos, A. C., & Leite, J. P. (2004). Contraversive pushing in non-stroke patients. J Neurol, 251(11), 1324-1328.

Santos-Pontelli, T. E., Pontes-Neto, O. M., de Araujo, D. B., Santos, A. C., & Leite, J. P. (2011). Neuroimaging in stroke and non-stroke pusher patients. Arq Neuropsiquiatr, (in press).

Sharpe, J. A. (2003). What's up, doc? Altered perception of the haptic, postural, and visual vertical. Neurology, 61(9), 1172-1173.

Shepherd, R. B., & Carr, J. A. (2005). New aspects for the physiotherapy of pushing behaviour, D. Broetz and H.-O. Karnath, Neurorehabilitation 20 (2005), 133-138. NeuroRehabilitation, 20(4), 343-345.

Talairach, J., Tournoux, P. (1988). Co-planar stereotaxic atlas of the human brain. Thieme Medical Publishers, New York.

Ticini, L. F., Klose, U., Nagele, T., & Karnath, H. O. (2009). Perfusion imaging in Pusher syndrome to investigate the neural substrates involved in controlling upright body position. PLoS One, 4(5), e5737.

Trousselard, M., Barraud, P. A., Nougier, V., Raphel, C., & Cian, C. (2004). Contribution of tactile and interoceptive cues to the perception of the direction of gravity. Brain Res Cogn Brain Res, 20(3), 355-362.

Tyson, S. F., Hanley, M., Chillala, J., Selley, A., & Tallis, R. C. (2006). Balance disability after stroke. Phys Ther, 86(1), 30-38.

Van der Werf, Y. D., Witter, M. P., Uylings, H. B., & Jolles, J. (2000). Neuropsychology of infarctions in the thalamus: a review. Neuropsychologia, 38(5), 613-627.

Wilde EA, McCauley SR, Kelly TM, Levin, H.S., Pedroza, C., Clifton, G.L., Valadka, A.B., Robertson, C.S., & Moretti, P. (2010). Feasibility of the Neurological Outcome Scale for Traumatic Brain Injury (NOS-TBI) in adults. J Neurotrauma. 27, 975-981.

Wityk, R.J., Pessin, M.S., Kaplan, R.F., & Caplan, L.R. (1994). Serial assessment of acute stroke using the NIH Stroke Scale. Stroke, 25, 362-365.

Wulf, G., Hoss, M., & Prinz, W. (1998). Instructions for Motor Learning: Differential Effects of Internal Versus External Focus of Attention. J Mot Behav, 30(2), 169-179.

Zazulia, A.R., Diringer, M.N., Derdeyn, C.P., & Powers, W.J. (1999). Progression of mass effect after intracerebral hemorrhage. Stroke, 30, 1167-1173.

# 14

# Neurosonological Evaluation of the Acute Stroke Patients

Giovanni Malferrari and Marialuisa Zedde
*Department of Neurology-Stroke Unit-Arcispedale Santa Maria Nuova, Reggio Emilia*
*Italy*

## 1. Introduction

Stroke is a condition with an high mortality rate and a relevant burden of disability and social costs. Indeed it is the third cause of death and the first cause of disability in western countries. About 80% of strokes is ischemic and due to the occlusion of a large or small cerebral artery. Therefore the rationale of thrombolysis is the reopening of the occluded vessel within a short time window from symptoms onset, mainly by using iv rtPA but also by using local delivery of rtPA and/or mechanical disruption of the thrombus. The basic assumption is simple and clear: a large vessel was abruptly occluded and the corresponding brain territory was deprived of oxygenated blood and nutrients. The brain metabolism during ischemia is flow- and time-dependent; there are precise perfusional thresholds for maintaining membrane pump activity; therefore the cell integrity and the duration of neuronal life is related to the time from the vessel occlusion, in a variable combination of individual ischemic tolerance and activation of the collateral circulation. The irreversibly damaged brain tissue is known as ischemic core and the suffering, but still viable, tissue is known as penumbra. The penumbra to core ratio is affected by several factors, but it is widely recognized that both occlusive pattern and time from symptoms onset are strong predictors of the presence of as much viable tissue as needed for the success of the reperfusion treatment. The clinical data and the neurological severity scales, as NIHSS (National Institute of Health Stroke Scale), do not reliably predict if there is a large vessel occlusion and for which extent in single cases. The clinical presentation can be the same for a very proximal large arterial occlusion and for a small perforating artery involvement, but the recanalization rate is strictly dependent on the occlusive pattern. Therefore, because the recanalization is a strong predictor of a good outcome, the prognosis depends on it and it can be early inferred by the diagnosis of the occlusive pattern.

All efforts should be made to achieve the diagnosis of vessel occlusion ad brain perfusion condition as early as possible, in order not only to predict the prognosis but also to tailor the treatment.

In acute stroke time is brain, and therefore the diagnostic steps should be reliable, fast and not time consuming. Ultrasound techniques have these features for other body districts, also for extracranial vessels, but their use for the examination of the intracranial circulation has been hampered for many years, because of the attenuation effect of the skull. In the last twenty years this limitation has been demonstrated to be passed by neurosonological

techniques, Transcranial Doppler (TCD) and Transcranial Colour Coded Duplex Sonography (TCCS). Both these tools are safe, reliable, bedside executable, fast, not expensive and repeatable. Because of these advantages, neurosonology represents an ideal tool to diagnose patients with a focal neurological deficit of suspected vascular origin, particularly in an emergency setting. Furthermore the repeatability and the safety make transcranial Doppler the most suitable tool for monitoring the recanalization, both during a thrombolytic treatment and spontaneously.
In the following sections mainly TCCS will be mentioned and discussed, first because of the undeniable advantage of the B-mode visualization of the brain structures and vascular landmarks, and second because the expertise of our group with this technique and the related literature contributes. In a similar manner our attention will be focused on the anterior circulation stroke.

## 2. Ultrasound examination of cerebroafferent vessels: Extracranial carotid axis

Ultrasound examination of the extracranial carotid artery (common and internal carotid artery) is a useful and standardized technique and it represents, in patients with a focal neurological symptom, the ideal screening tool for the identification of carotid stenosis and occlusion and the selection of lesions amenable to surgical or endovascular treatment. Atherosclerosis is a relevant cause of transient ischemic attack and stroke, but also non atherosclerotic conditions, like spontaneous cervical artery dissection and arteritis, can be diagnosed and followed-up. In acute stroke patients the involvement of the extracranial carotid axis is the cause of the cerebrovascular event quite in 18%, being the majority of vessel lesions in the intracranial circulation and sometimes both in extracranial and intracranial circulation (Malferrari G et al. 2007). For both atherosclerotic and non-atherosclerotic diseases, the ultrasound findings and the diagnostic criteria has been compared to the neuroradiological findings and criteria in the literature, whereas Digital Subtraction Angiography (DSA) is considered the gold standard.

### 2.1 Atherosclerotic carotid stenoocclusion

Atherosclerotic involvement of the extracranial carotid artery is not the main cause of vascular lesions in acute stroke patients. It has been reported in about 18% of patients in a 6 hours time window, whereas the intracranial large vessel stenoocclusion accounts for 52.8%. There are two main mechanisms by which the carotid atherosclerotic disease may lead to cerebral infarction: first, an embolic mechanism, as an artery to artery embolism from the plaque rupture; second, an hemodynamic mechanism, because of the blood flow reduction downstream the stenoocclusion. The first one is linearly related to the severity of the carotid stenosis, increasing as the stenosis increases, but the second one is not related to the severity of the stenosis and it depends on multiple factors, as the cerebrovascular reserve, the collateral circulation failure, the time course of the vessel lesion, etc. In many situations the global risk of cerebrovascular events is related to a combination of the two abovementioned mechanisms, because in a territory with an hemodynamic failure, also the clearance of emboli is worse (Caplan L et al. 1998). Ultrasound techniques are suitable to identify carotid lesions and there are several studies in the literature, comparing ultrasound techniques with neuroradiological techniques, but they were conducted mainly in a non acute setting. Very few studies or case series are published, using both neuroradiological and neurosonological techniques, in the setting of acute stroke, and the main target of these studies was the intracranial disease. Therefore we are somewhat obliged to translate the reliability data of the non acute phase to the acute phase. This process is make easier by the high accuracy of neurosonological grading of carotid stenosis in a symptomatic patient (Chapell F et al., 2009; Wardlaw et al. 2006).

The overall accuracy of ultrasound examination of the internal carotid artery versus neuroradiological techniques was the subject of several studies and the following figure (from Wardlaw et al. 2006, modified) shows the results of a meta-analysis of them for the 70-99% range with the NASCET system.

| | DUS | CTA | MRA | CEMRA |
|---|---|---|---|---|
| 70-99% stenosis | | | | |
| Sensitivity<br>95% CI | 0.89<br>(0.85-0.92) | 0.77<br>(0.68-0.84) | 0.88<br>(0.82-0.92) | 0.94<br>(0.88-0.97) |
| Specificity<br>95% CI | 0.84<br>(0.77-0.89) | 0.95<br>(0.91-0.97) | 0.84<br>(0.76-0.97) | 0.93<br>(0.89-0.96) |

DUS: Doppler UltraSound
CTA: Computed Tomography Angiography
MRA: Magnetic Resonance Angiography
CEMRA: Contrast Enhanced Magnetic Resonance Angiography

Fig. 1. Sensitivity and specificity for the diagnosis of a severe carotid stenosis (ultrasound versus neuroradiological techniques) of non-invasive diagnostic techniques compared to DSA

In the acute setting, even more than in a post-acute management, the main objective is the diagnosis or the exclusion of carotid lesion amenable to surgical or endovascular treatment, according to the current guidelines. Therefore it is relevant to assess the reliability of ultrasound techniques for 70-99% stenosis. In the above cited meta-analysis 41 studies (2541 patients, 4876 arteries) from 1980 to 2004 were included, comparing non-invasive imaging with intra-arterial angiography. The conclusion of this meta-analysis agrees with the common clinical practice of using first-line non-invasive tests, as DUS, for diagnosing 70–99% stenosis. For lesser degrees of stenosis (50–69%) the accuracy of non-invasive techniques is not so high, but again, if surgical indication is well documented for symptomatic carotid stenosis > 70%, the benefit is discussed and very narrow, also for high risk patients, for lesser degrees of stenosis. This categorization is internationally made using the angiographic NASCET grading system (NASCET coll. 1991) and non-invasive imaging techniques should have validated their diagnostic and grading criteria versus the NASCET system.

The ultrasound grading criteria were stated in the Consensus Conference of American Academy of Radiology in 2003 (Grant et al. 2003), but neuroradiological techniques have less shared criteria, based on caliper measurements and ratios, rather than the subjective visual impression. Unfortunately, an implementation of their use in the clinical practice, outside the clinical trials and the evaluation of a central reader, is needed, because the visual impression could be useful only for excluding very tight stenosis, but not for achieving a precise grading (U-King-Im et a. 2007).

In the next figures the grading systems of carotid stenosis and the ultrasound diagnostic criteria are shown.

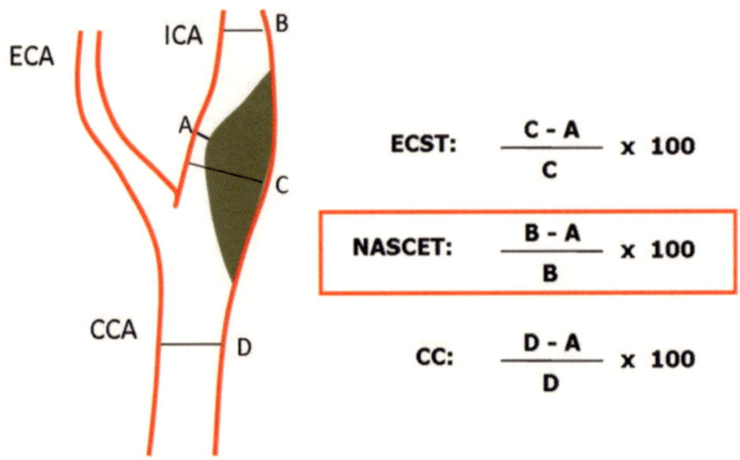


CCA: commobn carotid artery
ICA: internal carotid artery
ECA: external carotid artery
ECST: European Carotid Surgery Trial
NASCET: North American Symptomatic Carotid Endarterectomy Trial
CC: Common Carotid

Fig. 2. Schematic drawing of the grading systems of carotid stenosis (NASCET system in the red box)

| DEGREE OF STENOSIS | PRIMARY CRITERIA ICA PSV (cm/sec) | STIMA PLACCA (%) | ADDITIONAL CRITERIA ICA/CCA PSV ratio | ICA EDV (cm/sec) |
|---|---|---|---|---|
| Normal | < 125 | None | < 2 | < 40 |
| < 50% | < 125 | < 50 | < 2 | < 40 |
| 50-69% | 125-230 | ≥ 50 | 2-4 | 40-100 |
| ≥ 70% | > 230 | ≥ 50 | > 4 | > 100 |
| Near occlusion | High, low or not detectable | Visible | Variable | Variable |
| Occlusion | Not detectable | Visible, lumen not detectable | Not applicable | Not applicable |

Fig. 3. DUS criteria from Grant et al. 2003. These criteria have a 92% sensitivity and a 97% specificity for diagnose a carotid stenosis > 70%

In acute stroke evaluation the finding of a severe carotid stenosis should raise the question of identifying intracranial artery-to-artery embolization as a tandem lesion, in large or small vessels. Sometimes the intracranial occlusion can be missed by imaging, both for spontaneous recanalization and spreading of the clot fragments in the distal vessels, and for the very distal localization, witnessed by the localization of infarcts in the distal cortex of the cerebral hemispheres or in the gray-to white matter junction.

If there is a significant hemodynamic finding in carotid arteries in patients with acute stroke within 6 hours, it would be often an acute carotid occlusion or a near occlusion. An acute carotid occlusion may occur for the acute complication of a plaque rupture, as a thrombus above the plaque, regardless the previous presence of a mild stenosis, considering only atherosclerosis. The cause of an acute carotid occlusion may be atherosclerosis, cardiac embolism or dissection, because a carotid plaque is not always clearly detectable. Another possibility is the downstream extension of a thrombus in the petrous or intracranial segment of the internal carotid artery, e.g. from an acute complication of intracranial atherosclerosis. The follow-up of the vessel lesion, if surgically or endovascular untreated, can help to define the diagnosis, because time, morphology and rate of recanalization vary, depending on the cause of the occlusion.
Near occlusion is defined as a stenosis in the range 95-99% with distal reduction of vessel size and flow limitation, typically without the increase of flow velocity of the lesser degrees of stenosis (Bartlett et al. 2006; Thanvi and Robinson 2007).

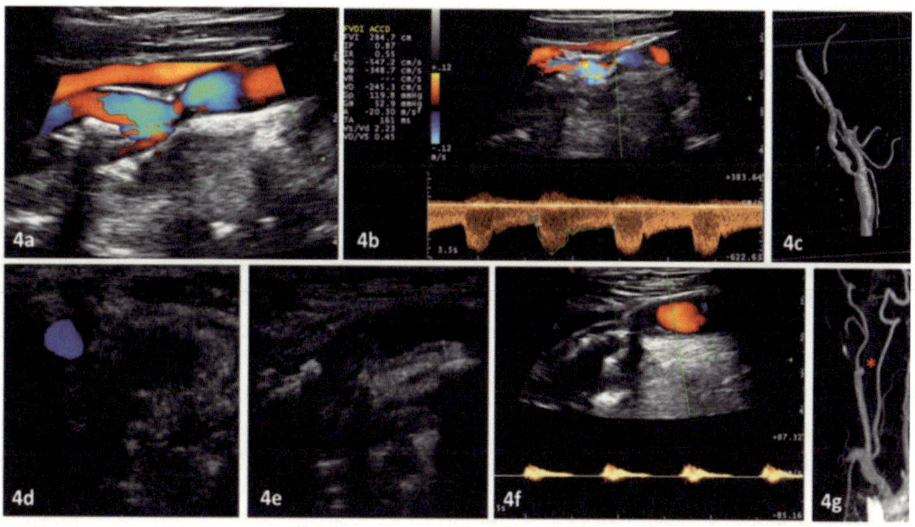


4a ICA stenosis in power mode; 4b ICA stenosis with the flow waveform; 4 c corresponding 3D reconstruction from CTA; 4d ICA occlusion with hypoechoic luminal thrombus in transverse scanning at the carotid bifurcation (ECA in blue); 4 e corresponding longitudinal scanning in B-mode with the highly hyperechoic plaque and the superimposed organized thrombus; 4g corresponding MRA with the lacking ICA (red asterisk).

Fig. 4. Ultrasound hemodynamic findings of the extracranial carotid axis.

Finally, the ultrasound examination of carotid artery allows to recognize an indirect sign of the hemodynamic involvement of the petrous and/or intracranial segment of the same artery. Indeed, if a middle cerebral artery stenosis or occlusion does not lead to changes in the upstream flow of the carotid artery, because of the distribution of the resistances in the polygon of Willis, a severe stenosis or occlusion of the intrapetrous segment of the internal carotid artery or at the siphon level, has an identifiable consequence on the waveform of the internal carotid artery, as decreased systolic and diastolic flow velocities, increased systolic-diastolic ratio of the flow velocity, and disappearance of the diastolic component of velocity waveform, depending of the increased resistance to the flow downstream. The more characteristic finding of this situation is the so-called "stump flow" in the extracranial internal carotid artery. A summary of the main ultrasound hemodynamic findings is shown in the fig. 4, compared to neuroradiological imaging.

## 2.2 Carotid dissection

Another cause of stroke, mainly in young patients, is the arterial dissection. It can occur both in extracranial and in intracranial arteries, it is frequently spontaneous and it can start from the intimal or from the adventitial layer of the vessel wall. In the first case the more frequent evolution is a carotid stenosis or occlusion and a potential cerebral damage due not only to hemodynamic factors, but also to artery-to-artery embolism from the clot superimposed on the intimal interruption; in the second case there is a greater likelihood of pseusoaneurysmal evolution with or without rupture (Fusco and Harrigan 2011). Even in a spontaneous dissection, it is often reported a history of trivial or repetitive trauma (1/4 of cases). The gold standard for diagnosis is DSA, but often, when the vessel is partially involved or the mural hematoma is not hemodynamic, magnetic resonance angiography with T2 weighed sections and fat suppression can be almost as much sensitive than DSA. The role of ultrasound examination is discussed, because of the missing petrous carotid segment and of the inability to image or find indirect signs of non-hemodynamic intracranial arterial lesions. The extracranial internal carotid artery is well imaged by ultrasound and therefore a pathologic process is well detectable, if it is located at the carotid bulb and at the origin of internal carotid artery. Unfortunately, a spontaneous extracranial carotid dissection occurs more frequently in the distal segment of the internal carotid artery and sometimes a focal, partial, non-hemodynamic process can be missed by ultrasound examination (Goyal and Derdeyn 2009). Therefore for a reliable evaluation of the sensitivity and specificity of colour-coded duplex ultrasound diagnosis of carotid dissection, it should be taken into account that two different subpopulations exist:

- patients with signs and symptoms of cerebral ischemia in the carotid territory, and
- patients with other complaints or signs (e.g. Horner sign) but without cerebral ischemia.

In the first group, where it can be easily expected an hemodynamic carotid lesion (stenosis or occlusion), the reliability of ultrasound technique is very high. Indeed in a study on 177 young patients with signs of cerebral ischemia in the carotid artery territory, examined by colour duplex ultrasound and MRA, sensitivity, specificity, and positive and negative predictive values for ultrasound diagnosis of spontaneous internal carotid artery dissection, causing carotid territory ischemia, was 96%, 94%, 92%, and 97%, respectively (Benninger et al. 2006).

In the second group, where partial non-hemodynamic arterial lesions are often present, the reliability of ultrasound technique is lower. In patients with isolated Horner syndrome nearly 1/3 of spontaneous internal carotid artery dissection does not have any hemodynamic sign, and therefore was missed by ultrasound (Arnold et al. 2008). Considering both hemodynamic and direct signs, the sensitivity of ultrasound for diagnosis of spontaneous internal carotid artery dissection reaches 90% (Alecu et al. 2007).

In an ultrasound semeiological approach, direct signs of a vessel dissection are the visualization of the intimal flap and/or the intramural hematoma; indirect signs are the hemodynamic relevance of the vessel disease, as stenosis without significant atheromatosis and occlusion by acute thrombosis, or signs of distal stenoocclusion from the flow waveform, as stump flow. Unfortunately the identification of a intimal flap or an intramural hematoma is not a frequent finding, although diagnostic of the dissection (fig. 5).

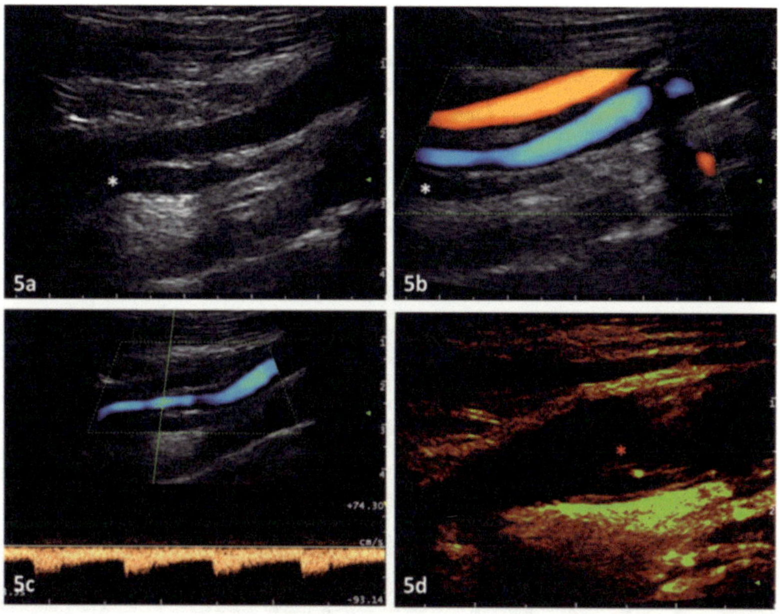


5a-c are images from the same patient; B-mode (a) and Power-mode (b) longitudinal scanning of ICA with a mural hematoma (white asterisk) without hemodynamic consequences (flow waveform in c). 5d: intimal flap (red asterisk) at the carotid bulb.

Fig. 5. Direct ultrasound findings of carotid dissection.

Ultrasound techniques are also suitable for the monitoring of recanalization in patients with carotid artery dissection, because this disease has an highly dynamic course and it is possible, during days and weeks, to image both recanalization and reocclusion or pseudo-aneurysmal evolution (fig. 6). In a recent study (Nedeltchev et al 2009), of 268 spontaneous internal carotid artery dissections the vessel hemodynamics at presentation was: 7.5% with 50% stenosis, 11.6% with 51% to 80% stenosis, 34.3% with 81% to 99% stenosis, and 46.6% with an occlusion. The sonological follow-up showed normal findings (complete healing of the vessel without residual signs of the dissection on the wall) in 60%, 50% stenosis in 10%, 51% to 80% stenosis in 1%, 81% to 99% stenosis in 10%, and occlusion in 19% of the vessels.

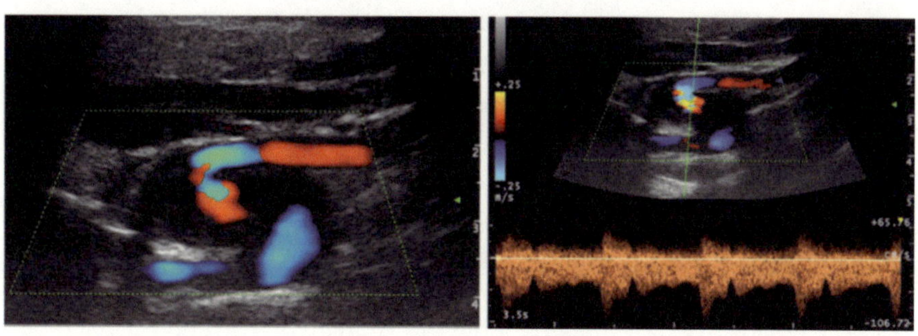

Fig. 6. Pseudo-aneurysmal evolution of a spontaneous internal carotid artery dissection. In the left side Power-mode longitudinal scanning of distal ICA with a partially thrombosed wall enlargement; in the right side corresponding waveform with a minor focal flow acceleration (aliasing in the Colour-mode)

The serial ultrasound examination allowed to define the timing of recanalization: indeed the rate of complete recanalization was 16% at 1 month, 50% at 3 months, and 60% at 6 and 12 months. Therefore the recanalization process occurs mainly within the first six months, regardless the treatment. The main factor that was related to a reduced recanalization rate, was an initial occlusion of the dissected vessel, whereas the absence of stroke symptoms and the presence of local manifestations and signs as the unique clinical presentation, were associated with an increased rate of complete recanalization.

## 3. Intracranial vessels: TCCS examination

TCCS is a reliable, safe and bedside tool to image intracranial circulation, mainly in acute stroke patients. The natural course of intracranial vessel occlusion is highly dynamic within hours and days and therefore a tool at least so much dynamic is needed in order to monitor the recanalization process.
A basic TCCS scanning is obtained from the temporal bone window in the mesencephalic axial plane, showing the full circle of Willis, as in the figure 7.

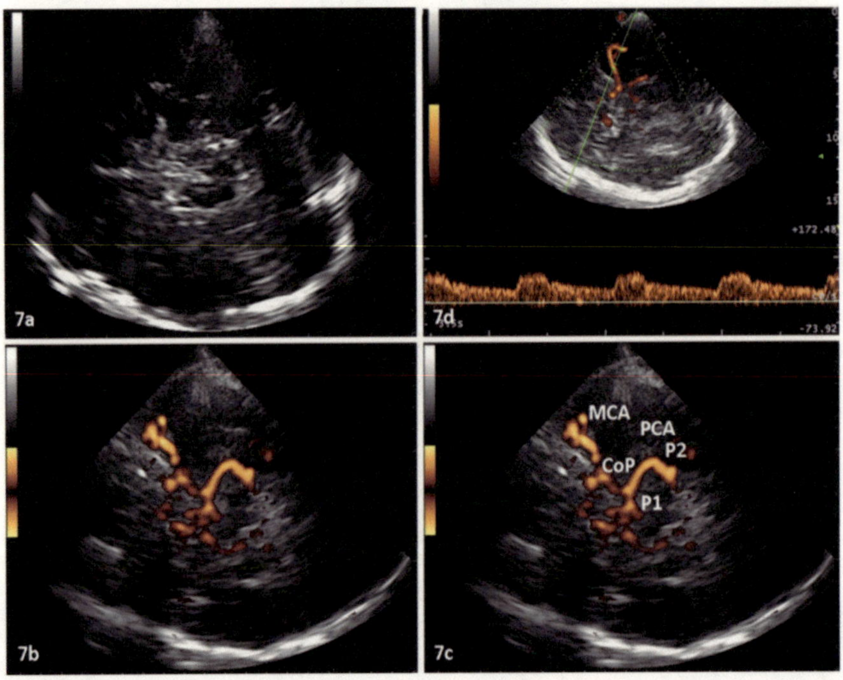


a. B-mode evaluation in gray scale with the butterfly shaped midbrain at the midline; b. corresponding Power-mode with the main vessels of the circle of Willis, tagged in c; d. waveform of the flow spectrum of ipsilateral M1 MCA (normal pattern).

Fig. 7. TCCS axial scanning from the temporal bone window, mesencephalic plane.

TCCS is a very reliable tool for imaging large intracranial vessels and for diagnosing their occlusion in the acute phase. The current guidelines about its application in clinical practice are not updated from 2004 (Sloan et al. 2004), but further data are now available from clinical studies in acute stroke patients, comparing neurosonology with neuroradiology and documenting the usefulness for monitoring the recanalization and enhance clot lysis. The clinical indications for TCCS are basically the same of TCD for imaging of large intracranial vessels, but TCCS has the clear advantage to image the brain parenchyma and the intracranial structures, allowing also the application in neurodegenerative disease (mainly extrapiramidal disorders), the diagnosis and monitoring of hemorrhagic parenchymal transformation after treatment, the perfusional evaluation of the microcirculation, etc. The sensitivity and specificity of TCCS is not lesser than the ones of TCD and the established indication for TCD in acute stroke are also applicable to TCCS.

In a recent systematic review (Alexandrov et al. 2010) of TCD application, for patients with acute ischemic symptoms in anterior or posterior circulation who had cranial CT or MRI, the authors stated that "TCD can identify patients with proximal arterial occlusions both in anterior and posterior circulation who have the worst prognosis and can benefit the most from intravenous thrombolysis or rescue intraarterial therapies".

### 3.1 Advantages and limitations of neurosonology

Neurosonological tools, both TCD and TCCS are reliable and useful in acute stroke patients and have several comparative studies with MRA, CTA or DSA. The advantage of neurosonology in this setting are:

- the virtual absence of contraindications (because of the rarity of adverse reactions against ultrasound contrast agents, whose use is mandatory in about 10% of patients without a suitable temporal bone window) (Baumgartner et al. 1997, Kunz et al. 2006)
- the bedside feasibility
- the very low time consumption with a dedicated examination pathway and a fast-track scanning protocol for extracranial and intracranial arteries, lasting lesser than 15 minutes (Alexandrov et al. 1999)
- the high reliability for the early diagnosis of large artery proximal occlusions in acute stroke patients before thrombolysis; in the above cited article 69% of thrombolysis-eligible patients had a proximal occlusion on TCD (Alexandrov et al. 1999)
- the high reliability for obtain functional and hemodynamic data; in 26% of 130 patients, TCD provided relevant informations, that helped to refine the severity of a stenosis and determine stroke pathogenesis, in addiction to DSA (Alexandrov et al. 1999)
- the repeatability during thrombolytic treatment, to monitor recanalization and help to select patient for a rescue strategy (Saqqur et al. 2005)
- the low cost of examination

Disadvantages are mainly the operator-dependency, but it is notable that all diagnostic techniques somewhat depend on technical skills and expertise of operators, as documented by the intraoperator discordance in grading an extracranial carotid artery stenosis on NASCET study. The early diagnosis of a large vessel occlusion has a great impact on the prognosis of patient and on the choice of the proper treatment. Also in studies with an extended time window for thrombolysis up to 9 hours, because of the mismatch evaluation, only patients with residual large vessel occlusion shown a positive response to treatment and a significant improvement of disability scores (Hacke et al. 2009). Similarly persisting occlusions after reperfusion treatment have worse outcome and this information could be useful to address patients to intra-arterial clot removal or, in some cases, hemicraniectomy.

Sensitivity and specificity of neurosonological diagnosis of intracranial steno-occlusion is very high also compared to DSA (Sloan et al. 2004) (Fig. 8)

| | Sensitivity (%) | Specificity (%) |
|---|---|---|
| Anterior Circulation | 70-90 | 90-95 |
| Posterior Circulation Occlusion | 50-80 | 80-96 |
| MCA | 85-95 | 90-98 |
| ICA, VA, BA | 55-81 | 96 |

Fig. 8. Reliability of neurosological techniques vs DSA for diagnosis of intracranial occlusions

It can be noted that the specificity is globally very high, i.e. a negative transcranial examination can reliably exclude a large vessel occlusion, and also the sensitivity for MCA lesion is very good and it is relevant, because most strokes occur in the MCA territory through an MCA main stem occlusion or stenosis.

The reliability of this technique is also very high in the follow-up of stroke, during the monitoring of recanalization (Fig. 9) (Sloan et al. 2004)

| | Sensitivity (%) | Specificity (%) |
|---|---|---|
| Complete Occlusion | 50 | 100 |
| Partial Occlusion | 100 | 76 |
| Recanalization | 91 | 93 |

Fig. 9. Reliability of neurosological techniques vs DSA for monitoring recanalization of intracranial occlusions

Also for monitoring the recanalization process the global reliability of TCD is high, and even higher for partial than for complete occlusion. This last feature is well understood if the extremely high dynamicity and temporal resolution of ultrasound techniques is kept in mind, because the serial use of DSA has forcedly time intervals of several hours or days between the successive examinations, and so it is easier to lose the partial recanalization step between occlusion and complete reopening of the vessel. Neurosonological techniques can be applied every minute or hour and therefore also a small variation in vessel patency is well recognized.

Another partial limitation of TCCS (and even more of TCD) is the incomplete evaluation of the internal carotid artery, because of the inability to image the petrous segment. This is a partial limitation, since an hemodynamic lesion in this segment can be inferred by indirect sign, both in extracranial and intracranial ICA, if it is an acute process. The C5-C1 segment of internal carotid artery, according to angiographic terminology, can be explored by TCCS combining the axial and coronal access (Eggers et al. 2009).

### 3.2 TCCS: How to perform the examination and the consensus statements

TCCS is increasingly used in acute stroke patients, but it should pay for being ten years younger than TCD; therefore there are not clinical shared guidelines, as for TCD, but recently guidelines for its application in clinical trials on acute stroke have been published (Nedelmann et al 2009). Before these guidelines, there was not a systematic consensus on how TCCS examination should be performed in acute stroke patients. Furthermore standardized recommendations are needed to compare the results of TCCS studies from several centres. Therefore a systematic review of the literature on TCCS in acute stroke was performed and the resulting manuscript was corrected and commented by a panel of

international experts with previous publications in the field of TCCS in acute stroke and finally collegially revised.
The examination procedure was carefully described, choosing a basic and comparable insonation modality for the anterior circulation stroke. The main examination plane is the axial transtemporal mesencephalic one (fig. 7), showing a good visualization of the circle of Willis (Malferrari et al. 2007, Wong 2003, Valaikiene et al 2008). A useful information to compare TCCS planes with the corresponding images from neuroradiological techniques, is that the transcranial axial insonation plane is usually different from the axial plane displayed with MR and CT imaging. There are also parenchymal and bone landmarks to identify the vessels and make easier to compare the oblique transcranial images with the neuroradiological images of CT or MR. The transtemporal bone window in the axial insonation plane allows to recognize the main branches of the Willis circle:

- sphenoidal (M1) and insular (M2) segments of the middle cerebral artery
- precommunicating (A1) segment of the anterior cerebral artery
- distal intracranial part of the ICA
- precommunicating (P1) and postcommunicating (P2) segments of the posterior cerebral artery

Also the use of the coronal plane can be useful to localize and distinguish both vessel segments and normal from pathologic conditions (Valaikiene et al 2008).
All segments of all visible arteries should be investigated, not only by Colour- or Power-mode, but especially by spectral Doppler sonography (Zipper and Stolz 2002, Baumgartner 2004, Krejza and Baumgartner 2004).
The way to examine the entire circle of Willis by TCCS, makes unnecessary the orbital bone window, conventionally used by TCD for the exploration of the ophtalmic artery and its branches, as stated in the above cited consensus (Nedelmann et al. 2009) (Fig. 10).

| | |
|---|---|
| *Consensus Statement 1* | An adequate interpretation of intracranial findings always requires careful assessment of the extracranial vasculature, because obstructive disease of extracranial vessels may significantly influence or severely compromise intracranial hemodynamics. |
| *Consensus Statement 2* | The standard extracranial protocol in the acute stroke setting does not necessarily include evaluation of the ophthalmic artery or supraorbital arteries. In case of relevant ICA pathology, an inverted flow direction in the ophthalmic artery does not provide further information beyond a complete ICA examination. In case of insufficient temporal bone window, evaluation of ophthalmic artery flow direction may be of additional value. |

Fig. 10. Statements 1 and 2 from Nedelmann et al 2009

About the main limitation of transcranial Doppler, i.e. the poor acoustic window, the Consensus carefully examined it. Also this review of the literature agreed with the known rate of 10% of patients with cerebrovascular diseases, where the insonation of the basal cerebral arteries is incomplete (Seidel et al. 1995; Kenton et al. 1997; Krejza et al. 2007). In this case the intravenous administration of an ultrasound contrast agent dramatically improves the insonation and therefore increases the number of conclusive ultrasound studies, allowing an adequate diagnosis in 80% to 90% of those patients with insufficient bone window before the contrast agent injection (Zunker et al. 2002; Postert et al. 1999;

Gerriets et al. 1999; Baumgartner et al. 1995; Goertler et al. 1998; Nabavi et al. 1998; Kunz et al. 2002). The shared criterion for defining sufficient the temporal bone window is the adequate displaying of the ipsilateral proximal branches of the circle of Willis, in both Colour- or Power-mode and spectral Doppler. This raises the question of the evaluation of the quality of the insonation window in a case of T-occlusion diagnosis. The Consensus Conference examined also the indication for ultrasouns contrast agents (UCA) in acute stroke in the setting of clinical trials and the Consensus Statement 3 shows the achieved agreement (Fig.11).

***Consensus Statement 3***

UCA should be used in the setting of clinical trials:

- In case of an insufficient temporal acoustic bone window: insufficient signal intensity, or absent visibility of the proximal branches of the circle of Willis.
- In cases in which UCA are given at baseline, follow-up examinations should also be performed with UCA. This is important because measured flow velocities may be higher when using UCA (Baumgartner et al. 1997; Khan et al. 2000)
- Because of varying availability of UCA in different countries and because of a lack of studies with direct comparison of the different UCA, there are no specific recommendations on the type of UCA. In view of the current literature, application of multiple small boli or continuous intravenous infusion increases the length of the diagnostically useful time window.

Fig. 11. Statements 3 from Nedelmann et al 2009

Another intuitive difference between TCD and TCCS is the possibility of achieving an angle-corrected flow waveform and angle-corrected flow velocity measurements. The relevance of this item comes from the anatomic course of intracranial arteries; indeed the angle between the ultrasound beam and the major intracranial arteries is not the same in each segment of the same artery and between similar segments of the arteries of both sides, mainly in acute stroke patients, because of the time changing mass effect of the ischemic lesion (Eicke et al. 1994). The diagnostic criteria for intracranial stenosis with their velocity threshold are different between TCD and TCCS, because of the angle-corrected measurements with TCCS. Angle corrected threshold have an higher sensitivity to detect arterial narrowing because of stenosis or vasospasm (Baumgartner et al. 1999), and they do not cause a decreased intrarater or interrater reproducibility, as compared to non-corrected measurements (Baumgartner et al. 1994; Maeda et al. 1990; Stolz et al. 2001). These considerations lead to the Consensus Statement 4 and 5 about angle-corrected measurements (Fig. 12).

The focus of this discussion about angle correction is its usefulness to examine patients in the acute phase of stroke, mainly MCA stroke, because the diagnosis of a distal M1 MCA or MCA branches occlusion involves the evaluation of flow velocity differences between MCA of the affected side and MCA of the contralateral side. This is because branch occlusions of MCA cannot be directly imaged by ultrasound and only indirect signs on the flow waveform could be searched, as a reduction of the M1 flow velocity compared to the contralateral side. In the literature there is a prospective TCD study, angiography-controlled, defining the so called asymmetry index without angle correction for the diagnosis of branch occlusions (Zanette et al. 1989). According to this study it is possible to diagnose a condition of multiple MCA branch occlusions (> 3). There is only another study in the literature, addressing this item by contrast-enhanced TCCS and a comparison with angiography (Ogata et al. 2005). Its results were that an end-diastolic velocity of <26 cm/sec within the M1 segment of MCA, associated with an end-diastolic ratio of < 2.5 between the contralateral and the ipsilateral M1 MCA identified branch occlusion; instead a >2.5 ratio indicated M1 occlusion. The main limitation of this study are the small sample of patients and the lack of specifications on how the criteria relate to the number of affected MCA branches. Another known pitfall is the use of contrast agents, because of the potential increase of flow velocity by 10% to 20% as compared to those assessed without contrast agents (Baumgartner et al. 1997; Khan et al. 2000). Finally it is possible that only the criterion "end-diastolic ratio < 2.5", but not the criterion "end-diastolic MCA velocity < 26 cm/sec" could be useful and exported to non-enhanced TCCS. The definite statement of the Consensus Conference about the diagnosis of MCA branch occlusion is shown in the fig. 13.

| | |
|---|---|
| ***Consensus Statement 4*** | To prevent inadequate measurements, angle correction should only be applied to velocity measurements when the sample volume can be located in a sufficiently long vessel segment that allows sufficient tracing of the main flow vector (Zipper et al. 2002; Giller et al. 1994).<br>In case of a stenosis being located in a curved arterial segment, angle correction should be omitted, and the ultrasound probe should be repositioned to obtain the smallest insonation angle possible. |
| ***Consensus Statement 5*** | In case of angle-corrected measurements, the correction angle or additional values of uncorrected velocities (that can be calculated from angle corrected velocities and the correction angle) should be provided in publications. This may help to further define the value of angle correction. |

Fig. 12. Statements 4 and 5 from Nedelmann et al 2009

| | |
|---|---|
| ***Consensus Statement 6*** | To date, 2 studies have been published that investigated hemodynamics of the M1 segment in MCA branch occlusion. Its solid evaluation requires normal extracranial and contralateral findings as a prerequisite. Angle-corrected TCCS may allow a more accurate approach to detection of MCA branch occlusion. However, the studies discussed were small and one of them used contrast-enhanced TCCS.<br>Therefore, no recommendation can be made regarding which of the criteria should be used in the setting of clinical trials until validation of this specific issue is conducted in a larger study. |

Fig. 13. Statements 6 from Nedelmann et al 2009

Angle-corrected measurements are more precise in the acute phase, because, in the presence of a large brain lesion, tissue edema may dynamically modify, expanding and decreasing, mainly within the first hours-days. Therefore a huge lesion in the MCA territory can displace the MCA and vary its course (Krejza et al. 2001) (example in fig. 14). The resulting change of the insonation angle on the affected side is not only different hour by hour or even minute by minute, but also it may lead to a wrong interpretation of the inter-hemispheric differences in flow velocity measurements. However this item requires other dedicated studies and settings to solve the doubts.

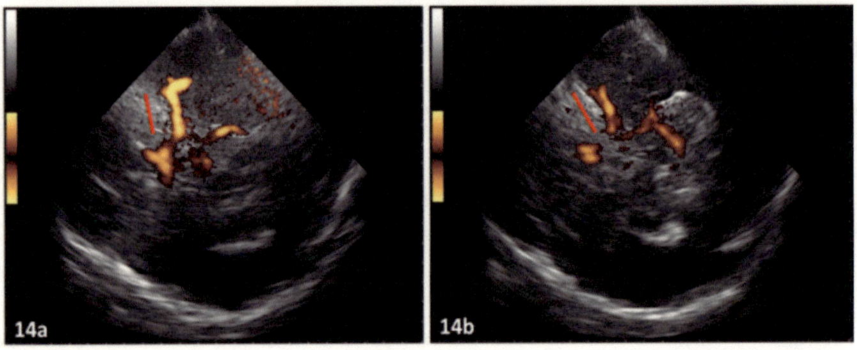


a. left side transtemporal insonation; b. right side transtemporal insonation. The red lines show the left and right MCA course.

Fig. 14. TCCS of a patient with acute ischemic stroke in the right MCA territory.

### 3.3 Scales and measurements in neurosonology

Both in clinical trials and in clinical practice, the course of recanalization has been followed by ultrasound, using shared classification, for achieving a common language and easily compare the results of different centres. The first classification was derived from the angiographic classification, the so-called TICI (Thrombolysis in Cerebral Infarction) scale, which in turn was created beginning from the corresponding coronarographic reperfusion grading system, TIMI (Tomsick 2007). It was called TIBI (Thrombolysis In Brain Ischemia) score and was based on Doppler waveform; it has been widely used for the assessment of initial hemodynamics and recanalization phenomena (Alexandrov, Wojner, Grotta 2004; Demchuk et al. 2001; Molina et al. 2006). Because of the waveform-based being of the scale, it was used primary for TCD examination, and then it was transferred to TCCS, always using only the Doppler spectrum as criterion. TIMI and TICI, being angiography-based, were assumed to assess both features of flow restoration or revascularization: reopening of the originally occluded artery and restoration of effective flow or reperfusion into the distal arterial bed of the originally occluded artery. These two concepts are related each to other but not exactly the same phenomenon, because the reopening of an occluded artery does not mean automatically the restoration of an effective perfusion status in the downstream circulation, due to the duration of ischemia, the efficiency of the collateral circulation, the microembolic load, the viability of tissue, etc. Therefore, also a complete recanalization of the primarily occluded vessel may be associated to variable patterns of distal patency and perfusion/reperfusion ratios (Tomsick 2007).

The TIBI grading system refers only to recanalization process, and not to reperfusion of cerebral tissue. It is a valid and widely used tool to assess recanalization, both for TCD and for TCCS. It is shown in Fig. 15 with some examples of the Doppler spectra corresponding to each grade.

As shown in the fig. 15, this scale comprises 6 different degrees of flow abnormalities. The application of this grading system in clinical practice and in trials is sometimes difficult and there is a broad range of subjectivity, mainly in attributing grade 2 and 3. For this reason in some multicentre trials about ultrasound enhanced thrombolysis, a preliminary training was performed to guarantee the comparability of results. To avoid partially this subjectivity, flow grades are frequently separated into 3 major categories (Burgin et al. 2000), as in the angiographic classification (Fig. 16). These categories are:

- MCA main stem occlusion (TIBI 0–1)
- partial recanalization (TIBI 2–3)
- complete recanalization (TIBI 4–5)

| TIBI Flow Grade | Definition | Example |
|---|---|---|
| **Grade 0**<br>**ABSENT FLOW** | Absent flow signals are defined by the lack of regular pulsatile flow signals despite varying degrees of background noise | 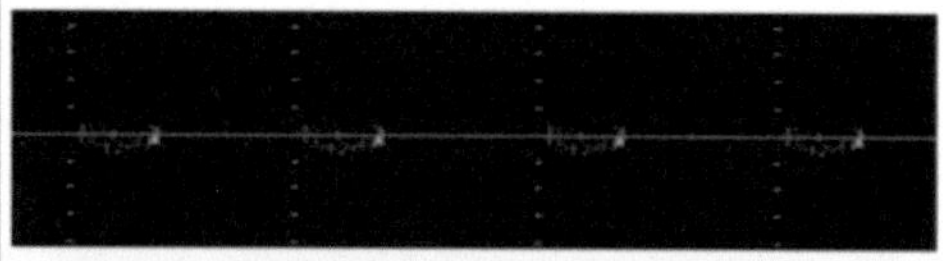 |
| **Grade 1**<br>**MINIMAL FLOW** | - systolic spikes of variable velocity and duration<br>- absent diastolic flow during all cardiac cycles<br>- reverberating flow | 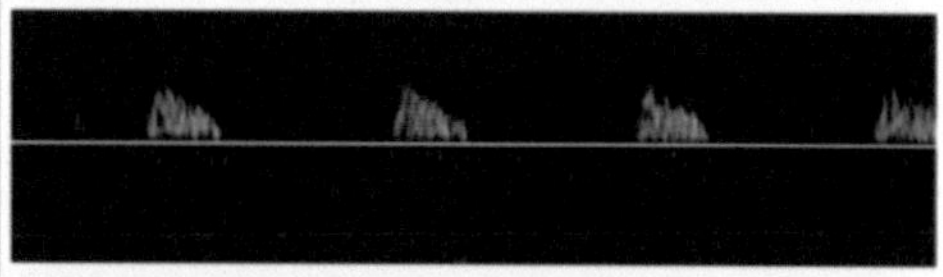 |
| **Grade 2**<br>**BLUNTED FLOW** | - flattened systolic flow acceleration of variable duration compared to control<br>- positive end diastolic velocity and pulsatility index < 1.2 | 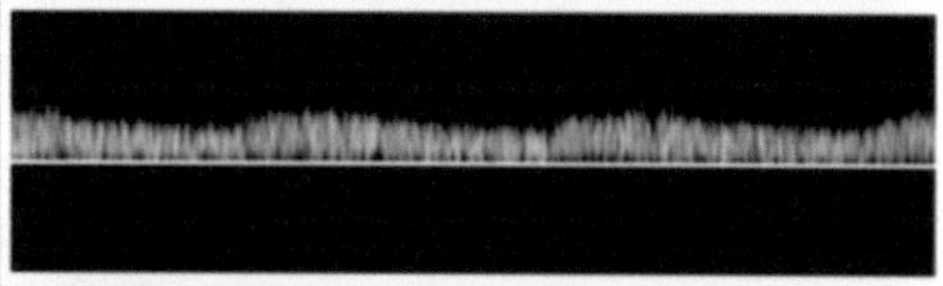 |
| **Grade 3**<br>**DAMPENED FLOW** | - normal systolic flow acceleration<br>- positive end diastolic velocity<br>- decreased mean flow velocities by 30% compared to control | 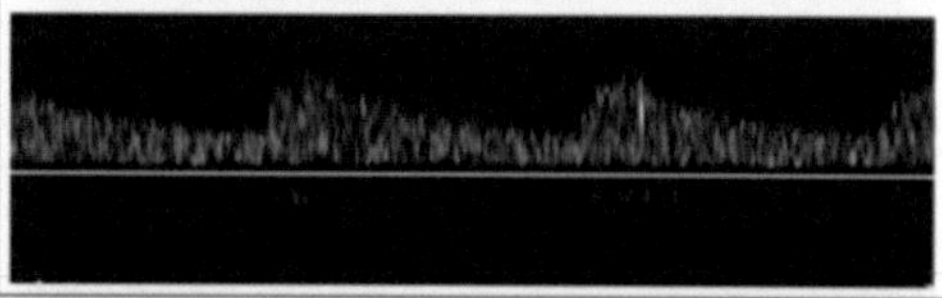 |
| **Grade 4**<br>**STENOTIC FLOW** | - MFV of >80 cm/s and velocity difference of >30% compared to the control side or<br>- if both affected and comparison sides have MFV <80 cm/s due to low end-diastolic velocity, MFV >30% compared to the control side and signs of turbulence | 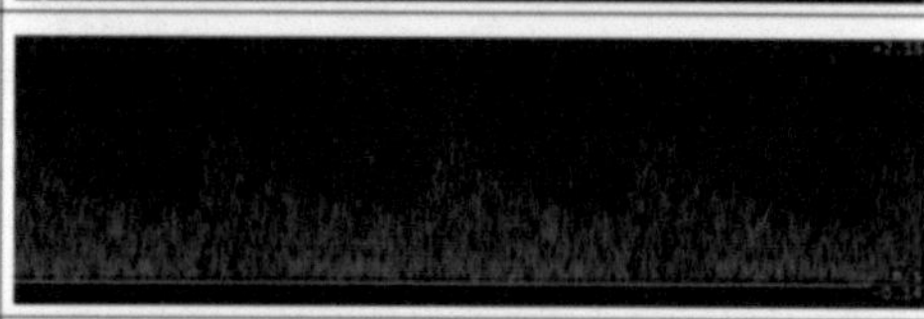 |
| **Grade 5**<br>**NORMAL FLOW** | - <30% mean velocity difference compared to control<br>- similar waveform shapes compared to control | 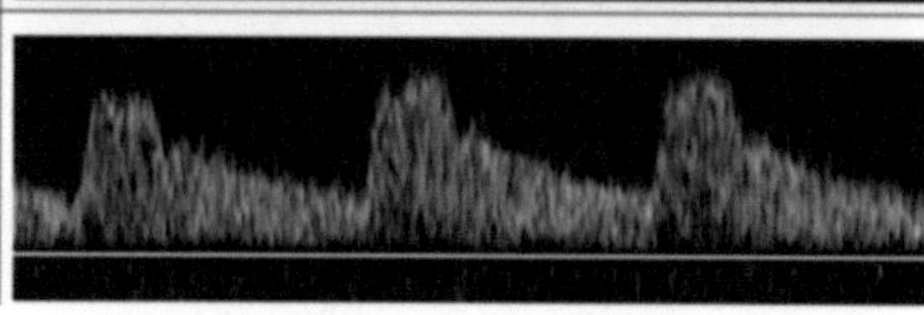 |

Fig. 15. TIBI flow grading system (adapted from Malferrari and Zedde 2008 and Malferrari 2010)

The relevance of this subclassification is that all categories has been externally validated by DSA. But, if this purpose is praiseworthy, it should also considered that only twenty-five patients were examined, half the cases were evaluated by DSA, and the time interval between the two examinations, TCD and DSA, was not short. Indeed TCD was performed at 12+16 hours and angiography at 41+57 hours after stroke onset; only 52% of studies were performed within 3 hours (Burgin et al. 2000). Although this limitations, the authors found that recanalization on TCD had the following accuracy parameters compared with angiography:

- sensitivity 91%
- specificity 93%
- positive predictive value (PPV) 91%

- negative predictive value (NPV) 93%.

As previously stated in the discussion about guidelines (Sloan et al. 2004), to predict partial occlusion (TICI grade II), TCD had an high reliability (sensitivity of 100%, specificity of 76%, PPV of 44%, and NPV of 100%). Also, TCD predicted the presence of complete occlusion on DSA (TICI grade I) with lower, but yet high reliability (sensitivity of 50%, specificity of 100%, PPV of 100%, and NPV of 75%). The conclusions of the authors were that TCD flow signals correlated with angiographic occlusive pattern (Burgin et al. 2000).

| TICI | TIBI |
|---|---|
| **Grade 0** **COMPLETE OCCLUSION** | **Grade 0** No detectable Doppler shift distal to the occlusion site |
| | **Grade 1** Absent end-diastolic flow and a short systolic spyke |
| **Grade 1** **PARTIAL OCCLUSION** | **Grade 2** Delayed systolic flow acceleration and a MFV < 30 cm/sec |
| | **Grade 3** Pulsatile signal with normal acceleration, MFV decrease of > 30% compared to normal side, and positive end diastolic flow |
| **Grade 2** **COMPLETE RECANALIZATION** | **Grade 4** Low resistance flow with a significant focal velocity increase; may also be seen in hyperemia |
| | **Grade 5** Low resistance flow with no significant difference in velocities compared to the normal side |

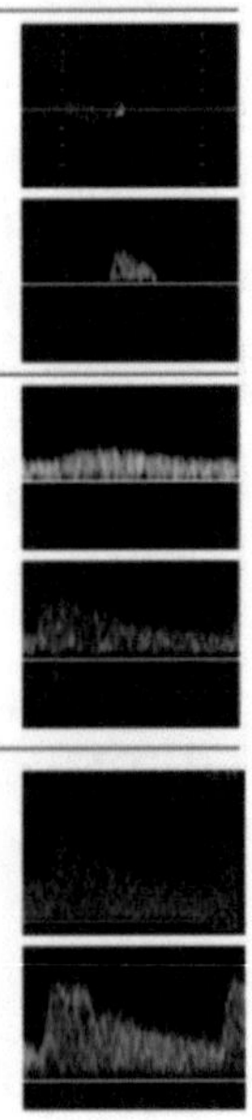

Fig. 16. TIBI flow grading grouping, according to TICI scale (modified from Burgin et al 2000)

The difficulty in differentiation between TIBI grades 1 to 3 (minimal flow, blunted flow, dampened flow) and the limitation of the above cited DSA comparative study (Burgin et al. 2000) raised some questions about the usefulness and the comparability of this grading system in clinical practice. Therefore the authors of the Consensus Conference (Nedelmann et al 2009) noted that, because of the relevant effect of the upstream and downstream arterial status, flow patterns graded by TIBI could not only reflect partial recanalization of the M1 MCA, but also include different hemodynamic situations in a combination of upstream and downstream steno-occlusions (e.g. extracranial or intracranial ICA occlusion, and obstruction of MCA branches). A TIBI flow grade of 2 or 3 may be seen for example in extracranial carotid steno-occlusion without intracranial artery disease, not only during MCA recanalization process.

Based on these considerations, an evolution of the TIBI score into a TCCS-based grading system has been proposed and called COGIF (COnsensus on Grading Intracranial Flow obstruction) score (Nedelmann et al 2009) (Fig. 17).

The purpose of this scoring system is to avoid the interference of previous arterial disease, and it is exclusively based on known hemodynamic changes of the Doppler spectrum, occurring in the acute stage of stroke.

As TIBI score, also COGIF score can be applied for both baseline evaluation and assessment of the spontaneous or treatment-induced recanalization. The score comprise these major grades (fig. 17):

- vessel occlusion (grade 1)
- partial recanalization (grades 2 and 3)
- established perfusion (grade 4).

Each grade is partially different from TIBI corresponding grade, because of the attempt to strongly reduce the subjective interpretation of the Doppler spectrum, mainly for TIBI grades 1 to 3, which are also the ones more affected by downstream and/or upstream arterial status. Furthermore, although the COGIF score, as the TIBI score, is based on the Doppler spectrum for the grading, the first one was designed for TCCS, and then some morphologic findings may play a role in achieving the waveform and in the occlusive pattern diagnosis. This score was proposed in the Consensus Conference (Nedelmann et al. 2009) primary for clinical trials, in order to make easier and reliable the assessment of recanalization grades, but its use is yet under evaluation, because of the lack, at our knowledge, of published prospective studies or retrospective evaluations, using the COGIF score.

| COGIF GRADE | HEMODYNAMIC PATTERN | EXAMPLE |
|---|---|---|
| Grade 1 | No flow | 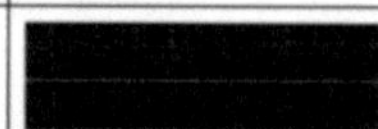 |
| Grade 2 | Low flow velocities without diastolic flow | 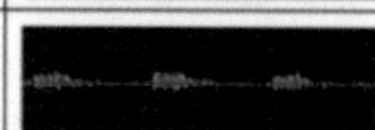 |
| Grade 3 | Low flow velocities with diastolic flow | 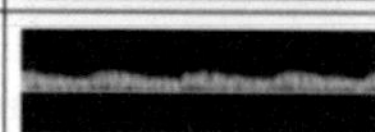 |
| Grade 4 | Established perfusion | |
| | a. Flow velocities equal to controlateral side | 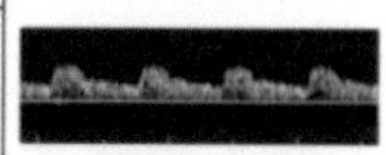 |
| | b. High focal flow velocities (i.e. stenosis) | 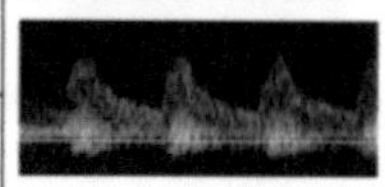 |
| | c. High segmental flow velocities (hyperperfusion) | |

Fig. 17. COGIF flow grading score: grading, hemodynamic features and examples (modified from Nedelmann et al 2009 and Malferrari et al 2010)

The COGIF score was designed to better follow the recanalization process with its dynamicity and potential alternation of recanalization and reocclusion. Therefore the time course of grades during serial TCCS examination was carefully encoded (Fig. 18).

## 4. Anterior circulation stroke

For this chapter anterior circulation stroke was described to show the usefulness and the role of sonological vascular imaging as a guide to treatment and to define the prognosis. Indeed the knowledge of vascular status in acute ischemic stroke have a clear prognostic relevance and it could be used also as a criterion to tailor the treatment and select the best reperfusion strategy for each patient, both in a single modality and in a sequential or

| HEMODYNAMIC CHANGE | EFFECT ON COGIF SCORE | EXAMPLE BASELINE | EXAMPLE CONTROL |
|---|---|---|---|
| 1. Reflow a. partial recanalization | Improvement by ≥ 1 grade |  | 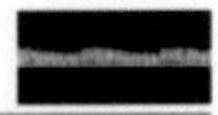 |
| b. complete recanalization | Improvement to grade 4 | 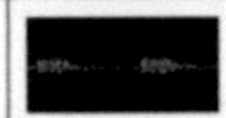 | 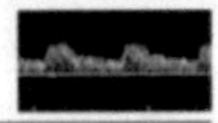 |
| 2. No change | None | 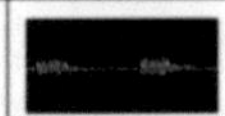 | 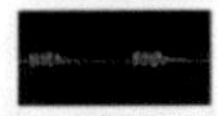 |
| 3. Worsening | Deterioration by ≥ 1 grade | 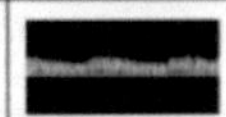 | 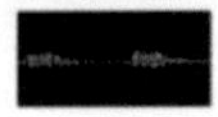 |

Fig. 18. Hemodynamic changed and COGIF flow grading score (modified from Nedelmann et al 2009)

combined modality. It has been undoubtedly accepted that the occlusive pattern at the presentation is closely related to the outcome of patient, as the recanalization of the primarily occluded vessel and its time course. Another strong predictor of the outcome is the perfusional status of the brain tissue in the downstream of the occluded vessel and it is evaluable mainly by using neuroradiological techniques, MR or CT, but also ultrasound imaging by TCCS and UCA injection may provide some informations about the cerebral perfusion in the MCA territory in acute stroke patients. The combination of the two findings, the occlusive pattern and the perfusional status, could provide a reliable classification of acute stroke patients in terms of the most adequate treatment to reverse the globally poor outcome (Malferrari and Zedde 2008). The following sections are mainly focused on occlusive pattern diagnosis, monitoring of recanalization and perfusional imaging, from the point of view of ultrasound techniques application.

### 4.1 Occlusive pattern diagnosis

The main studies from which intravenous thrombolysis with recombinant tissue plasminogen activator (rtpA) for stroke achieved an evidence of efficacy (total amount of 2889 patients) (NINDS group 1995; Hacke et al. 1995; Hacke et al. 1998; Clark et al. 1998; Clark et al 2000) did not provide any information about the status of extra- and intracranial vessels before treatment. Therefore it could be hypothesized that a great amount of patients treated with rtPA had a situation of extracranial and intracranial patent vessels. Indeed there is a clearly demonstrated relation between the stroke subtype, according to the Oxfordshire Community Stroke Project Classification (OCSPC), and the occlusive pattern on TCD: Partial or Total Anterior Circulation Strokes (PACIs and TACIs respectively), as expected, are more frequently associated with large vessel disease, as compared with lacunar infarcts (LACIs), where only few patients had an intracranial vessel
lesion (Mead et al. 2000). This last subgroup belongs to Parent Artery Disease (PAD), with the same prognosis of patients with large artery disease.

The relation between the occlusive pattern and the outcome has been demonstrated by several studies, and then it is possible to say that "severe arterial stenosis/occlusion in the early arterial study was highly related with 90-day mortality in an unselected series of patients with stroke" (Ois et al. 2007). This is right non only for severe stroke but also for mild stroke, and it is not related to the imaging technique used. Therefore, if possible, all attempts should be made to diagnose a large-artery intracranial occlusion before

thrombolysis by using neuroradiological techniques or neurosonological ones (TCD or TCCS) (Malferrari and Zedde 2008), without delaying the treatment.
The assumption for this imaging is the close link between the clot burden (i.e. the occlusive pattern) and the extent of brain lesion (i.e. the perfusional status), strongly suggesting the need of diagnosing presence and site of vessel occlusion in the acute phase of stroke. The advantages of neurosonology has been detailed in the previous sections, as widespread availability, easiness of use, the possibility of a repeated bedside examination and monitoring of recanalization, an highest reliability.
Another main advantage of the knowledge of the occlusive pattern before treatment is the possibility of predicting the success of the reperfusion strategy in terms of recanalization rate, because it has been known from the old and recent literature that each occlusive pattern is associated with a different response to rtPA administration (Ringelstein et al. 1992; Trouillas et al. 1998). In the NINDS trial (NINDS group 1995) the subgroup of patients with combined occlusion of ICA and MCA (tandem occlusion) had lesser benefit from thrombolysis than patients with isolated MCA occlusion, particularly in case of branch occlusions, although the clinical presentation and the severity score was the same in the two groups. Another series of 139 patients shown the same results (Del Zoppo et al. 1992), and so on a small study designed for the evaluation of tandem occlusion prognosis (Rubiera et al. 2006) and several studies demonstrated a poor recanalization rate in T-type occlusion (Arnold et al. 2003).
Then there are several occlusive patterns from which it could be expected a different response to thrombolysis: "...the patients presented with similar severity of hemiplegia, but the severity of perfusion deficit and recovery were dramatically different. TCD allows early differentiation of patency and natural history of MCA thromboembolic events. This may have important implications in the decision for thrombolytic therapy..." (Alexandrov et al. 2000).
The neurosonological examination by TCD and TCCS can help in the early diagnostic work-up of patients with acute ischemic stroke (Iannuzzi et al. 1995; Lee et al. 1996; Razumovsky et al. 1999; Alexandrov et al 1999; Garami et al 2003); two studies addressed the reliability of the combined application of ultrasound examination of extracranial and intracranial arteries in acute stroke patients, respectively by TCD and TCCS (Alexandrov et al. 1999; Malferrari et al 2007). This strategy allows to identify the vascular occlusive pattern eligible for treatment (accuracy near to 100%) (IMS study investigators 2004) and a fast-track ultrasound examination protocol has been proposed to diagnose the presence and site of vessel lesion bedside (Alexandrov et al. 1999; Molina et al. 2002; Feldberg et al. 2002), achieving a sensitivity, specificity, positive predictive value and negative predictive value near to 100% (Feldberg et al. 2002; Grant et al. 2003; Demchuk et al. 2001; Burgin et al. 2001; El-Mitwalli et al. 2002; Christou et al 2001).
The occlusive pattern diagnosis was categorized as shown in fig. 19.
There are validated diagnostic criteria for occlusive pattern in acute stroke, both for TCD (Demchuk et al. 2000) and by TCCS (Malferrari et al. 2007) (fig. 20).
Therefore TCD and TCCS are a non-invasive, rapid, reproducible, bedside, reliable tool, to provide useful data on cerebral circulation and then to select patients for reperfusion treatment. Indeed "Ultrasound and other non-invasive tests should be available for the diagnosis of carotid, vertebral artery and intracranial artery stenosis and occlusion" in the acute phase of stroke (European Perspective on Stroke Management, Kjellstrom et al 2007).

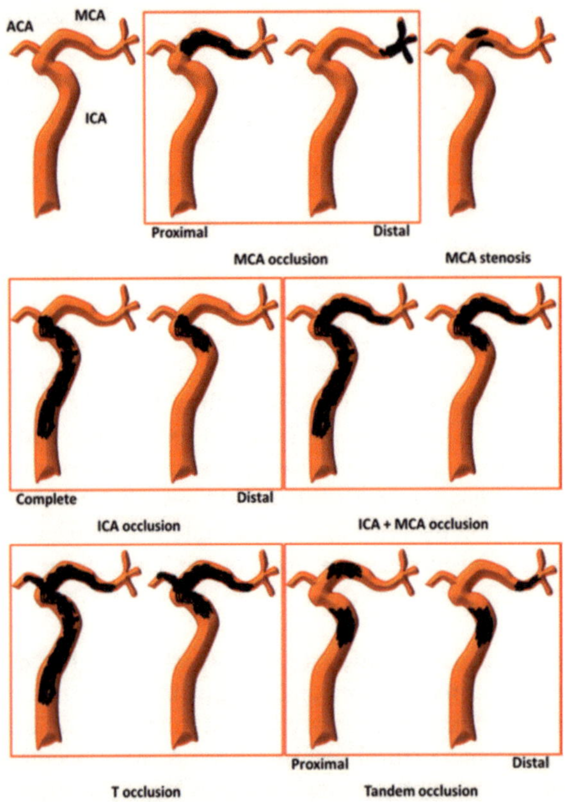


Fig. 19. Occlusive pattern in acute stroke patients.

The step following the diagnosis of occlusive pattern is the assignment of the TIBI or COGIF score, because of the need of a baseline value for monitoring the recanalization. The link between the grading score and the occlusive pattern diagnosis is globally weak, because a single score value matches several occlusive patterns.

Therefore the proposal of the COGIF score (Nedelmann et al. 2009) was associated to the careful analysis of each grade of the score, made by the same authors, both for the diagnosis of arterial occlusion and for the follow-up of recanalization, but mainly for the first one.

The grade 1 (no flow) corresponds to TIBI grade 0 and describes the main spectral finding seen in M1 MCA occlusion (comprising T-occlusion and its variants). The main diagnostic criterion of the M1 MCA occlusion is the absence of a Colour or Power-mode Doppler flow signal and its Doppler spectrum at the proximal MCA main stem (Malferrari et al 2007; Malferrari and Zedde 2008; Malferrari 2010). The absence of Doppler signals may also be caused by an insufficient acoustic bone window, and therefore for a reliable diagnosis of occlusion a sufficient visualization of the other ipsilateral arteries (A1 ACA, C1 ICA, posterior cerebral artery) is requested; sometimes the identification of contralateral arteries of the anterior circulation is also requested (Fig. 21).

The difficulties in the evaluation of MCA versus T occlusions by TCCS born from the lack of angiographically validated criteria. The mostly used diagnostic criterion of carotid T occlusion is detailed in fig. 20, i.e. the absence of colour Doppler flow signal and its Doppler spectrum in M1 MCA, intracranial ICA, and the ipsilateral A1 ACA (Fig. 22). The reliability of this diagnosis is increased by the simultaneous visualization of the deep middle cerebral vein, the ipsilateral A2 ACA, or the contralateral anterior circulation (Nedelmann et al 2009).

| | **Intracranial Occlusion Criteria by TCD** | **Intracranial Occlusion Criteria by TCCS** |
|---|---|---|
| **M1 MCA occlusion** | Abnormal Transcranial In Brain Ischemia (TIBI) flow signals were found at a depth of > 45 mm through a temporal bone window, which allow insonation of other intracranial arteries | When no Doppler signal could be obtained in the lateral fissure while the anterior and posterior cerebral arteries (P1 or P2 segment) were sufficiently assessable (Georgiadis et al. 2004) |
| **M2 MCA occlusion** | Abnormal TIBI flow signals were found at a depth of < 45 mm or when there were on average > 21% lower mean flow velocities in the ispilateral than in the controlateral M1 MCA, using the Asymmetry Index or Zanette Index (Zanette et al. 1989; Thomassen et al 2005) | Distal occlusions of the MCA (M2) were diagnosed using the interhemispheric asymmetry index with the known threshold of 21% (Zanette et al. 1989) for nonagle-corre4cted measurements and the criterion of end-diastolic ratio < 2.5 between sides for angle-corrected measurements (Ogata et al. 2004) |
| **Terminal ICA occlusion** | Abnormal TIBI flow signals were found at a depth of 60 to 70 mm | Whenever a high-resistance signal pattern was recorded on the proximal ICA and if no or minimal signals from M1 and A1 segments were found |
| **Tandem proximal ICA/MCA occlusion** | When abnormal TIBI signals at depths 30 to 65 mm were found with signs of collateralization of flow through anterior, posterior communicating, or ophthalmic arteries | Tandem occlusion was classified when there was an occlusion of the extracranial ICA on ECD-SAV, and according to sonographic intracranial criteria previously published by Alexandrov and colleagues (El-Mitwalli et al. 2002) |
| **T-type occlusion** | | According to the following criteria: (1) absent flow signal of the MCA, ACA, or distal ICA; (2) sufficient temporal bone window, as demonstrated by flow signals in the ipsilateral PCA or contralateral MCA; and (3) resistance profile with increased systolic and decreased end-diastolic velocities (EDV) in the extracranial ipsilateral ICA and CCA. The third criterion was applied only in the absence of < 70% stenosis or occlusion of the extracranial ICA (Georgiadis et al. 2004). |
| **M1 MCA stenosis** | Focal mean flow velocity increase of >30% compared with the controlateral MCA | Intracranial stenosis of the proximal and distal MCA were diagnosed according to Baumgartner's criteria (Baumgartner et al. 1999) |

Fig. 20. Diagnostic criteria of occlusive pattern in acute stroke patients by TCD and TCCS.

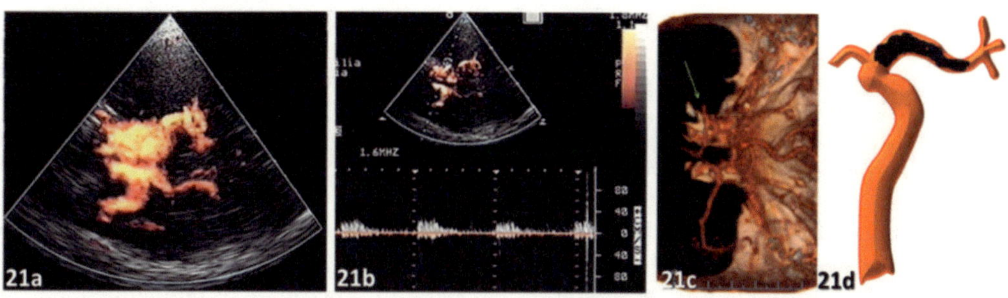


Fig. 21. An example of MCA occlusion by TCCS, compared to CT angiography.

a. TCCS from the temporal bone window in Power-mode with UCA administration: it is well visible the lack of signal in ipsilateral M1 MCA with the sparing of the other vessel of the circle of Willis; b. corresponding Doppler spectrum at MCA origin, with TIBI 2 score and COGIF 2 score; c Tridimensional reconstruction of the intracranial circulation by CT angiography of the same patient with the lack of M1 MCA (green arrow); d schematic drawing of the occluded artery, as in Fig. 19.

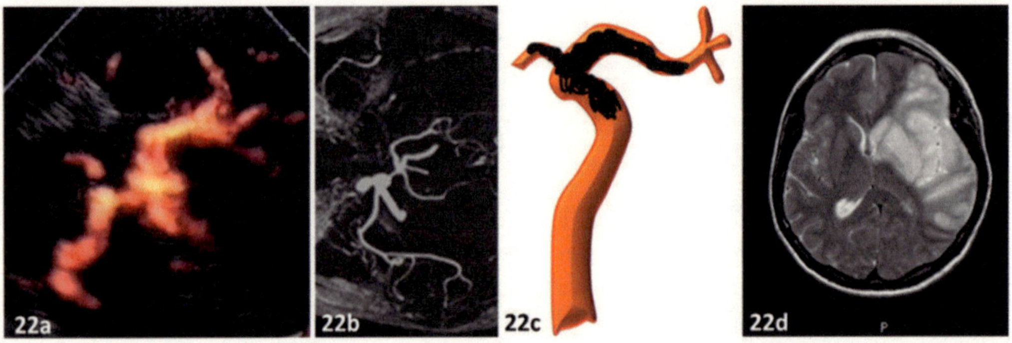


Fig. 22. An example of T occlusion by TCCS, compared to intracranial MR angiography.

a. TCCS from the temporal bone window in Power-mode with UCA administration: it is well visible the lack of signal in ipsilateral M1 MCA, C1 ICA and A1 ACA with the sparing of the posterior cerebral artery and the contralateral anterior circulation; b. MR angiography of the intracranial circulation of the same patient with the corresponding findings; c. schematic drawing of the occluded artery, as in Fig. 19; d. final cerebral infarction at MRI.
In the Consensus Conference these considerations raised other two statements about the diagnostic criterion of T occlusion (Fig. 23).

| | |
|---|---|
| ***Consensus Statement 7*** | If these criteria are fulfilled, it is not necessary to further confirm these diagnoses by use of UCA. A minimal quality standard requires the use of UCA only if insonation conditions are unsatisfactory and a reliable diagnosis is not possible otherwise (see Consensus Statement 3). |
| ***Consensus Statement 8*** | Diagnosis of a carotid T occlusion should be additionally confirmed by presence of decreased flow velocities, in particular end-diastolic, or oscillating flow, in the ipsilateral cervical ICA and common carotid artery in comparison to the contralateral side. |

Fig. 23. Consensus Statements 7 and 8 from Nedelmann et al. 2009

### 4.2 Monitoring of recanalization

As previously outlined, a main prognostic factor in acute stroke patients, treated with rtPA, is the timing of vessel patency restoration. If there have been discussions about the usefulness of vascular imaging before thrombolysis to diagnose the occlusive pattern, there is no doubt that the monitoring of recanalization is useful and widely recommended; for this purpose TCD or TCCS is the preferred technique, because of the known advantages and time resolution. These features make neurosonology a reliable and irreplaceable tool for continuous, real-time monitoring of the beginning, speed, timing and degree of arterial recanalization during thrombolysis (Alexandrov et al. 1999; Malferrari et al 2008). The relation between time of recanalization and outcome is well explained by the attempt of achieve, through the reopening of the occluded artery, the as early as possible restoration of blood flow mainly in the penumbra (Alexandrov et al 2001; Molina et al. 2004). The residual blood flow signals classification TIBI was described and validated by Alexandrov and coworkers (Demchuk et al 2000b, 2001; Molina et al. 2002) (fig. 15). This classification has been demonstrated to be useful, because the degree of residual flow signals predicts the likelihood of recanalization (Labiche et al. 2003). Patients with TIBI 1 to 3 have a likelihood of recanalization twice more higher than patients with TIBI 0 grade, irrespectively to the occlusion site. This is probably due to the consideration that the detectable residual flow (TIBI 1-3) ensues a better delivery of rtPA to thrombus than the condition of no flow (TIBI 0). Furthermore, an early improvement of blood flow on TCD or TCCS, within 30 min after rt-PA bolus, is related to an higher likelihood of achieving a final complete recanalization and a better outcome (Alexandrov et al. 2001). Then it has been demonstrated that neurosonological technique may distinguish patients who will benefit from thrombolysis, from patients who probably don't. This last subgroup has a poor outcome and the early knowledge of this status could allow to select more aggressive or rescue strategies to achieve the recanalization of the occluded vessel (Saqqur et al. 2006; Sekoranja et al. 2006; Ribo et al. 2006).

In studies defining the impact of recanalization time od an occluded MCA on outcome by TCD monitoring during rtPA treatment (Alexandrov et al. 2001), the timing of arterial reopening was classified into:

- sudden (sudden reappearance of normal flow signal or low resistance stenosis, within 60 s)
- stepwise (flow signal improvement into 1-29 min)
- slow (reappearance of flow signal after 30 min).

In the stepwise group the mean recanalization time of onset was after 17 min from rt-PA bolus and it was complete after 35 min. The complete recanalization was more rapid (mean 10 min) than the partial one (mean 30 min) and recanalization time positively correlated with a favourable clinical outcome. This was also demonstrated in tandem ICA and MCA occlusions (Kim et al. 2005). The slow recanalization pattern and the confimation of TIBI 3 at the end of rtPA administration were poor prognostic factors, related to the persistence of a distal occlusion (Demchuk et al. 2001).

Another useful application of neurosonological examination in the acute stroke, combined with a perfusional approach, is the potential identification of patients treatable beyond the 3 h time window (Ribo et al. 2005).

As expected according to the previous considerations, the time of tPA-induced recanalization, monitored by TCD (Delgado-Mederos et al. 2007) is a strong predictor of the evolution of ischemic lesion at diffusion-weighted imaging (DWI)-MRI (Kidwell et al. 2000; Fiehler et al. 2004) and of the clinical outcome; slow recanalization pattern correlates with greater lesion size and poorer short- and long-term outcomes than sudden and stepwise patterns (Malferrari and Zedde 2008).

DIAS study (Duplex-Sonographic Assessment of the Cerebrovascular Status in Acute Stroke), a German multicentre study, was designed to evaluate the vascular status within 6 h from symptoms onset and to monitor the recanalization after thrombolysis or best medical therapy (Gerriets et al. 2000). Only one of the twelve patients with T occlusion not treated with thrombolysis shown a late spontaneous reperfusion. Also another relevant multicentre study, the NAIS (Study Project of the Neurosonology Research Group of the World Federation of Neurology) (Allendoerfer et al. 2006) had the aim of monitoring the vascular status within 6 h from symptoms onset and differentiating the several occlusive pattern in extra- and intracranial circulation. Only 32% of the included patients shown a significant extracranial carotid disease and the conclusion of the authors was that it is unlikely that the success of thrombolysis is independent from vascular status, with a statistical significant difference in recanalization between proximal and distal MCA occlusion. Furthermore the "sudden pattern" of recanalization, isolated MCA occlusion, embolic origin of MCA occlusion, are prognostic factors for favourable outcome in patients treated with rtPA within 3 hours and monitored by TCD (Molina et al. 2004 b).

As previously mentioned, the recanalization rate is related to the occlusive pattern. In controlled angiographic trials of intravenous thrombolysis the partial or complete recanalization rate of a previously occluded MCA, is not higher than 25% (Del Zoppo et al. 1998). Trials with intra-arterial thrombolysis had a better recanalization rate (Furlan et al 1999): for example in the PROACT II trial (121 patients), the rate of complete recanalization was 20% and the rate of partial recanalization was 46%, but the median symptom to needle time was 5.3 h and the recanalization, when it occurred, was achieved at > 7 hours from stroke onset.

The sequential bridged strategy of i.v. followed by i.a. thrombolysis, is promising and could be more efficient than each of both single technique, joining the benefit of the rapid administration of i.v. rtPA with the higher recanalization rate of the i.a. treatment (Lewandowski et al. 1999; Flaherty et al. 2005; Lee et al. 2004; Zaidat et al. 2002; Sekoranja et al. 2006).

Several studies described the role of TCD and TCCS as a useful tool for the diagnosis of MCA occlusion and the monitoring of its recanalization and the prognostic value of early arterial recanalization, identified by TCD, was reaffirmed in terms of good outcome at 3 months (Labiche et al. 2003) for:

- 50% of patients with a complete recanalization
- 44% of patients with a partial recanalization
- 22% of patient without recanalization

In this study 20% of patients with proximal MCA occlusion who do not recanalize within 30 min is dead at 3 months.

In the Eligible study (Malferrari et al. 2007; Malferrari and Zedde 2008) the subgroup of patients with MCA stenosis or occlusion had the highest recanalization rate and distal MCA lesions shown a better and earlier recanalization and a significantly lower mortality rate than proximal ones, being patent nearly 50% at 3–6 h, as in the NAIS study (Allendoerfer et al. 2006). The authors conclude that "in acute stroke patients the early identification of a MCA stenosis or occlusion, mainly distal MCA lesions, is a strong predictor of good functional outcome at 3 months". The known differences in the speed and rate of recanalization are probably related to the clot age and composition, because rtPA has a better penetration in fibrin-rich thrombi, likely more recent and embolic, than in platelet-rich thrombi, whose lysis is often slow and partial, with clot fragments moving to the distal smaller vessels and prolonging ischemia (Molina et al. 2004 b; Malferrari and Zedde 2008).

A revision of the data from CLOTBUST study to find out the relationship among the presence and site of vessel lesion and the rate of complete recanalization and clinical recovery was recently made (Saqqur et al. 2007), and its findings were not different from the results of the ELIGIBLE study (Malferrari et al. 2007; Malferrari and Zedde 2008):

- Distal MCA occlusion had an OR of 2 for complete recanalization (44.2%, CI 95: 1.1 to 3.1, P < 0.005)
- Proximal MCA occlusion had an OR of 0.7 (30%, CI 95: 0.4 to 1.1, P < 0.13)
- Terminal ICA had an OR of 0.1 (5.9%, CI 95: 0.015 to 0.8, P < 0.015)
- Tandem cervical ICA/MCA had an OR of 0.7 (27%, CI 95: 0.3 to 1.9, P < 0.5)
- Basilar artery had an OR of 0.96 (30%, CI 95: 0.2 to 4, P < 0.9).

In this study patients with TIBI 0 grade had less probability of complete recanalization than patients with TIBI 3 (ORadj: 0.256, CI 95: 0.11 to 0.595, P < 0.002).
In the CLOTBUST study (Alexandrov et al. 2004 b) the continuous TCD monitoring (i.e. exposure to ultrasound) was a positive predictor for complete recanalization (ORadj: 3.02, CI95: 1.396 to 6.514, P < 0.005). NIHSS score < 2 at 24 h was achieved in 22% of patients, so categorized in terms of the occlusive pattern:

- distal MCA occlusion 33%
- tandem cervical ICA/MCA occlusion 24%
- proximal MCA occlusion 16%

It is notable that none of the patients with T occlusion had dramatic recovery (0%) (P < 0.003).
Modified Rankin Scale score <1 was achieved in 35% of patients, so categorized in terms of the occlusive pattern:

- distal MCA occlusion 52%
- proximal MCA occlusion 25%
- tandem cervical ICA/MCA occlusion 21%
- T occlusion 18%

The likelihood of a good long-term outcome was twice higher for patients with distal MCA occlusion than for patients with proximal MCA occlusions (OR: 2.1, CI 95: 1.1 to 4, P < .025). The authors conclude that the "clinical response to thrombolysis is influenced by the site of occlusion" and "patients with no detectable residual flow signals as well as those with terminal internal carotid artery occlusions are least likely to respond early or long term" (Alexandrov et al. 2004b; Saqqur et al. 2007).
Also the Eligible study (Malferrari et al. 2007) shown that the clinical recovery at both 24 h and 3 months is influenced by the site of occlusion.
CLOTBUST (Alexandrov et al. 2004b; Saqqur et al. 2007), NAIS (Allendoerfer et al. 2006) and ELIGIBLE (Malferrari et al. 2007; Malferrari and Zedde 2008) studies demonstrated the high predictive value of neurosonology for identifying proximal MCA occlusion. The CLOTBUST authors (Alexandrov et al. 2004b; Saqqur et al. 2007) proposed TCD as a screening tool for i.v./i.a. thrombolysis. A similar proposal has been made for TCCS by an interesting but small clinical study (Sekoranja et al. 2006), where the patients with partial or complete MCA recanalization at 30 min from the onset of i.v. thrombolysis showed an higher rate of positive outcome at 24 h and at 3 months than patients with none recanalization. In this latter subgroup the subsequent i.a. thrombolysis with the residual amount of rtPA was performed and provided a substantial benefit. Therefore, 56% of patients treated with combined i.v./i.a. thrombolysis achieved a good outcome at 3 months (mRS 0-2), compared with 22% of a previous study (Labiche et al. 2003) in patients with no recanalization with i.v. thrombolysis.
As in the TCD studies (Saqqur et al. 2005), this TCCS experience (Sekoranja et al. 2006) found that TIBI classification, defined by TCCS, was reliably related with the corresponding TIMI angiographic grades. Therefore neurosonological techniques, both TCD and TCCS, can

be "a suitable noninvasive tool for selecting patient with persistent arterial occlusions despite initial i.v. rtPA treatment with an i.v. /i.a. protocol" (Saqqur et al. 2005).

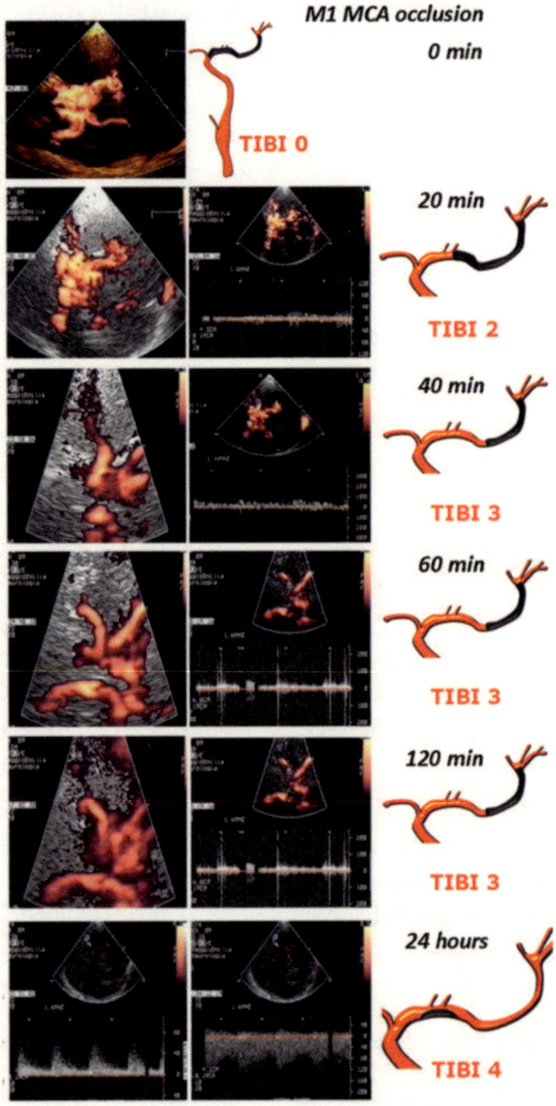


Fig. 24. From top to bottom a sequential TCCS examination of a patient with MCA occlusion and contraindication to thrombolysis. In the right side the corresponding drawings (adapted from Malferrari 2010) and TIBI flow grades.

This is mainly true for vascular occlusive patterns known and accepted for being prognostically poor, i.e. tandem occlusions of ICA and proximal MCA and T occlusions (Fig. 14). It has been known that tandem occlusions of ICA and proximal MCA have a poorest response to i.v. thrombolysis and are associated with an early (within 7 days) mortality rate, as high as 18%, but also 80% of the survivors have a severe disability (mRS > 2) (Rubiera et

al. 2006). T occlusions have similar, if not poorer, mortality and disability rates and a recanalization rate of 31% at 3 days with i.v. thrombolysis (almost all were late or slow recanalizations) (Linfante et al. 2002). This is because of the broader clot burden with lesser collateral circle (Jansen et al. 1995; von Kummer et al. 1995; Christou et al. 2002).
An example of a slow recanalization process is in Fig. shown in Fig. 24.
After the literature review about clinical practice, it is useful to consider the TCCS score, COGIF (Nedelmann et al. 2009) for the potential pitfalls of the recanalization monitoring in clinical trials, i.e. for grade > 2.
Grades 2 and 3 define the low flow situation and it may be determined by different pathological conditions. Low-flow phenomena in the M1 MCA are a main feature of a partial recanalization or T occlusion or tandem pattern, because of an upstream or downstream obstruction (i.e., distal main stem or MCA branch occlusions). The differentiation of these conditions from partial recanalization is well addressed by the Consensus Conference, as summarized in Fig. 25.

| | |
|---|---|
| ***Upstream occlusion*** 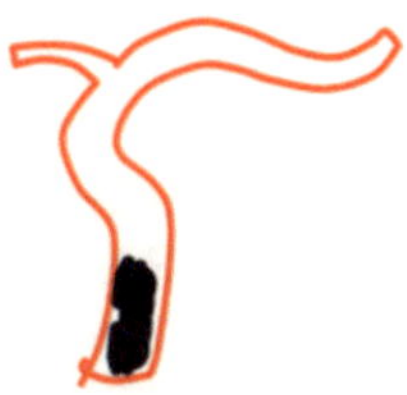 | A hemodynamically compromising ICA lesion can reduce downstream flow velocities in the MCA without MCA or intracranial ICA disease. Such a lesion can also produce compensatory increased flow velocities in the contralateral hemisphere, thereby increasing the asymmetry index. To ascribe an intracranial flow reduction to intracranial pathology, an upstream obstruction of the ICA an has to be ruled out. |
| ***Downstream occlusion (braches occlusion)*** 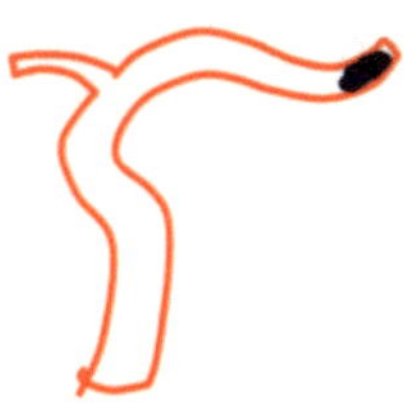 | The diagnosis of MCA branch occlusions is based on the calculation of the asymmetry index. This index should only be calculated if the supplying carotid arteries and the contralateral MCA can be assessed without relevant stenosis or occlusion. |

Fig. 25. The influence of upstream and downstream occlusions on low-flow status in COGIF score (modified, from Nedelmann et al. 2009)

In the COGIF score, low-flow velocities without diastolic flow (grade 2: residual flow), are distinguished from complete obstruction (grade 1: no flow), because residual flow signals are associated with improved results of thrombolysis (Labiche et al. 2003; Saqqur et al. 2008). The grade 4 (established perfusion) comprises different hemodynamic situations: normal flow (4a), stenotic flow (4b), and high-flow velocities in hyperperfusion (4c). This grouping was determined by the thought that distinguishing high-flow velocities from normal-flow velocities is not so relevant for defining a reestablishment of sufficient hemispheric perfusion.
About the differentiation between grade 4 b and 4 c the statement 9 is well explicative (fig. 26).

| | |
|---|---|
| ***Consensus Statement 9*** | In a prospective study, TCCS data were correlated with digital subtraction angiography. Criteria based on this study allowed for the reliable assessment of > 50% and < 50% basal cerebral artery diameter narrowing. They should be applied for the detection and follow-up of intracranial stenoses.<br>However, these criteria have not been validated in the setting of acute stroke. Reactive hyperperfusion may possibly lead to overestimation of the degree of intracranial stenosis. |

Fig. 26. Consensus Statement 9 (from Nedelmann et al. 2009)

### 4.3 Perfusional ultrasound imaging

As previously mentioned at the beginning of this section, both vascular and perfusional informations are relevant to define the prognosis of acute stroke patients and the success of treatment, because the reopening of the occluded vessel is not equal to the reperfusion of the affected brain tissue. Neuroradiological imaging, with the concept of core/penumbra mismatch, raised some questions about the reliability and the usefulness of these data before thrombolysis, but there are several logistic limitation to the wide use of this techniques, besides some contraindications (to the technique, as for patients with pacemakers in MRI, or to the contrast medium, as for CT). Ultrasound techniques, namely TCCS with UCA administration and harmonic imaging, are safe and bedside executable, but their reliability for evaluating the brain perfusional status has not been demonstrated and there are not validated thresholds for core (brain tissue irreversibly harmed and not salvageable by any treatment) and penumbra (brain tissue surrounding the core and hypoperfused, likely not irreversibly harmed, and therefore potentially salvageable by reperfusion). Although these limitations, TCCS can help the clinician to decide in the acute stroke setting, where other techniques are not available or reliable (as for patients with severe arterial disease on both sides).

The purpose of this imaging strategy is the selection of patients for reperfusion treatment, i.v. or i.a., in order to improve its safety and efficacy, decreasing the hemorrhagic complications. This strategy could theoretically lead to overcome the concept of a fixed time window.

In clinical practice, there are two established imaging techniques to distinguish core from penumbra, MRI and contrast CT. The first technique diagnoses the core by using DWI and the penumbra by using perfusion-weighted imaging (PWI); the second one uses CT cerebral blood volume imaging for the core and PWI for the penumbra.

Also ultrasound techniques allow to perform a perfusional study of the brain parenchyma, depicting the blood flow in the microcirculation (Malferrari and Zedde 2008). This non-invasive tool can assess the perfusion deficits in acute stroke patients, although the lack of validated threshold in comparison with conventional neuroradiological methods.

The optimization of this concept was achieved by routine use of second generation UCA (for European countries, because UCA are not approved for neurosonological application in the USA) and harmonic imaging, that allow a real time dynamic study of cerebral circulation. It is possible to achieve an early visualization of the estimated size of the ischemic area in the acute phase, with minimal or no signs at the basal unenhanced CT (Seidel et al. 2004; Wiesman et al. 2004; Meyer-Wiethe et al. 2007). Ultrasound perfusion, like perfusional studies by CT and MRI, is based on dilution theory and allows to obtain wash-in and washout curves into selected areas of cerebral parenchyma or ROIs (Region of Interest) (Malferrari and Zedde 2008) (Fig. 27).

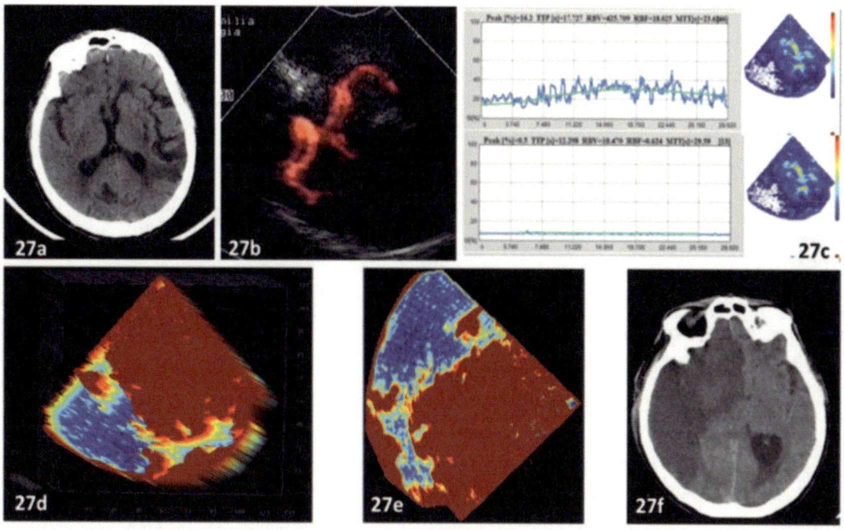


Fig. 27. An example of Ultrasound Perfusional Imaging.

a. unenhanced brain CT at the baseline; b. TCCS from the right temporal window with a diagnosis of a T occlusion; c. ultrasound perfusional curves (normal hemisphere in the upper half and flattened curves of the affected hemisphere in the lower half); d. tridimensional perfusional map with a broad area of hypoperfusion (blue); e. 90° rotated bidimensional map to make easier to compare it with the CT; f. 24 hours unenhanced brain CT with a perfectly corresponding ischemic lesion.

Another recent application of TCCS is the monitoring of the hemorrhagic transformation after thrombolysis for acute stroke of the anterior circulation (Seidel et al. 2009). An example of this application is showed in Fig. 28.

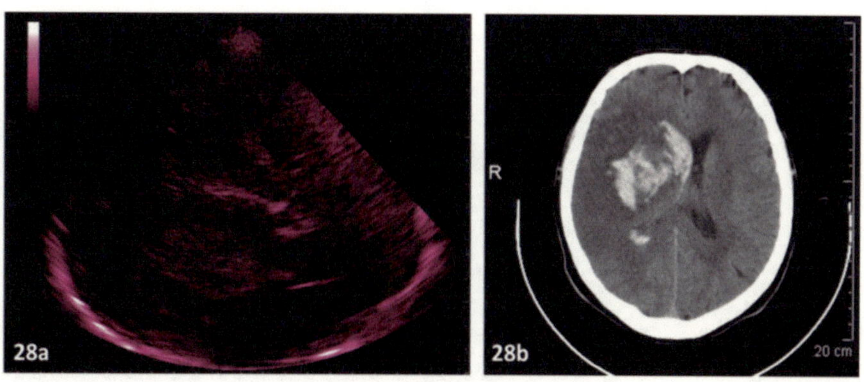


Fig. 28. Parenchymal haemorrhage after thrombolysis.

a. TCCS from the left temporal window, showing the rounded hyperechoic hemorrhagic lesion in the contralateral hemisphere; b. corresponding unenhanced brain CT.

## 5. Focus on intracranial stenosis

Intracranial atherosclerosis is an often neglected cause of stroke but it represents the first cause of ischemic stroke in the world (Gorelick et al. 2008). Not only atherosclerosis may cause an intracranial stenosis, but it is certainly the most frequent cause and also in the white population, in patients with multiple vascular risk factors.

Some relevant aspects of intracranial large artery disease, as recently stated and summarized (Gorelick et al. 2008), are:

- the magnitude of the public health problem;
- the risk of stroke and other cardiovascular diseases associated with intracranial occlusive disease;
- the etiology;
- medication and non-medication approaches to treatment and prevention;
- gaps in our understanding of intracranial occlusive disease and possible next steps to unravel enigmas related to this disorder.

The evaluation of the intracranial atherosclerosis and stenosis has addressed in the literature mainly in the setting of the post-acute phase and the diagnostic criteria for all techniques are not directly applicable in the acute phase; for example the TCCS criteria (Baumgartner et al. 1999) were selected and validated in a stable situation, because of the frequent presence of a transient intracranial stenosis (TIBI grade 4 and COGIF grade 4b) during the recanalization process of an occluded intracranial artery; therefore it is not possible to define criteria for a dynamically changing situation and the persistence of the stenosis days and weeks after the acute phase may more reliably indicate the intracranial atherosclerosis as the cause of the cerebrovascular event (Nedelmann et al. 2009; Malferrari et al. 2007; Malferrari et al. 2008).

Because of these considerations, the diagnosis of intracranial stenosis is not a main item in the ultrasound monitoring of the acute phase of ischemic stroke. Nevertheless it is useful to outline a neglected aspect of intracranial stenosis, as previously mentioned, i.e. the PAD subgroup (patients with clinical and radiological manifestations of lacunar infarction as a result of intracranial large artery atherosclerosis, mainly in MCA, located near the origin of perforating branches and therefore occluding them by direct clot growth of artery-to-artery embolism) (Bang et al. 2002) (Fig. 29).

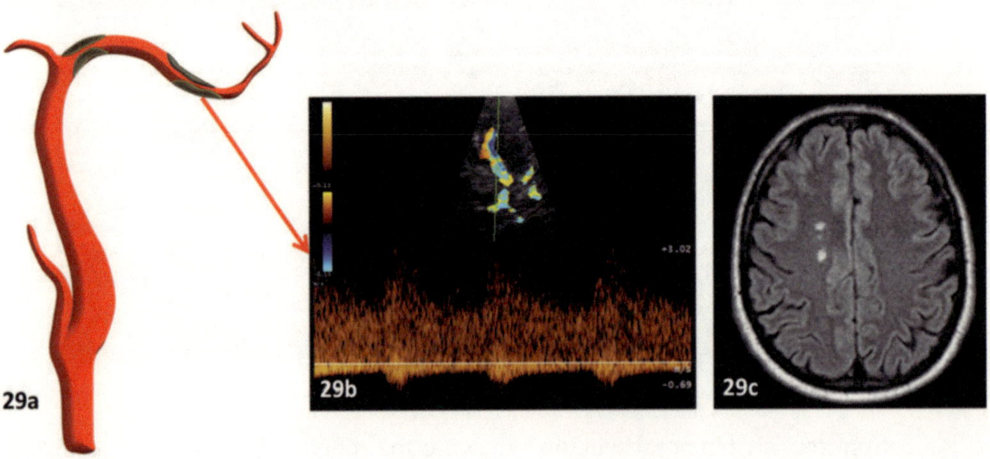


Fig. 29. PAD example.

a. schematic drawing of proximal and distal atherosclerosis of M1 MCA; b. corresponding TCCS from the right temporal window, with the Doppler spectrum and a clear increase of the flow velocity; c. MRI with ischemic lesions in the centrum semiovale of lacunar size.

## 6. Ultrasound-assisted thrombolysis

In the last decade a considerable amount of experimental and pilot clinical studies on stroke patients addressed the matter of ultrasound-assisted thrombolysis. The in vitro experience and the studies on animal models demonstrated that ultrasounds at frequencies in the 20 KHz -1 MHz range, lower than the ones usually available for diagnostic purposes, can potentiate the action of endogenous or exogenous tPA (Malferrari and Zedde 2008), leading to design a human study with a specific therapeutic ultrasound machine (Daffershofer et al. 2005) with the premature stop of the enrolment because of the increased rate of hemorrhage. This study caused a mild slowdown in the TCCS application on this field, although the good results of the above-mentioned CLOTBUST study with TCD (Alexandorv et al. 2004b).

The phenomena by which ultrasounds enhance thrombolysis is the increased delivery of rtPA into the fibrin clot and the breaking of the tight binding of fibrin itself, therefore providing a greater surface for thrombolytic drugs action, by cavitation, starting from the tissue and blood microbubbles (Alexandrov 2009).

The association of the UCA administration provides a great amount of right-sized microbubbles and then makes easier the clot fragmentation by the cavitation and thermal effects of ultrasound waves. This process happens by using the same ultrasound machines available for clinical purposes and the frequencies of the diagnostic transcranial doppler (1-2 MHz) (Malferrari and Zedde 2008). Microbubbles lower the ultrasound-induced cavitation threshold and dramatically increase the lytic action of ultrasounds. Several microbubbles has been used in experimental studies and some kind of not commercially available microbubbles also for human studies (Molina et al. 2009). The CLOTBUST study (Alexandrov et al. 2004b) evaluated the combined effect of rtPA administration within 3 h from symptom onset and TCD continuous monitoring at 2 MHz (diagnostic parameters), achieving a recanalization rate of 36% and an hemorrhagic transformation rate of 9%, not significantly different in comparison with the hemorrhagic rate of non-monitored patients. Other authors used TCCS for the same purposes with a diagnostic setting, with or without rtPA administration, confirming these findings (Cintas et al. 2002; Eggers et al. 2008).

The data about ultrasound-enhanced thrombolysis has been recently analysed in a meta-analysis (Tsivgoulis et al. 2010) and the results were comforting, regarding the safety of sonothrombolysis with high frequency ultrasounds, with or without UCA. This modality of sonothrombolysis "is associated with a nearly 3-fold increased likelihood of complete recanalization and 2-fold higher likelihood of functional independence at 3 months" (Tsivgoulis et al. 2010).

The limitations are certainly the small number of patients included, particularly in sonothrombolysis studies using TCCS, and other studies are needed.

## 7. Conclusion

Neurosonology is a safe, reliable and useful technique for evaluate acute stroke patients It may provide relevant information about the prognosis and guide the selection of the most adequate treatment for each patient. The recent development of intrinsic therapeutic perspectives, as ultrasound-enhanced thrombolysis, make even more recommendable its use in this setting.

## 8. References

Alecu C, Fortrat J, Ducrocq X, et al. Duplex scanning diagnosis of internal carotid artery dissections. A case control study. Cerebrovasc Dis 2007; 23:441–447

Alexandrov AV, Demchuk AM, Wein TH, Grotta JC. Yield of Transcranial Doppler in Acute Cerebral Ischemia. Stroke. 1999;30:1604-1609

Alexandrov A, Demchuk AM, Felberg RA, et al. High rate of complete recanalization and dramatic clinical recovery during rt-PA infusion when continuously monitored with 2-MHz transcranial Doppler monitoring. Stroke 2000; 31: 610-614

Alexandrov AV, Burgin SW, Demchuk AM, El-Mitwalli A, Grotta JC. Speed of intracranial clot lysis with intravenous tissue plasminogen activator therapy: sonographic classification and short-term improvement. Circulation 2001; 103: 2897–2902

Alexandrov AV, Wojner AW, Grotta JC. CLOTBUST: Design of a randomized trial of ultrasound-enhanced thrombolysis for acute ischemic stroke. J Neuroimaging. 2004;14:108 –112

Alexandrov AV, Molina CA, Grotta JC, et al. for the CLOTBUST Investigators. Ultrasound-Enhanced Systemic Thrombolysis for Acute Ischemic Stroke. N Engl J Med 2004; 351: 2170-8 (b)

Alexandrov AV. Ultrasound enhancement of fibrinolysis. Stroke. 2009; 40 (3Suppl): S107–S110

Alexandrov AV, Sloan MA, Tegeler CH, Newell DN, Lumsden A, Garami Z, Levy CR, Wong LKS, Douville C, Kaps M, Tsivgoulis G, for the American Society of Neuroimaging Practice Guidelines Committee, Practice Standards for Transcranial Doppler (TCD) Ultrasound. Part II. Clinical Indications and Expected Outcomes, J Neuroimaging 2010;20:1-10.

Allendoerfer J, Goertler M, von Reutern GM, for the Neurosonology in Acute Ischemic Stroke (NAIS) Study Group. Prognostic relevance of ultra-early doppler sonography in acute ischaemic stroke: a prospective multicenter study. Lancet Neurol 2006; 5:835–40

Arnold M, Nedeltchev K, Mattle HP, et al. Intra-arterial thrombolysis in 24 consecutive patients with internal carotid artery T occlusion. J Neurol Neurosurg Psychiatry 2003; 74: 739-742

Arnold M, Baumgartner RW, Stapf C, Nedeltchev K, Buffon F, Benninger D, Georgiadis D, Sturzenegger M, Mattle HP, Bousser MG, Ultrasound Diagnosis of Spontaneous Carotid Dissection With Isolated Horner Syndrome, Stroke. 2008;39:82-86

Bang OY, Heo JH, Kim JY, Park JH, Huh K, Middle Cerebral Artery Stenosis Is a Major Clinical Determinant in Striatocapsular Small, Deep Infarction, Arch Neurol. 2002;59:259-263

Bartlett ES, Walters TD, Symons SP, and Fox AJ, Diagnosing Carotid Stenosis Near-Occlusion by Using CT Angiography AJNR Am. J. Neuroradiol. 2006; 27(3): 632 - 637

Baumgartner RW, Mathis J, Sturzenegger M, Mattle HP. A validation study on the intraobserver reproducibility of transcranial color-coded duplex sonography velocity measurements. Ultrasound Med Biol. 1994;20:233–237.

Baumgartner RW, Arnold M, Gönner F, Staikow I, Herrmann C, Rivoir A, Müri RM, Contrast-Enhanced Transcranial Color-Coded Duplex Sonography in Ischemic Cerebrovascular Disease. Stroke. 1997;28:2473-2478

Baumgartner RW, Mattle HP, Schroth G. Assessment of 50% and 50% intracranial stenoses by transcranial color-coded duplex sonography. Stroke. 1999;30:87–92.

Baumgartner RW. Transcranial color duplex sonography in cerebrovascular disease: a systematic review. Cerebrovasc Dis. 2003;16:4–13

Benninger DH, Georgiadis D, Gandjour J, Baumgartner RW. Accuracy of Color Duplex Ultrasound Diagnosis of Spontaneous Carotid Dissection Causing Ischemia. Stroke. 2006;37:377-381

Burgin WS, Malkoff M, Felberg RA, Demchuk AM, Christou I, Grotta JC, Alexandrov AV. Transcranial Doppler ultrasound criteria for recanalization after thrombolysis for middle cerebral artery stroke. Stroke. 2000;31:1128 -1132

Burgin WS, Wojner AW, Demchuk AM, et al. Validity and reliability of the Thrombolysis In Brain Infarction [TIBI] flow grades. Stroke 2001; 32: 324

Caplan LR, Hennerici M. Impaired clearance of emboli (washout) is an important link between hypoperfusion, embolism, and ischemic stroke. Arch Neurol. 1998; 55: 1475–1482

Chappell FM, Wardlaw JM, Young GR, Gillard GH, Roditi GH, Yip B, Pell JP, Rothwell PM, Brown MM, Gough MJ, Randall MS, Carotid Artery Stenosis: Accuracy of Noninvasive Tests—Individual Patient Data Meta-Analysis, Radiology 2009; 251:493–502

Christou I, Felberg RA, Demchuk AM, et al. Accuracy parameters of a broad diagnostic battery for bedside transcranial Doppler to detect flow changes with internal carotid artery stenosis or occlusion. J Neuroimaging 2001; 11: 236 -242

Christou I, Felberg RA, Demchuk AM, et al. Intravenous tissue plasminogen activator and flow improvement in acute ischemic stroke patients with internal carotid artery occlusion. J Neuroimaging 2002; 12: 119 -123.

Cintas P, Le Traon AP, Larrue V. High rate of recanalization of middle cerebral artery occlusion during 2 MHz transcranial colour-coded continuous monitoring without thrombolytic drug. Stroke 2002; 33: 626–628

Clark WM, Wissman S, Albers GW, Jhamandas JH, Madden KP, Hamilton S. Recombinant tissue-type plasminogen activator (Alteplase) for ischemic stroke 3 to 5 hours after symptom onset. The ATLANTIS Study: a randomized controlled trial. Alteplase Thrombolysis for Acute Noninterventional Therapy in Ischemic Stroke. JAMA 1999; 282: 2019–2026

Clark WM, Albers GW, Madden KP, Hamilton S. Thrombolytic therapy in acute ischemic stroke study investigators. The rtPA (alteplase) 0- to 6-hour acute stroke trial, part A (A0276g): results of a double-blind, placebo-controlled, multicenter study. Stroke 2000;31: 811- 816

Daffertshofer M, Gass A, Ringleb R, et al., Transcranial Low- Frequency Ultrasound-Mediated Thrombolysis in Brain Ischemia: Increased Risk of Hemorrhage With Combined Ultrasound and TissuePlasminogen Activator: Results of a Phase II Clinical Trial. Stroke 2005; 36; 1441-1446

Del Zoppo G, Poek K, Pessin MS, et al. Recombinant Tissue Plasminogen Activator in Acute Thrombotic and Embolic Stroke. Ann Neurol 1992; 32: 78-86

Del Zoppo GJ, Higashida RT, Furlan AJ, Pessin MS, Rowley HA, Gent M, for the PROACT investigators. PROACT: a phase II randomized trial of recombinant pro-urokinase by direct arterial delivery in acute middle cerebral artery stroke. Prolyse in Acute Cerebral Thromboembolism. Stroke 1998; 29: 4–11

Delgado-Mederos R, Rovira A, Alvarez-Sabın J, et al. Speed of tPA-Induced Clot Lysis Predicts DWI Lesion Evolution in Acute Stroke. Stroke 2007; 38: 955-960

Demchuk AM, Christou I, Wein TH, et al. Accuracy and criteria for localizing arterial occlusion with transcranial Doppler. J Neuroimaging 2000; 10: 1-12

Demchuk AM, Christou I, Wein TH, et al. Specific transcranial Doppler flow findings related to the presence and site of arterial occlusion. Stroke 2000;31:140–146 (b)

Demchuk AM, Burgin WS, Christou I, et al. Thrombolysis In Brain Infarction [TIBI] transcranial Doppler flow grades predict clinical severity, early recovery, and mortality in patients treated with intravenous tissue plasminogen activator. Stroke 2001; 32: 89 -93

Eggers J, König IR, Koch B, Händler G, Seidel G. Sonothrombolysis with transcranial color-coded sonography and recombinant tissue-type plasminogen activator in acute middle cerebral artery main stem occlusion: results from a randomized study. Stroke. 2008; 39: 1470–1475

Eggers J, Pade O, Rogge A, Schreiber SJ and Valdueza JM, Transcranial Color-Coded Sonography Successfully Visualizes All Intracranial Parts of the Internal Carotid Artery Using the Combined Transtemporal Axial and Coronal Approach, American Journal of Neuroradiology 2009;30:1589

Eicke BM, Tegeler CH, Dalley G, Myers LG. Angle correction in transcranial Doppler sonography. J Neuroimaging. 1994;4:29 -33

El-Mitwalli A, Saad M, Christou I, Malkoff M, Alexandrov AV. Clinical and sonographic patterns of tandem internal carotid artery/middle cerebral artery occlusion in tissue plasminogen activator-treated patients. Stroke 2002; 33: 99 -102

Felberg RA, Okon NJ, El-Mitwalli A, Burgin WS, Grotta JC, Alexandrov AV. Early Dramatic Recovery During Intravenous Tissue Plasminogen Activator Infusion Clinical Pattern and Outcome in Acute Middle Cerebral Artery Stroke. Stroke 2002; 33: 1301-1307

Fiehler J, Knudsen K, Kucinski T, et al. Predictors of apparent diffusion coefficient normalization in stroke patients. Stroke 2004;35: 514 -519

Flaherty ML, Woo D, Kissela B, et al. Combined IV and intraarterial thrombolysis for acute ischemic stroke. Neurology 2005; 64:386–388

Furlan A, Higashida R, Wechsler L, et al. Intra-arterial prourokinase for acute ischemic stroke. The PROACT II study: a randomized controlled trial. Prolyse in Acute Cerebral Thromboembolism. JAMA 1999; 282:2003-2011

Fusco MR, Harrigan MR, Cerebrovascular Dissections—A Review Part I: Spontaneous Dissections, Neurosurgery 2011; 68:242–257

Garami Z, Calleja S, Labiche L, et al. Yield of urgent carotid scanning in acute cerebral ischemia. Stroke 2003;34:266

Georgiadis D, Oehler J, Schwarz S, Rousson V, Hartmann M, Schwab S. Does acute occlusion of the carotid T invariably have a poor outcome? Neurology 2004; 63: 22–26

Gerriets T, Seidel G, Fiss I, Modrau B, Kaps M. Contrast-enhanced transcranial color-coded duplex sonography: efficiency and validity. Neurology. 1999;52:1133–1137

Gerriets T, Postert T, Goertler M, et al.; for the DIAS (Duplex Sonography in Acute Stroke) Study Group. DIAS I: Duplex-Sonographic Assessment of the Cerebrovascular Status in Acute Stroke. A Useful Tool for Future Stroke Trials. Stroke 2000;31:2342-2345

Giller CA. Is angle correction correct? J Neuroimaging. 1994;4:51–52.

Goertler M, Kross R, Baeumer M, Jost S, Grote R, Weber S, Wallesch CW. Diagnostic impact and prognostic relevance of early contrastenhanced transcranial color-coded duplex sonography in acute stroke. Stroke. 1998;29:955–962.

Gorelick PB, Wong KS, Bae HJ, Pandey DK, Large Artery Intracranial Occlusive Disease. A Large Worldwide Burden but a Relatively Neglected Frontier, Stroke. 2008;39:2396-2399

Grant EG, Benson CB, Moneta GL, Alexandrov AV, Baker JD, Bluth EI, Carroll BA, Eliasziw M, Gocke J, Hertzberg BS, Katanick S, Needleman L, Pellerito J, Polak JF, Rholl KS, Wooster DL, Zierler E, Carotid Artery Stenosis: Gray-Scale and Doppler US Diagnosis—Society of Radiologists in Ultrasound Consensus Conference; Radiology 2003; 229:340–346

Hacke W, Kaste M, Fieschi C, et al. Intravenous thrombolysis with recombinant tissue plasminogen activator for acute hemispheric stroke: The European Cooperative Acute Stroke Study (ECASS). JAMA 1995; 274: 1017–1025

Hacke W, Kaste M, Fieschi C, et al. Second European-Australasian Acute Stroke Study Investigators. Randomised double-blind placebo-controlled trial of thrombolytic therapy with intravenous alteplase in acute ischaemic stroke (ECASS II). Lancet 1998; 352:1245–1251.

Hacke W, Furlan AJ, Al Rawi Y, et al. Intravenous desmoteplase in patients with acute ischaemic stroke selected by MRI perfusion-diffusion weighted imaging or perfusion CT (DIAS-2): a prospective, randomised, double-blind, placebo-controlled study. Lancet Neurol. 2009;2:141-150

Kenton AR, Martin PJ, Abbott RJ, Moody AR. Comparison of transcranial color-coded sonography and magnetic resonance angiography in acute stroke. Stroke. 1997;28:1601–1606.

Khan HG, Gailloud P, Bude RO, Martin JB, Szopinski KT, Khaw C, Rufenacht DA, Murphy KJ. The effect of contrast material on transcranial Doppler evaluation of normal middle cerebral artery peak systolic velocity. Am J Neuroradiol. 2000;21:386–390

Kjellström T, Norrving B, Shatchkute A. Helsingborg Declaration 2006 on European Stroke Strategies. Cerebrovasc Dis 2007; 23:229–241

Kidwell C, Saver J, Mattiello J, et al. Thrombolytic reversal of acute human cerebral ischemic injury shown by diffusion/perfusion magnetic resonance imaging. Ann Neurol 2000; 47: 462- 469

Kim YS, Garami Z, Mikulik R, Molina CA, Alexandrov AV, for the CLOTBUST Collaborators. Early Recanalization Rates and Clinical Outcomes in Patients With Tandem Internal Carotid Artery/Middle Cerebral Artery Occlusion and Isolated Middle Cerebral Artery Occlusion. Stroke 2005; 36: 869-871

Krejza J, Mariak Z, Babikian VL. Importance of angle correction in the measurement of blood flow velocity with transcranial Doppler sonography. Am J Neuroradiol. 2001;22:1743–1747

Krejza J, Baumgartner RW. Clinical applications of transcranial color-coded duplex sonography. J Neuroimaging. 2004;14:215–225

Krejza J, Swiat M, Pawlak MA, Oszkinis G, Weigele J, Hurst RW, Kasner S. Suitability of temporal bone acoustic window: conventional TCD versus transcranial color-coded duplex sonography. J Neuroimaging. 2007;17:311–314

Kunz A, Hahn G, Mucha D, Muller A, Barrett KM, von Kummer R, Gahn G. Echo-enhanced transcranial color-coded duplex sonography in the diagnosis of cerebrovascular events: a validation study. Am J Neuroradiol. 2006;27:2122–2127.

Jansen O, Von Kummer R, Forsting M, Hacke W, Sartor K. Thrombolytic therapy in acute occlusion of the intracranial internal carotid artery bifurcation. AJNR Am J Neuroradiol 1995;16:1977–1986

Iannuzzi A, Wilcosky T, Mercuri M, Rubba P, Bryan FA, Bond MG. Ultrasonographic correlates of carotid atherosclerosis in transient ischemic attack and stroke. Stroke 1995; 26: 614–619

IMS Study Investigators. Combined intravenous and intra-arterial recanalization for acute ischemic stroke: the Interventional Management of Stroke Study. Stroke 2004; 35: 904 -911

Labiche LA, Malkoff M, Alexandrov AV. Residual flow signals predict complete recanalization in stroke patients treated with TPA. J Neuroimaging 2003; 13: 28 -33

Lee DH, Gao FQ, Rankin RN, Pelz DM, Fox AJ. Duplex and color Doppler flow sonography of occlusion and near occlusion of the carotid artery. Am J Neuroradiol 1996; 17: 1267–1274

Lee KY, Kim DI, Kim SH et bal. Sequential combination of intravenous recombinant tissue plasminogen activator and intra-arterial urokinase in acute ischemic stroke. Am J Neuroradiol 2004;25:1470–1475

Lewandowski C, Frankel M, Tomsick T, et al. for the EMS Bridging Trial investigators. Combined intravenous and intra-arterial rtPA vs intra-arterial therapy of acute ischemic stroke: Emergency Management of Stroke [EMS] Bridging Trial. Stroke 1999; 30:2598–2605

Linfante I, Llinas RH, Selim M, et al. Clinical and vascular outcome in internal carotid artery vs middle cerebral artery occlusions after intravenous tissue plasminogen activator. Stroke 2002; 33:2066–2071

Maeda H, Etani H, Handa N, Tagaya M, Oku N, Kim BH, Naka M, Kinoshita N, Nukada T, Fukunaga R. A validation study on the reproducibility of transcranial Doppler velocimetry. Ultrasound Med Biol. 1990;16:9 -14.

Malferrari G, Bertolino C, Casoni F, Zini A, Sarra VM, Sanguigni S, Pratesi M, Lochner P, Coppo L, Brusa G, Guidetti D, Cavuto S, Marcello N. The ELIGIBLE study: ultrasound assessment in acute ischemic stroke within 3 hours. Cerebrovasc Dis. 2007;24:469–476.

Malferrari G, Zedde M, Marcello N, Role of Ultrasound Vascular Imaging in the Acute Phase of Stroke, Vascular Disease Prevention, Vol. 5, No. 4. (November 2008), pp. 252-269

Malferrari (Editor), Neurosonological examination in acute stroke patients. A pocket guide. Grandi ed. 2010

Manu S. Goyal and Colin P. Derdeyn, The diagnosis and management of supraaortic arterial dissections, Current Opinion in Neurology 2009, 22:80–89

Mead GE, Wardlaw JM, Dennis MS, et al. Relationship between pattern of intracranial artery abnormalities on transcranial Doppler and Oxfordshire community stroke project clinical classification of ischemic stroke. Stroke 2000; 31: 714-719

Meyer-Wiethe K, Cangür H, Schindler A, Koch C, Seidel G. Ultrasound perfusion imaging: determination of thresholds for the identification of critically disturbed perfusion in acute ischemic stroke: a pilot study. Ultrasound in Med. & Biol 2007; 33: 851–856

Molina CA, Alvarez-Sabín J, Montaner J, et al. Thrombolysis-Related Hemorrhagic Infarction A Marker of Early Reperfusion, Reduced Infarct Size, and Improved Outcome in Patients With Proximal Middle Cerebral Artery Occlusion. Stroke 2002; 33:1551-1556

Molina CA, Alexandrov AV, Demchuk AM, Saqqur M, Uchino K, Alvarez-Sabın J. Improving the predictive accuracy of recanalization on stroke outcome in patients treated with tissue plasminogen activator. Stroke 2004; 35: 151–156

Molina CA. et al. ,Differential pattern of tissue plasminogen activator induced middle cerebral artery recanalization among stroke subtypes. Stroke 2004; 35: 486-490 (b)

Molina CA, Ribo M, Rubiera M, Montaner J, Santamarina E, Delgado-Mederos R, Arenillas JF, Huertas R, Purroy F, Delgado P, Alvarez-Sabin J. Microbubble administration accelerates clot lysis during continuous 2-MHz ultrasound monitoring in stroke patients treated with intravenous tissue plasminogen activator. Stroke. 2006;37:425–429

Molina CA, Barreto AD, Tsivgoulis G, Sierzenski P, Malkoff MD, Rubiera M, Gonzales N, Mikulik R, Pate G, Ostrem J, Singleton W, Manvelian G, Unger EC, Grotta JC, Schellinger PD, Alexandrov AV, Transcranial ultrasound in clinical sonothrombolysis (TUCSON) trial. Ann Neurol. 2009;66:28 -38

Nabavi DG, Droste DW, Kemeny V, Schulte-Altedorneburg G, Weber S, Ringelstein EB. Potential and limitations of echocontrast-enhanced ultrasonography in acute stroke patients: a pilot study. Stroke. 1998;29:949–954

NASCET Collaborators. Beneficial effect of carotid endarterectomy in symptomatic patients with high-grade carotid stenosis. N Engl J Med. 1991;325:445-453

Nedelmann M, Stolz E, Gerriets T, Baumgartner RW, Malferrari G, Seidel G, Kaps M, for the TCCS Consensus Group, Consensus Recommendations for Transcranial Color-Coded Duplex Sonography for the Assessment of Intracranial Arteries in Clinical Trials on Acute Stroke, Stroke. 2009;40:3238-3244

Nedeltchev K, Bickel S, Arnold M, Sarikaya H, Georgiadis D, Sturzenegger M, Mattle HP, Baumgartner RW, Recanalization of Spontaneous Carotid Artery Dissection, Stroke. 2009;40:499-504

NINDS (National Institute of Neurological Disorders and Stroke) rt-PA Stroke Study Group. Tissue plasminogen activator for acute ischemic stroke. N Engl J Med 1995; 333: 1581–1587

Ogata T, Kimura K, Nakajima M, Naritomi H, Minematsu K. Diagnosis of middle cerebral artery occlusive lesions with contrast-enhanced transcranial color-coded real-time sonography in acute stroke. Neuroradiology. 2005;47:256 -262

Ois A, Cuadrado-Godia E, Jimenez-Conde J, et al. Early Arterial Study in the Prediction of Mortality After Acute Ischemic Stroke. Stroke 2007; 38: 2085-2089

Postert T, Braun B, Meves S, Koster O, Przuntek H, Weber S, Buttner T. Contrast-enhanced transcranial color-coded sonography in acute hemispheric brain infarction. Stroke. 1999;30:1819 –1826.

Razumovsky AY, Gilliard JH, Bryan RN, Hanley DF, Oppenheimer SM. TCD, MRA, MRI in acute cerebral ischemia. Acta Neurol Scand 1999; 99: 65–76

Ribo M, Molina CA, Rovira A, et al. Safety and Efficacy of Intravenous Tissue Plasminogen Activator Stroke Treatment in the 3- to 6-Hour Window Using Multimodal Transcranial Doppler/MRI Selection Protocol. Stroke 2005; 36: 602-606

Ribo M, Alvarez-Sabın J, Montaner J, et al. Temporal Profile of Recanalization After Intravenous Tissue Plasminogen Activator Selecting Patients for Rescue Reperfusion Techniques. Stroke 2006;37: 1000-1004

Ringelstein EB, Biniek R, Weiller C, Ammeling B, Nolte PN, Thron A. Type and extent of hemispheric brain infarctions and clinical outcome in early and delayed middle cerebral artery recanalization. Neurology 1992; 42: 289-298

Rubiera M, Ribo M, Delgado-Mederos R, et al. Tandem Internal Carotid Artery/Middle Cerebral Artery Occlusion An Independent Predictor of Poor Outcome After Systemic Thrombolysis. Stroke 2006; 37: 2301-2305.

Saqqur M, Shuaib A, Alexandrov AV, Hill MD, Calleja S, Tomsick T, Broderick J, Demchuk AM., Derivation of transcranial Doppler criteria for rescue intra-arterial thrombolysis: multicenter experience from the Interventional Management of Stroke study. Stroke. 2005;36:865-8.

Saqqur M, Uchino K, Demchuk AM, et al. for CLOTBUST Investigators. Site of Arterial Occlusion Identified by Transcranial Doppler Predicts the Response to Intravenous Thrombolysis for Stroke. Stroke 2007; 38: 948-954

Saqqur M, Tsivgoulis G, Molina CA, Demchuk AM, Shuaib A, Alexandrov AV. Residual flow at the site of intracranial occlusion on transcranial Doppler predicts response to intravenous thrombolysis: a multicenter study. Cerebrovasc Dis. 2008;27:5–12

Sekoranja L, Loulidi J, Yilmaz H, et al. Intravenous vs Combined (Intravenous and Intra-Arterial) Thrombolysis in Acute Ischemic Stroke A Transcranial Color-Coded Duplex Sonography–Guided Pilot Study. Stroke 2006; 37: 1805-1809

Seidel G, Kaps M, Gerriets T. Potential and limitations of transcranial color-coded sonography in stroke patients. Stroke. 1995;26:2061–2066

Seidel G, Karsten Meyer W, Grit B, et al. Ultrasound Perfusion Imaging in Acute Middle Cerebral Artery Infarction Predicts Outcome. Stroke 2004; 35: 1107-1111

Seidel G, Cangür H, Albers T, Burgemeister A, Meyer-Wiethe K., Sonographic evaluation of hemorrhagic transformation and arterial recanalization in acute hemispheric ischemic stroke, Stroke. 2009 Jan;40:119-23

Sloan MA, Alexandrov AV, Tegeler CH, Spencer MP, Caplan LR, Feldmann E, Wechsler LR, Newell DW, Gomez CR, Babikian VL, Lefkowitz D, Goldman RS, Armon C, Hsu CY, Goodin DS. Assessment: transcranial Doppler ultrasonography: report of the Therapeutics and Technology Assessment Subcommittee of the American Academy of Neurology. Neurology 2004 May 11;62(9):1468-81.

Stolz E, Babacan SS, Bodeker RH, Gerriets T, Kaps M. Interobserver and intraobserver reliability of venous transcranial color-coded flow velocity measurements. J Neuroimaging. 2001;11:385–392

Thanvi B and Robinson T, Complete occlusion of extracranial internal carotid artery: clinical features, pathophysiology, diagnosis and management, Postgrad. Med. J., February 1, 2007; 83: 95 - 99

Thomassen L, Waje-Andreassen U, Naess H, Aarseth J, RussellD. Doppler ultrasound and clinical findings in patients with acute ischemic stroke treated with intravenous thrombolysis. European Journal of Neurology 2005; 12: 462–465

Tomsick T, TIMI, TIBI, TICI: I Came, I Saw, I Got Confused, American Journal of Neuroradiology 28:382-384, February 2007

Trouillas P, Nighoghossian N, Derex L, et al. Thrombolysis with intravenous rtPA in a series of 100 cases of acute ischemic carotid territory stroke: determination of etiological, topographic and radiological outcome factors. Stroke 1998; 29: 2529-2540

Tsivgoulis G, Eggers J, Ribo M, Perren F, Saqqur M, Rubiera M, Sergentanis TN, Vadikolias K, Larrue V, Molina CA, Alexandrov AV, Safety and Efficacy of Ultrasound-Enhanced Thrombolysis. A Comprehensive Review and Meta-Analysis of Randomized and Nonrandomized Studies. Stroke. 2010;41:280-287

U-King-Im JM, Graves MJ, Cross JJ, Higgins NJ, Wat J, Trivedi RA, Tang T, Howarth SPS, Kirkpatrick PJ, Antoun NM, Gillard JH, Internal Carotid Artery Stenosis: Accuracy of Subjective Visual Impression for Evaluation with Digital Subtraction Angiography and Contrast-enhanced MR Angiography; Radiology 2007; 244:213–222

Valaikiene J, Schuierer G, Ziemus B, Dietrich J, Bogdahn U, Schlachetzki F. Transcranial color-coded duplex sonography for detection of distal internal carotid artery stenosis. Am J Neuroradiol. 2008;29:347–353.

von Kummer R, Holle R, Rosin L, Forsting M, Hacke W. Does arterial recanalization improve outcome in carotid territory stroke? Stroke 1995;26:581–587

Wardlaw JM, Chappell FM, Best JJK, Wartolowska K, Berry E, on behalf of the NHS Research and Development Health Technology Assessment Carotid Stenosis Imaging Group, Non-invasive imaging compared with intra-arterial angiography in the diagnosis of symptomatic carotid stenosis: a meta-analysis, Lancet 2006; 367: 1503–12

Wardlaw JM, Carotid imaging for secondary stroke prevention in routine practice, International Journal of Stroke Vol 3, February 2008, 20–32

Wiesmann M, Meyer-Wiethe K, Albers T, Seidel G. Parametric Perfusion Imaging with Contrast-Enhanced Ultrasound in Acute Stroke. Stroke 2004; 35: 508-513

Wong KS, Li H. Long-term mortality and recurrent stroke risk among Chinese stroke patients with predominant intracranial atherosclerosis. Stroke. 2003;34:2361–2366.

Zaidat OO, Suarez JI, Santillan C, et al. Response to intra-arterial and combined intravenous and intra-arterial thrombolytic therapy in patients with distal internal carotid artery occlusion. Stroke 2002; 33: 1821–1826

Zanette EM, Fieschi C, Bozzao L, Roberti C, Toni D, Argentino C, Lenzi GL. Comparison of cerebral angiography and transcranial Doppler sonography in acute stroke. Stroke. 1989;20:899 -903

Zipper SG, Stolz E. Clinical application of transcranial colour-coded duplex sonography-a review. Eur J Neurol. 2002;9:1– 8

Zunker P, Wilms H, Brossmann J, Georgiadis D, Weber S, Deuschl G. Echo contrast-enhanced transcranial ultrasound: frequency of use, diagnostic benefit, and validity of results compared with MRA. Stroke. 2002; 33:2600 –2603.

# 15

# Is There a Place for Clinical Neurophysiology Assessments in Synucleinopathies?

M. Onofrj, L. Bonanni, A. Thomas, L. Ricciardi, F. Ciccocioppo,
D. Monaco V. Onofrj and F. Anzellotti
*University G.d'Annunzio of Chieti-Pescara*
*Italy*

## 1. Introduction

Parkinson Disease (PD), Dementia with Lewy Bodies (DLB) and Multiple System Atrophy (MSA) are characterized by deposition of Lewy Bodies (LB), consisting of eosinophilic intracellular (intraneural in PD and DLB and intraglial in MSA) inclusions of α-synuclein and allowing the three disorders to be categorized as synucleinopathies. The identification in the last two decades of specific clinical features of synucleinopathies has been a major breakthrough in Neurology, as it prompted a reconsideration of diagnostic and therapeutic approaches to dementia and parkinsonism. The recognition of synuclein and ubiquitin markers in dementia resulted in the reclassification of patients previously considered as affected by Alzheimer Disease (AD) and Vascular Dementia (VaD), and there is now agreement that DLB is the second most common cause of dementia in elderly population: its prevalence is reported to be in the 25-43% range in different studies.

DLB is clinically characterized by the presence of prominently dysexecutive dementia (frontal lobe or subcortical dementia according to earlier classification [1]), cognitive fluctuations, consisting of remitting-relapsing episodes of blunted conscience reaching levels of stupor, by the occurrence of visual hallucinations and delusions, by parkinsonian motor signs and hypersensitivity to neuroleptic treatment, ranging from worsening of parkinsonism to the possible lethal neuroleptic-malignant syndromes [2]. Yet, variances of presentation and overlapping symptoms with AD and Fronto-Temporal lobe Degeneration (FTD), could be misleading in the process of addressing a clinical diagnosis with consequent therapeutic risks(e.g. introducing neuroleptic treatments in patient with DLB), or economic costs (e.g. addressing patients with DLB to treatment protocols dedicated to AD patients, based on vaccines or antibodies against β amyloid proteins, a neuropathological feature of AD).

It is evident the stringent need for improvement of reliable diagnostic tools (u.e. biomarkers) to differentiate the diseases associated with dementia. In 2010 the National Institute of Health, NIH, held a symposium focused on the development of possible biomarkers for DLB. Among the different suggested biomarkers, neurophysiological assessments were reconsidered, as a large amount of neurophysiological studies had been devoted to AD and PD, whose characteristics are shared by DLB.

We contributed to several studies on this argument along the years, and in the present chapter we discuss the role of clinical neurophysiological studies in DLB in comparison with other disorders. The essential background of our original studies laid in the fact that most historical studies were performed when the DLB clinical entity was unknown and therefore some of the past results were marred by absent recognition of this clinical entity.

## 2. Synucleinopathies: Dementia with lewy bodies

Synucleinopathies comprise a diverse groups of neurodegenerative proteinopathies that share common pathological lesions composed of aggregates of conformational and posttranslational modifications of alpha-synuclein in selected populations of neurons and glia. Abnormal filamentous aggregates of misfolded alpha-synuclein protein are the major components of LB, dystrophic (Lewy) neurites and the Papp–Lantos filaments in oligodendroglia and neurons linked to degeneration of affected brain regions. The synucleinopathies (see table 1) include Lewy Body disease (Parkinson Disease (PD), DLB, Multiple System Atrophy (MSA)) and neurodegeneration with brain iron accumulation type I, (NBIIA), formerly Hallervorden–Spatz disease. The pathological diagnosis of Lewy body disease is established by validated consensus criteria based on semi-quantitative assessment of subcortical and cortical LB as their common hallmarks. They are accompanied by subcortical multisystem degeneration with neuronal loss and gliosis with or without AD pathologic features. LB deposition also occur in numerous other disorders, including pure autonomic failure, neuroaxonal dystrophies and their presence is also evident in various amyloidoses and tauopathies. MSA, a sporadic, adult-onset degenerative movement disorder of unknown cause, is characterized by alpha-synuclein–positive glial cytoplasmic and rare neuronal inclusions throughout the central nervous system associated with striato-nigral degeneration, olivopontocerebellar atrophy and involvement of medullar and spinal autonomic nuclei. In NBIIA alpha-synuclein is present in axonal spheroids and glial and neuronal inclusions. While the identity of the major components of LB suggests that a pathway leading from normal soluble to abnormal misfolded filamentous proteins is central for their pathogenesis, regardless of the primary disorder, there are conformational differences in alpha-synuclein between neuronal and glial aggregates, showing no uniform mapping for its epitopes. Despite several cellular and transgenic models, it is not clear whether inclusion body formation is an adaptive/neuroprotective or a pathogenic reaction process generated in response to different, mostly undetermined, functional triggers linked to neurodegeneration. From a clinicopathological point of view, recognizable differences appear along the spectrum of the synucleinopathies. In fact PD is characterized by subcortical and rare cortical LB associated with degeneration of the dopaminergic nigrostriatal and other subcortical systems while more extensively distributed LB accompanied by striatonigral degeneration and variable extents of AD pathologic states typify DLB which, depending on the severity and extent of neuritic AD pathologic conditions, can be divided into two subgroups: "pure" DLB and DLB variant of AD. Finally, LB may also occur in AD, which is defined by the presence of neocortical neuritic pathologic findings (β amyloid plaques and neurofibrillary tangles). Among the synucleinophaties DLB represents the second most frequent cause of dementia in the elderly after AD [3].

| SYNUCLEINOPHATIES | LESION/COMPONENTS | LOCATION |
|---|---|---|
| PARKINSON'S DISEASE | LB/DYSTROPHIC NEURITIS | INTRACYTOPLASMIC |
| LEWY BODY DEMENTIA | LB/DYSTROPHIC NEURITIS | INTRACYTOPLASMIC |
| LEWY BODY VARIANT OF ALZHEIMER DISEASE | LB/DYSTROPHIC NEURITIS<br>Aβ-PLAQUES<br>TANGLES PHF/TAU | INTRACYTOPLASMIC<br>EXTRACELLULAR<br>INTRACELLULAR |
| PURE AUTONOMIC FAILURE | LB | INTRACYTOPLASMIC |
| ALZHEIMER'S DISEASE | PLAQUES (Aβ AMYLOID)<br>TANGLES PHF/TAU<br>LB/α-SYNUCLEIN | EXTRACELLULAR/ INTRACYTOPLASMIC |
| MULTIPLE SYSTEM ATROPHY | CYTOPLASMATIC GLIAL INCLUSION | INTRACYTOPLASMIC |
| HALLERVORDEN-SPATZ DISEASE | LB/CYTOPLASMATIC GLIAL INCLUSION | INTRACYTOPLASMIC |
| NEUROAXONAL DYSTROPHY | AXONAL SPHEROIDS | |
| AMYOTROPHIC LATERAL SCLEROSIS | UBIQUITIN, INCLUSION SOD 1, LB | INTRANUCLEAR, INTRACYTOPLASMIC |
| OTHER:<br>DOWN SYNDROME<br>MOTOR NEURON DISEASE | | INTRACYTOPLASMIC |

Table 1. Sinucleinophaties and LB location.

The central clinical feature of DLB is progressive dementia prominently characterized, in the early phases of the disease, by deficits in attention, executive function and visuospatial ability, at difference with AD where memory impairment is the main early feature of dementia. Fluctuations in attention and alertness, recurrent complex visual hallucinations and parkinsonism represent the core features for the diagnosis. Suggestive clinical features are REM sleep behavior disorder, severe sensitivity to neuroleptics and low dopamine transporter uptake in the basal ganglia demonstrated by single photon emission computerized tomography (SPECT) or Positron Emission Tomography (PET) imaging. Supportive features are often present and are represented by repeated falls and syncopes, transient and unexplained loss of consciousness, severe autonomic dysfunction (e.g., orthostatic hypotension, urinary incontinence), hallucinations in other modalities than visual, systematized delusions, depression, relative preservation of medial temporal lobe structures on CT or MRI scans, generalized low uptake on SPECT/PET perfusion scans with low occipital activity, abnormally low uptake on $^{123}$I-metaiodobenzilguanidine ($^{123}$I-MIBG) myocardial scintigraphy [2].

In this last revision of criteria for the diagnosis of DLB, electroencephalography (EEG) abnormalities with transient slow waves or sharp waves were also reported as supportive features for the diagnosis[2,4].

We performed a prospective study evaluating the incidence and characteristics of EEG abnormalities in patients affected by AD, DLB and PD with Dementia at their first presentation in a tertiary clinic, not later than 1 year from the onset of dementia [5]. Supportive elements for the diagnosis came from Clinical Assessment of Fluctuations (CAF) scale, polysomnography (PSG) and Mayo Sleep Questionnaire for the assessment of REM sleep Behaviour Disorder (RBD). CAF is a neuropsychological test [6] able to evidence, on the basis of patient and caregivers interviews, the presence of fluctuating consciousness. The questionnaires are able to discriminate 85% of DLB patients, as confirmed by autopsy [7]. Cognitive fluctuations are considered a clinical feature typical of DLB, described in 70-80% of these patients, only in 14-20% of AD patients and in 15-30% of VaD subjects [8].

## 3. Visual Evoked Potentials (VEPs)

PD and parkinsonism are associated with a variety of visual signs and symptoms summarized in table 2.

| OCULAR ASPECT | CHANGE IN PD | REFERENCES |
|---|---|---|
| **PRIMARY FUNCTION**<br>VISUAL ACUITY<br>VISUAL FIELD<br>COLOR VISION | POOR, ESPECIALLY AT LOW CONTRAST<br>INCREASE IN GLAUCOMATOSE VISUAL FIELD DEFECTS<br>VISION BLURRED FOR COLOURED STIMULI/PROGRESSIVE DETERIORATION | Repka et al., 1996<br>Bayer et al., 2002<br>Price at al., 1992/<br>Diederich et al., 2002 |
| **EYE MOVEMENTS**<br>SACCADIC GAZE<br>SACCADIC EYE MOVEMENT<br>SMOOTH PURSUIT<br>OPTOKINETIC NYSTAGMUS | SLOWER THAN NORMAL<br>HYPOMETRIA<br>AFFECTED EARLY IN DISEASE PROCESS<br>ABNORMAL IN SOME PATIENTS | Shibasaki et al., 1999<br>Crawford et al., 1989<br>Bares et al., 2003<br>Shibasaki et al., 1999 |
| **BLINK REFLEX**<br>FREQUENCY<br>HABITUATION | REDUCED<br>NOT OBSERVED | Garland et al., 1952<br>Garland et al., 1952 |
| PUPIL REACTIVITY<br>CONTRACTION AMPLITUDE<br>LIGHT REFLEX | REDUCED<br>LONGER LATENCY | Biousse et al., 2004<br>Miceli et al., 1991 |
| **VEP**<br>FLASH ERG<br>PATTERN ERG<br>CORTICAL VEP<br>CHROMATIC VEP | REDUCED AMPLITUDE OF b WAVE with PHOTIC E SCOTOPIC STIMULI<br>REDUCED AMPLITUDE, DELAYED P50<br>DELAYED P100, CHANGING TO NORMAL WITH L-DOPA<br>INCREASED LATENCY AND REDUCED AMPLITUDE | Gottlob et al., 1987<br>Gottlob et al., 1987<br>Bodis-Wallner et al., 1982<br>Sartucci et al., 2006 |
| **COMPLEX VISUAL FUNCTION**<br>VISUO-SPATIAL ORIENTATION<br>VISUAL HALLUCINATIONS | SEVERE IMPAIRMENT<br>IMPAIRED<br>CHRONIC IN 30-60% TREATED CASES | Davidsdottir et al., 2005<br>Trick et al., 1994<br>Diederich et al., 2005 |

Table 2. Abnormal visual symptoms in PD

Recent epidemiological studies have shown an association between visual impairments and visual hallucinations in patients with PD [9]. Neuropsychological studies have revealed visuoperceptual impairments in PDD and DLB patients with visual hallucinations [10]. Additionally, recent radiological studies have demonstrated decreased blood flow in the posterior temporal and occipital regions in hallucinatory PD and DLB patients [11]. Taking these findings together, it is possible to speculate that visual information processing functions are selectively impaired in DLB and PDD.

Impairment of achromatic as well as chromatic vision in PD has been extensively proven using clinical, psychophysiological and electrophysiological methods (ERGs and VEPs) and attributed to dopaminergic deficiency at the retina level.

Some studies demonstrated a significant difference between PD patients and well matched control subjects in the amplitude of VEP, of flash (ERG) and pattern electroretinogram (PERG: retinal response evoked by viewing an alternating checkerboard or grating) [12]. The VEP, PERG and flash ERG originate from different parts of the retina and central nervous system and reflect different physiological processes. The changes in these potentials in PD may reflect the widespread nature of the biochemical disorder affecting both retina and central nervous system. Indeed PD patients have also been shown to have abnormal auditory evoked potentials [13]. Abnormal VEPs were described in patients with PD: the percentage of VEP delays and the amount of latency increments detected in PD patients are dependent on the spatial frequency (that is a parameter of the stimulating pattern). The VEP latency increases as a function of increasing spatial frequency [14] in normal subjects, and our results [15] show that this latency increase is enhanced in PD and also when dopamine blockers are administered. Delayed responses, consisting of increased latencies of the P100 component evoked by patterned stimuli of degree to 7.5′ elements (spatial frequency of 0.5 to 4 cycles per degree) were observed in PD patients and the delays disappeared together with clinical symptoms when L-Dopa was administered [15,16,17]. The evidence of VEP delays in PD were concomitant with the identification of dopaminergic cells (amacrine and horizontal cells) in the retina, both evidences reciprocally supporting the idea that the cause of delays was dependent on retinal dopamine cell deficiencies. In these studies retinal and occipital visual evoked potentials and event-related potentials (P300) have been recorded in normal human subjects before and after the administration of the dopaminergic receptor antagonist, haloperidol, and/or the dopaminergic precursor L-DOPA. The data show that either retinal or occipital visual potentials and P300 are delayed by haloperidol. These findings are consistent with the hypothesis that haloperidol in healthy subjects mimics the electrophysiological abnormalities observed in PD. On the other hand, L-Dopa does not generally modify these latencies in controls, while it is known to decrease the same parameters in PD patients. This is in accord with the involvement of a specific mechanism in the recovery observed in PD patients during L-Dopa therapy. Data confirm that the alterations of visual and cognitive potentials observed in PD are closely related to the impairment of dopaminergic transmission. The results of our study [15] on haloperidol administration in non-PD patients showed that this dopamine receptor blocking drug increased the latency of VEPs obtained with 2 and 4 cpd stimuli, while the effect on 0.5 cpd and 1 cpd VEPs was less consistent. This finding supports the hypothesis that dopamine modifies the processing of VEPs by acting at the synaptic level. The specific sensitivity of VEP changes to the spatial frequency of stimulation in PD and haloperidol treated subjects, which is evident in our results, might suggest that the VEP abnormalities found in our study are dependent on the impairment of dopaminergic neural structures which regulate spatial frequency sensitivity. VEP findings were robustly confirmed in studies performed in animal models of PD [18, 19]. Despite the interest for the finding, only few confirmative studies were provided [15-17], most studies come from few laboratories devoted to this experimental approach. Guidelines for the use of VEPs in clinical practice only rarely suggested a role of VEPs in PD studies and VEPs were finally confined to the assessment of Multiple Sclerosis. Although the increased latency of the VEP in multiple sclerosis has in general been attributed to demyelination in the visual pathways, other mechanisms such as humoral factors, synaptic malfunction or changes in dendritic potentials may play a part. Such mechanisms may also be relevant to central nervous system disorders other than multiple sclerosis which have abnormal VEPs. Although the major clinical manifestations of PD involve the motor systems and the responsible pathology is located in the basal ganglia, there is evidence of more widespread disease, both pathologically, electrophysiologically and clinically. Only two studies explored the possible use of VEPs for the assessment of DLB [20,21] yet no comparison were presented with other forms of dementia. In MSA the visual system is believed to be spared and dopamine deficiency has been hypothesized to be less pronounced than in PD [22], even though the data in the literature are scarce and not unanimous and nothing on retinal dopamine content has been reported. Little information is available on VEPs and PERGs in MSA patients [22]. The main interest for studying responses elicited by patterns with pure chromatic contrast is that they allow recording of specific responses from colour-opponent pathways, anatomically and physiologically distinct from the achromatic ones at the retinal as well as the geniculate and cortical levels. A more recent study [23] showed that PERGs are virtually unaffected in MSA, whereas in early PD they are clearly impaired, suggesting different pathogenic retinal mechanisms and a useful simple tool for distinguishing MSA from PD. The strongest objection against the use of VEPs for the assessment of synucleinopathies derived from the technical constraints of VEP recordings: VEPs are altered by abnormalities of optic nerve and visual pathways, VEPs recordings require the adequate collaboration of patients who must focus attention on stimuli [24-26], VEP variable (amplitude, latency) are dependent on laboratories settings and must be adjusted according to each laboratory statistics of distribution.

The characteristic of VEP cannot be simply shared by different laboratories and differences in equipments might sustain variability which are far wider than variability observed in patient and control populations.

With the introduction of digital and led stimulating screen this condition worsened rather than improving [27].

In the age range of AD, DLB and PDD optic and visual abnormalities (cataracts, maculopathies, retinopathies, ischemic lesions) are frequent and might mislead possible diagnoses. In DLB, fluctuations of cognition (i.e. defective attention and collaboration to the task) are common and might impair the diagnostic yield of VEP recordings. It has been suggested that the discrepancies between different reports on VEP in Parkinson's disease may be due to the greater sensitivity of grating patterns compared to checkerboard patterns and, if so, this might in part account for our normal PD VEP latencies. The grating subtense used is about one third of that for the checkerboard, and the retinal field stimulated is predominantly foveal for the grating whereas for the checkerboard it extends beyond the perimacula. This could explain the observed differences rather than the pattern form, per se. We suggest that VEP recordings might still represent a "niche" research tool, but do not provide sufficient robustness in order to constitute a biomarker.

## 4. P 300 abnormalities

In an event related potential (ERP) the P300 is a positive deflection peaking at approximately 300 ms after a stimulus. It is supposed to be an endogenous response, mainly depending on the processing of stimulus context, involving registration, evaluation and memory of stimuli, and categorization (decision/closure) and impinging on attention and arousal [28]. P300 can reliably be elicited with relatively simple paradigms, such as the "oddball paradigm", which requires the detection of a rare ("target") stimulus within a train of frequent irrelevant "non target" stimuli. Other complex paradigms include the administration of multiple stimuli, dichotic stimuli, multisensory modalities, in order to evaluate responses evoked from anterior brain regions. We recently performed a P300 study on patients with DLB in comparisons with patients with AD matched for dementia severity and age and with age matched control subjects [29] to look for differences of P300 responses in the two dementia subtypes and for possible correlations between P300 recordings and EEG, as abnormal EEG variability was described in DLB [5].

P300 responses were recorded with Ag/AgCl electrodes from 19 derivations corresponding to Fp1, Fp2, F3, F4, C3, C4, P3, P4, O1, O2, F7, F8, T3, T4, T5, T6, Cz, Fz, Pz positions of the 10-20 International System with supplementary A1 and A2 derivations. Care was taken to avoid recordings if variations of body temperature, recent food ingestion, or previous-night sleep disturbances were present [30]. A classical auditory "oddball" paradigm was used. The stimuli were 500 Hz and 1000 Hz tones, designated as the "non-target" and "target" stimuli, respectively, and delivered by STIM System Headphones. Patients were instructed to count only "target" stimuli, aloud in a preliminary trial and mentally in subsequent trials. The presentation ratio of "non target/target" tones for training was 4/1-8/1 and during recording purposes 5/1. The intensity of the tone was 75 dBnHL, the duration of the stimulus was 150 ms (rise-fall and the plateau times 5 and 140 ms, respectively). The presentation rate was random with a minimum inter-stimulus interval of 1.1 seconds and a maximum interval of 4 seconds. Digital filters was set at 0.15 Hz and 100 Hz, and averaged with a dwell time of 0.5 ms, 2000 Hz sampling rate, 100 ms of pre-stimulus baseline recording. An artifact rejection system was calibrated on four supplementary derivations placed on eyebrows and inferior orbital ridges; the rejection system blocked the acquisition when eye movement exceeded 100 uV. As the mean reference is known to distort P300 distribution one earlobe was used as online reference, with offline averaging with the other earlobe [31].

In each recording session, the correspondence between the counted and delivered stimuli was checked as described in previous studies [32] and stored on the hard disk. Sets where two or more targets had not been recognized or sets impaired by attention defects or false recognitions were discarded from analysis.

In each patient and control 120 responses to non-target and target stimuli were averaged in a single Final Average (FA). Four Sub-Averages (SA) of only 30 responses to target stimuli were preliminarily obtained in order to assess reliability of P300 among the recording sessions. Finally, inter-subject Grand Averages (GA) were obtained in DLB, AD and control groups. N100, N200, and P200 were detected at the Fz, Cz and Pz electrode for each subject separately. Peak latencies of each component were measured from stimulus onset to the point of maximum voltage in the range of 50-150 ms and 150-250 ms respectively. P300 was identified, in a time window of 300-500 ms, according to the operating definition based on its scalp distribution (central-parietal amplitude gradient), probability and sequence of preceding components. For every electrode location the following P300 variables were analyzed: amplitude (voltage difference between pre-stimulus baseline and the largest positive-going peak of the ERP waveform within a latency range of 300-500 ms), latency (time from the stimulus onset to the point of maximum positive amplitude within 300-500 ms time window: latencies were considered delayed if the peak latency was at least 2SD longer than the controls mean value. 2SD was chosen because previous studies showed that more restrictive criteria, 3SD from the mean, are insensitive to detect differences between controls and patients populations [33]), inter-electrode (Fz-Cz; Fz-Pz; Cz-Pz) latency and amplitude distribution gradients (difference in latency or amplitude of P300 responses between each pair of leads). The use of 3SD in defining normative limits for P300 was discharged as being at risk of excluding an excessive number of patients from investigative categorization. Studies on P300 scalp distribution and topography showed that peak latency changes across the scalp i.e., it is shorter over anterior cortical regions and longer over parietal areas [34], which allows to identify an earlier anterior, and a late posterior P3 component. Whether anterior and posterior P3 components recorded with a simple oddball paradigm originate from the same generators as those proposed for the P3a and P3b components obtained with the three-stimuli "novel" paradigm is yet unclear, however studies evaluating P3 scalp distribution suggested that early P3 component and late P3 component have separate origins: anterior superior temporal gyrus [35], prefrontal cortex [36], and anterior cingulate or supplementary motor area [37] for the early component vs temporo-parietal junction for the late one [38]. P300 studies in dementia were originally based on recordings from midline scalp derivations (the three leads Fz, Cz, Pz). Recordings in patients with dementia were compared with normative data obtained through P300 measurements in age-matched control populations. In demented patients, comparisons between ranges of different widths evidenced that, for P300 latency, the 2SD criterion had the greatest sensitivity in the detection of dementia [39]. Thus, if recordings in patients exceeded the 95% odds ratio, corresponding to normal mean±2SD, these recordings were considered abnormal and related to the cognitive disorder. By inference, delayed P300 latencies (by 2SD) or reduced P300 amplitudes were considered features of dementia, and thus useful diagnostic tools [40]. Based on this method, several studies found delays or amplitude decreases of P300 recorded from posterior (Pz) derivations in patients with putative AD [41], subcortical dementia [42], metabolic disorders [43] e PDD [44]. Yet, dementia categorization in the last ten years has been revolutionized by the identification of DLB, representing from 25 to 43% of all dementia cases. Therefore, one can assume that a discrete percentage of patients classified as AD patients in earlier studies, were instead affected by DLB. Because of cognitive ERPs were less investigated in DLB than other types of dementia, we examined the rates and qualitative features of P300 abnormalities in DLB vs AD patients. As EEG abnormalities are prevalent and linked to variability in DLB, the possible identification of correlations with EEG frequencies might support or challenge recent hypotheses suggesting that P300 is, or is not, the result of EEG phase resetting, due to orientation of attention to stimuli [45]. As our P300 recordings were obtained from a multielectrode montage covering the scalp, we could extend our analysis to further measurements, including topographic distribution of P300. Earlier topographical studies on P300 distribution were focused on AD patients, yet the same possible diagnostic flaws underlined above could be reported for topographic studies, and results were in some cases inconclusive with abnormal distributions described in anterior or in posterior derivations

[34], in the, supposedly, same kind of patients. The "classic" evaluation method was however encouraged by methodological guidelines [30] even after that topographic studies had been developed. The numerous clinical P300 studies suggest that this ERP component, elicited by auditory, visual, olfactory or somatosensory stimuli may be clinically useful as an index of such cognitive functions as attention and working memory. This assumption suggests that specific alterations should be found in DLB, where the cognitive disturbance is mainly characterized by fluctuating alterations of arousal and vigilance. Due to frontal dysexecutive dysfunction, DLB patients would be expected to express prevalent alterations of the anterior P3 component with a fronto-central scalp topography, whereas AD patients, with their early hypometabolism in the temporo-parietal junction, would be expected to show prevalent alterations in the parietal P3b response. If we restrict P300 measurements to classic assessment of P300 latencies in posterior (parietal) derivations, our study [32] shows that delayed latency and reduced amplitude, present in both dementia groups, can distinguish DLB from AD group, even though it is not possible to infer the applicability of these measures to an individual patient-to-patient analysis. The use of an active task did not allow us to investigate possible differences between groups in the mismatch negativity response, but we made sure that patients kept constant their attention during recordings, as P300 amplitude is sensitive to the amount of attention resources engaged during the task. In every group, N200 latencies were correlated with P300 latencies, confirming previous studies that showed prolonged N200 and P300 latencies in patients with dementia [46]. Topographical analysis of P300 recordings including all scalp leads did not add information about possible differences between patient groups, confirming that study of P300 topography could be limited to midline electrodes. Topographical differences, as latency distribution gradient, emerged and showed that P300 is different in DLB as compared to AD (figure 1): DLB patients had a more delayed P300 in anterior than in posterior derivations, while in all but two AD patients the latency was increased in posterior leads as compared to anterior leads, same as in controls. The normal latency distribution gradient consisting of increased latency in posterior leads as compared to anterior leads was reversed in DLB. Also the amplitude distribution gradients were reversed and thus different in DLB patients compared to AD or controls. The amplitude of P300 was prominent in frontal leads in DLB and in parietal leads in AD and controls. The finding of reversed amplitude gradient, with higher amplitude in frontal leads and smaller amplitude in posterior leads in DLB patients is apparently counterintuitive, as reduced amplitudes would be expected in a disease characterized by early frontal lobe involvement. Yet, delayed P300 latencies are also prominent in anterior leads of DLB patients and the two findings together seem compatible with the early frontal involvement of DLB. These findings suggest abnormal activity in anterior cortical areas of DLB patients, as compared with AD and controls. The correlation between P300 frontal delay and neuropsychological test scores exploring frontal lobe functions (FAB, NPI) supports this hypothesis. A possible interpretation might suggest that, in the early course of their disease, DLB patients need to increase efforts in frontal areas involved in recognition-attention tasks. P300 amplitude increment with delayed latency is correlated to increments of encoding loads in experimental paradigms [47].

An alternative hypothesis could be that altered topographical P300 distribution in DLB represents a constant interference of the frontal P3a component, which is normally evoked by "novel" stimuli. According to this hypothesis DLB patients might produce frontal P300 component as the target stimuli will be interpreted as novel because DLB patients could not act and decide on these stimuli (i.e. match and encode in the target category). Further

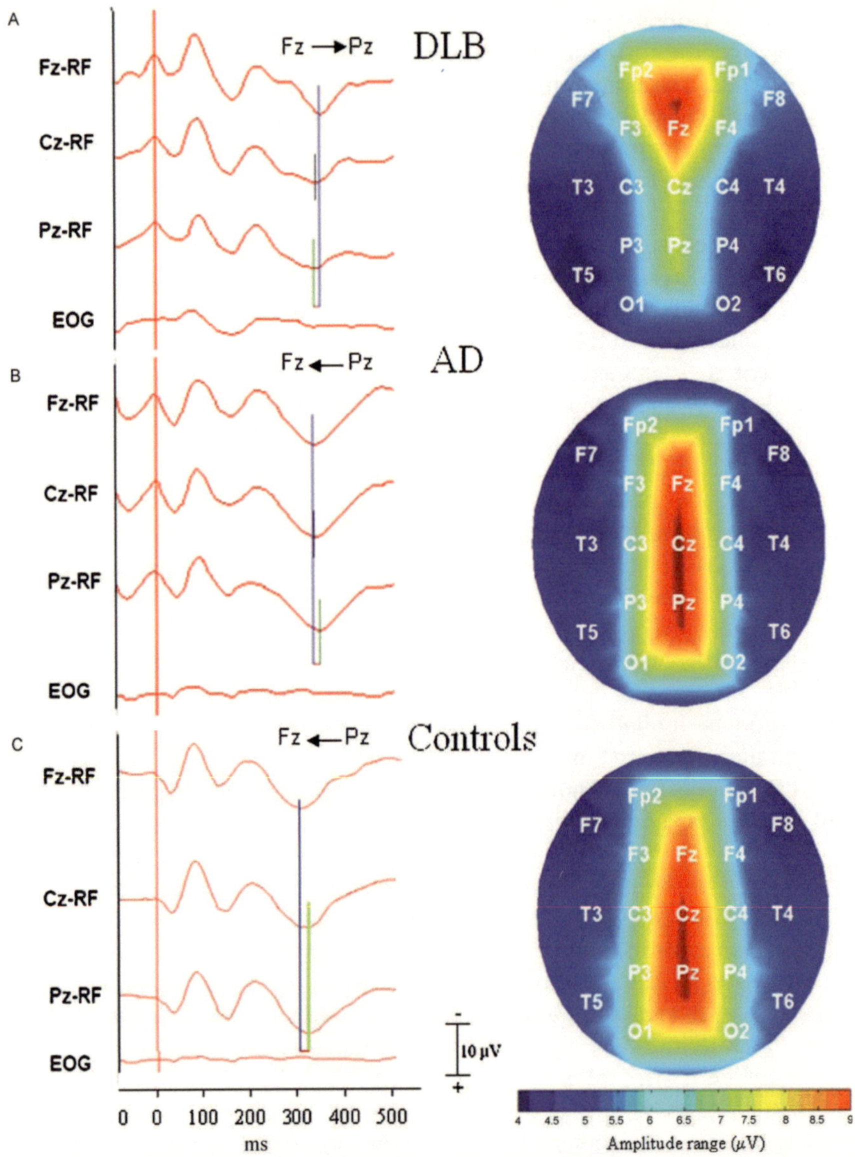


Fig. 1. Grand averages and amplitude maps of P300 response in the three groups of subjects. A. Left. Grand averages of P300 responses in the DLB group. Vertical lines mark peak latency. U-shaped bars mark the difference in latency between Fz and Pz leads, same or shorter latency in Pz. Right. Amplitude map of P300 distribution throughout the scalp (at the maximum amplitude recorded) in DLB group. Notice anterior-to-posterior (reversed) amplitude distribution gradient. B. Left. Grand Averages of P300 responses in AD group. Vertical lines mark peak latency. U-shaped bars mark the difference in latency between Fz and Pz leads, longer in Pz. Right. Amplitude map of P300 distribution throughout the scalp (at the maximum amplitude recorded) in the AD group. Notice a posterior to anterior amplitude distribution gradient. C. Traces and distribution in controls. EOG: electrooculogram; DLB: Dementia with Lewy Bodies; AD: Alzheimer's Disease.

studies, in which infrequent distractor stimuli, will be inserted into the sequence of target and non target stimuli, should be carried out in order to evaluate the P3a and P3b components in AD and DLB patients. Indeed novel stimuli produce P3a component that is generally largest over the anterior and central recording sites and reflects frontal lobe function. On the other hand temporo-parietal pathway contributes to P300 from the target stimuli (P3b). Anyhow, the clinical utility of P300 recordings in differentiating DLB from AD was evidenced, in the patient populations with reliable P300 response, by sensitivity reaching 70% and specificity of 97%. Due to high specificity, when a reliable P300 is recorded in a patient with early dementia, and its gradients of latency and of amplitude across the scalp are reversed, i.e. anterior-to-posterior instead of the normal posterior to anterior distribution, P300 might have value to address diagnosis of DLB. Conversely, finding that P300 responses, although delayed and with reduced amplitude compared to controls, reach maximum amplitude and longer latencies in posterior leads suggests that the diagnosis of DLB is unlikely. The study of correlations between P300 recordings and neuropsychological test scores showed that increased latency and reduced amplitude were correlated with test scores assessing the presence of frontal lobe dysfunction (FAB), behavior abnormalities (NPI), fluctuating cognition (CAF). Topographical redistribution of P300 latency and amplitude, evidenced as distributions gradients were correlated with the presence of fluctuating cognition (positive CAF scores), typical symptom of DLB patients (figure 2). These correlations evidenced that the differences between groups are related to dementia and not to neuropsychiatric differences. A correlation between the performance of frontal lobe function in standardized neuropsychological tests and maximal P300 scalp distributions were also found in a previous study on a group of old adults [48]. Specifically, subjects who showed frontal-maximal P3 had lower performance than those elderly subjects who showed posterior-maximal scalp topographies. P300 measurements were also correlated with EEG descriptors (figure 2): latency and amplitude anterior to posterior distribution gradients were correlated with the DFP pre-alpha and with abnormal CSA patterns (CSA Patterns 2 to 4, see next on the test), typical of DLB, confirming the specificity of topographical redistribution of P300 in DLB patients.

## 5. Blink reflex abnormalities

Patients with PD exhibit a reduced frequency of blinking leading to a staring appearance [49]. Reduced blink rate can cause an abnormal tear film, dry eyes and reduced vision. A characteristic ocular sign may be the blink reflex, elicited by a light tap on the glabella above the bridge of the nose: successive taps in normal individuals produce less and less response as the reflex habituates but in PD subjects the blink reflex does not disappear on repeated tapping. Habituation may improve after treatment with L-dopa or amantadine. Blink duration and excitability appear to be increased in PD and as in VEP latency may reflect loss of dopamine neurons [50]. The electric Blink Reflex (BR) is a neurophysiological technique exploring pontine structures through a reflex arc connecting nuclei of the 5th to the nuclei of the 7th cranial nerve. The Blink reflex consists of three separate responses: R1, R2, R3. The first one is generated in the trigemino-facial reflex arc, the second and third one are generated in polysynaptic pathways involving the brainstem reticular formation [51]. Clinically, the BR is used to evaluate brainstem lesions and it has been applied in clinical and neurophysiological studies of brainstem lesions and neurodegenerative disorders [52-54].

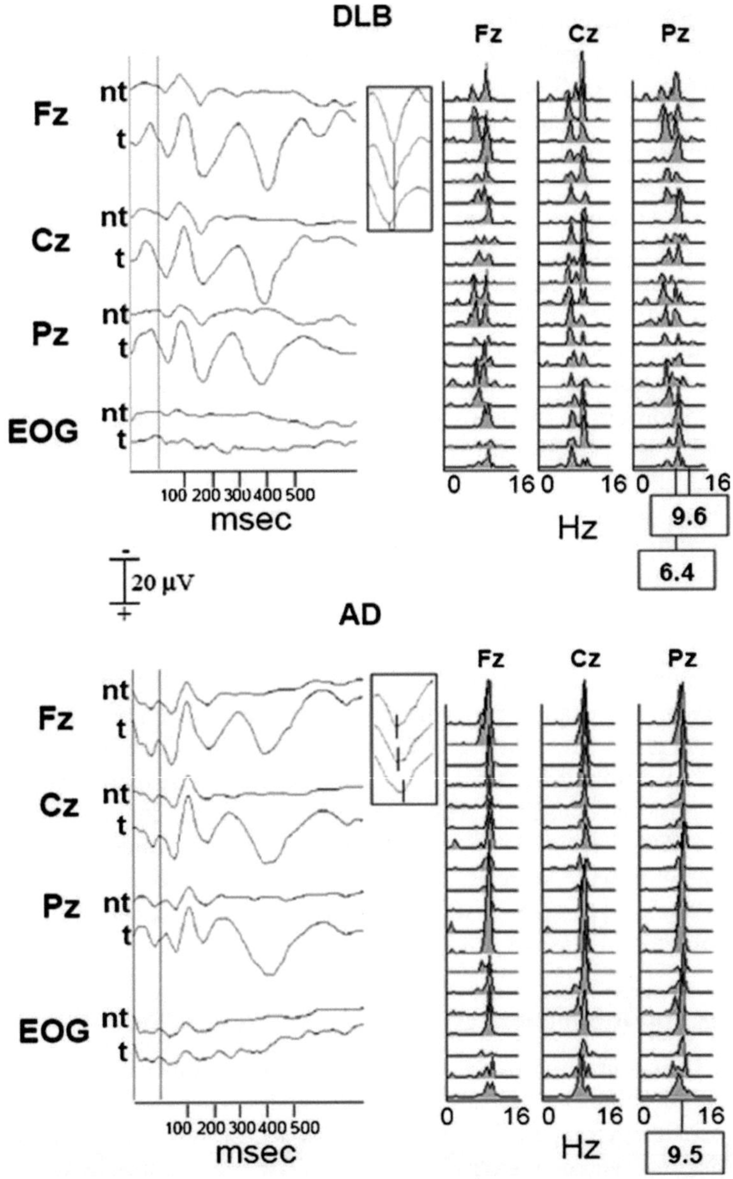


Fig. 2. Examples of P300 and CSA traces in one DLB and one AD patient. Top. Example of recordings in a DLB patient. Left. P300 recording. P300 response appears delayed (420 ms) with no latency inter-electrode distribution gradient and has a higher amplitude in frontal derivations (26.7 uV) compared to posterior derivations (21.0 uV) (inset, U-shaped bars mark the anterior-to-posterior (reversed) latency distribution gradient in the responses to target stimuli). Fz: frontal derivation, Cz: central derivation, Pz: posterior derivation, EOG: ocular derivation. Nt: non-target stimuli, t: target stimuli. Right. Quantitative EEG of the same patient represented as Compressed Spectral Array (CSA), i.e. arrays of traces are the representation of EEG power distribution in consecutive 2-second epochs. Peaks of power (amplitude) are found in variable frequencies shifting from alpha (9.6 Hz) to pre-alpha (6.4

Hz), corresponding to EEG CSA pattern 2 observed only in DLB patients [5]. Bottom. Example of neurophysiological recordings in an AD patient. Left. P300 recording. P300 response is delayed (410 ms) with posterior to anterior latency distribution gradient. Amplitude is higher in posterior derivations (14.9 uV) compared to anterior derivations (14.5 uV) (inset, I-shaped lines mark peak latencies in the responses to target stimuli). Fz-RF: frontal derivation, Cz-RF: central derivation, Pz-RF: posterior derivation, EOG: ocular derivation. Right. CSA of the same patient, with stable alpha dominant frequency at 9.5 Hz. EOG: electrooculogram; nt: non target stimuli, t: target stimuli; DLB: dementia with Lewy bodies; AD: Alzheimer's disease.

We performed a study of the blink reflex in patients with PD, DLB, MSA, AD and Progressive Supranuclear Palsy (PSP).
The subjects were comfortably sitting on an armchair in a quiet room, with eyes gently closed. The recordings took place in a temperature-controlled room (at about 25°C) in half-light. The cathode was placed over the supraorbital foramen and the anode 2cm rostrally. Surface electrodes were placed on the inferior part of the orbicularis oculi muscles on each side, recording ipsilateral R1, and ipsilateral and contralateral R2 and R3. Ground electrode was placed under the chin. Stimuli of 0,1ms of duration with intensity of 5-10 mA elicited stable R1 in repeated trials. Because surface electrodes lay only few centimetres away from the cathode, R1 tended to overlap the stimulus artifact, which could last more than 10ms. A special amplifier with a short blocking time (0.1ms) and low internal noise (0.5 uV at a bandwidth of 2kHz) minimized the problem of stimulus artifact. Signals were amplified and filtered (bandwidth 20-2000Hz), to avoid habituation the interstimuli intervals must be of at least 7 sec, 5-10 responses per site were elicited and stored. BR recording were previously described in MSA, PSP and PD patients: all reports showed R2 latencies inside the 2 SD of the mean and only evidenced enhancement or inhibition of R1-R2 in excitability-duration curve paradigms [52,53,55] in untreated PD. Recently we studied the BR in parkinsonism [56]: in all PD, MSA, PSP and AD patients we found normal R1 and R2 latencies inside the 2SD of the control mean independently of the presence of RBD. Only in DLB patients we found R2 latencies clustering in the upper limits of normality or definitely above the limits (figure 3). All findings were statistically significant. Thus, BR recordings might reveal brainstem dysfunction in DLB, but not in other parkinsonisms where different yet definite brainstem abnormalities are also described. According to the pathophysiological hypothesis [6] our data suggested that in DLB the brainstem is the site of initial lesions, consisting of α-synuclein deposits. Synucleinopathy is ascending from the brainstem, progressively involving the lower brainstem and inducing the appearance of REM Sleep Behaviour Disorder (RBD), then the mesencephalus, inducing the occurrence of parkinsonism and finally involving limbic structures, inducing hallucinations and psychosis, and cortical areas, inducing cognitive disorders. R2 latency delay might be attributed to the ascending synucleinopathy inducing the appearance of RBD, but our findings suggest that this possible correlation is controversial, as normal R2 latencies were observed in PD and MSA patients presenting with RBD, while delayed R2 latencies were recorded in 5 DLB patients who did not present with RBD. Our findings suggest instead that R2 latency delay in DLB is independent of the presence of RBD. The correlation with scores assessing cognitive fluctuations suggests that R2 abnormalities might evidence dysfunction of reticular brain stem pathways involved in vigilance regulation.

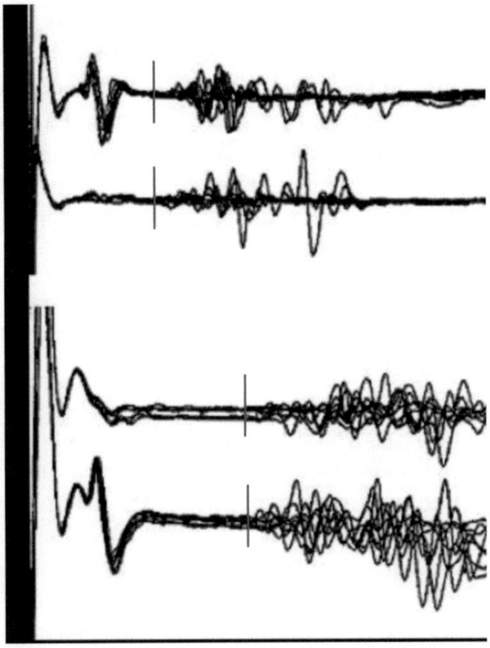

Fig. 3. Example of a blink response in a control subject (top: about 30msec) and in a patient with DLB (bottom: about 45msec). Note the delayed R2 response in the DLB patient in both the ipsilateral and contralateral recordings.

Current interpretations of BR neurophysiology [51,57] suggest that R2 abnormality should be ascribed to disruption of the afferent pathway when it is evident in ipsilateral and contralateral responses to stimuli of one side and efferent when the abnormality is observed in ipsilateral or contralateral responses of only one side, independently of the site of stimulation. Only in 3 of the DLB patients presenting with R2 delays, discrepant latencies on the two sides of stimulation were found [8], yet ipsilateral and contralateral responses were always overlapping, thus it is likely that the afferent pathway is prominently involved in DLB. In a successive study we tested the supposition that BR alterations present in DLB patients are sensitive to cholinergic modulation. It is known indeed, that choline acetyltransferase enzyme levels are lower in DLB compared with AD [58] whereas high muscarinic receptor density has been found in DLB [59]. Alterations of this cortical network are the pathophysiological correlate of cognitive impairment and attention deficit in DLB and are accompanied by abnormal electrocortical arousal [8,60] with alteration of electroencephalogram, event-related potential and choice reaction time. Administration of donepezil has been shown to significantly improve cognitive scores as well as electroencephalogram and event-related potential alterations in patients with fluctuating cognition [12] as a result of improvement of attentional participation in tested activities [60-63]. So we assessed whether BR alterations present in DLB patients are sensitive to cholinergic modulation [64]. We evaluated 26 patients affected by DLB and 20 patients affected by AD: for each patient, we performed BR recordings before and after 1 and 2 weeks of treatment with donepezil. The correlation between R2 abnormalities and score assessing cognitive fluctuations suggest that R2 latency delay might evidence dysfunctions of brain stem reticular pathways involved in vigilance regulation. The administration of donepezil significantly improved BR response in DLB patients, with a mean reduction of 8.2%. R2 mean latency reduction was highly correlated with R2 mean latency delay at baseline, with a 46% of patients showing no difference between R2 mean latency at baseline and after treatment. Thus, the reduction of R2 latency was evident only in patients who had delayed R2 at baseline. A possible explanation is a "bottom effect" of R2 mean latency reduction, meaning that the correction of brain stem dysfunction by ChEI treatment is mostly evident when the alteration of subcortical cholinergic networks is so conspicuous to be evidenced by a BR response alteration. Another possible explanation is that 2 subpopulation of DLB patients can be recognized: responders and not responders to ChEI treatment. No correlation between R2 latency reduction and MMSE scores was found, as expected because of the short test-retest interval and learning effect [65]. However, at baseline, a high correlation between R2 abnormalities and CAF and ODFA scores was found, suggesting that responders are those patients with the worst grade of cognitive fluctuations. In our study, CAF scores were not significantly modified by the 2-week treatment, again as expected, because CAF scores track behaviors, reported by caregivers, of the last month. However, ODFA scores were significantly different after treatment compared with baseline. Our study suggests therefore that ChEI effect is mediated by correction of dysfunction of the brain stem reticular pathways involved in vigilance regulation. A previous study [66] had shown the correlation between improvement of attentional activities and improvement of neuropsychological scores after ChEI therapy and the finding was confirmed by following reports [60,62,67]. The lack of BR response alterations and subsequent absence of R2 latency modification by ChEI in AD patients suggest that due to the lower cholinergic functioning in DLB, a greater potential improvement from these drugs than that seen in AD might be expected, at least in the early phases of DLB pathophysiology, when a prevalent brain stem involvement is called into cause [6]. Furthermore, the presence of fewer neurofibrillary tangles and neuritic plaques and of less neuronal loss in DLB than AD [68,69] suggests that neurons in DLB are more viable than those in AD and could be more responsive to cholinergic stimulation [70-72]. These data suggest that the presence of alterations of neurophysiological responses tracking brain stem reticular formation might also predict the response to ChEI in DLB, as concluded in previous studies [67,73] about the efficacy of ChEI on cognitive impairments and psychiatric symptoms, and foster further studies on the long-term effect of ChEI and identification of responders.

## 6. Quantitative eeg:qeeg

Quantitative Electroencephalography (QEEG) is the measurement, using digital technology, of electrical patterns at the surface of the scalp which primarily reflect cortical activity or "brainwaves". A multi-electrode recording of brain wave activity is recorded and converted into numbers by a computer. These numbers are then statistically analysed and are converted into a colour map of brain functioning. Digital EEG techniques have grown rapidly in both technology and popularity since the early 1980's for recording, reviewing and storing EEG data. Compared to other systems, QEEG is a non-invasive procedure and offers a superior temporal (time) resolution compared with fMRI, SPECT and PET imaging techniques. MEG systems, though providing a high temporal and spatial resolution, are a relatively expensive means of monitoring the brain as compared with QEEG. Recently we had designed a QEEG study in a cohort of patients affected by early AD and DLB, whose diagnoses were confirmed by laboratory methods and by a 2-year follow-up, which allowed confirming or discarding earlier diagnoses, and thus reaching the best possible level of certainty on the classification of these two disorders [5]. As specific EEG abnormalities reflecting the presence of cognitive fluctuations (superimposition of pre-alpha/theta activity on alpha dominant frequency, or of theta/delta activity on dominant pre-alpha frequency) were evidenced in early DLB [5,74-76] while alpha dominant activity was more stable in early AD [1], we evaluated possible correlations between P300 and EEG characteristics in AD and DLB. Several electroencephalographic studies on dementia were performed in the years preceding the identification of DLB as a widespread cognitive disorder. Slowing of the rhythms and reduced coherence among brain regions, increased theta and delta activity, in parallel with reduction of alpha and beta rhythms were observed in patients affected by putative AD [76]: computerized EEG spectral analysis showed an increase in delta and theta power in AD patients compared to controls mainly in the left temporal area. EEGs were recorded with Ag/AgCl disk scalp electrodes placed on 19 derivations corresponding to Fp1, Fp2, F3, F4, C3, C4, P3, P4, O1, O2, F7, F8, T3, T4, T5, T6, Cz, Fz, Pz positions of the 10-20 International System with supplementary A1, A2 derivations. Derivations were grouped in order to define 5 scalp regions: anterior (Fz, Fp2, F7, Fp1, F3, F4, F8), central (T3, C3, Cz, C4, T4), posterior (T5, P3, Pz, P4, T6, O1, O2) and peripheral (Fp1, Fp2, F8, T4, T6, O1, O2, T5, T3, Fz) or internal (F3, F4, Fz, C3, Cz, C4, P3, Pz, P4). Reference was the mean (mean reference) of recordings from all scalp leads, A1, A2 signals were also stored for digitalized derivation reconstruction. Ground was placed at FpZ. Impedance was below 5 KOhm. The patients were seated in a quiet room on a comfortable armchair, awake with closed eyes under continuous control (Video EEG); wakefulness of the patients was verified every 2 min by asking to open eyes and checking block reactions; 2 supplementary derivations monitored electro-oculography (vertical and horizontal), two derivations monitored possible interference of tremor and two pairs of additional bipolar recording channels for the respiration and electrocardiogram were applied. EEG was acquired as a continuous signal for 30 min and visually inspected for current clinical interpretation or detection of artifacts and stored in order to be epoched in off-analysis setting as series of 2 seconds-long epochs. EEGs interpreted with classical visual inspection, corresponding to categories reported in previous literature [77,78] were defined as Classic Interpretation Methods (CIM) in results. The computer collected 10 minutes of EEG recorded with closed eyes, digitized at 1024 Hz with a low filter at 0.5 Hz and high filter at 70 Hz (decay constant 12 dB) with a 50 Hz notch filter in each channel. Blocks of artifact-free 2 seconds-long epochs appearing consecutively for 20-40 sec were selected off-line by visual inspection after pre-programmed automatic blink reduction and muscle and tremor artifact rejection system and were compared with the remaining artifact-free epochs in order to avoid possible discrepancies among acquired sets. A total of 90 epochs per patient were processed by an automatic transforming program present in the NEUROSCAN SynAmps System performing a fast Fourier Transform on each second of EEG acquisition, allowing a frequency sensitivity=0.05 Hz. The obtained spectra values were then processed in order to compute a mean Power Spectrum (mPS) for each epoch and for each channel and expressed in square uV ($uV^2$). The mPS was divided automatically into 4 frequency bands (1-3.9 Hz [delta], 4-5.5 Hz [theta], 5.6-7.9 Hz [fast theta or pre-alpha], 8-12 Hz [alpha]). These bands were defined after the post hoc analysis with the purpose to facilitate identification of differences, in the description of results, as statistical differences were evidenced when theta band was halved in two parts (4-5.5 Hz, theta and 5.6-7.9 Hz pre-alpha). Fast Fourier transform-QEEG program expressed power values automatically after a log transform (log[x/(1-x)]) and indicated the Dominant Frequency (DF) of the entire power spectrum of each epoch, i.e. the specific frequency where the maximum power for a single epoch or a sum of multiple epochs was contained. Mean Relative Power Spectra (mRPS: percentage of the global mPS of each frequency band) were computed and log transformed [79] to normalize the data, automatically calculated and expressed in numeric percentages for each one of the single epochs obtained from each scalp derivation. EEG power spectra were represented as scalp maps of band amplitudes measured on the 180 sec total analysis (Total Power) and analyzed as Mean Frequency (MF), indicating the average frequency for the 90 epochs, and as mean frequency variability (MFV), representing changes of mean frequency during the 90 epochs. Single channel power spectra were also represented as Compressed Spectral Arrays (CSA) showing the sequences of absolute or relative power spectra in each one of the 90 analysed epochs. mRPS from all the scalp derivations were averaged in order to obtain a single Global Mean RPS representative of the frequency band powers in each patient expressing the average distribution of powers recorded from all the derivations. Eventually, in each epoch, mean band power in each of the three groups of patients (AD, DLB, PDD) as well as in the control group was then computed by averaging the values of subjects in each group.

Our EEG study [5] completed and detailed results of a preliminary study performed with Magneto-Encephalography (MEG) recordings [80] suggesting that activities in parietal and occipital areas differentiate early DLB from early AD. MEG technique excluded a reference effect, showed differences in reactivity of alpha rhythms between groups of patients, and explored coherence: therefore the present study was focused on waking-closed eyes condition and on methods evidencing differences. The different EEG variables analysed in our study showed some distinct and specific patterns in patients affected by DLB or PDD with cognitive fluctuations (PDDF). When EEGs were interpreted with the classic visual inspection methods, absent alpha in posterior derivations was observed in 63.9% of DLB and in none of AD patients. In PDD absent alpha was observed in 25.7% of patients (all from PDDF group). Intermittent delta and sharp transients, described in previous studies [2,4,9], occurred more frequently in DLB patients compared to AD (13.9% vs 2.5% and 5.6% vs 2.5%) yet these findings were rare, and therefore scarcely useful for diagnostic purposes. Visual inspection was not sufficient to evidence other differences which were observed with QEEG methods: the first relevant finding was the identification of slow activities in posterior derivations, with a frequency of 5.6-7.9 Hz, which were observed in all DLB patients and significantly separated DLB patients from AD. This activity was defined pre-alpha because it was suppressed by eye opening. Two studies [81,82] quantified EEG characteristics during polisomnography (PSG) in patients with RBD and DLB/PDD and indicated differences with controls in the same EEG frequency band. QEEG was analyzed with different methods. Total power and mRPS showed that pre-alpha activity on posterior derivations expressed the highest statistical difference between AD or PDD without cognitive fluctuations (PDDNF) and DLB or PDDF patients ($p<0.01$). The study of MFV showed that variability of EEG activity was the second most relevant finding leading to the identification of specific EEG patterns in DLB or PDDF ($p<0.001$) as reported in a previous study [83]. The variability of the EEG frequencies in relaxed waking conditions was best evidenced by using the CSA method of representation, showing that dominant frequencies (DF) in DLB were either in the pre-alpha band or varied across time with pseudocyclic patterns of delta-theta/pre-alpha or theta-pre-alpha/alpha, differentiating DLB or PDDF patients from AD or PDDNF patients. CSA representation had only been previously used to assess coma or anaesthesia levels [83], and in the present study it allowed to evidence changes of EEG activities in single derivations. It allowed therefore to evaluate local variability, at contrary with total QEEG analyses and MF evaluations, and to evidence that significant differences among groups of patients were prevalent in posterior leads. CSA showed that changes of dominant activity could be separated in five patterns, salient at visual inspection of the sequence of traces: one, with dominant stable alpha, was only observed in early AD and in 54.3% of PDD (PDDNF), while the other patterns, differently grading the dominant frequency variability and pre-alpha presence, were only observed in posterior derivations of early DLB and PDDF. The abnormal patterns consisted either of a stable dominant activity at 5.6-7.9 Hz, encountered in 25% of DLB and 11.4% of PDD, but never in AD, or of unstable activities, all encompassing the presence of the 5.6-7.9 Hz activity and significant variations of the dominant frequency across time. When these EEG abnormalities are observed in a patient with initial signs of cognitive decline, i.e. MMSE<24, they support a diagnosis of DLB. Therefore our study clarifies and quantifies the suggestion that EEG might support the diagnosis [2]. When EEGs were recorded two years later [5], further alterations were observed which differentiated groups of patients, even though the administration of current therapies could have partly marred the results. In DLB patients and in 74.3% of PDD patients EEGs were similar, with a stable pre-alpha activity or unstable DF across time, with variability above 3 Hz, consisting of the presence of unstable alpha, pre-alpha, theta and delta activities. In 72.5% of AD patients and in 25.7% of PDD patients DFV was below 3 Hz and alpha activity was present. At follow-up patterns 2-4 were observed prominently in posterior derivations of DLB and PDDF patients, while only 27.5% of AD patients presented with similar EEG abnormalities. Pattern 5 was observed at follow-up in patients with severe cognitive deteriorations (5 DLB, 2 AD, 3 PDD), suggesting therefore that this degraded pattern is aspecific. In our experience we recorded pattern 5 activity also in cases of severe Progressive Supranuclear Palsy and Fronto-temporal dementia. In conclusion we would add two further considerations. First, PDD in its early course can be apparently separated in two different groups: one with fluctuating cognition elements and EEG pattern abnormalities akin to the ones observed in early DLB and a group with normal EEG akin to the AD patients and without fluctuating cognition. With follow-up, however, the majority of PDD patients (74.3%) presents with the same EEG abnormalities characterizing DLB. The presence of two different clusters in early PDD suggests that the distribution of neuropathological abnormalities might have different patterns in different patients, cumulating however across time to show, at follow-up, clinical and EEG patterns similar to the ones observed in DLB. Second, in AD we found less EEG abnormalities than previously reported [76]. We suggest that this finding depends on patients selection methods used in our study. In this study the selection was focused on elements of fluctuating cognition (CAF-ODFA scales) and presence of RBD, prominently

characterizing DLB [2]: the occurrence of positive CAF scores and of RBD during follow-up supported the categorization of patients. Patients diagnosed as affected by AD, who did not show evidence of fluctuating cognition or RBD, had rare EEG abnormalities. Yet, recent reports [84] showed that power spectra abnormalities in AD patients are characterized only by an increase in theta and a decrease in alpha and beta rhythms at rest and mostly limited to the temporal, and centro-parietal regions, or showed that entropy of EEG, expressing the irregularity and variability of EEG patterns, is reduced, rather than increased, in AD.
In conclusion, the definite presence of EEG abnormalities early in the course of DLB, with a core feature evidencing marked variability of dominant frequencies in posterior derivations, occurring every few seconds, or with the substitution of alpha with frequencies at 5.6-7.9 Hz, suggests that centers regulating EEG rhythms in parieto-occipital areas are affected in the early course of this disease.

## 7. Other investigations and future prospectives

Syncope associated to orthostatic hypotension, urinary incontinence and constipation is common symptoms in demented patients, mainly in DLB and in PDD. AD and FTD show less frequently autonomic dysfunction. There are non invasive tests including standard cardiovascular tests, $^{123}$I-MIBG cardiac scintigraphy, urodynamic tests, gastrointestinal motility studies, sweating reflexes and pupillary responses that assess autonomic dysfunction in these patients.
$^{123}$I-MIBG is an analogue of the sympathomimetic amine guanethidine, which is used to determine the location, integrity, and function of postganglionic noradrenergic neurons [85]. Patients with PD can exhibit reduced cardiac $^{123}$I-MIBG-derived radioactivity without other evidence of autonomic failure, whereas those with DLB can have reduced cardiac $^{123}$I-MIBG-derived radioactivity without evidence of parkinsonism [86]. $^{123}$I-MIBG may have the potential to differentiate PD from other causes of parkinsonism. For example, MSA and PSP pose a difficult diagnostic challenge.
In PD and DLB, LB are encountered in extracranial tissues, notably in autonomic ganglia [87]. Cardiac sympathetic degeneration can be demonstrated early in the disease process before motor symptoms. In 2005, the DLB Consortium concluded that diminished uptake of $^{123}$I-MIBG on cardiac scintigraphy was a "supportive" clinical feature that required more study [2].
Positron emission tomography (PET) utilizes biologically active molecules in micromolar or nanomolar concentrations that have been labelled with short-lived positron-emitting isotopes. The physical characteristics of the isotopes and the molecular specificity of labeled molecules, combined with the high detection efficacy of modern PET scanners, provide a sensitivity for human in vivo measurement of indicator concentrations that is several orders of magnitude higher than with the other imaging techniques. Whereas the very short half-lives of $O^{15}$ (2 min) and $C^{11}$ (20 min) limit their use to fully equipped PET centres with a cyclotron and radiopharmaceutical laboratory, $F^{18}$ labelled tracers (half-life 110 min) can be produced in specialized centres and distributed regionally to hospitals running a PET scanner only. Clinical use of PET is now well established in clinical oncology and it is therefore becoming widely available in major hospitals. In addition to its use in research, brain PET also provides diagnostically relevant information mainly in neurodegenerative disorders, focal epilepsy and brain tumors. In dementia, the measurement of cerebral

glucose metabolism by 18F-2-fluoro-2-deoxy-Dglucose (FDG) and specific molecular imaging techniques involving tracers for amyloid and major neurotransmitters are of diagnostic interest. Brain PET using FDG is a firmly established technique for demonstration of regional functional impairment in neurodegenerative disease. AD is associated with typical regional impairment of posterior cortical association areas that allow very early diagnosis before clinical manifestation of dementia and monitoring of progression and treatment effects. DLB additionally involves metabolic impairment of the primary visual cortex. Predominant impairment of the frontal and anterior temporal regions is seen in FTD, primary progressive aphasia and semantic dementia. New perspectives are opened by tracers for imaging amyloids, which appear to be very sensitive for detecting even preclinical AD cases, although confirmation of the specificity remains to be demonstrated. Tracers for measuring local AChE activity and the binding capacity of nicotinic and serotoninergic receptors address neurotransmitter deficits in dementia. Impairment of dopamine synthesis that is characteristic for DLB can be demonstrated by 18F-fluorodopa PET. Pittsburgh compound-B (PIB)-PET imaging is a sensitive and specific marker for underlying β amyloid deposition and represents an important investigative tool for examining the relationship between amyloid burden, clinical symptoms and structural and functional changes in dementia. Amyloid imaging may also be useful for selecting patients for anti-amyloid therapies. However, studies have identified PIB-positive cases in otherwise healthy older individuals (10–30%), limiting diagnostic specificity. Development of biomarkers for investigating other aspects of dementia pathology, i.e. soluble β amyloid, tau protein, synuclein deposition and brain inflammation would further inform our understanding and assist in studying disease-modifying and preventive treatments in dementia. Both DLB and PDD are characterized at autopsy by the presence of subcortical and/or cortical Lewy bodies. It has been well established that often there is also a substantial burden of amyloid pathology, though, compared to AD, plaques are more often diffuse than dystrophic neurites [88]. A limited number of PET studies have examined the amyloid burden in DLB and PDD in vivo [89] and showed that in DLB mean brain PIB uptake was significantly higher than in controls, while uptake in PDD was comparable to controls and PD without dementia. In particular, 85% of DLB patients had significantly increased amyloid load in one or more cortical regions, whereas 83% of PDD patients had 'normal' PIB uptake. None of the PD patients showed any evidence of increased cortical amyloid deposition. A report by Gomperts and colleagues [90] revealed that cortical amyloid burden as measured by PIB was higher in DLB than in PDD, but similar to AD. The findings suggest that global cortical amyloid burden is high in DLB but low and infrequent in PDD. An increased amyloid burden could contribute to the rapid progression of dementia in DLB [89] while it may also play a role in the timing of dementia relative to the motor symptoms of Parkinsonism in DLB and PDD [88,90]. Either PET or SPECT can be employed to provide functional imaging of the nigrostriatal dopaminergic system in vivo. SPECT has the advantage of being more readily available and somewhat easier to organize and undertake, and the majority of the reported studies of imaging of the dopaminergic system in DLB have been SPECT studies, even though PET has produced equivalent results [91]. The first ligand used in SPECT was [123I]-2b-carbomethoxy-3b-(4-iodophenyl) tropane (b-CIT). Subsequently, [123I] N-x-flouropropyl-2b-carbomethoxy- 3b-(4-iodophenyl) nortropane (FP-CIT) became available. FP-CIT was preferable because the time interval between injection and scanning was just 3 hours, making the procedure possible on a single outpatient visit. Both ligands are cocaine analogues, which bind the dopamine reuptake and transporter molecule found in the presynaptic cell membrane of dopamine producing nigrostriatal nerve terminals in the striatum (caudate and putamen). Reduced binding reflects dysfunction or loss of nerve terminals, usually associated with loss of the neuronal cell bodies in the substantia nigra. Clearly, the test is not specific with regard to the nature of the pathology in the substantia nigra, but Lewy body pathology is the commonest cause of major bilateral loss of substantia nigra neurones, with loss of about 50% of neurones being necessary before parkinsonism becomes clinically detectable [92]. These studies show consistently and convincingly that in subjects with a clinical diagnosis of probable DLB, there is reduced binding of ligand in the putamen and caudate, and that in AD, the ligand binding is not significantly different from controls, suggesting strongly that FP-CIT SPECT would be effective in distinguishing DLB cases from AD cases when the distinction cannot be confidently made on clinical grounds. FP-CIT scans were abnormal in DLB cases without parkinsonism, as well as in cases with parkinsonism [93].

The weakness of all the studies is that the diagnoses of DLB and AD were clinical, and therefore subject to error. An autopsy diagnosis has to be the gold standard, notwithstanding the uncertainties involved in the neuropathological diagnosis of both AD and DLB and the difficult issue of the coexistence of neuropathological features in both disorders. In applying the consensus clinical diagnostic criteria for probable DLB proposed by the consortium on DLB at their first international workshop, the greatest accuracy when compared with subsequent autopsy diagnosis was achieved by the Newcastle upon Tyne group (83% sensitivity, 95% specificity). The estimated sensitivity and specificity of FP-CIT SPECT scan abnormality for a diagnosis of DLB versus AD will obviously be affected by the extent to which patients are wrongly categorized clinically. Ideally every patient with dementia deserves a diagnosis as accurate as possible. Accordingly, in any patient whose dementia diagnosis is uncertain and who could possibly have DLB a dopamine transporter SPECT scan should be considered. Most such patients will fulfill clinical diagnostic criteria for "possible DLB" (dementia plus one core feature; or dementia plus one or more "suggestive" features, obviously excluding abnormal dopamine transporter scan which is currently one of the suggestive features). The effectiveness of FP-CIT in contributing to the diagnosis of DLB has recently been convincingly shown [94]. Most patients with clinically typical DLB do not need a FP-CIT scan. However, there are patients who fulfill diagnostic criteria for probable DLB, but are also affected by complicating medical issues such as cerebrovascular disease or are on medication with extrapyramidal adverse effects, and in such situations, a dopamine transporter scan can clarify the diagnosis. Finally, there are patients who have mild cognitive impairment (not dementia) and in addition have features raising the possibility of DLB (such as visual hallucinations, fluctuating cognition, and neuroleptic sensitivity). In these cases, recurrent delirium may be a concern, leading to repeated investigations. An abnormal FP-CIT scan can be diagnostically helpful and possibly cost worthy.

Although there is a large and increasing body of knowledge on the genetic, molecular and cellular mechanisms of neurodegenerative disorders, the exact cause is unknown, except for a few rare genetic variants. Neurophysiological understanding could guide early differential diagnosis, and may suggest new ways to monitor treatment response. Since a few years the availability of whole-head MEG systems has expanded the scope of such studies. MEG can record brain activity directly, and has several advantages compared to conventional EEG recordings. In contrast to EEG, MEG is hardly affected by the skull, and does not require a reference electrode. Therefore, MEG may provide a more accurate image of ongoing brain activity. In addition, significant advances have been made in neuroscience concerning the understanding of oscillatory and synchronized brain activities. In particular it is now assumed that synchronization of neural activity between different brain regions may reflect functional interactions between these regions [95]. Such synchronization processes can be measured at the level of the scalp with EEG and even better with MEG. Interesting patterns of abnormal oscillatory activity and interregional synchronization have now been described in various brain disorders, including PD and AD [96].

One of the first MEG studies in PD was aimed at auditory evoked magnetic fields [97]; they suggest that this might reflect the combined effect of basal ganglia disease and auditory cortex degeneration. MEG studies were stimulated by the observation that PD may be associated with an increase in EEG coherence in the beta band, possibly due to the failure of a normal basal ganglia/thalamic drive to the cortex [98]. These changes were reversible after either dopaminergic treatment or deep brain stimulation. Functional connectivity was studied in the same large cohort of non-demented PD patients mentioned above using the synchronization likelihood [99]. In untreated, early phase PD patients a diffuse increase in functional connectivity in the lower alpha band was found. This abnormally high connectivity extended to other frequency bands, in particular the theta, upper alpha and beta bands, with progression of the disease. Disease severity was associated with abnormal connectivity in theta and beta bands. Cognitive perseveration was correlated with inter-hemispheric alpha band synchronization. In contrast to spectral changes, functional connectivity in PD does respond to treatment with L-dopa. Again, changes in demented PD patients are qualitatively different from those in non-demented PD patients. Demented PD patients showed a loss of functional connectivity, especially between the frontal and temporal areas within each hemisphere, and between the temporal areas of both hemispheres, in the alpha band [100]. Connectivity changes in dementia thus are on the decrease rather than on the increase trend, and a distribution that is more fronto-temporal compared to the central dominance of connectivity changes in non-demented PD. The overall pattern of connectivity changes in demented PD shows a similarity patterns found in studies on AD [101]. Although the number of MEG studies in PD is still very small, a consistent pattern of changes in local band power and interregional synchronization is becoming clear. Slowing of background activity (increased theta; decreased beta) and increased alpha band connectivity occur early in non-demented, drug naïve PD patients; with disease progression the spectral changes keep constant, whereas increased connectivity extends to other bands. Dopamine affects connectivity, but does not influence power. With the advent of dementia, slowing occurs in different frequency bands (increased delta power; loss of alpha power), and lower rather than higher connectivity is seen mainly in the alpha band. Changes in demented PD may be reversible after cholinergic rather than dopaminergic treatment. This characteristic pattern of progressive neurophysiological changes in non-demented and demented PD patients could reflect the progressive involvement of different neurotransmitter systems, as well as subcortical and cortical Lewy body pathology, during the course of the disease [102].

The advent of whole-head MEG systems, and the improvements in the understanding of oscillatory and synchronized brain activity, have opened up the way to study disturbances

in large-scale brain networks in neurodegenerative disorders such as PD and AD. Many MEG studies, most of which were conducted in the last five years, have confirmed and extended findings from previous EEG work. It is becoming clear that PD and AD show characteristic patterns of abnormal brain function, both locally as manifested by changes in spectral power, as well as at the scale of functional networks, manifested by changes in interregional synchronization. These changes may reflect abnormalities in specific networks and neurotransmitter systems, and could become useful in differential diagnosis and treatment monitoring. While MEG may be superior to EEG especially for functional connectivity studies, its high cost and the impossibility to combine it directly with structural MRI remain important obstacles. In this respect the development of ultra low field MRI (ULF MRI) could be a very interesting new approach [103]. If this technology can be further developed high quality integrated structural and functional studies of brain networks may become feasible. However, improvements on the acquisition side alone may not be sufficient for a better understanding of normal and disturbed brain networks. There is a urgent need for a proper theoretical framework for the analysis and interpretation of the data obtained with advanced functional imaging techniques. One attempt to deal with this problem is the application of graph theory to functional neuroimaging data [104]. This approach provides a theoretical framework for describing the structure and function of complex networks.
Further studies along these lines, could help to advance our knowledge of disrupted brain networks in neurodegenerative disease.

## 8. References

[1] McKhann GM, Albert MS, Grossman M, Miller B, Dickson D, Trojanowski JQ; Work Group on Frontotemporal Dementia and Pick's Disease. Clinical and pathological diagnosis of frontotemporal dementia: report of the Work Group on Frontotemporal Dementia and Pick's Disease. Arch Neurol. 2001 Nov;58(11):1803-9.

[2] McKeith IG, Dickson DW, Lowe J, Emre M, O'Brien JT, Feldman H, Cummings J, Duda JE, Lippa C, Perry EK, Aarsland D, Arai H, Ballard CG, Boeve B, Burn DJ, Costa D, Del Ser T, Dubois B, Galasko D, Gauthier S, Goetz CG, Gomez-Tortosa E, Halliday G, Hansen LA, Hardy J, Iwatsubo T, Kalaria RN, Kaufer D, Kenny RA, Korczyn A, Kosaka K, Lee VM, Lees A, Litvan I, Londos E, Lopez OL, Minoshima S, Mizuno Y, Molina JA, Mukaetova-Ladinska EB, Pasquier F, Perry RH, Schulz JB, Trojanowski JQ, Yamada M; Consortium on DLB. Diagnosis and management of dementia with Lewy bodies: third report of the DLB Consortium. Neurology. 2005 Dec 27;65(12):1863-72. Review.

[3] Ince PG, McKeith IG. Dementia with Lewy bodies. In: Dickson DW, et al, editors. Neurodegeneration: The molecular pathology of dementia and movement disorders. Basel: International Society of Neuropathology Press; 2003. p 188–199.

[4] Bonanni L, Thomas A, Onofrj M. Diagnosis and management of dementia with Lewy bodies: third report of the DLB Consortium. Neurology 2006;66:1455.

[5] Bonanni L, Thomas A, Tiraboschi P, Perfetti B, Varanese S, Onofrj M. EEG comparisons in early Alzheimer's disease, dementia with Lewy bodies and

Parkinson's disease with dementia patients with a 2-year follow-up. Brain. 2008 Mar;131(Pt 3):690-705.

[6] Walker MP, Ayre GA, Cummings JL, Wesnes K, McKeith IG, O'Brien JT, Ballard CG. The Clinician Assessment of Fluctuation and the One Day Fluctuation Assessment Scale. Two methods to assess fluctuating confusion in dementia. Br J Psychiatry 2000;177:252-56.

[7] Ballard CG, Aarsland D, McKeith I. Fluctuations in attention: PD dementia vs DLB with parkinsonism. Neurology 2002;59:1714-20.

[8] Walker MP, Ayre GA, Cummings JL, Wesnes K, McKeith IG, O'Brien JT, Ballard CG. Quantifying fluctuation in dementia with Lewy bodies, Alzheimer's disease, and vascular dementia. Neurology 2000;54:1616-25.

[9] Doe´ de Maindreville A, Fe´nelon G, Mahieux F. Hallucinations in Parkinson's disease: a follow-up study. Mov Disord 2004;20:212–217.

[10] Mosimann UP, Mather G, Wesnes KA, O'Brien JT, Burn DJ, McKeith IG. Visual perception in Parkinson disease dementia and dementia with Lewy bodies. Neurology 2004;63:2091–2096.

[11] Oishi N, Udaka F, Kameyama M, Sawamoto N, Hashikawa K, Fukuyama H. Regional cerebral blood flow in Parkinson disease with nonpsychotic visual hallucinations. Neurology 2005;65: 1708–1715.

[12] Nightingale S, Mitchell KW, Howe JW. Visual evoked cortical potentials and pattern electroretinograms in Parkinson's disease and control subjects. Journal of Neurology, Neurosurgery, and Psychiatry 1986;49:1280-1287.

[13] Gawal MJ, Das P, Vincent S, Clifford Rose F. Visual and auditory evoked responses in patients with Parkinson's disease. J Neurol Neurosurg Psychiatry 198 1;44: 227-32.

[14] Skrandies W. Scalp potential fields evoked by grating stimuli: effects of spatial frequency and orientation. Electroencephalogr Clin Neurophysiol 1984;58: 325-32.

[15] Onofrj M, Ghilardi MF, Basciani M, Gambi D. Visual evoked potentials in parkinsonism and dopamine blockade reveal a stimulus-dependent dopamine function in humans. J Neurol Neurosurg Psychiatry. 1986;49:1150-9.

[16] Bhaskar PA, Vanchilingam S, Bhaskar EA, Devaprabhu A, Ganesan RA Effect of L-dopa on visual evoked potential in patients with Parkinson's disease. Neurology. 1986;36:1119-21.

[17] Stanzione P, Fattapposta F, Tagliati M, D'Alessio C, Marciani MG, Foti A, Amabile G. Dopaminergic pharmacological manipulations in normal humans confirm the specificity of the visual (PERG-VEP) and cognitive (P300) electrophysiological alterations in Parkinson's disease. Electroencephalogr Clin Neurophysiol Suppl. 1990;41:216-20.

[18] Onofrj M, Bodis-Wollner I, Ghilardi MF, Marx M, Glover A. Pattern vision in monkeys with Parkinsonism: a stimulus specific effect of MPTP on retinal and cortical responses. In: Markey SP, Castagnoli N, Trevor A, Kopin IJ eds. "MPTP: a Neurotoxin Producing a Parkinsonian Syndrome". California: Academic Press.

[19] Onofrj M, Bodis-Wollner I. Dopamine deficiency causes delayed visual evoked potentials in rats. Ann Neurol 1982;11:484-90.

[20] Devos D, Tir M, Maurage CA, Waucquier N, Defebvre L, Defoort-Dhellemmes S, Destée A. ERG and anatomical abnormalities suggesting retinopathy in dementia with Lewy bodies. Neurology. 2005;65:1107-10.

[21] Kurita A, Murakami M, Takagi S, Matsushima M, Suzuki M. Visual hallucinations and altered visual information processing in Parkinson disease and dementia with Lewy bodies. Mov Disord. 2010;25:167-71.

[22] Delalande I, Hache J, Forzy G et al Do visual-evoked potentials and spatiotemporal contrast sensitivity help to distinguish idiopathic Parkinson's disease and multiple system atrophy? Mov Disord 1998;13:446–452.

[23] Sartucci F, Orlandi G, Bonuccelli U, Borghetti D, Murri L, Orsini C, Domenici L, Porciatti V. Chromatic pattern-reversal electroretinograms (ChPERGs) are spared in multiple system atrophy compared with Parkinson's disease. Neurol Sci. 2006;26:395-401.

[24] Guidelines for calibration of stimulus and recording parameters used in clinical electrophysiology of vision. Brigell M, Bach M, Barber C, Moskowitz A, Robson J; Calibration Standard Committee of the International Society for Clinical Electrophysiology of Vision. Doc Ophthalmol. 2003;107:185-93.

[25] Wu Z, Lai Y, Xia Y, Wu D, Yao D. Stimulator selection in SSVEP-based BCI. Med Eng Phys. 2008;30:1079-88.

[26] Tartaglione A, Pizio N, Bino G, Spadavecchia L, Favale E. VEP changes in Parkinson's disease are stimulus dependent. J Neurol Neurosurg Psychiatry 1984;47: 305-7.

[27] Husain AM, Hayes S, Young M, Shah D. Visual evoked potentials with CRT and LCD monitors: when newer is not better. Neurology. 2009;13;72:162-4.

[28] Linden DE. The P300: where in the brain is it produced and what does it tell us? Neuroscientist 2005;6:563—76.

[29] Polich J, Kok A. Cognitive and biological determinants of P300: an integrative review. Biol Psychol 1995;41:103—46.

[30] Duncan C, Barry R, Connolly J, Fischer C, Michie P, Näätänen R, et al. Event-related potentials in clinical research: Guidelines for eliciting, recording, and quantifying mismatch negativity, P300, and N400. Clin Neurophysiol 2009;120:1883-908.

[31] Onofrj M, Fulgente T, Nobilio D, Malatesta G, Bazzano S, Colamartino P, et al. P3 recordings in patients with bilateral temporal lobe lesions. Neurology 1992;42:1762-77.

[32] Bonanni L, Franciotti R, Onofrj V, Anzellotti F, Mancino E, Monaco D, Gambi F, Manzoli L, Thomas A, Onofrj M. Revisiting P300 cognitive studies for dementia diagnosis: Early dementia with Lewy bodies (DLB) and Alzheimer disease (AD). Neurophysiol Clin. 2010;40:255-65.

[33] Polich J, Ladish C, Bloom FE. P300 assessment of early Alzheimer's disease. Electroenceph Clin Neurophysiol 1990;77:179-89.

[34] Onofrj MC, Ghilardi MF, Fulgente T, Nobilio D, Bazzano S, Ferracci F, et al. Mapping of event-related potentials to auditory and visual oddball paradigms. Electroencephalogr Clin Neurophysiol 1990;41(Suppl):183-201.

[35] Alho K, Winkler I, Escera C, Huotilainen M, Virtanen J, Jaaskelainen IP, et al. Processing of novel sounds and frequency changes in the human auditory cortex: magnetoelectroencephalographic recordings. Psychophysiology 1998;35:211-24.

[36] He B, Lian J, Spencer KM, Dien J, Donchin E. A cortical potential imaging analysis of the P300 and novelty P3 components. Hum Brain Mapp 2001;12:120-30.

[37] Dien J, Spencer KM, Donchin E. Localization of the eventrelated potential novelty response as defined by principal components analysis. Cognit Brain Res 2003;17:637-50.

[38] Polich J. Updating P300: an integrative theory of P3a and P3b. Clin Neurophysiol 2007;118:2128-48.

[39] Filipovic SR, Vladimir S, Kostic VS. Utility of auditory P300 in detection of presenile dementia. J Neurol Sci 1995;131:150-5.

[40] Syndulko K, Hansch EC, Cohen SN, Pearce JW, Goldberg Z, Montan B, et al. Long-latency event-related potentials in normal aging and dementia. Adv Neurol 1982;32:279-85.

[41] Golob EJ, Ringman JM, Irimajiri R, Bright S, Schaffer B, Medina LD, et al. Cortical event-related potentials in preclinical familial Alzheimer disease. Neurology 2009;73:1649-55.

[42] Goodin DS, Aminoff MJ. Electrophysiological differences between subtypes of dementia. Brain 1986;109:1103-13.

[43] Pfefferbaum A, Rosenbloom M, Ford JM. Late event-related potential changes in alcoholics. Alcohol 1987;4:275- 81.

[44] Stanzione P, Semprini R, Pierantozzi M, Santilli AM, Fadda L, Traversa R, et al. Age and stage dependency of P300 latency alterations in non-demented Parkinson's disease patients without therapy. Electroencephalogr Clin Neurophysiol 1998;108:80-91.

[45] Fuentemilla L, Marco-Pallarés J, Grau C. Modulation of spectral power and of phase resetting of EEG contributes differentially to the generation of auditory event-related potentials. Neuroimage 2006;30:909-16.

[46] Sumi N, Harada K, Fujimoto O, Taguchi S, Ohta Y, Nan-no H, et al. Inter-peak latency of auditory event-related potentials (P300) in cases of aged schizophrenia and Alzheimer-type dementia. Psychogeriatrics 2001;1:64-8.

[47] Shucard JL, Tekok-Kilic A, Shiels K, Shucard DW. Stage and load effects on ERP topography during verbal and spatial working memory. Brain Res 2009;1254: 49-62.

[48] Fabiani M, Friedman D, Cheng JC. Individual differences in P3 scalp distribution in older adults, and their relationship to frontal lobe function. Psychophysiology 1998;35:698 Coles.

[49] Biousse V, Skibell BC, Watts RL, Loupe DN, Drews-Botsch C, Newman NJ. Ophthalmologic features of Parkinson's disease. Neurology 2004; 62: 177–180.

[50] Peshori KR, Schicatano EJ, Gopalaswamy R, Sahay E, Evinger C. Aging of the trigeminal blink system. Exp Brain Res 2001; 136: 351– 363.

[51] Cruccu G, Iannetti GD, Marx JJ, Thoemke F, Truini A, Fitzek S, et al. Brainstem reflex circuits revisited. Brain. 2005;128:386-94.

[52] Valls-Sole´ J, Valldeoriola F, Tolosa E, et al. Distinctive abnormalities of facial reflexes in patients with progressive supranuclear palsy. Brain 1997;120:1877–83.
[53] Valls-Sole´ J. Neurophysiological characterization of parkinsonian syndromes. Neurophysiol Clin 2000;30:352–67.
[54] Braak H, Del Tredici K, Rub U, et al. Staging of brain pathology related to sporadic Parkinson's disease. Neurobiol Aging 2003;24:197–211.
[55] Kimura J. Disorder of interneurons in parkinsonism. The orbicularis oculi reflex to paired stimuli. Brain 1973; 96:87-96.
[56] Bonanni L, Anzellotti F, Varanese S, et al. Delayed blink reflex in dementia with Lewy bodies. J Neurol Neurosurg Psychiatry 2007;78:1137-1139.
[57] Cruccu G, Deuschl G. The clinical use of brainstem reflexes and hand-muscle reflexes. Clin Neurophysiol 2000;111:371-87.
[58] Samuel W, Alford M, Hofstetter CR, et al. Dementia with Lewy bodies versus pure Alzheimer disease: differences in cognition, neuropathology, cholinergic dysfunction, and synapse density. J Neuropathol Exp Neurol 1997;56:499-508.
[59] Teaktong T, Piggott MA, McKeith IG, et al. Muscarinic M2 and M4 receptors in anterior cingulate cortex: relation to neuropsychiatric symptoms in dementia with Lewy bodies. Behav Brain Res 2005;161:299-305.
[60] Onofrj M, Thomas A, Iacono D, et al. The effects of cholinesterase inhibitor are prominent in patients with fluctuating cognition: a part 3 study of the main mechanism of cholinesterase inhibitors in dementia. Clin Neuropharmacol 2003;26:239-251.
[61] Thomas A, Iacono D, Bonanni L, et al. Donepezil, rivastigmine, vitamin E in Alzheimer's disease: a combined P300 event related potentials-neuropsychological tests evaluation over 6 months. Clin Neuropharmacol 2001;1:31-42.
[62] Onofrj M, Thomas A, Luciano AL, et al. Donepezil versus vitamin E in Alzheimer's disease part 2: mild versus moderate-severe Alzheimer's disease. Clin Neuropharmacol 2002;4:207-215.
[63] Cummings JL. Cholinesterase inhibitors: a new class of psychotropic compounds. Am J Psychiatry 2000;57:613-620.
[64] Anzellotti F, Bonanni L, Iorio E, Di Baldassarre F, D'Andreagiovanni A, Monaco D, Thomas A, Onofrj M. Delayed blink reflex in dementia with Lewy bodies is sensitive to cholinergic modulation. Clin Neuropharmacol. 2008;31:231-7.
[65] Galasko D, Abramson I, Corey-Bloom J, et al. Repeated exposure to the Mini-Mental State Examination and the Information-Memory-Concentration Test results n a practice effect in Alzheimer's disease. Neurology 1993;43:1559-1563.
[66] Shea C, MacKnight C, Rockwood K. Donepezil for treatment of dementia with Lewy bodies: a case series of nine patients. Int Psychogeriatr 1998;10: 229-238.
[67] McKeith IG, Grace JB, Walker Z, et al. Rivastigmine in the treatment of dementia with Lewy bodies: preliminary findings from an open trial. Int J Geriatr Psychiatry 2000;15:387-392.
[68] Lippa CF, Smith TW, Swearer JM. Alzheimer's disease and Lewy body disease: a comparative clinicopathological study. Ann Neurol 1994;35: 81-88.

[69] Lippa CF, Johnson R, Smith TW. The medial temporal lobe in dementia with Lewy bodies: a comparative study with Alzheimer's disease. Ann Neurol 1998;43: 102-106.
[70] Wild R, Pettit T, Burns A. Cholinesterase inhibitors for dementia with Lewy bodies. Cochrane review, The Cochrane Collaboration. The Cochrane Library 2007, Issue 1.
[71] Bohnen NI, Kaufer DI, Ivanco LS, et al. Cortical cholinergic function is more severely affected in parkinsonian dementia than in Alzheimer Disease: an in vivo positron emission tomographic study. Arch Neurol 2003;60:1745-1748.
[72] Perry EK, Irving D, Kerwin JM, et al. Cholinergic transmitter and neurotrophic activities in Lewy body dementia: similarity to Parkinson's and distinction from Alzheimer Disease. Alzheimer Dis Assoc Disord 1993;7:69-79.
[73] Tiraboschi P, Hansen LA, Alford M, et al. Cholinergic dysfunction in disease with Lewy bodies. Neurology 2000;54:407-411.
[74] Ballard C, O'Brien J, Gray A, Cormack F, Ayre G, Rowan E, et al. Attention and fluctuating attention in patients with dementia with Lewy bodies and Alzheimer disease. Arch Neurol 2001;58:977-82.
[75] Roks G, Korf ES, van der Flier WM, Scheltens P, Stam CJ. The use of EEG in the diagnosis of dementia with Lewy bodies. J Neurol Neurosurg Psychiatry 2008;79:377-80.
[76] Coben LA, Danziger WL, Berg L. Frequency analysis of the resting awake EEG in mild senile dementia of Alzheimer type. Electroencephalogr Clin Neurophysiol 1983;55:372–80.
[77] Barber PA, Varma AR, Lloyd JJ, Haworth B, Snowden JS, Neary D. The electroencephalogram in dementia with Lewy bodies. Acta Neurol Scand 2000;101:53-6.
[78] Briel RCG, McKeith IG, Barker WA, Hewitt Y, Perry RH, Ince PG, Fairbairn AF. EEG findings in dementia with Lewy bodies and Alzheimer's disease. J Neurol Neurosurg Psychiatry 1999;66:401-3.
[79] Rodriguez G, Copello F, Vitali P, Perego G, Nobili F. EEG profile to stage Alzheimer's disease. Clin Neurophysiol 1999;110:1831-7.
[80] Franciotti R, Iacono D, Della Penna S, Pizzella V, Torquati K, Onofrj M, Romani GL. Cortical rhythms reactivity in AD, LBD and normal subjects: A quantitative MEG study. Neurobiol Aging 2006;27:1100-9.
[81] Fantini ML, Gagnon JF, Petit D, Rompre S, Decary A, Carrier J, Montplaisir J. Slowing of electroencephalogram in rapid eye movement sleep behavior disorder. Ann Neurol 2003;53:774-80.
[82] Massicotte-Marquez J, Carrier J, Decary A, Mathieu A, Vendette M, Petit D, Montplaisir J Slow-wave sleep and delta power in rapid eye movement sleep behavior disorder. Ann Neurol 2005;57:277-82.
[83] Karnaze DS, Marshall LF, Bickford RG. EEG monitoring of clinical coma: the compressed spectral array. Neurology 1982;32:289-92.
[84] Mattia D, Babiloni F, Romigi A, Cincotti F, Bianchi L, Sperli F, Placidi F, Bozzao A, Giacomini P, Floris R, Grazia Marciani M. Quantitative EEG and dynamic

susceptibility contrast MRI in Alzheimer's disease: a correlative study. Clin Neurophysiol 2003;114:1210-6.
[85] Braune S, Reinhardt M, Bathmann J, Krause T, Lehmann M, Lucking CH. Impaired cardiac uptake of meta-[123i]iodobenzylguanidine in Parkinson's disease with autonomic failure. Acta Neurol Scand. 1998;97:307–314.
[86] Courbon F, Brefel-Courbon C, Thalamas C, et al. Cardiac MIBG scintigraphy is a sensitive tool for detecting cardiac sympathetic denervation in Parkinson's disease. Mov Disord. 2003;18:890–897.
[87] Wakabayashi K, Takahashi H. Neuropathology of autonomic nervous system in parkinson's disease. Eur. Neurol. 1997;38(Suppl 2):2–7.
[88] Ballard C, Ziabreva I, Perry R, et al. 2006. Differences in neuropathologic characteristics across the Lewy body dementia spectrum. Neurology 67: 1931–1934.
[89] Edison P, Rowe CC, Rinne JO, et al. 2008. Amyloid load in Parkinson's disease dementia and Lewy body dementia measured with [11C]PIB positron emission tomography. J Neurol Neurosurg Psychiatr 79: 1331- 1338.
[90] Gomperts SN, Rentz DM, Moran E, et al. 2008. Imaging amyloid deposition in Lewy body diseases. Neurology 71: 903–910.
[91] Gilman S, Koeppe RA, Little R, et al. Striatal monoamine terminals in Lewy body dementia and Alzheimer's disease. Ann Neurol 2004;55:774–780.
[92] Fearnley JM, Lees AJ. Ageing and Parkinson's disease: substantia nigra regional selectivity. Brain 1991;114:2283–2301.
[93] McKeith I, O'Brien J, Walker Z, et al. Sensitivity and specificity of dopamine transporter imaging with 123I-FP-CIT SPECT in dementia with Lewy bodies: a phase III, multicentre study. Lancet Neurol 2007;6:305–313.
[94] O'Brien JT, McKeith IG, Walker Z, et al. Diagnostic accuracy of 123I-FP-CIT SPECT in possible dementia with Lewy bodies. Br J Psychiatry 2009;194:34–39.
[95] Varela F, Lachaux JP, Rodriguez E, Martinerie J. The brainweb: phase synchronization and large-scale integration. Nat Rev Neurosci 2001;2:229–39.
[96] Uhlhaas PJ, Singer W. Neural synchrony in brain disorders: relevance for cognitive dysfunctions and pathophysiology. Neuron 2006;52:155–68.
[97] Pekkonen E, Ahveninen J, Virtanen J, Teräväinen H. Parkinson's disease selectively impairs preattentive auditory processing: an MEG study. Neuroreport 1998;9: 2949–52.
[98] Silberstein P, Pogosyan A, Kuhn AA, Hotton G, Tisch S, Kupsch A, et al. Corticocortical coupling in Parkinson's disease and its modulation by therapy. Brain 2005;128:1277–91.
[99] Stoffers D, Bosboom JLW, Deijen JB, Wolters ECh, Stam CJ, Berendse HW. Increased cortico-cortical functional connectivity in early-stage Parkinson's disease: an MEG study. Neuroimage 2008;41:212–22.
[100] Bosboom JL, Stoffers D, Wolters ECh, Stam CJ, Berendse HW. MEG resting state functional connectivity in Parkinson's disease related dementia. J Neural Transm. 2009;116:193-202.

[101] Stam CJ, Jones BF, Manshanden I, van Cappellen van Walsum AM, Montez T, Verbunt JPA, et al. Magnetoencephalographic evaluation of resting-state functional connectivity in Alzheimer's disease. Neuroimage 2006;32:1335–44.
[102] Berendse HW, Stam CJ. Stage-dependent patterns of disturbed neural synchrony in Parkinson's disease. Parkinsonism Relat Disord 2007;13:S440–5.
[103] Zotev VS, Matlashov AN, Volegov PL, Savukov IM, Espy MA, Mosher JC, et al. Microtesla MRI of the human brain combined with MEG. J Magn Reson 2008;194:115–20.
[104] Reijneveld JC, Ponten SC, Berendse HW, Stam CJ. The application of graph theoretical analysis to complex networks in the brain. Clin Neurophysiol 2007;118:2317–31.

# 16

# How fMRI Technology Contributes to the Advancement of Research in Mental Imagery: A Review

Marta Olivetti Belardinelli[1,2], Massimiliano Palmiero[3] and Rosalia Di Matteo[2,4]
[1]*Department of Psychology, "Sapienza" University of Rome*
[2]*ECONA, Interuniversity Centre for Research on Cognitive Processing in Natural and Artificial System*
[3]*Department of Internal Medicine and Public Health, University of L'Aquila*
[4]*Department of Neuroscience & Imaging, "G. d'Annunzio" University, Chieti*
*Italy*

## 1. Introduction

Mental imagery involves the generation of images using information stored in long-term memory, as opposed to the extemporaneous registration of information by our senses, giving rise to introspective experiences, such as 'seeing with the mind's eye', 'hearing with the mind's ear', 'smelling with the mind's nose'. In the past four decades, there has been much debate regarding the extent to which key elements of perception rely upon mental images versus propositional knowledge of sensory principles. Two contrasting approaches were developed i.e. perceptual and propositional theories. According to the perceptual approach, mental imagery is supported by mechanisms and processes involved in the actual perception. It functions as a modal analogue of that which is perceived by the senses (Kosslyn et al., 2006). Thus, mental images resemble perceptual information, e.g., visual images preserve both pictorial and spatial properties. According to the propositional approach, mental imagery is supported by abstract symbols of the sort used in a language-like system. It functions as an a-modal description of the external world (Anderson & Bower, 1973; Pylyshyn, 1981, 2002, 2003). In particular, mental images rely on a code, structured by rules and relationships, rather than on mere verbal descriptions. Therefore, these mental images are epiphenomena of thought: instead of exhibiting the sensory aspects that determine their analogical nature, they are affected by "cognitive permeability," or the tacit knowledge of physical laws in the external world (Pylyshyn, 1981, 2002).
These perspectives have primarily been investigated using visual imagery as a reference modality. After many years of behavioral research, the debate reached an impasse, as empirical evidence could only be explained by considering one of the two competitive approaches at a time (Kosslyn, 1980). The advent of neuroimaging techniques, particularly fMRI, offered the scientific community a new opportunity to solve the imagery debate. Unlike previous neuroimaging techniques, fMRI is capable of isolating many simultaneous and coordinated brain events with high spatial resolution. This facilitates the delineation of

brain anatomy, which increases sensitivity while maintaining selectivity. In comparison to Positron Emission Tomography (PET), fMRI offers increased statistical power for two reasons: first, the activation maps from multiple individuals do not need to be averaged, and the spatial transformation is not necessary, providing an enormous advantage in terms of signal-to-noise ratios (Watson et al., 1993); second, scanning can easily be extended over time.

Because of these advantages, fMRI has been used extensively to identify brain structures uniquely involved in cognitive functions, included mental imagery. This accordingly makes fMRI more suitable than PET and Single Photon Emission Computer Tomography (SPECT) for examining the extent to which imagery and perception share overlapping cortical areas in the functioning of various sensory modalities. In exploring this issue, researchers aimed to clarify whether imagery involves the activation of primary sensory cortices in visual, auditory, tactile, olfactory, gustatory, motor, and proprioceptive modalities. The present review is therefore aimed at investigating the status of fMRI research in all imagery modalities, with separate sections for each imagery modality, followed by collective conclusions.

## 2. Visual iImagery

Visual imagery relies on the "mind's eye" and has traditionally been associated with the visual buffer (Kosslyn, 1980) or the visuo-spatial sketchpad of working memory (Baddeley & Loogie, 1992). In particular, Kosslyn (1980, 1994) proposed that visual imagery of a known object is generated from a semantic representation that accesses stored visual information about the object. This visual information is then loaded into a short-term "visual buffer", which functions as a coordinate space that temporarily maintains and manipulates information. Though some constraints are present, research has found that visual mental images can be rotated (Shepard & Metzler, 1971), scaled (Larsen & Bundesen, 1978), scanned (Kosslyn et al., 1978), transformed in shape and color (Dixon & Just, 1978), and inspected (Thompson et al., 2008).

Although these studies appeared to lead to the conclusion that visual imagery and visual perception share common mechanisms and processes, fMRI was used to clarify that the recruitment of the primary visual cortex (calcarine fissure - BA 17) may vary according to different factors. In a previous review Kosslyn & Thompson (2003) suggested that this contradiction in the literature may be accounted for by the fact that the primary visual cortex can be activated when the sensitivity of the neuroimaging technique is high (e.g., using fMRI rather than PET), and when inspecting details of visual mental images with high resolution to visualize shapes rather than spatial patterns. Amedi et al. (2005) later demonstrated that deactivating the auditory cortex, as measured by BOLD functional magnetic resonance imaging, may differentiate between visual imagery and visual perception. During visual imagery, the deactivation of the auditory cortex is negatively correlated with the activation of the visual cortex as well as with scores on the subjective Vividness of Visual Imagery Questionnaire (VVIQ) (Marks, 1973). When using fMRI, however, primary visual cortex activity correlated with the reported vividness of visual images when participants were instructed to visualize themselves or another person either bench pressing or stair climbing (Cui et al., 2007), or imagining concrete objects (e.g., to see a bucket) (Olivetti et al., 2009).

Under specific circumstances visual mental images seem to involve neural mechanisms recruited by visual perception, as evidenced by the fact that the lateral geniculate nucleus is activated during visual imagery (Chen et al., 1998). Ganis et al. (2004) clarified, however, that when participants were instructed to either imagine or see faint drawings of simple objects, and then judge specific aspects of the drawings, such as 'taller than wider', visual imagery and visual perception recruited similar neural machinery, especially in frontal and parietal regions. Though the calcarine cortex was activated in both conditions, this spatial overlap was neither complete nor uniform.

The spatial overlap observed during imagery and perception does not necessarily imply that the corresponding representations are qualitatively similar to each other. Reddy et al. (2010) accordingly explored the extent to which it is possible to establish which item participants were imaging, as well as the comparability between representations evoked during imagery and visual perception. Participants were instructed to both imagine and see stimuli belonging to four object categories: food, tools, faces, buildings. By using pattern classification techniques, which test each classifier (perceptual or imagery) on the other condition, authors were capable to decode category information from ventro-temporal cortex in both imagery and perceptual conditions, but only during actual viewing from visual primary area. Using the same logic, Stokes et al. (2009) found similar results, revealing that imagery of the letter X versus the letter O could be decoded from the lateral occipital complex.

## 3. Auditory imagery

Intons-Peterson (1992, p. 46) defined auditory imagery as "the introspective persistence of an auditory experience, including one constructed from components drawn from long-term memory, in the absence of direct sensory instigation of that experience". This type of imagery runs auditory traces from prior experiences (e.g., someone's voice, environmental sounds, melodies) through the "mind's ear". In this section, the fMRI studies on auditory verbal imagery will be presented first, followed by auditory imagery of environmental sounds, and musical imagery will be discussed last.

### 3.1 Auditory verbal imagery

Auditory verbal imagery can occur spontaneously or deliberately when recalling the sound of our own voice or someone else's voice. Within the frame of working memory, auditory verbal imagery has been associated with the operation of the phonological loop sub-system (Baddeley & Loogie, 1992). Two components have been discerned: a short-lived store that represents material in phonological form (inner ear), and an articulatory rehearsal process (inner voice) that is used to recode and refresh decaying representations into the phonological store (Smith et al., 1995).

By using fMRI, Shergill et al. (2001) found that there is a lack of activation in the primary auditory cortex (Heschel gyrus - BA 41/42) during auditory verbal imagery. Relative to the baseline condition (listening to each word carefully), first person imagery (imagining sentences of the form "I like..." in ones' own voice) showed no activation in the auditory cortex, while second and third person imagery (imagining sentences of the form "You like...." and "He likes...." in voices that participants had heard on a tape) showed activation in the secondary auditory cortex (BA 22), namely in the superior temporal gyrus. Jancke &

Shah (2004) also showed that the primary auditory cortex was not activated during auditory verbal imagery. Relative to the resting condition, imagining hearing a syllable (e.g., Ka, Ta, Pa) yielded activation in the bilateral superior temporal gyri, including the planum temporale, and the dorsal bank of the superior temporal sulcus. By exploring the fMRI correlates of auditory verbal imagery associated with the phonological processing of words, Aleman et al. (2005) confirmed the lack of activation of the primary auditory cortex. Participants were presented with bi-syllabic words and were required to indicate the syllable that carried the stress, discriminating between weak-initial words and strong-initial words. In the perceptual condition, words were delivered by headphones, whereas in the imagery condition, words were presented on a screen and participants were instructed to imagine hearing the word being spoken by another person. Results revealed that both perceptual and imagery conditions activated the bilateral supplementary motor area, bilateral post-central gyrus, bilateral insula, the left inferior frontal gyrus (Broca's area), the posterior left superior temporal sulcus/superior temporal gyrus, and the left intra-parietal sulcus/superior parietal lobule. Kim et al. (2008) reported a deactivation in the left superior temporal cortex (BA 22/42) and anterior cingulated cortex during auditory verbal imagery of another's remarks expressed toward self, which were derogatory in content, relative to auditory verbal imagery of another's remarks expressed toward self, which were non-derogatory and neutral in content. In addition, activation was found in both medial frontal cortex, left inferior frontal cortex, both pre-central gyrus, both inferior parietal lobule, right occipital-temporal cortex, left occipital cortex, both posterior insula, and both amigdala.

### 3.2 Auditory imagery of environmental sounds

This type of auditory imagery can occur spontaneously or deliberately when recalling the sound produced by environmental objects or auditory sources, such as the ringing of the phone, the shot of a gun, or sound produced by animals. In this direction, Olivetti Belardinelli et al. (2004a) investigated the neural correlates of mental imagery in different sensory modalities, including the auditory modality, by contrasting imagery sentences (e.g., hearing a shot) with abstract sentences (e.g., the power of reason). Relative to the abstract condition, there was no activation found in the primary auditory cortex during auditory imagery. There was, however, activity in the left middle temporal gyrus (BA 22/37), left inferior temporal gyrus (BA 37), left inferior-middle frontal gyrus, left inferior parietal lobule, and left insula. Using the same methodology, Olivetti Belardinelli et al. (2009) found a bilateral activation in the Heschl's gyrus comparing high-vivid participants with low-vivid participants in generating auditory images of environmental sounds, and in the right hemisphere of the same gyrus regressing the vividness scores of auditory images onto the bold signal. These activations, however, were not significant at the corrected threshold for multiple comparisons. Significant activations were found in the left middle frontal gyrus, right angular gyrus, right posterior cingulate, and left lingual gyrus. Authors explained the lack of significant modality-specific activation in the Heschl's gyrus in the light of the interference of the scanner noise on the auditory image formation process, which may have led to signal decrease solely in the primary auditory cortex, as showed by Gaab et al. (2007). Nonetheless, Bunzeck et al. (2005) used the fMRI technique and did not find any activation of the primary auditory cortex during imagery of familiar complex environmental sounds, either. Compared to watching a silent scrambled movie of familiar scenes (control condition), watching familiar scenes and listening to the corresponding sounds (perception condition) yielded activations in the bilateral Heschl's gyrus, superior temporal gyrus, and left fusiform gyrus, and planum temporale. In contrast, the imagery condition consisted of watching the same movies presented in the perception condition but without the appropriate sounds, which had to be imagined by the participants. This condition elicited bilateral hemodynamic responses only in the right superior temporal gyrus, including the bilateral planum temporale.

### 3.3 Musical imagery

Musical imagery is a type of auditory imagery that relies upon the capacity to mentally conceptualize songs, tunes, and general musical input. Musical imagery processes the tempo, temporal extension (Halpern, 1988), pitch (loudness) (Intons-Peterson Russell & Dressel, 1992), and timbre (sound quality of different instruments or voices) of real music (Pitt & Crowder, 1992). The first event-related fMRI study showed activation in the bilateral primary and secondary auditory areas in the superior temporal gyri when participants imagined a single computer-generated note (Yoo et al., 2001). The results also revealed significant activation in the medial and inferior frontal gyri, precuneus, middle frontal gyri, superior temporal gyri, and anterior cingulate gyri. This suggests that fMRI may be sensitive at least to the activation caused by simple internally generated sounds. This study, however, had no control conditions or task validation, and did not isolate timbre. Halpern et al. (2004) examined musical imagery of timbre relative to the visual imagery control. They found that the former activated the posterior temporal cortex, but not the primary auditory cortex, whereas the perception condition (judgments of the timbres of sounds) activated primary and secondary auditory areas with some right-sided asymmetry.

No activation was found in the primary auditory cortex during musical imagery, even in musicians. Langheim et al. (2002) asked to musicians to imagine musical performances for 30 seconds alternated with resting periods. Relative to the resting condition, musical imagery activated supplementary motor and pre-motor areas, right superior parietal lobule, right inferior frontal gyrus, bilateral mid-frontal gyri, and bilateral lateral cerebellum. Yet, Lotze et al. (2003) did not find any activation of the primary auditory cortex when asking amateurs and professional violinists to mentally perform Mozart's "Violin concerto in G major" (KV216). During the musical imagery condition, professionals recruited the supplementary motor area, the superior premotor cortex, anterior areas (Larsell's lobule HVI) in the left cerebellar hemisphere, and bilateral superior parietal areas. Latter Zatorre et al. (2010) carried out two fMRI experiments with musicians. Participants were presented with the first few notes of a familiar tune (Experiment 1) or its title (Experiment 2), followed by a string of notes that was either an exact or an inexact reversal. The task was to judge whether the second string was correct or not by mentally reversing all its notes, which required both maintenance and manipulation of the represented string. During the reversal process, neither experiment showed activation of the primary auditory cortex, but both showed activation of the superior parietal lobe (intraparietal sulcus). Ventrolateral and dorsolateral frontal cortices were also activated, consistent with the memory load required during the task. Authors interpreted these results in the context of other mental transformation tasks, such as mental rotation in the visual domain, which are known to recruit the intraparietal sulcus region.

Kraemer et al. (2005) conducted the only fMRI study that showed activation in the primary auditory cortex. In this study, participants were asked to listen to excerpts of songs with lyrics and instrumentals with no lyrics. Each piece of music was pre-rated by subjects as either familiar or unknown. Short sections of music (lasting for 2–5 s) were extracted at different points during the soundtrack and replaced with silent gaps. Participants were instructed to continue imaging the musical selection. Results revealed that imaging the continuation of familiar songs induced greater activation in auditory association areas than imaging the continuation of unknown songs (in both songs with lyrics and without lyrics). Moreover, when familiar songs contained no lyrics, cortical activity extended into the left primary auditory cortex. However, authors revealed that neural activation during lyrics were in the auditory association areas, whereas with instrumental music, neural activity extended to the primary auditory cortex.

## 4. Tactile imagery

Tactile imagery can be considered part of the haptic system, based on sensors in skin, muscles, tendons, and joints (Klatzky et al., 1991). Similar to other modalities, Craig & Rollman (1999) included the tactile sense as part of the working memory system, characterized by 3 different processing stages: retention up to 500 ms after stimulus offset; vivid recollections of uncategorized stimulus information, with interfering tasks affecting process until approximately 5 s after stimulus offset. The rehearsal mechanisms would last up to 30 seconds after stimulus offset (Burton & Sinclair, 2000).

Few fMRI studies were conducted to clarify the neural correlates of tactile imagery (Falgatter et al., 1997). Querleux et al. (1999) found that during the imagination of tactile stimulation, activation was mostly localized in the ipsilateral somato-sensory cortex (post-parietal gyrus - BA 1/2/3). During a period of tactile perception, there was a strong activation in the contra-lateral cortex. Yoo et al. (2003) demonstrated that the left primary (post-central gyrus - BA 1/2/3) and left secondary somatosensory areas (frontal operculum, area 43) were activated when participants imagined a tactile stimulation on the back of the right hand, relative to resting condition. Although the left primary and secondary somatosensory areas were modulated by the mental imagery of tactile sensation, a significant portion of the activation occurred solely during the actual perception. In Yoo et al. (2003), tactile imagery also selectively activated the inferior parietal lobule. Olivetti Belardinelli et al. (2004a) found activation in the inferior parietal lobule, but not in the primary or secondary somatosensory cortex, during the imagination of tactile properties of objects when verbally cued (e.g., to touch something grainy), as compared to the abstract condition. Yet, Olivetti Belardinelli et al. (2009) demonstrated that the primary somatosensory cortex (right parietal post-central gyrus - BA 2), as well as the right post-central gyrus (BA 5) were more activated in high-vivid participants compared to low-vivid participants. In other words, the level of vividness of tactile imagery can modulate the activation of primary somatosensory cortex. This study also revealed that the inferior occipital cortex (BA 18) was strongly activated in high-vivid participants.

## 5. Motor imagery

Motor (or kinaesthetic) imagery is the result of first-person kinaesthetic information processing, as people feel themselves executing a given action (Jeannerod, 1995). This experience is called internal imagery or first-person perspective, which is different from the representation of the external imagery or third person perspective, in which information processing involves the visualization of spatial components of the perceived world (Ruby & Decety, 2001).

Various studies using fMRI have yielded contrasting results regarding the involvement of primary motor cortex during motor imagery. On one hand, the first studies revealed bilateral supplementary motor area and pre-motor activations, without an increase in signal intensity in the primary motor cortex (pre-central gyrus - BA 4) or somatosensory cortex during self-paced complex finger movements (Rao et al., 1993) or sequential finger opposition movements (Tyszka et al., 1994). However, using stance and locomotion (walking and running) imagery condition (Jahn et al., 2004), complex imagery actions (e.g., running) (Olivetti Belardinelli et al., 2004a), mental training-related changes on a finger-tapping task (Nyberg et al., 2006), and fingers or objects movements imagery task (Lorey et al., 2010), there was no reported activity in the primary motor cortex. Even when participants were instructed to imagine using a common tool, such as the brush for an action related to the hair, activity was observed in the pre-motor cortex, posterior part of the parietal cortex, and cerebellum, but not in the primary motor cortex (Higuchi et al., 2007). On the other hand, there was activity in the primary motor cortex more reduced for motor imagery than for actual performance (Fieldman et al., 1993). In particular, the primary motor cortex was activated during the mental execution of movements with either the left or right hand (Dechent et al., 2004; Lotze et al., 1999; Porro et al., 1996; Roth et al., 1996), when participants were instructed to imagine a right-hand self-paced button press sequence before (novel condition) and after (skilled condition) one week of intensive physical practice (Lacourse et al., 2005), when participants imagined dancing Tango after five training days (Sacco et al., 2006), when participants were instructed to imagine complex everyday movements (e.g., eating a meal, swimming) (Szameitat et al., 2007), or situations involving actions cued by appropriate motor phrases (e.g., to cut) (Tomasino et al., 2007). Sharma, Jones, Carpenter, & Baron (2008) likewise revealed that both the anterior and posterior primary motor area can be bilaterally activated when imaging a finger opposition sequence (2, 3, 4, 5; paced at 1 hz). According to these authors, the role of the primary motor area and its subdivisions may be non-executive, perhaps related to spatial encoding. Recently, Olivetti Belardinelli et al. (2009) demonstrated that primary motor cortex can be activated in high-vivid participants rather than in low-vivid participants, but did not confirm the same activation when motor imagery vividness was regressed onto the BOLD signal, showing activation for only the left pre-central gyrus (BA 6), the right medial frontal gyrus (BA 6), and the inferior parietal lobule. Nevertheless, even considering the studies showing the activation of the primary motor area during motor imagery, it should be noted that the majority of these experiments did not employ electrophysiological monitoring to exclude muscle contractions during scanning. To exclude this possible confounding factor, Takashi et al. (2003) employed electromyographic monitoring within the scanner while participants performed sequential finger-tapping movements in response to visually presented number stimuli in either a movement or an imagery mode of performance. Results revealed that the movement condition activated the primary sensory and motor areas, parietal operculum, anterior cerebellum, caudal pre-motor areas, and area 5 that had mild-to-moderate imagery-related activity, whereas the motor imagery condition yielded the activation of the pre-central sulcus at the level of middle frontal gyrus (BA 6/44), and the posterior superior parietal cortex/pre-cuneus (BA 7), and bilateral cerebellum. Moreover, activity of the

superior pre-central sulcus and intra-parietal sulcus areas, predominantly on the left, was associated with the accuracy of the imagery task performance.
However, the fMRI approach based on "effective connectivity" between network components, defined as the influence of one neural system over another, clarified the issue of the primary motor cortex activation during motor imagery. In particular, Solodikin et al. (2004) demonstrated the connectivity between the supplementary motor area and the primary motor cortex during motor imagery. By using structural equation modelling to estimate the effective connectivity networks underlying motor execution, visual mental imagery, and kinesthetic mental imagery with specified regions of interests, Solodikin et al., (2004) showed that the inputs from the supplementary motor area and lateral–dorsal pre-motor cortex to the primary motor cortex had a suppressing effect during motor imagery. These results suggest a physiological mechanism encompassing the prevention of overt movements. Using Dynamic Causal Modeling, Kasess et al. (2008) confirmed that the activity of the primary motor cortex was heavily suppressed by the supplementary motor area during motor imagery, namely imagine pressing buttons on a small panel, first with the index finger, then the middle finger, and again with the index finger, as rapidly as possible. Then, by using the Granger Causality Mapping method, Chen et al. (2009) found forward and backward connectivity between the supplementary motor area and the contra-lateral primary motor cortex during both the left- and right-hand motor imagery (finger tapping sequences cued by pictures). Gao et al. (2011) extended these results revealing the influence of the brain asymmetry of right-handedness on effective connectivity networks: left dorsal pre-motor cortex, inferior parietal lobule, and superior parietal lobule were identified as causal sources in both motor imagery and motor execution.

## 6. Olfactory imagery

Olfactory mental images can be defined as short-term memory representations of olfactory events that give rise to the experience of smelling with the "mind's nose" (Rinck et al., 2009). However, experimental evidence about the existence of olfactory imagery is controversial given that it is not clear whether an olfactory mental image is semantically or perceptually mediated, or whether it reflects the influence of explicit knowledge of olfactory principles rather than a specific mode of operation of odour imagery (Elmes, 1998; Herz, 2000). Using fMRI, Levy et al. (1999), and Henkin & Levy (2002) found a substantial overlap in the areas activated by real and imagined stimuli (ripe banana and peppermint), although all activations were reduced in the imagery condition. However, given the lack of anatomical details, it is not possible to draw reliable conclusions from these two studies. Later, Olivetti Belardinelli et al. (2004a) found activation in the left insula, but not in the primary olfactory area, when the olfactory imagery condition was contrasted with the abstract condition. The lack of activity in the primary olfactory cortex was also observed when high-vivid participants were contrasted with low-vivid participants (Olivetti Belardinelli et al., 2009). In Olivetti et. al.'s studies, the olfactory-specific modality activations likely were not found because of the difficulty in generating vivid images of smells, especially when they are verbally cued (Herz, 2000). This is confirmed by Zelano et al. (2009), who found that remembering nameable odorants was reflected in sustained activity in prefrontal language areas, and remembering unnameable odorants was reflected in sustained activity in primary olfactory cortex. In other words, only smells dissociated from their verbal label were eligible to activate the primary olfactory cortex.

In the past few years, the role of the piriform cortex during olfactory imagery was reconsidered according to two points of view: retrieval-related processes and expertise. First, it was surmised that piriform cortex activation reflects retrieval-related olfactory "imagery" processes (Elmes, 1998; Bensafi et al., 2003). Because odour imagery was shown to elicit sniffing (Bensafi et al., 2003), which in turn can elicit activation in piriform cortex (Sobel et al., 1998), it is possible that the piriform activity indicates odour imagery associated with sniffing. In an fMRI study, Bensafi et al. (2007) evoked hedonic-specific activity in piriform cortex by asking participants to sniff during the perception and imagination of a pleasant odour (strawberry) and an unpleasant odour (rotten eggs). In particular, activity induced by imagining odours mimicked that induced by perceiving real odours, and for both real and imagined odours, unpleasant stimuli induced greater activity than pleasant stimuli in the left frontal portion of piriform cortex and left insula. Regarding the expertise issue, it was also surmised that experience with odours plays a key role for the reorganization of brain regions involved in olfactory imagery. In fact, Plailly et al. (2011) revealed that expertise plays a key role: olfactory imagery activated the primary olfactory (piriform) cortex, as well as the orbitofrontal cortex, and the hippocampus during the creation of mental images of odours by professional perfumers.

## 7. Gustatory imagery

Gustatory imagery refers to the ability to generate mental images of tastes. Although gustatory imagery is involved in food craving, or the "irresistible urge to consume" (Tiggemenn & Kemps, 2005), which in turn may have implications for clinical and non-clinical population, relatively little experimental research has been devoted to this imagery system. It is also uncertain whether proper gustatory mental imagery can be evoked, and to what extent images of tastes activate the primary gustatory cortex. In an fMRI study, Kobayashi et al. (2004) instructed their participants to perceive (water stimuli) and imagine several tastes (grapefruit, candy, pudding, coffee, lemon, banana, beer, sugar). Images were verbally cued by written words, by spoken language, and by using pictures. In general, results revealed that gustatory imagery can activate the primary gustatory cortex (anterior insula/frontal operuculm), especially the left side, sharing common parts of neural substrates with gustatory perception. Authors also clarified that the middle and superior frontal gyri were not activated by gustatory perception, but they participated in the generation of gustatory images, plausibly mediating the top-down control of retrieving gustatory information from the storage of long-term memories. The activation of the anterior insula and the middle frontal gyri during gustatory imagery (the spicy taste, the tart taste, etc) were confirmed also by Olivetti Belardinelli et al. (2004a) relative to an abstract condition, and by Olivetti Belardinelli et al. (2009) according to the level of vividness of participants. Finally, Kikuki et al. (2005) revealed that when participants concentrated on pickled plums (umeboshi), a traditional Japanese food with a strong and sour taste, activations were observed weakly in the right insula, but more strongly in the bilateral opercula, the bilateral orbitofrontal cortices, and the left Broca's area.

## 8. Proprioceptive imagery

Proprioceptive processing is part of the haptic system. In particular, proprioceptive imagery involves the ability to generate organic images based on body sensations, such as the sensations of hungry, thirsty, cold, drunkenness, etc. Very few fMRI studies were devoted to proprioceptive imagery. Olivetti Belardinelli et al. (2004a) did not show any activation of the primary somatosensory cortex during proprioceptive imagery, whereas Olivetti Belardinelli et al. (2009) revealed that high vivid participants activated the right post-central gyrus (BA 2/3) during proprioceptive imagery in comparison with low-vivid participants.

## 9. Conclusions

Compared to previous neuroimaging techniques, fMRI technology has generally improved our understanding of neural networks involved in mental imagery in all sensory modalities. The higher sensitivity of fMRI allowed researchers to better differentiate between primary and secondary sensory cortices, whereas the extreme flexibility of scanning procedures allowed the implementation of different imagery paradigms, which likewise has implications for the imagery debate issue.

Several, several conclusions can be made from the fMRI literature reviewed above. First, the involvement of the primary sensory cortices varies according to the imagery modality investigated, and may be modulated by different factors, such as the individual differences in generating mental images or expertise, tasks, types of paradigms, or analyses employed. Second, the activation of the secondary sensory cortices in all imagery modalities is more consistent, as well as the recruitment of pre-frontal areas or associative cortices, the former plausibly participating in the top-down processes which are executed for retrieving information from long-term memory, the latter facilitating supra-modal processing of sensory information. This picture is partially in contrast with the perceptual approach, which assumes that mental images correspond with percepts and events also in terms of both mechanisms and processes used. It also supports the propositional approach, which assumes an amodal format for all types of mental images. Indeed, when generating mental images, the human brain seems to rely mostly on secondary sensory cortices rather than primary ones, clearly indicating that imagery and perception rely on overlapping but dissociable neural networks.

Looking separately at the relevant fMRI literature on imagery modalities, more detailed information can be obtained. First, fMRI showed that under specific conditions, visual imagery corresponds to the isolated activation of visual cortical areas, including the primary one, with concurrent deactivation of irrelevant sensory processing (Amedi et al., 2005). However, the overlap between visual imagery and visual perception is more consistent in the frontal and temporal cortices (Ganis et al., 2004) or ventro-temporal cortex (Reddy et al., 2010), rather than in the occipital cortex. The insights for visual imagery cannot be simply generalized, given the different sensory characteristics of percepts, as well as the roles that each imagery system can play in the cognitive system.

Indeed, fMRI literature showed that auditory verbal imagery relies mostly on the secondary auditory cortex, left inferior frontal cortex, supplementary motor area, and inferior parietal areas, rather than the primary auditory cortex. The former regions were found to be involved in the verbal perception domain: particularly, left pre-frontal areas mediate phonological recoding (Thierry et al., 1999), whereas the supplementary motor area is important for silent articulation or inner speech, and posterior superior temporal gyrus or temporo-parietal junction are involved in the acoustic-phonetic feature-based processing (Scott & Johnsrude, 2003).

Moreover, auditory imagery of environmental sounds never yielded activation in the primary auditory cortex. Even when the sparse temporal sampling technique was used to ensure that the acoustic scanner noise did not lead to interferences with the auditory perception and imagery conditions, the primary auditory cortex was not activated (Bunzeck et al., 2005). This pattern of results shows that when imaging environmental sounds the top-down process is initiated mostly by the inferior frontal gyrus and insular regions, and manages to activate only secondary auditory areas.

Still, the fMRI literature on musical imagery, with the exception of Kraemer et al. (2005), showed no activation of the primary auditory cortex, even when enrolling musicians. Given the pattern of activation yielded by musical imagery, an associative network independent of primary sensory-motor and auditory activity is likely representing the cortical elements most intimately linked to music production. In addition, considering that both amateurs and professional musicians did not report any activation in the primary auditory cortex, and that motor areas were not recruited, either, during musical imagery involving mental performances, it is highly probable that these areas become tightly coupled with executed activities during musical training. Finally, given that musical imagery in professional musicians revealed more anterior cerebellar activations, it is possible to conclude that musical imagery involves the recruitment of stored movement programs of sequential finger movements (Lotze et al., 2003).

The extent to which the primary motor cortex is involved in motor imagery remains unclear. However, recent fMRI studies have highlighted the importance of the supplementary motor area, which seems to be involved in suppressing the activity of the primary motor cortex, and consequently, movements that are not intended to be performed. This would mean that motor imagery and motor execution do not rely on the same neural network.

Regarding olfactory imagery, fMRI results are in line with behavioral findings: if images of smells are cued by verbal labels it is hard to detect the activation of the primary olfactory cortex. On the contrary, if odors are perceptually encoded, it is possible to find activation in the piriform cortex when generating images of smells. However, the activity in the olfactory primary cortex was found to be modulated by the hedonic pattern of stimuli to be imagined, and by expertise in generating or using olfactory images. This means that olfactory imagery may activate olfactory areas under specific conditions, basically when people really evoke images of smells.

The literature on gustatory, tactile, and proprioceptive imagery is more consistent. All three of these modalities seem to rely on the primary sensory cortices. Nevertheless, given the scarcity of studies carried out on these imagery systems, especially on the proprioceptive imagery, any conclusion would be premature.

In conclusion, fMRI technique has helped to clarify the neural circuits of mental imagery, but a lot a work needs to be still done. For example, the role of certain cortical areas remains unclear, as does the connectivity among cortices in mental imagery. Research is trying to clarify this issue in respect to the motor imagery modality, but it should also be addressed in respect to the others. It is also important to explore the common cortical networks involved in all imagery modalities to clarify the extent to which mental imagery relies on non-sensory cortices. Indirectly, this information would contribute to improve our understanding of the imagery debate, as having access to the common areas shared by all imagery modalities provides an understanding of the extent to which imagery involves propositional encoding. Currently, only Olivetti Belardinelli et al. (2001, 2004b) have attempted to investigate this issue. Though there has been some difference in terms of anatomical extension, results revealed that the generation of images in all sensory modalities activated the left inferior temporal cortex (including the left fusiform gyrus) and the bilateral inferior parietal lobule.

The left inferior temporal area has been associated with semantic processing (Thompson-Schill et al., 1999), and visual mental imagery (D'Esposito et al., 1997), whereas the inferior parietal lobule was linked to supra-modal transformation of information (Jordan et al., 2001). In light of the imagery debate, these results showed that the generation of mental imagery in different sensory modalities may involve visual appearance and to some extent semantic processing. Afterwards, Palmiero et al. (2009) found that, relative to the resting condition, all imagery modalities showed activity in the pre-central gyri (BA 6), likely involving pre-motor feed-forward control during imagery generation. However, it is important to develop techniques that allow researchers to be sure that images are really generated by participants in the scan. Indeed, in most studies, it is assumed that participants generated mental images, resulting in cortical activations that may reflect the lack of generation of images. It is also essential to better differentiate between pure imagery-based representations and memory-based representations, which may engage different neural networks. Finally, the inter-modal issue should also be addressed. Thus, given the above literature, it seems that mental images are mapped on the human brain according to the request of the psychological system, with implications for both thinking and performance.

## 10. References

Aleman, A., Formisano, E., Koppenhagen, H., Hagoort, P., de Haan, E.H.F. & Kahn, R.S. (2005). The functional neuroanatomy of metrical stress evaluation of perceived and imagined spoken words. *Cerebral Cortex*, Vol.15, No.2, (2005), pp. 221-228, ISSN 1047-3211

Amedi, A., Malach, R., & Pascual-Leone, A. (2005). Negative BOLD differentiates visual imagery and perception. *Neuron*, Vol. 48, No.5, (December 2005), pp. 859–872, ISSN 0896-6273

Anderson, J.R., & Bower, G.H. (1973). *Human associative memory*. Winston & Sons, ISBN 0-8058-3824-4, Washington DC, USA

Baddeley, A.D. & Logie, R. (1992). Auditory imagery and working memory. In *Auditory Imagery*, D. Reisberg, (Ed.), 179-197, Lawrence Erlbaum Associates, Inc. Publishers, ISBN 0-8058-2292-5, New Jersey, USA

Bensafi, M., Sobel, N., Khan, R.M. (2007). Hedonic-specific activity in piriform cortex during odor imagery mimics that during odor perception. *Journal of Neurophysiology*, Vol.98, (October 2007), pp. 3254–3262, ISSN 0022-3077

Bensafi, M., Porter, J., Pouliot, S., Mainland, J., Johnson, B., Zelano, C., Young, N.,Bremner, E., Aframian, D., Khan, R., & Sobel, N. (2003). Olfactomotor activity during imagery mimics that during perception. *Nature Neuroscience*, Vol.6, No.11, (October 2003), pp. 1142–1144, ISSN 1097-6256

Bunzeck, N., Wuestenberg, T., Lutz, K., Heinze, H.J., & Jancke, L. (2005). Scanning silence: Mental imagery of complex sounds. *NeuroImage*, Vol.26, No.4, (May 2005), pp. 1119-1127, ISSN 1053-8119

Burton, H, & Sinclair, R.J. (2000). Attending to and remembering tactile stimuli: A review of brain imaging data and single-neuron responses. *Journal Clinical Neurophysiology*, Vol.17, No.6, (November 2000), pp. 575-591, ISSN 0736-0258

Chen, W., Kato, T., Zhu, X.H., Ogawa, S., Tank, D.W., & Ugurbil, K. (1998). Human primary visual cortex and lateral geniculate nucleus activation during visual imagery. *NeuroReport*, Vol.9, No.16, (November 1998), pp. 3669–3674, ISSN 0959-4965

Chen, H., Yang, Q., Liao, W., Gong, Q., & Shen, S. (2009). Evaluation of the effective connectivity of supplementary motor areas during motor imagery using Granger causality mapping. *NeuroImage*, Vol.47, No.4, (October 2009), pp.1844-1853, ISSN 1053-8119

Craig, J.C, & Rollman, G.B. (1999). Somesthesis. *Annual Review of Psychology*, Vol.50, No.1, (February 1999), pp. 305-331, ISSN 0066-4308

Cui, X., Jeter, C.B., Yang, P.D., Montague, R., & Eagleman, D.M. (2007). Vividness of mental imagery: Individual variability can be measured objectively. *Vision Research*, Vol. 47, No.4, (February 2007), pp. 474–478, ISSN 0042-6989

Dechent, P., Merboldt, K.D., & Frahm, J. (2004). Is the human primary motor cortex involved in motor imagery? *Cognitive Brain Research*, Vol.19, No.2, (April 2004), pp. 138–144, ISSN 0006-8993

D'Esposito, M., Detre, J.A., Aguirre, G.K., Stallcup, M., Alsop, D.C., Tippet, L.J., & Farah, M. J. (1997). A functional MRI study of mental image generation. *Neuropsychologia*, Vol.35, No. 5 (May 1997), pp. 725-730, ISSN 0028-3932

Djordjevic, J., Zatorre, R.J., Petrides, M., Boyle, J.A., & Jones-Gotman, M. (2005). Functional neuroimaging of odor imagery. *Neuroimage*, Vol.24, No.3, (February 2005), pp.791–801, ISSN 1053-8119

Dixon, P., & Just, M.A. (1978). Normalization of irrelevant dimensions in stimulus comparisons. *Journal of Experimental Psychology: Human Perception and Performance*, Vol.4, No.1, (Febraury 1978), pp.36-46, ISSN 0096-1523

Elmes, D.G. (1998). Is there an inner nose? *Chemical Senses*, Vol.23, No.4, (1998), pp.443–445, ISSN 0379-864X

Fieldman, J.B., Cohen, L.G., Jezzard, P., Pons, T., Sadato, N., Turner, R., LeBihan, D. & Hallet, M. (1993). Proceeding of 12th Annual Meeting of the Society of Magnetic Resonance in Medicine Functional neuroimaging with echo-planar imaging in humans during execution and mental rehearsal of a simple motor task. *Proceeding of 12th Annual Meeting of the Society of Magnetic Resonance in Medicine*, p. 1416, New York USA, August, 14-20.

Gaab, N., Gabrieli, J.D., & Glover, G.H. (2007). Assessing the influence of scanner background noise on auditory processing. II. An fMRI study comparing auditory processing in the absence and presence of recorded scanner noise using a sparse design. *Human Brain Mapping*, Vol.28, No.8, (August 2007), pp.721-732, ISSN 1097-0193

Ganis, G., Thompson, W.L. & Kosslyn, S.M. (2004). Brain areas underlying visual mental imagery and visual perception: An fMRI study. *Cognitive Brain Research*, Vol.20, No.2, (July 2004), pp.226-241, ISSN 0006-8993

Gao, Q., Duan, X., & Chen, H. (2011). Evaluation of effective connectivity of motor areas during motor imagery and execution using conditional Granger causality. *NeuroImage*, Vol.54, No.2, (January 2011), pp.1280-1288, ISSN 1053-8119

Halpern, A.R. (1988). Mental scanning in auditory imagery for tunes. *Journal of Experimental Psychology: Learning, Memory and Cognition*, Vol.14, No.3, (July 1988), pp.434–443, ISSN 0278-7393

Halpern, A.R., Zatorre, R.J., Bouffard, M., & Johnson, J.A. (2004). Behavioural and neural correlates of perceived musical timbre. *Neuropsychologia*, Vol.42, No.9, (2004), pp.1281-1292, ISSN 0028-3932

Henkin, R.I., & Levy, L.M. (2002). Functional MRI of congenital hyposomia: brain activation to odors and imagination of odors and tastes. *Journal of Computer Assistant Tomography*, Vol.26, No.1, (Febraury 2002), pp.39–61, ISSN 0363-8715

Herz, R.S. (2000). Verbal coding in olfactory versus nonolfactory cognition. *Memory and Cognition*, Vol.28, No.6, (September 2000), pp.957-64, ISSN 0090-502X

Higuchi, S., Imamizu, H., & Kawato, M. (2007). Cerebellar activity evoked by common tool-use execution and imagery task: An fMRI study. *Cortex*, Vol.43, No.3, (April 2007), pp.350-358, ISSN 0010-9452

Jancke, L., & Shah, N.J. (2004). Hearing syllables by seeing visual stimuli. *European Journal of Neuroscience*, Vol.19, No.9, (May, 2004), pp.2603–2608, ISSN 0953-816X

Jahn, K., Deutschlander, A., Stephan, T., Strupp, M., Wiesmann, M., & Brandt, T. (2004). Brain activation patterns during imagined stance and locomotion in functional magnetic resonance imaging. *NeuroImage*, Vol.22, No.4, (August 2004), pp.1722–1731, ISSN 1053-8119

Jeannerod, M. (1995). Mental imagery in motor context. *Neuropshychologia*, Vol.33, No.11, (November 1995), pp.1419-1432, ISSN 0028-3932

Jordan, K., Heinze, H.J., Lutz, K., Kanawski, M. & Lanche, L. (2001). Cortical activations during the mental rotation of different visual objects. *NeuroImage*, Vol.13, No.1 (January 2001), pp.143-152, ISSN 1053-8119

Intons-Peterson, M.J. (1992). Components of auditory imagery. In *Auditory Imagery*, D. Reisberg, (Ed.), 179-197, Lawrence Erlbaum Associates, Inc. Publishers, ISBN 0-8058-2292-5, New Jersey, USA

Intons-Peterson, M.J., Russell, W. Dressel, S. (1992). The role of pitch in auditory imagery. *Journal of Experimental Psychology: Human Perception & Performance*, Vol.18, No.1, (Febraury 1992), pp. 233-240, ISSN 0096-1523

Kaas, A.L., van Mier, H. & Goebel, R. (2007). The neural correlates of human working memory for haptically explored object orientations. *Cerebral Cortex*, Vol.17, No.7, (July 2007), pp. 1637-1649, ISSN 1047-3211

Kasess, C.H., Windischberger, C., Cunnington, R., Lanzenberger, R., Pezawas, L., & Moser, E. (2008). The suppressive influence of SMA on M1 in motor imagery revealed by fMRI and dynamic causal modeling. *NeuroImage*, Vol.40, No.2, (April 2008), pp.828-837, ISSN 1053-8119

Kikuchi, S., Kubota, F., Nisijima, K., Washiya, S. & Kato, S. (2005). Cerebral activation focusing on strong tasting food: A functional magnetic resonance imaging study. *NeuroReport*, Vol.16, No.3, (Febraury 2005), pp.281-283, ISSN 0959-4965

Kim, Ji-W., Choi, E. Ae, Kim, J.J., Jeong, B.S., Kim, S. E., & Ki, S.W. (2008). The role of amygdala during auditory verbal imagery of derogatory appraisals by others. *Neuroscience Letters*, Vol.446, No.1, (November 2008), pp.1-6, ISSN 0304-3940

Klatzky, R.L, Lederman, S.J., & Matula, D.E. (1991). Imagined haptic exploration in judgements of objects properties. *Journal of Experimental Psychology: Learning, Memory and Cognition*, Vol.17, No.2, (March 1991), pp.314-322, ISSN 0278-7393

Kobayashi, M, Takeda, M., Hattori, N., Fukunaga, M., Sasabe, T., Inoue, N., Nagai, Y., Sawada T., Sadato, N., & Watanabe, Y. (2004). Functional imaging of gustatory perception and imagery: "top-down" processing of gustatory signals. *NeuroImage*, Vol.23, No.4, (December 2004), pp.1271-1282, ISSN 1053-8119

Kosslyn, S.M. (1980). *Image and mind.* Harvard University Press, ISBN 0-674-44365- 9, Cambridge, MA, USA

Kosslyn, S.M. (1994). *Image and brain: The resolution of the imagery debate.* MIT Press, ISBN 0262611244, Cambridge, MA, USA

Kosslyn, S.M., Ball, T.M., & Reiser, B.J. (1978). Visual images preserve metric spatial information: Evidence from Studies of image Scanning. *Journal of Experimental Psychology: Human, Perception and Performance,* Vol.4, No.1, (February 1978), pp.47-60, ISSN 0096-1523

Kosslyn, S.M., & Thompson, W.L. (2003). When is primary visual cortex activated during visual mental imagery? *Psychological Bulletin,* Vol.129, No.5, (September 2003), pp.723-746, ISSN 0033-2909

Kosslyn, S.M., Thompson, W.L., & Ganis, G. (2006). *The case for mental imagery.* Oxford University Press, ISBN 0195398971, New York, USA

Kraemer, D.J.M., Macrae, C.N., Green, A.E., & Kelley, W.M. (2005). Sound of silence activate auditory cortex. *Nature,* Vol.434, No.7030, (March 2005), pp.158, ISSN 1207-9596

Lacourse, M.G., Orr, E.L.R., Cramer, S.C. & Cohen, M.J.D. (2005). Brain activation during execution and motor imagery of novel and skilled sequential hand movements. *NeuroImage,* Vol.27, No.3, (September 2005), pp.505-519, ISSN 1053-8119

Langheim, F.J., Callicott, J.H., Mattay, V.S., Duyn, J.H., & Weinberger, D.R. (2002). Cortical systems associated with covert music rehearsal. *NeuroImage,* Vol.16, No.4, (August 2002), pp.901–908, ISSN 1053-8119

Larsen, A. & Bundesen, C. (1978). Size Scaling in Visual Pattern Recognition. *Journal of Experimental Psychology: Human Perception and Performance,* Vol.4, No.1, (February 1978), pp.1-20, ISSN 0096-1523

Levy, L.M., Henkin, R.I., Lin, C.S., Hutter, A., & Schellinge, D. (1999). Odor memory induces brain activation as measured by functional MRI. *Journal of Computer Assistant Tomography,* Vol.23, No.4, (August 1999), pp.487– 498, ISSN 0363-8715

Lorey, B., Pilgramm, S., Walter, B., Stark, R., Munzert, J., & Zentgraf, K. (2010). Your mind's hand: Motor imagery of pointing movements with different accuracy. *NeuroImage,* Vol.49, No.4, (February 2010), pp.3239-3247, ISSN 1053-8119

Lotze, M., Montoya, P., Erb, M., Hèulsmann, E., Flor, H., Klose, U., et al. (1999). Activation of cortical and cerebellar motor areas during executed and imagined hand movements: An fMRI study. *Journal of Cognitive Neuroscience,* Vol.11, No.5, (September 1999), pp.491–501, ISSN 0898-929X

Lotze, M., Scheler, G., Tan, H.R., Braun, C., & Birbaumer, N. (2003). The musician's brain: Functional imaging of amateurs and professionals during performance and imagery. *NeuroImage,* Vol.20, No.3, (November 2003), pp.1817–1829, ISSN 1053-8119

Nyberg, L., Eriksson, J., Larsson, A., & Marklund, P. (2006). Learning by doing versus learning by thinking: An fMRI study of motor and mental training. *Neuropsychologia,* Vol.44, No.5, (2006), pp.711-717, ISSN 0028-3932

Olivetti Belardinelli, M., Del Gratta, C., Di Matteo, R., De Nicola, A., Ferretti, A., Tartaro, A., Bonomo, L. & Romani, G.L. (2001). Sensory image generation: a comparison between different sensory modalities with fMRI. *Neuroimage,* Vol.13, No.6 (part 2), pp.394, ISSN 1053-8119

Olivetti Belardinelli M., Di Matteo R., Del Gratta C., De Nicola A., Ferretti A., Tartaro A., Bonomo L., & Romani G.L. (2004a). Inter-modal sensory image generation: An fMRI Analysis. *European Journal of Cognitive Psychology*, Vol.16, No.5, (September 2004), pp. 729-752, ISSN 2044-5911

Olivetti Belardinelli, M., Di Matteo, R., Del Gratta, C., De Nicola, A., Ferretti, A., & Romani, G.L. (2004b). Communalities between visual imagery and imagery in other modalities: An investigation by means of fMRI. In *Seeing, thinking and knowing*. A. Carsetti, (Ed.), pp. 203-218, ISBN 079235303X, Kluwer, Dordrecht

Olivetti Belardinelli, M., Palmiero, M., Sestieri, C., Nardo, D., Di Matteo, R., Londei, A., D'Ausilio, Ferretti, A., Del Gratta, C., & Romani, G.L. (2009). An fMRI investigation on image generation in different sensory modalities: The influence of vividness. *Acta Psychologica*, Vol.132, No.2, (October 2009), pp.190-200, ISSN 0001-6918

Palmiero, M., Olivetti Belardinelli, M., Nardo, D., Sestieri, C., Di Matteo, R., D'Ausilio, A., & Romani, G.L. (2009). Mental imagery generation in different modalities activates sensory-motor areas. *Cognitive Processing*, Vol.10, No.2, (September 2009), pp.268-271, ISSN 1612-4782

Pitt, M.A., & Crowder, R.G. (1992). The role of spectral and dynamic cues in imagery for musical timbre. *Journal of Experimental Psychology: Human Perception and Performance*, Vol.18, No.3, (August 1992), pp.728–738, ISSN 0096-1523

Plailly, J., Delon-Martin, C., & Royet, J.P. (2011). Experience induces functional reorganization in brain regions involved in odor imagery in perfumers. *Human Brain Mapping*, (in press) ISSN 1065-9471.

Porro, C. A., Francescato, M. P., Cettolo, V., Diamond, M. E., Baraldi, P., Zuiani, C., et al. (1996). Primary motor and sensory cortex activation during motor performance and motor imagery: A functional magnetic resonance imaging study. *Journal of Neuroscience*, Vol.16, No.23, (December 1996), pp. 7688–7698, ISSN 0270-6474

Pylyshyn, Z.W. (1981). The imagery debate: Analogue media versus tacit knowledge. *Psychological Review*, Vol.88, No.1, (January 1981), pp.16-45, ISSN 0033-295X

Pylyshyn, Z.W. (2002). Mental imagery: In search of a theory. *Behavioral & Brain Sciences*, Vol25, No.2, (April 1981), pp.157-238, ISSN 0140-525X

Pylyshyn, Z.W. (2003). *Seeing and visualizing: It's not what you think.* MIT Press, ISBN 0-262-66197-7, Cambridge, MA, USA

Querleux, B., Gazano, G., Mohen-Domenech, O., Jacquin, J., Burnod, Y., Gaudion, P., et al. (1999). Brain activation in response to a tactile stimulation: Functional magnetic resonance imaging (fMRI) versus cognitive analysis. *International Journal of Cosmetic Science*, Vol.21, No.2, (April 1999), pp.107–118, ISSN 0142-5463

Rao, S.M., Binder, J.R., Bandettini, P.A., Hammeke, T.A., Yetkin, F.Z., Jesmanowicz, A., Lisk, L.M., Morris, G.L., Mueller, W.M., Estkowski, L.D., Wong, E.C., Haughton, V.M. & Hyde, J.S. (1993). Functional magnetic resonance imaging of complex human movements. *Neurology*, Vol.43, No.11, (November 1993), pp. 2311-2318, ISSN 0028-3878

Reddy, L., Tsuchiya, N., & Serre, T. (2010). Reading the mind's eye: Decoding category information during mental imagery. *NeuroImage*, Vol.50, No.2, (April 2010), pp.818-825, ISSN 1053-8119

Rinck, F., Rouby, C., & Bensafi, M. (2009). Which format for odor images? *Chemical Senses*, Vol.34, No.1, (January 2009), pp.11-13, ISSN 0379 864X

Roth, M., Decety, J., Raybaudi, M., Massarelli, R., Delon-Martin, C., Segebarth, C., et al. (1996). Possible involvement of primary motor cortex in mentally simulated movement: A functional magnetic resonance imaging study. *NeuroReport*, Vol.7, No.7, (May 1996), pp.1280–1284, ISSN 0959-4965

Ruby, P. & Decety, J. (2001). Effect of subjective perspective taking during simulation of action: A PET investigation of agency. *Nature Neuroscience*, Vol.4, No.5, (May 2001), pp.546-550, ISSN 1097-6256

Sacco, K., Cauda, F., Cerliani, Mate, D., Duca, S., & Geminiania, G.C. (2006). Motor imagery of walking following training in locomotor attention: the effect of 'the Tango lesson'. *NeuroImage*, Vol.32, No.3, (September 2006), pp.1441-1449, ISSN 1053-8119

Scott, S.K., & Johnsrude, I.S. (2003). The neuroanatomical and functional organization of speech perception. *Trends of Neuroscience*, Vol.26, No.2, (September 2003), pp.100-107, ISSN 0166-2236

Sharma, N., Jones, P.S., Carpenter, T.A., & Baron, J.C. (2008). Mapping the involvement of BA 4a and 4p during motor imagery. *NeuroImage*, Vol.41, No.1, (May 2008), pp.92-99, ISSN 1053-8119

Shepard, R.N., & Metzler J. (1971). Mental rotation of three-dimensional objects. *Science*, Vol.171, No.3972, (Febraury 1971), pp.701-703, ISSN 0036-8075

Shergill, S.S., Bullmore, E.T., Brammer, M.J., Williams, S.C., Murray, R.M., & McGuire, P.K. (2001). A functional study of auditory verbal imagery. *Psychological Medecine*, Vol.31, No.2, (February 2001), pp.241- 253, ISSN 0033-2917

Smith, J.D., Wilson, M. & Reisberg, D. (1995). The role of subvocalization in auditory imagery. *Neuropsychologia*, Vol.33, No.11, (November 1995), pp.1433-1454, ISSN 0028-3932

Sobel, N., Prabhakaran, V., Desmond, J.E., Glover, G.H., Goode, R.L., Sullivan, E.V., & Gabrieli, J.D . (1998). Sniffing and smelling: Separate subsystems in the human olfactory cortex. *Nature*, Vol.392, No.6673, (March 1998), pp.282–286, ISSN 1207-9596

Solodkin, A., Hlustik, P., Chen, E.E., & Small, S.L. (2004). Fine modulation in network activation during motor execution and motor imagery. *Cerebral Cortex*, Vol.14, No.11, (November 2004), pp.1246–1255, ISSN 1047-3211

Stokes, M., Thompson, R., Cusack, R., Duncan, J. (2009). Top-down activation of shape specific population codes in visual cortex during mental imagery. *Journal of Neuroscience*, Vol.29, No.5, (February 2009), pp.1565-1572, ISSN 0270-6474

Szameitat, A.J., Shen, S., & Sterr, A. (2007). Motor imagery of complex everyday movements. An fMRI study. *NeuroImage*, Vol.34, No.2, (January 2007), pp.702–713, ISSN 1053-8119

Takashi, H., Immisch, I., Toma, K., Dymyan, M.A., Van Gelderen, P., & Hallet, M. (2003). Functional properties of brain areas associated with motor execution and imagery. *Journal of Neurophysiology*, Vol.89, No.2, (February 2003), pp.989-1002, ISSN 0022-3077

Thierry, G,. Boulanouar, K., Kherif, F., Ranjeva, J.P., & Demonet, J.F. (1999). Temporal sorting of neural components underlying phonological processing. *Neuroreport*, Vol.10, No.12, (August 1999), pp.2599-2603, ISSN 0959-4965

Thompson-Schill, S.L., Aguirre, G.K., D'Esposito, M., & Farah, M.J. (1999). A neural basis for category and modality specificity of semantic knowledge. *Neuropsychologia*, Vol.37, No.6, (June 1999), pp.671-676, ISSN 0028-3932

Thompson, W.L., Kosslyn, S.M., Hoffman, M.S., & van Der Kooij, K. (2008). Inspecting visual mental images: Can people "see" implicit properties as easily in imagery and perception? *Memory & Cognition*, Vol.36, No.5, (July 2008), pp.1024-1032, ISSN 0090-502X

Tiggemann, M., & Kemps, E. (2005). The phenomenology of food cravings: The role of mental imagery. *Appetite*, Vol.45, No.3, (December 2005), pp.305–313, ISSN 0195-6663

Tomasino, B., Werner, C.J., Weiss, P.H., & Fink, G.R. (2007). Stimulus properties matter more than perspective: An fMRI study of mental imagery and silent reading of action phrases. *NeuroImage*, Vol.36, No.2, (March 2007), pp.128-141, ISSN 1053-8119

Tyszka, J.M., Grafton, S.T., Chew, W., Woods, R.P. & Colletti, P.M. (1994). Parceling of mesial frontal motor areas during ideation and movement using functional magnetic resonance imaging at 1.5 Tesla. *Annual Neurolology*, Vol.35, No.6, (June 1994), pp.746-749, ISSN 0364-5134

Watson, J., Myers, R., Frackowiak, R., Hajnal, J., Woods, R., Mazziotta, J., Shipp, S., & Zeki, S. (1993). Area V5 of the human brain: Evidence from a combined study using positron emission tomography and magnetic resonance imaging. *Cerebral Cortex*, Vol.3, No.2, (April 1993), pp.79–94, ISSN 1047-3211

Yoo, S.S., Freeman, D.K., McCarthyll, J.J. & Jolesz, F.A. (2003). Neural substrates of tactile imagery: A functional MRI study. *NeuroReport*, Vol.14, No.4, (March 2003), pp.581-585, ISSN 0959-4965

Yoo, S.S., Lee, C.U., & Choi, B.G. (2001). Human brain mapping of auditory imagery: An event-related functional MRI study. *NeuroReport*, Vol.12, No.14, (October 2001), pp.3045–3049, ISSN 0959-4965

Zatorre, R.J., Halpern, A.R., & Bouffard, M. (2010). Mental reversal of imagined melodies: A role for the posterior parietal cortex. *Journal of Cognitive Neuroscience*, Vol.22, No.4, (April 2010), pp.775-89, ISSN 0898-929X

Zelano, C., Montag, G., Khan, R., & Sobel, N. (2009). A specialized odor memory buffer in primary olfactory cortex. *PLoS ONE*, Vol.4, No.3, (March 2009), pp.e4965, ISSN 1932-6203

# Part 5

## Post Traumatic Stress Disorder

# 17

# Stress Shaping Brains: Higher Order DNA/Chromosome Mechanisms Underlying Epigenetic Programming of the Brain Transcriptome

George S. Gericke
*BioSequences (Pty) Ltd,*
*South Africa*

## 1. Introduction

*"I believe there is little reason to question the presence of innate systems that are able to restructure a genome. It is now necessary to learn of these systems and to determine why many of them are quiescent and remain so over very long periods of time only to be triggered into action by forms of stress, the consequences of which vary according to the nature of the challenge to be met". Barbara Mc Clintock, (1978), as cited in (Jorgensen, 2004).*

Attempts to link specific neurobehavioural phenotypes with causative genes, a necessary step preceding the development of highly specific neuroimaging biomarkers for these phenotypes, have been spectacularly unsuccessful, although numerous significant gene candidates emerged during the process. Various family study approaches, including twin studies, sib pairs, 'trios' and so-called 'pure multiplex pedigrees' excluding comorbid disorders have been employed in various linkage and association study designs to determine the genes and proteins underlying the relevant disorders. Some genomewide association studies surprised investigators with the information that, when initially promising genomic coding region hotspots were supersaturated with markers at increasingly closer map distances, the results showed weakening of signals in targeted exonic areas, possibly indicating an influence outside these coding areas. The importance of epigenetics (including increasingly complex regulatory region and RNA metabolism gene expression-modifying mechanisms), gradually emerged during the course of molecular genetic 'brain and behaviour' studies. "Epigenetics is defined as mitotically or meiotically stable molecular processes that regulate genome activity independent of DNA sequence. The term 'heritable' has been included in the definition, but has been omitted recently since this implies generational inheritance by definition and therefore does not include all elements of epigenetics (Skinner, 2011). The brain represents a particular area of interest with regard to epigenetics, where it has been demonstrated that epigenetic modifications are not static, but dynamically change in response to external stimuli including synaptic activity (Crepaldi & Riccio, 2009). The increasing likelihood of the role played by transgenerational epigenetic influences in neurogenetics studies now also impacts on the tracking of neuropsychiatric disorder gene candidates in families, implying a requirement for analyses of both coding as well as noncoding polymorphisms and the manner in which these interact, as well as distinguishing between context dependent and germline dependent epigenetic changes (Crews, 2008).

The extensive comorbidity recorded in neuropsychiatric disorders and the acknowledgement of their role when devising candidate gene approaches has been a major challenge. Even though the importance of epistasis and gene pleiotropy are generally acknowledged, there is still no clear understanding of the mechanisms of comorbidity, and biomarker investigative choices thus often remain too simplistic.

The increasing application of sophisticated network dynamics analyses may provide the means to resolve these issues, and the problems posed by variable overlapping of disparate conditions in complex syndromes may soon be better understood by a 'diseasome' approach (Potkin et al., 2010; Barabási et al., 2011), as outlined below. While seemingly introducing even more variables, the aim of network medicine concepts is to actually reduce the noise arising from experiments producing vast amounts of data and organise the information existing in published and newly executed research, ranging from studies of single markers to massively parallel array sequencing experiments. Applying genetic data from genome-wide association studies in a gene network analytic approach, using brain imaging as a quantitative trait phenotype, can increase the statistical power to identify the molecular pathways in which risk genes participate (Potkin et al., 2010). These authors demonstrated the utility of a regulatory network approach by measuring correlations among transcript levels in the mouse and human postmortem tissue which allowed the derivation of an enriched gene set that identified several microRNA's that could be associated with negative symptom schizophrenia. Last but not least, there may be a belated resurgence of interest in the value of 'clinical experience' when discussing which phenotypes to analyse and how to identify the most appropriate research subjects by using experienced investigators within a specific field, rather than relying on massive amounts of data (and biospecimens) accrued by means of research questionnaires dealt with by inexperienced but willing junior research assistants.

This review deals only with the first step in the development of radioligands for imaging in neuropathology (i.e. understanding the clinical genetic context before the selection of disorder-relevant biomarkers). Once a suitable molecular biomarker candidate can be demonstrated, this needs to be followed by selection of leading compounds, radionuclide, labeled position, and synthesis methods; in vitro and in vivo evaluation including probability for imaging, selectivity, specificity, and species differences, and finally an evaluation of factors impinging on safety such as acute toxicity, mutagenicity and radiation dosimetry (Ishiwata, 2009). This does not mean that simpler biomarker identification approaches may not be effective, but it is proposed that a total understanding of the full scope of specific neurobehavioural problems and the mechanisms according to which they overlap can only be developed in this manner. An attempt will be made to integrate the fundamentals of an interface system in the brain with an evolutionary understanding of the mechanism that could give rise to a cluster of seemingly unrelated disorders. This approach may be useful as a model according to which some currently important facets regarding comorbidity can be placed in context.

## 2. Combining in vivo neuroimaging technologies with 'omics' biomarkers

Noninvasiveness of molecular imaging offers a potent advantage for monitoring endpoints of molecular medicine interventions. In particular, pharmaceutically-relevant neuroimaging endpoints based on disorder-specific biomarkers have great potential for better definition and stratification of preclinical study groups, and for providing direct biological measures of response (Waerzeggers et al., 2010). Not all biomarker molecules are suitable for radioimaging approaches, though many potentially interesting molecular biomarkers also appear to be suitable molecular imaging agents. Activatable molecular probes are designed to elicit a detectable change in signal upon enzymatic activity or in response to specific biomolecular interactions. In many cases, these unique characteristics allow for very high signal-to-background ratios compared with conventional targeted contrast agents and they open up the possibility of imaging intracellular targets (Garcia-Campayo et al., 2009).

Molecular biology now offers system-wide insights which have to be incorporated in the derivation of appropriate imaging biomarkers: '*Omics*' is a general term for a broad discipline of science for analysing interactions of biological information. These include studies of the genome, fragilome, transcriptome, proteome, metabolome, expressome, interactome etc. The main focus in these endeavours is on mapping information objects such as genes, proteins, and ligands, finding interaction relationships among the objects and engineering the networks to understand and manipulate the regulatory mechanisms. *Systems biology* integrates information from the various 'omics' subfields, and generates a more comprehensive 'interactome'.

Combined with the disciplines of molecular imaging and molecular medicine, systems biology approaches to understanding disease complexity promises to provide predictive, preventive and personalized medicine that are expected by many to be able to transform healthcare in the future. Continued development of these technologies and applications requires collaboration transcending traditional boundaries between disciplines - e.g. for suitable biomarker consideration, clinical molecular geneticists and radiochemists have to liaise to decide on the choice and molecular characteristics of biomarkers suitable for both laboratory assays as well as being able to bind radioligands. Using disorder specific biomarkers for both laboratory assays and radioimaging allows a two-pronged approach enabling both mass screening and targeted imaging.

## 3. Epigenetics and the brain – foetal programming

The observed foetal basis of some adult onset diseases requires both epigenetic and genetic factors to be involved in regulating developmental biology outcomes, as emphasized by Skinner (2011), who cites the now classical example of insulin resistance and obesity. Developmental studies of metabolic 'programming' suggest that insulin resistance may appear during early development in individuals born small for gestational age. Insulin resistance can promote obesity, which in turn, could sustain the state of insulin resistance in later life. Skinner et al. (2011) stresses that "the current paradigm of DNA mutational events promoting evolution is accurate, but the inclusion of epigenetics allows for a much higher degree of variability in the biological system to facilitate an adaptation event and epigenetic transgenerational inheritance is a novel concept with considerable experimental support in plant and mammalian studies. This insight, therefore, does not modify the fundamental Darwinian evolutionary paradigm, but adds a neo-Lamarckian component allowing a more diverse molecular mechanism" (Skinner 2011). The role of epigenetics in controlling neuronal functions that may ultimately underlie behavioural adaptations represents a strong emerging research theme (Nelson & Monteggia, 2011).

### 3.1 Context-dependent epigenetic modifications

Context-dependent epigenetic modifications refer to transmission within a generation (within an individual's own lifetime, including the interaction of parent and young), while germline-dependent epigenetic modifications deal with transmission across generations (Crews, 2008). The best examples of context-dependent epigenetic modifications are those that either have an effect early in life, such as exposure to endocrine disrupting compounds *in utero* or smoking during childhood and adolescence (known collectively as the foetal basis of adult disease, or foetal programming also alluded to above. In the first instance the onset of disease manifests later or the deleterious effects decline with time. However, "the extent to which the modification is perpetuated is by simple persistence of the environmental factors that bring about the epigenetic modification; that is, in each generation individuals are exposed to the same conditions. Hence, the environment can induce epialleles, but this environmentally induced epigenetic state can be reversed by a different environmental factor" (Crews, 2008). An example supplied by Crews (2008) of a context-dependent epigenetic modification on behaviour is considered to be exemplified by the study of Meaney and colleagues (Meany, 2001; Meaney & Syzf, 2005; Champagne, 2008). In a series of studies in rats, this group demonstrated that the nature and amount of care a pup receives from the mother modulates its reaction to stress in later life, largely through effects on the glucocorticoid receptor (GR) in the hippocampus. This maternal effect can cross generations, but its heritability depends upon the pup's experience in the first week of life. Crews (2008) mentions in his review that Meaney's group also recently documented that being reared by a high quality mother results in the expression of the transcription factor A (NGFI-A), a nerve growth factor-inducible protein, that binds to the first exon of the GR gene, resulting in increased expression of GR. High quality maternal care during this critical period demethylates NGFI-A and the acetylation of histones. Just as cross-fostering can reverse these molecular and behavioural changes, infusion of methionine, a histone deacetylase inhibitor, into the hippocampus can also reverse these events (Weaver et al., 2006).

Selective breeding cannot stabilize these brain–behaviour differences and, the effects of high and low quality mothering disappear after five generations indicating that it is not a germline-dependent epigenetic modification but a context-dependent epigenetic modification. The implications of the work are, however, still regarded as important: in humans it has been reported that rearing environment can overcome the influence of a polymorphism in the gene encoding the neurotransmitter-metabolizing enzyme monoamine oxidase A in the aetiology of violent behaviour (Caspi et al., 2003).

### 3.2 Germline-dependent epigenetic modifications

Germline-dependent epigenetic modifications "are fundamentally different from context-dependent epigenetic modification in that the epigenetic imprint has become independent of the original causative agent" (Crews, 2008). Here the epigenetic modification is transferred to subsequent generations because the change in the epigenome has been incorporated into the germline. Thus, the effect is manifest each generation without the need for re-exposure. The inheritance of environmentally induced phenotypes is the origin of the concept of epigenetics as conceptualized by Conrad Waddington in 1934. (Costa et al., 2004; Morange, 2009). In such instances the DNA methylation imprints of heritable epialleles are passed through to subsequent generations rather than being erased as occurs normally during gametogenesis and shortly after fertilization. Germline-dependent epigenetic modifications tend to be associated with one sex, an important aspect as many behaviours and affective disorders show sex differences (Crews, 2008). A comprehensive review of over 100 cases of transgenerational epigenetic inheritance have now reported the phenomena in a wide range of organisms including prokaryotes, plants, and animals (Jablonka et al., 2009). It appears that RNA plays a major role in germline dependent epigenetic modifications (Ashe & Whitelaw, 2007), an aspect which is relevant to links suggested to exist between chromosomal rearrangement at fragile regions, transgenerational transmission of certain behaviours and neurodevelopment.

### 3.3 Caveats of twin studies in disorders where epigenetics are important

Twin research findings clearly indicate how an appreciation of epigenetics is missing from an understanding of how different phenotypes can originate from the same genotype. Although epigenetically indistinguishable during the early years of life, monozygotic twins exhibit remarkable differences later in life in their overall content and genomic distribution of 5-methylcytosine DNA and histone acetylation, affecting their gene-expression profiles (Fraga et al., 2005). Epigenetic changes can result in a normal genotype suddenly being associated with a disease phenotype and genotypes associated with susceptibility to certain disorders may have reduced penetrance and subsequently develop as a normal phenocopy (Singh et al., 2004). Due to the indirect relationship between phenotype and genotype in epigenetics, finding a distinct set of genes that will be consistently linked with a particular neurobehavioural disorder phenotype on a worldwide basis may prove to be more difficult than originally envisaged.

## 4. The brain genome - environment interface: – stress as an evolutionary driver

Following Waddington's early epigenetic concept, biological stress could be stated to represent a dyshomeostatic influence which produces a diversifying biological response following which a novel variant may have a survival advantage, making it an essential driver of evolution. Evolutionary processes are strongly influenced by the competition for available energy, with the required physical or mental skills being passed to offspring of the most able competitors. Diversity is clearly an asset in this process. A broader repertoire of cognitively linked, novelty stress-based learning associated with a complex range of emotions and increased cognitive integration through higher interneuronal density in humans is suggested to have diversified novelty information management. Stress hormones participate in modulation of memory consolidation processes in both the amygdala and the hippocampus (Guterman et al., 2006).

It increasingly appears possible that stress management systems operating within non-pathological parameters are utilised to deal with 'novelty'. The physiological activity of stress hormones has been shown to play an important role in modulation of memory consolidation processes in both the amygdala and the hippocampus (Turner et al., 2008). Severe psychosocial stress in early life crossing the proposed physiological stress management system boundaries, can adversely impact brain development itself, and the literature on stress suggests that these changes also occur largely through the hypothalamic pituitary adrenocortical (HPA) axis (Loman and Gunnar, 2010). Steroid receptors function by binding to specific structural elements in the regulatory regions of target genes by recruitment of cofactors that modify histones and chromatin structure (Trapman & Dubbink, 2007). Global changes in epigenetic markers in response to fear conditioning have been demonstrated

(Lubin & Sweatt, 2007), and RNA-mediated chromatin-level silencing is increasingly implicated in development, stress responses, and natural epigenetic variation that may promote phenotypic diversity, physiological plasticity, and evolutionary change (Madlung & Comai, 2004). Epigenetic markers on the promoter regions of the Bdnf gene have been the most extensively studied, including alterations in histone acetylation, phosphorylation, methylation, and DNA methylation associated with memory behaviour (Gupta et al., 2010), as well as activity-dependent changes in DNA methylation (Nelson et al., 2008).

### 4.1 How it all comes together: A flexible networking "interface system"

The ability to alter development, physiology, growth, and behaviour in response to different environmental conditions represent critical assessments of both external and internal factors as a function of energy balance and environmental stress as well as physiological, developmental, and behavioural responses to these determinations (Crespi & Denver, 2005). What may have made humans unique, is an enormously increased feedback capability for constructive interaction between internal structures and extra-biological factors, self reflective evaluation and an improved ability to shape the environment, to such an extent that there is now an unprecedented information continuum between information captured in biological processes and the environment itself. In support of more holistic modelling, integrative biological concepts have also arisen, for instance the concept of a "neuro-immuno-endocrine system". It is additionally proposed here that the flexible disparate stress response mechanisms responsible for the storage of novel information should be considered as a combinatorially regulated "interface system". It can be expected that an evolutionary strategy would exploit the effect of integrating the different systems for the transmission of genetic information with systems relating to the external adaptation of the organism (Bengtsson, 2004). An interface can be defined as a point at which independent systems or diverse groups interact. Although such a proposed environmental interface system presumably consists of many more components than mentioned here, an example will be provided of a nonlinear brain system with flexible internal structural responses to environmentally induced perturbation i.e. the brain chromosomal 'fragilome' which appears to underly certain aspects of neuroplasticity and memory storage and which appears to be closely linked with the stress hormonal system and immunoglobulin DNA strand break and genomic rearranging phenomena. The essential important characteristic of the brain fragilome is that of genetic breakage and recombination offering a structural basis for genetic/neuronal diversification and storage of memories (Gericke, 2010).

Chromosomal fragile sites represent large heritable chromosomal regions that preferentially exhibit gaps or breaks after DNA synthesis is partially perturbed by stressors affecting the replication process (Arlt et al., 2006) and are classified as 'rare' or 'common', depending on their induction method and frequency within the population. Common fragile sites (CFS) are found in all individuals, are variable, extend over large regions and are associated with transcriptional activity (Sbrana et al., 1998).

Several of the currently known human CFS regions span large genes that extend from 700 kb to over 1.5 Mb of genomic sequence. Many of these genes have been functionally linked with neurological development. Chromosomal fragile sites (*in toto* represented by the fragilome), represent *in vitro* observed genomic regions with particular structural characteristics related to epigenetic plasticity, resulting in the creation of diversity through a process of controlled double strand breaks and imperfect mismatch repair shielded from and/or below an apoptotic risk threshold under physiological circumstances. This modular assembly process has been adapted from the immune paradigm at the expense of a risk for instability and/or malignant transformation when associated control mechanisms are not in place (such as tumour suppressor genes). It is suggested that the abilities for diverse recognition of externally derived information, a dynamic response of somatic hypermutation followed by genome rearrangement creating a template for memory formation, and entry into a terminally differentiated state are features common to both the brain and immune system. Chromosome breaks and the various resulting structural rearrangements (genetic instability) have mostly been viewed in a pathological context by researchers, but controlled chromosomal breakage and rearrangement leading to altered gene expression without adverse effects may have been necessary for the evolutionary and neurodevelopmental flexibility required by the human brain (Gericke, 2010).

Such chromosomal breakage relates to alterations in DNA higher order structures and studies of fragile sites at the level of chromosome organization reveal an unusual chromatin structure associated with fragile sites influencing formation of nucleosomes and the formation of nucleosome arrays (Wang, 2006). The study of epigenetics focuses on the relationship between chromatin structure and gene transcription. DNA is commonly packaged into nucleosomes and wrapped tightly around a core of histone (H) proteins. Modifications that regulate chromatin structure influence transcriptional activity, in part, through effects on transcription factor binding. the environmental regulation of histone methylation states. Chromatin remodeling and gene transcription are linked in that transcriptional activation associates with chromatin states that enhance the probability of subsequent transcriptional activity, providing a feed-forward loop. (Cordero et al., 2006, Murr, 2010; Hayashi et al., 2011). Recent observations reveal that histones are removed and replaced to enable or restrict, respectively, access of the transcription machinery to regulate transcription. The ultimate goal of some epigenetic modifications might well turn out to be the regulation of histone occupancy on the DNA (Williams et al., 2008). CFS-associated duplication and deletion altering AT tract length and DNA flexibility have been linked with variation in nucleosomal architecture (Cosgrove & Walberger, 2005). AT-rich repeats mediate recombination events in non-homologous chromosomes during meiosis (Jackson et al., 2003) and due to a modification of binding factor characteristics, CFS have been proposed to contribute to epigenetic sensitive phenotypes (Woynarowski, 2004), a phenomenon which has been suggested to include neurobehavioral effects (Garofalo et al.,1993; Gericke et al., 1995, Gericke 1998, 2006, 2010; Simonic & Gericke 1996; Simonic & Ott, 1996; Savelyeva et al., 2006).

### 4.2 Developmental cytogenetic instability in the mammalian brain

"As many of the examples of epigenetic inheritance are mediated by position effects, the possibility exists that chromosome rearrangements may be one of the driving forces behind evolutionary change by exerting position effect alterations in gene activity, an idea first articulated by Richard Goldschmidt in 1940 in his book "The Material Basis of Evolution"(Reprinted in 1982).

The emerging evidence suggests that Goldschmidt's controversial hypothesis deserves a serious reevaluation" (Varmuza, 2003). Recent findings of rearranged and aneuploid chromosomes in brain cells suggest an unexpected link between developmental chromosomal instability and brain genome diversity (Yurov et al., 2007), (Yang et al., 2003). In humans, previously unrecognized large-scale double-stranded DNA breaks are now known to occur under normal circumstances in early postmitotic and differentiating neurons (Gilmore et al., 2000). In general, accumulation of DNA breaks in differentiating cells cannot be attributed to a decrease in the DNA repair efficiency. Poly(ADP)ribose synthesis often follows the DNA breakage in differentiating cells. It has been hypothesized that DNA fragmentation is an epigenetic tool for regulating the differentiation process (Sjakste & Sjakste, 2007). Genomes of developing and adult neurons can be different at the level of whole chromosomes (Rehen et al., 2005). Not only breakage and rearrangement and associated structural sequelae, but also large scale chromosomal ploidy alterations seem to have been recruited as a diversifying process, similar to processes involved in genetic diversification in plants. Metaphase chromosome spreads from whole brains of the teleost *Apteronotus leptorhynchus* revealed an euploid complement of 22 chromosomes in only 22% of the cells examined. Together with the recent discovery of aneuploidy in the adult mammalian brain, investigations suggest that the loss or gain of chromosomes might provide a mechanism to regulate gene expression during development of new cells in the adult vertebrate brain (Rajendran et al., 2007),(Yurov et al., 2005). Both neurons and non-neuronal cells can be aneuploid as a normal feature of the human brain (Rehen et al., 2005).

One possible consequence of nervous system aneuploidy is altered gene expression through loss of heterozygosity (Kaushal et al., 2003). Aneuploid neurons were found to be functionally active and demonstrate that functioning neurons with aneuploid genomes form genetically mosaic neural circuitries as part of the normal organization of the mammalian brain (Kingsbury et al., 2005). The average aneuploidy frequency has been found to be 1.25-1.45% per chromosome, with the overall percentage of aneuploidy tending to approach 30-35%. Furthermore, such mosaic aneuploidy appears to be exclusively *confined to the brain* (Yurov et al., 2007) and it is probably crucial to contain the extensive rearrangement processes in brain cells in order to prevent this extent of breakage and ploidy alterations from creating havoc in other mitotically active cells. This appears to be different from altered chromosomal breakage which can be demonstrated in peripheral blood and may reflect more widespread gene expression changes.

### 4.3 Protocadherin genetic rearrangement in the brain

Both the immune system and the brain evolved from a cell adhesion system. Evidence of the importance of DNA rearrangement in essential neurogenic processes also highlighted recent discoveries of genes encoding neuronal adhesion protocadherins which display structural similarity to immunoglobulins. Cadherin-related neuronal receptor/protocadherin transcript variance has also been linked with chromosomal variations in the nucleus of differentiated neurons (Yagi, 2003). Together with cytoskeletal proteins, such as tubulin, microtubule-associated proteins, and intermediate filament proteins, the neural adhesive protocadherins with immunoglobulin-like functional features and extracellular matrix glycoproteins are associated with dynamic structural remodelling in the nervous system (Miyate & Hatton, 2002; Chun 1999). Some brain protocadherins are specific to the hominoid lineage (Durand et al, 2006) and single nucleotide polymorphisms in the protocadherin-alpha and -beta genes are possible contributors to variation in human brain function (Pedrosa et al., 2008). Furthermore, different codons in the mammalian protocadherin ectodomains are under diversifying selection. These diversified residues likely play an important role in combinatorial interactions, which could provide the staggering diversity required for neuronal connections in the brain (Miki et al., 2005).

While lymphocytes express a single receptor molecule specifically directed against an outside stimulus, in contrast, each neuron has three specific recognition sites, each expressing a different protocadherin. In this way, 4,950 different neurons arising from one stem cell form a neuronal network in which homophilic contacts can be formed in 52 layers, permitting an enormous number of different connections between neurons (Wu, 2005). At the single-cell level, protocadherin-alpha mRNAs are regulated monoallelically, supporting the idea that diversified protocadherin molecules contribute to neural circuit development and provide individual cells with their specific identity (Hilschmann et al., 2001). The neocortical genomic response to stress is relayed via hormones and reactive oxygen/nitrogen species signaling, thereby implicating the mitochondrial genome and bioenergetic metabolism (Wallace, 2010), which is suggested to represent an extension of dynamic genomic changes in parallel to the immune recombination and neural rearrangement (protocadherin) histories and fragile site events (Gericke, 2006) of a particular individual.

## 5. Stress memory and immune-like rearrangement in the human brain

Doubts have more recently been raised whether gene transcription activated by dendritic calcium signals is sufficient to consolidate long-term functional alterations associated with memory consolidation. An alternative genomic hypothesis of memory suggests that acquired information is persistently stored within individual neurons through modifications of DNA, and that these modifications serve as the carriers of elementary memory traces. The emerging idea is therefore that lifelong behavioural memory storage may involve lasting changes in the physical, three-dimensional structure of DNA itself and chromatin alterations are emerging as a key epigenetic mechanism in the process in conjunction with use-dependent synaptic plasticity (Levenson & Sweatt, 2006; Delcuve et al., 2009). The expression of immune recombination activating genes in key stress-induced memory regions in the brain suggests the adoption by the brain of this ancient pattern recognition and memory system to establish a structural basis for long-term memory through controlled chromosomal breakage at highly specific genomic regions. Fundamentally unstable processes with narrow safety margins (controlled chromosomal breakage) thus appear to underlie pattern recognition and memory consolidation in both the immune system and brain.

Unusual genetic mechanisms for diversifying recognition proteins may be a widespread characteristic of animal immunity and may have paved the way for adaptation for management of neural sensory information (Litman et al., 2005). Stress reactions form part of neuroendocrine influences that also modulate immune function. The appearance of a lymphocyte-based recombinatorial system of anticipatory immunity in vertebrates approximately 500 mya facilitated developmental and morphological plasticity in addition to the advantage conferred by the ability to recognize a larger portion of the antigenic world (Pancer & Cooper, 2006). A prototypic example of epigenetic-facilitation in memory retention pertains to memory T-cells of the mammalian immune system (reviewed in Nakayama & Yamashita (2008)). Numerous epigenetic mechanisms such as histone modifications and DNA methylation modulate gene expression and thus play a role in T-cell survival and maintenance of T-cell function in various differentiated states. These processes underlie the formation of persistent immunological memory cells in response to transient environmental stimuli (reviewed in Nakayama & Yamashita (2008). Thus, like immune T-cells, it is plausible that epigenetic mechanisms such as methylation of the cytosine base are changeable and occur in post-mitotic neurons to mediate neuronal function. However, unlike epigenetic mechanisms in the immune system, chromatin modifications in the CNS are greatly understudied. Lymphoid cells purposely introduce DNA double strand breaks into their genome to maximize the diversity and effector functions of their antigen receptor genes (Rooney & Chaudhuri, 2004). Recombinase activation gene RAG-1 directed V(D)J recombination affecting only specific recognition sequences allows the immune system to encode memories of a vast array of antigens. Research findings provide a formal demonstration that certain CFS can function as signals for RAG complex targets (Raghavan et al., 2001). Conversely, CFS were found to be enriched for genes associated with the immune response (Re et al., 2006). RAG proteins have been proposed to contribute to chromosomal translocations in general (Chatterji et al., 2004), suggesting that these may be involved in immune-like stress induced rearrangement processes following breakage at CFS. Rag1 positive-cells mainly appear in the amygdalae, hypothalamus, thalamus and hippocampus at developmental stage (Sun et al., 2007). The RAG-1 gene is also localized to neurons in the hippocampal formation and related limbic regions that are involved in spatial learning and memory as well as other parameters of neurobehavioural performance (Cushman et al., 2003). While the role of RAG-1 in learning and memory in humans still has to be determined, it remains attractive to propose that their localization in relevant anatomical areas in the brain, the importance of epigenetics changes and the postulated role of chromosomal rearrangement make this an interesting area for future studies.

### 5.1 CFS, RAG genes and transposable elements (TE's)

It has been motivated_that the recombination system that carries out rearrangements may be a significant evolutionary force, perhaps not limited to rearrangements only at antigen-receptor loci (Roth 2000) (Chuzhanova et al., 2009). Genomic changes in V-gene structure, created by RAG recombinase acting on germline recombination signal sequences, led variously to the generation of fixed receptor specificities, pseudogene templates for gene conversion, and ultimately to Ig sequences that evolved away from Ig function (Hsu et al., 2006). RAG1 and RAG2, like the adaptive immune system itself, are found exclusively in jawed vertebrates, and are thought to have entered the vertebrate genome by horizontal transmission as components of a transposable element (Schatz, 2004). Such dynamicity allows extensive genome repatterning during transient stress phases (including oxidative stress signaling), during which some epigenetic features, such as DNA methylation, are relaxed, thus allowing transposable element (TE) amplification. Analysis of genomic rearrangement breakpoint regions has revealed specific TE repeat density patterns, suggesting that TEs may have played a significant role in chromosome evolution and genome plasticity. Hairpin DNA structures formed in palindromes (such as associated with CFS) are intermediates in V(D)J recombination and are formed by a chemical mechanism very similar to the early steps of transpositional recombination and retroviral integration. RAG proteins are able to capture exogenous target DNA molecules and carry out authentic transposition of signal ends into these targets.

Genomic instability has been indicated to involve epigenetic activation of mobile elements dispersed throughout the human genome (Stribinskis & Ramos, 2006). Barbara McClintock originally proposed that mobile elements restructure host genomes as an adaptive response to environmental challenge (McClintock, 1987; Dai et al., 2007). Retrotransposons are mobile genetic elements that can be amplified to high copy number and are considered to be an important source of genetic diversity (Grandbastien, 2004). Hypomethylation associated with genomic stress largely affects the intergenic and intronic regions of the DNA, particularly repeat sequences and transposable elements, and is believed to result in chromosomal instability and hypomethylation of regulatory DNA sequences activates transcription of protooncogenes, retrotransposons, as well as genes encoding proteins involved in genomic instability (Glover, 2006; Wilson et al., 2007). Retroelements represent evolutionary forces that establish and hone target gene networks of transcription factors in a species-specific manner. LTR class I endogenous retrovirus (ERV) retroelements impact considerably the transcriptional network of human tumour suppressor protein p53. A total of 1,509 of approximately 319,000 human ERV LTR regions have a near-perfect p53 DNA binding site. Human ERV p53 sites are likely part of the p53 transcriptional program and direct regulation of p53 target genes (Wang et al., 2007). Recent findings showed that key cell cycle checkpoint genes are important for genome stability at fragile sites. Altered sequences arising from chromosomal rearrangement and associated transposable element (TE) upregulation during 'cognitive stress' may result in neurospecific immune-like sequelae involving CFS as key participating regions. DNA double-strand break repair proteins were recognized 20 years ago as a major target of autoantibodies. Dysregulation of these processes can be considered to increase the risk for subsequently developing systemic inflammatory disorders through a central immunologically modified state and sensitization for increased stress responses in susceptible individuals. Because early changes may include misregulation of resident inflammatory myelomonocytic cells in the developing brain, this could be associated with prenatal–neonatal brain pathologies and neurobehavioural deficits (Dietert & Dietert, 2008).

### 5.2 CFS represent a network stress response

When data on CFS expression were analysed in a network context, it appeared that chromosomal fragile site associated genes function as part of a highly conserved stress response network (Re et al., 2006). The regulatory genome supplies an enormous computational capability with the capacity to process in parallel a vast number of regulatory inputs, comprising many thousands of processing units in the form of cis-regulatory modules. The interconnected cis-regulatory modules that control regulatory gene expression create a network that is the underlying mechanism of specification and illustrate the information processing that is done by the regulatory sequences (Ben-Tabou de-Leon & Davidson, 2007). AT islands in CFS have been shown to function as nuclear matrix attachment regions (MARs) both in vitro and in vivo (Jackson et al., 2003), which constitute the functional coordinate system for genomic regulatory regions (Liebich et al., 2002). DNA duplexes of AT islands are prone to base unpairing due to their unusual flexibility characteristics, which are necessary MAR attributes. Recent studies on the molecular mechanisms involved show that proteins of the nuclear envelope participate in regulation of transcription on several levels, from direct binding to transcription factors to induction of epigenetic histone modifications [Skalai et al., 2007]. MARs organize chromosomal loops in the interphase nucleus, are about 200 bp long, AT-rich, contain topoisomerase II consensus sequences and other AT-rich sequence motifs; often reside near cis-acting regulatory sequences, and their binding sites are abundant (greater than 10,000 per mammalian nucleus) (Blasquez et al., 1998). Cis-elements can be defined to include the repeat sequence units, the length and purity of the repeat tracts, the sequences flanking the repeat, as well as the surrounding epigenetic environment, including DNA methylation and chromatin structure (Cleary & Pearson, 2003). Contacts between cis-acting sequences through the formation of chromatin loops form the most basic level of organization that impedes or permits access of factors to the genes (Dillon, 2006). It is suggested that this links to developmental remodelling of neuronal connectivity and differential network connectivity has been suggested to form the basis for species-specific network connections as key drivers of evolutionary change (Boldogkoi 2004). The behavioural phenotype manifests itself as an emergent property of such networks (Anholt, 2004).

### 5.3 Chromosomal breakage and network assembly, gene duplication and gene copy number variation

Analyses support a nonrandom model of chromosomal evolution associated with both recurrent small-scale duplication and large-scale evolutionary rearrangements (Hinsch & Hannenhalli, 2006). Similarly, the human brain appears to have developed anatomically by the divergent modification of pre-existing parts (Striedter, 1998) and new areas may have evolved as a result of processes likely to be linked with underlying extensive duplication of transcription factors (Babu et al., 2004) or genes. The functional characterization through analysis of the ontology of genes located at connected fragile sites clearly highlights that a great proportion of genes with significant annotated terms are involved in innate and adaptive immune responses and in particular in pathways characteristic of activated T lymphocytes (Re et al., 2006). From these findings it has been proposed that correlated breakage at fragile sites may originate in proliferating lymphocytes from a co-regulated modified expression of fragile genes; in this view the genes identified by ontological analysis may be new fragile genes; chromatin changes and DNA replication alteration at or near these genes would be produced by cellular processes connected with their co-regulation performed through still unknown mechanisms. This is supported by the observation that a number of the analysed cytokine-related genes show actual functional interactions in lymphocytes or other cell types (Re et al., 2006). Duplicate genes rapidly diverge in their expression profiles in the network and contribute to maintaining network robustness as compared with singletons (Chung et al., 2006) and according to modelling analyses, duplication plays an important role in feed-forward loop evolution (Cordero et al., 2006). Gene copy number variation has been considered to underlie a significant proportion of normal human variation including differences in cognitive, behavioural, and psychological features (Lee & Lupski, 2006).

Dynamic interactions between components of living cells (e. g., proteins, genes) exist on genomic, transcriptomic, proteomic and metabolomic levels. The levels themselves are heavily interconnected, resulting in complex networks of different interacting biological entities (Bosman et al., 2007). Some novel data suggest that a large amount of genetic variation exists in the regulatory region of genes within populations. In addition, comparison of homologous DNA sequences of various species shows that evolution appears to depend more strongly on gene expression than on the genes themselves. Furthermore, it has been demonstrated in several systems that genes form functional networks, whose products exhibit interrelated expression profiles. Finally, it has been found that regulatory circuits of development behave as evolutionary units (Boldogkoi 2004).

These data demonstrate that (1) Instead of individual genes, gene networks (GNs) are responsible for the determination of traits and behaviours. (2) The primary source of microevolution is considered to be the intraspecific polymorphism in GNs and not the allelic variation in either the coding or the regulatory sequences of individual genes. (3) GN polymorphism is generated by the variation in the regulatory regions of the component genes and not by the variance in their coding sequences. (4) Evolution proceeds through continuous restructuring of the composition of GNs rather than fixing of specific alleles or GN variants (Boldogkoi 2004).

Unlike most optimization methods working from a single point in the decision space and employing a transition method to determine the next point, in a densely interconnected system genetic algorithms work from an entire "population" of points simultaneously, trying many directions in parallel and employing a combination of several genetically-inspired methods to determine the next population of points (Cantu-Paz & Goldberg, 1999). These aspects are likely to have been linked with evolutionary recruitment of an increasing number of gene promoters as members of progressively intricate gene expression networks employing different patterns of expression of stable household genes. Such principles may reflect the human ability to *combine and recombine* highly differentiated actions, perceptions, and concepts in order to construct larger, more complex, and highly variable units in a variety of behavioural domains including language, social intelligence, tool-making, and motor sequences (Gibson, 2002). It has been suggested that speech development and visual interpretation is characterized by multipart representations formed from elementary canonical parts (e.g., phonemes in speech, geons in visual perception) (Corballis, 1992), and in such new combinations similarly later gave rise to the introduction of iconic symbols used in art, writing and reading when information management became too complex for gestures and oral traditions.

## 6. Analytical challenges in building complex disease investigative models – network dynamics

The reductionistic approaches which have been successful in the early history of human genetics dealt with so-called 'single gene disorders' (increasingly a challenged concept), and currently fail to uncover the information required for insight into complex gene environment interaction such as required for studies in 'brain and behaviour'. Furthermore, bioenergetic metabolism as related to mitochondrial genetics (including both mitochondrial genes and nuclear genes involved with bioenergetic crosstalk) (Wallace, 2010) as well as epigenetic modification of DNA regulatory structures are considered to be increasingly important in neuroplasticity. Most of the gene identification studies have assayed for only one type of epigenetic marker. The problem of not evaluating the entire array of epigenetic modifications at specific gene promoters, along with the fact that most available gene chips fail to cover a large portion of the genome, means current technology has not yet reached the levels needed to fully assess the gene expression changes responsible for mediating many of the epigenetically-associated phenotypes in the adult brain.

### 6.1 Understanding the interactome

An excellent review of the topic was recently published in Nature Genetics (Barabási et al., 2011). The potential complexity of the human interactome (all the interactions between biological entities in cells and organisms considered as a whole), is daunting. The past decade has seen an exceptional growth in human specific molecular interaction data. Network based approaches to human disease have multiple biological and clinical implications. Networks operating in biological, technological or social systems are not random, but are characterized by a core set of organizing principles. Proteins that are involved in the same disease show a high propensity to interactly directly with each other. Thus, each disease may be linked to a well defined neighbourhood of the interactome, often referred to as a 'disease module', representing a group of network components that together contribute to a cellular function and disruption which results in a particular disease phenotype.

### 6.2 Mapping complex conditions with multiple comorbid disorders through a 'diseasome' approach

Similarly, the systematic mapping of the network based dependencies between pathophenotypes and their disease modules has culminated in the concept of the 'diseasome' which represents disease maps whose nodes are diseases and whose links represent various molecular relationships between the disease associated cellular components (Barabási et al., 2011). Understanding such links not only helps us understand how different phenotypes, often addressed by different medical subdisciplines are linked at the molecular level but can also help us to comprehend why certain groups of diseases arise together. Diseasome - based approaches can be expected to aid drug discovery, in particular when it comes to the use of approved drugs to treat molecularly linked diseases. Single target drugs can be expected to correct some dysfunctional aspects of the disease module, but they could also alter the activity of molecules that are situated in the neighbourhood of the disease module, leading to detectable side effects. Analysis of drug target networks demonstrated that many drugs are palliative, that is they do not target the actual disease associated proteins, but proteins in their network neighbourhood. Finally, using network analytic capabilities, safer and more focused multi-target combinations can be designed e.g. for anti-inflammatory or anticancer drug combinations (Barabási et al., 2011).

## 7. Interface system pathology – pain hypersensitivity (fibromyalgia syndrome) as a diseasome

Epidemiological evidence suggests that an adverse prenatal environment permanently 'programs' physiology and increases the risk of cardiovascular, metabolic, neuroendocrine and psychiatric disorders in adulthood. Prenatal stress or exposure to excess glucocorticoids might provide the link between foetal maturation and adult pathophysiology (Turner et al., 2008). In a variety of animal models, prenatal stress, glucocorticoid exposure and inhibition (or knockout of) 11beta-hydroxysteroid dehydrogenase type 2 (11beta-HSD2)--the foetoplacental barrier to maternal glucocorticoids--reduce birth weight and cause increases in adult blood pressure, glucose levels, hypothalamic-pituitary-adrenal (HPA) axis activity and anxiety-related behaviours. In humans, mutations in the gene that encodes 11beta-hydroxysteroid dehydrogenase type 2 are associated with low birth weight. Babies with low birth weight have higher plasma cortisol levels throughout life, which indicates HPA-axis programming. In human pregnancy, severe maternal stress affects the offspring's HPA axis and is associated with neuropsychiatric disorders; moreover, maternal glucocorticoid therapy alters offspring brain function (Turner et al., 2008). Genetic variation in HPA axis genes was associated with programming might reflect permanent changes in the expression of specific transcription factors, including the glucocorticoid receptor; tissue specific effects reflect modification of one or more of the multiple alternative first exons or promoters of the glucocorticoid receptor gene. Intriguingly, some of these effects seem to be inherited by subsequent generations that are unexposed to exogenous glucocorticoids at any point in their lifespan from fertilization, which implies that these epigenetic effects persist (Turner et al., 2008). The Fibromyalgia Syndrome (FMS) can be viewed from a certain perspective as a chronic pain/inflammation problem arising subsequent to a hypersensitized pain and/or stress memory in genetically predisposed individuals probably as early as intrauterine life. First degree relatives have a significantly increased risk to develop FMS. Foetal programming is expected to result in severe pathophysiological hyperreactivity when exposed to subsequent stressful stimuli. This, and much other contemporary research implies that foetal and perinatal stress could have long lasting sequelae in adult life and that it also involves inappropriate immune upregulation. The 'at risk' FMS genotype may represent a risk for several non-classical FMS outcomes as central stress induced hypersensitisation appears to cause subsequent susceptibility to posttraumatic stress disorder-like phenomena, chronic pain syndromes, mood disorders and several other adult onset diseases. These effects often include, but are not limited to, anxiety, depression, ADHD, substance use disorders, and tobacco dependence as well as a dramatically increased risk for a variety of mental disorders (Bhadra & Petersel, 2010; González et al., 2010; Natelson 2010). There may exist cross reactions between various emotional stress and pain responses which involve both the immune and nervous systems. These share quite similar processes for pattern recognition and memory consolidation, and may represent a useful perspective from which to regard aetiological relationships between conditions consistently occurring as comorbid disorders.

### 7.1 Chromosomal fragility in chronic fatigue/fibromyalgia syndrome (FMS)

In 1995, during research on chromosomal fragile sites at the University of Pretoria, my cytogenetics collaborator, Ingrid Simonic, found an increased expression of common aphidicolin-inducible chromosomal fragile sites in FMS/"chronic fatigue" patients as opposed to unaffected intrafamilial controls (Fig 1) (Simonic & Gericke, Unpublished data).

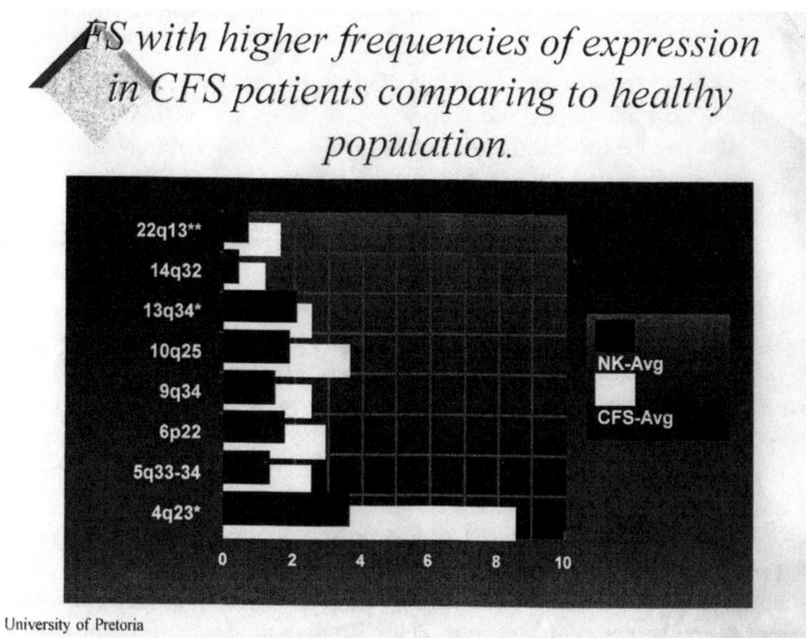


Fig. 1. Higher frequencies of some aphidicolin-induced common chromosomal fragile sites in FMS/chronic fatigue individuals versus first degree controls.

The involved sites included areas harbouring NF-KB genes, which are pro-neuroinflammatory factors (Fig 2). Several studies indicate that the nuclear factor-kappa B (NF-kappaB) -activation cascade plays a crucial role not only in immune esponses, inflammation, and apoptosis but also in the development and processing of pathological pain (Niederberger & Geisslinger, 2008). This could represent one aspect of a FMS diseasome.

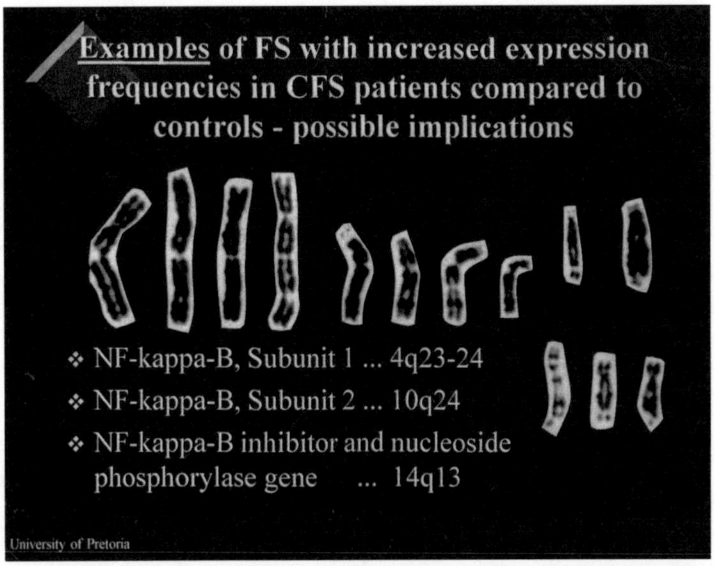


Fig. 2. Examples of induced chromosomal fragile sites in regions harbouring NF-KB genes.

### 7.2 A diseasome overlap with Persian Gulf War syndrome?

Chronic fatigue syndrome (CFS) and Persian Gulf War Ilness (PGI)/Persian Gulf War Syndrome (PGWS) and Fibromyalgia syndrome (FMS) are overlapping symptom complexes without objective markers or known pathophysiology according to the literature. When the cerebrospinal fluid proteome was examined to find proteins that were differentially expressed in this CFS-spectrum of illnesses compared to control subjects an identical set of central nervous system, innate immune and amyloidogenic proteins in cerebrospinal fluids were identified in two independent cohorts of subjects with overlapping CFS, PGWS and fibromyalgia. Although syndrome names and definitions were different, the proteome and presumed pathological mechanism(s) appear to be shared (Baraniuk et al., 2005). PGWS may be a syndrome especially occurring in FMS susceptible genotypes when exposed to specific genotoxicants or the stress of warfare. Of the 130 veterans who were evaluated clinically, 103 had unexplained fatigue, and 44 veterans met the 1994 U.S. Centers for Disease Control criteria for CFS (Mc Cauley et al., 2002). The number of Gulf War veterans who have developed the so-called Gulf War syndrome has risen to about one-third of the 800,000 U.S. forces deployed, and unknown proportions of those involved in the subsequent wars. Uncounted civilians and personnel of other nations that fought in Iraq and other wars since 1991 have also been afflicted (Bertell, 2006). Particulate depleted uranium (DU), widely suspected as one of the prime causes of PGWS associated pathologies, compounds were demonstrated to induce time and concentration-dependent cytotoxic (producing a toxic

effect on cells) and clastogenic (causing disruption or breakages of chromosomes) effects in human lung cells. The types of aberrations seen with treatment of particulate DU are consistent with those induced by other carcinogenic metals (Wise et al., 2007). Tests of 5 Gulf War Veterans in 2007 analysed by Wayne State University Medical staff revealed the 5 Veterans studied have severe chromosome damage. The damage uncovered is 10 times the level found in the normal population. The chromosome damage is similar to that seen when exposed to alpha radiation and could be related to depleted uranium munitions exposure.
In another study by Urnovitz et al., (1999), sera from Persian Gulf War veterans contained polyribonucleotides (amplicons) that ranged in size from 200 to ca. 2,000 bp. Sera from controls did not contain amplicons larger than 450 bp. DNA sequences were derived from two amplicons unique to veterans. These amplicons, which were 414 and 759 nucleotides, were unrelated to each other or to any sequence in gene bank databases. The amplicons contained short segments that were homologous to regions of chromosome 22q11.2, an antigen-responsive hot spot for genetic rearrangements. Many of these short amplicon segments occurred near, between, or in chromosome 22q11.2 Alu sequences. These results suggest that genetic alterations in the 22q11.2 region, possibly induced by exposures to environmental genotoxins during the Persian Gulf War, may have played a role in the pathogenesis of the Gulf War Syndrome. However, the data did not exclude the possibility that other chromosomes also may have been involved (Urnovitz et al., 1999). The fragile site-like nature of all of the breakpoint sites involved in translocations with the recurrent site on 22q11.21, suggests a mechanism based on delay of DNA replication in the initiation of these chromosomal rearrangements (Gotter et al., 2007). This breakpoint is located between two AT-rich inverted repeats that form a nearly perfect palindrome (a typical common fragile site structural characteristic (Politi et al., 2010). It remains remarkable that a known interface between environmental and genomic stress, the DNA double strand break, leading to altered transcriptional activity of genes suggested here to be involved with key PWGS-associated disorders, have not been considered before as a comprehensive study approach for PGWS.. Standard cytogenetic analyses will be inadequate, and a stringently controlled study of in vitro induced breakage is proposed in war veterans and unexposed controls, including first degree relatives.

## 8. Conclusion

Garcia-Campayo and co-workers (2009) took the optimistic view that imaging can take advantage of developments straight from routine individual biomarkers to multiple-scale biomarker profiles. "Imaging should predict treatment response, look at stratification for specific treatment modalities, and look at the characterization of an individual patient" (Garcia-Campayo et al., 2009). Browning et al., 2011 recently reviewed the debate about the nature of somatoform disorders (such as fibromyalgia) and posed the question: "Is there evidence of altered neural function or structure that is specifically associated with somatoform disorders?" These authors described studies reporting neuroimaging findings in patients with a somatoform disorder or a functional somatic syndrome (such as fibromyalgia) and found a "relatively mature literature on symptoms of pain" (and less developed literatures on conversion and fatigue symptoms). (Browning et al., 2011). Both the hippocampus (Emad et al., 2008; Wood et al., 2009; Fayed et al., 2010) and amygdala (Lutz et al., 2008; Burgmer et al., 2009; Valdés et al., 2010) have been implicated in FMS. To summarize, the literature suggests that early life is a period of increased vulnerability, although the effects of stress may be difficult to detect for years (as seems to be the case with the hippocampus); stress-induced changes in amygdala (initial increases in activity and growth) are apparent earlier in life and more robustly than the hippocampus (decreases in growth), and later in life, when hippocampal changes are finally apparent, the initial amygdala volume increases may ultimately change to volumetric decreases (although it may remain hyperactive). Thus, through a combination of connectivity and volumetric studies, it would be possible to, in children as young as two years old, and extending through adulthood, examine the structural and functional networks that underlie the embedding of adversity.These brain areas represent important neuroanatomical structural markers that could be linked to the proposed stress memory interface pathways modifying the effects of early experiences on the developing human brain.

### 8.1 Genetic and clinical implications

The clinical hypothesis that needs to be investigated further is that foetal programming by intrauterine stress leads to stress hypersensitivity during later life insults in genetically susceptible individuals. The genetic susceptibility mechanism may be based on disruption of a stress hormone-immune recombination-brain fragilome 'interface' pathway together with modifying polymorphic variation in the more fixed associated genetic building bricks anywhere along this pathway (e.g. HPA axis and glucocorticoid genetic variation). Furthermore, such a complex set of changes should be analyzable according to modern integrative genetics analyses. The ability to correlate dynamic changes in cellular ROS levels with mitochondrial metabolism and neuronal network activity is already a promising step towards a detailed mechanistic understanding of redox- and ROS-mediated signalling in normal and diseased brain function (Funke et al., 2011), and this can be expected to contribute significantly to imaging of programmed stress disorders.

In order to gain further insight into human genomic flexibility and its role in individual neurodevelopment, as well as neurological and neurobehavioural disorder phenotypes, current cytogenetic information about fragile genomic regions needs to be augmented by techniques such as innovative next generation sequence variation data, transcriptomic data, epigenomic data and analysis of the interactome to circumvent previous problems in this regard. Assigning genes to context-dependent and potentially overlapping 'transcription modules' in fragile regions will provide functional predictions for numerous genes as had been done in yeast to identify relations between modules (Re et al., 2006) and present a global view on the proposed interface system transcriptional networks. CFS characteristics may underly many previous analytic dilemmas in assessing the neurogenetic response to the environment. For instance, megabase-long satellite sequences and CFS-associated contiguous segmental duplications hamper both physical and fine scale genetic mapping. Links with miRNA, altered methylation and the origin of copy number variation now indicate that CFS region characteristics may be part of chromatinomic mechanisms that are increasingly linked with neuroplasticity and memory. RNA is centrally involved in directing various epigenetic processes considered to occur in neurons, implying that the transcriptional state of the cell is the primary determinant of epigenetic memory. Changes in a small number of RNA regulatory proteins may thus generate a great diversity of biological outcomes.

The stage is now set to integrate transgenerational psychological stress research with, *inter alia* fragilomic and epigenomic studies and the extensive amount of available neuroanatomic imaging findings in prototypical antenatally programmed stress disorders. The aim would be to initiate the research and design of suitable imaging biomarkers to elucidate the role of stress pathways of an interface system (hormones, antibodies and fragile sites) during physiological learning and memory processes, how such stress shapes the developing brain, and what spectrum of disorders may result when physiological activity thresholds are exceeded and pathological processes start appearing.

*"Data integration itself is not an end: it is designed to generate novel hypotheses and help to test them"* (Hawkins et al., 2010).

## 9. Acknowledgement

I wish to thank Dr Ingrid Simonic, who significantly contributed to a better understanding of the potential role of chromosomal fragile sites in complex multifactorial disorders in our earlier research.

## 10. References

Anholt, RR. (2004). Genetic modules and networks for behavior: lessons from Drosophila. *Bioessays* 26(12):1299–306.

Arlt, MF., Durkin SG., Ragland RL.,& Glover TW. (2006). Common fragile sites as targets for chromosome rearrangements. *DNA Repair (Amst)* Sep 8;5(9-10):1126-35.

Ashe, A., Whitelaw E. (2007). Another role for RNA: a messenger across generations. Trends Genet 23(1):8-10.

Babu, MM, Luscombe, NM, Aravind, L, Gerstein, M., & Teichmann, SA. (2004). Structure and evolution of transcriptional regulatory networks. *Curr Opin Struct Biol* 14(3):283–91.

Barabási, AL., Gulbahce, N., & Loscalzo, J. (2011). Network medicine: a network-based approach to human disease. *Nat Rev Genet* 12(1):56-68.

Baraniuk, JN., Casado, B., Maibach, H., Clauw, DJ., Pannell, LK., & Hess, S. (2005). A chronic fatigue syndrome - related proteome in human cerebrospinal fluid. *BMC Neurology* 5:22

Bengtsson, BO. (2004). Modelling the evolution of genomes with integrated external and internal functions. *J Theor Biol* 21;231(2):271-8.

Ben-Tabou de-Leon, S., Davidson, EH. (2007); Gene regulation: gene control network in development. *Annu Rev Biophys Biomol Struct* 36:191.

Bertell, R. (2006). Depleted uranium: all the queations about DU and Gulf War syndrome are not yet answered. *Int J Health Serv* 36(3):503-20.

Bhadra, P., Petersel, D. (2010). Medical conditions in fibromyalgia patients and their relationship to pregabalin efficacy: pooled analysis of Phase III clinical trials. *Expert Opin Pharmacother* 11(17):2805-12.

Blasquez, VC., Sperry, AO., Cockerill, PN., & Garrard WT. (1989). Protein:DNA interactions at chromosomal loop attachment sites. *Genome* 31(2):503–9.

Boldogkoi, Z. (2004). Gene network polymorphism is the raw material of natural selection: the selfish gene network hypothesis. *J Mol Evol* 59(3):340–57.

Bosman, DW., Blom, EJ., Ogao, PJ., Kuipers OP., & Roerdink JB. (2007). MOVE: a multi-level ontology-based visualization and exploration framework for genomic networks. *In Silico Biol* 7(1):35-59.

Browning, M., Fletcher, P., & Sharpe, M. (2011). Can neuroimaging help us to understand and classify somatoform disorders? A systematic and critical review. *Psychosom Med* 73(2):173-84.

Burgmer, M., Gaubitz, M., Konrad, C., Wrenger, M., Hilgart, S., Heuft, G., & Pfleiderer, B. (2009). Decreased gray matter volumes in the cingulo-frontal cortex and the amygdala in patients with fibromyalgia. *Psychosom Med* 71(5):566-73.

Cantu-Paz, E., Goldberg, DE. (1999). On the scalability of parallel genetic algorithms. *Evol Comput* 7(4):429-49.

Caspi, A., Sugden, K., Moffitt, TE., Taylor, A., Craig, I., Harrington, I., McClay, J., Mill, J., Martin, I., Braithwaite, A., & Poulton, R. (2003). Influence of life stress on depression: moderation by a polymorphism in the 5-HTT gene, *Science* 301:386–389.

Champagne, FA. (2008). Epigenetic mechanisms and the transgenerational effects of maternal care. *Front. Neuroendocrinol* 29:386–397.

Chun, J. (1999). Developmental neurobiology: a genetic Cheshire cat? *Curr Biol. Ser* 9;9(17):R651-4.

Corballis, MC. (1992). On the evolution of language and generativity. *Cognition* 44(3):197-26.

Cordero, OX., Hogeweg, P. (2006). Feed-forward loop circuits as a side effect of genome evolution. *Mol Biol Evol* 23(10):1931–6.

Cosgrove, MS., Wolberger, C. (2005). How does the histone code work? *Biochem Cell Biol* 83(4):468-76.

Costa, E., Grayson, DR., Veldic, M., & Guidotti, A. (2004). Neurochemical basis for an epigenetic vision of synaptic organization. *Int Rev Neurobiol* 59:73-91.

Chatterji, M., Tsai, CL., & Schatz, DG. (2004). New concepts in the regulation of an ancient reaction: transposition by RAG1/RAG2. *Immunol Rev* 200:261–71.

Chung, WY., Albert, R., Albert, I., Nekrutenko, A., & Makova, KD. (2006). Rapid and asymmetric divergence of duplicate genes in the human gene coexpression network. *BMC Bioinformatics* 7:46.

Chuzhanova, N., Chen, JM., Bacolla, A., Patrinos, GP., Férec, C., Wells, RD., & Cooper, DN. (2009). Gene conversion causing human inherited disease: evidence for involvement of non-B-DNA-forming sequences and recombination-promoting motifs in DNA breakage and repair. *Hum Mutat* 30(8):1189-1198

Cleary, JD., Pearson, CE. (2003). The contribution of cis-elements to disease-associated repeat instability: clinical and experimental evidence. *Cytogenet Genome Res* 100(1–4): 25–55.

Crepaldi, L., Riccio, A. (2009). Chromatin learns to behave. *Epigenetics* 4(1):23-6.

Crespi, EJ., Denver, RJ. (2005). Ancient origins of human developmental plasticity. *Am J Hum Biol* 17(1):44-54.

Crews, D. (2008). Epigenetics and its implications for behavioral neuroendocrinology. *Front Neuroendocrinol* 29(3):344-57.

Cushman, J., Lo J., Huang, Z., Wasserfall, C., & Petitto, JM. (2003). Neurobehavioral changes resulting from recombinase activation gene 1 deletion. *Clin Diagn Lab Immunol* 10(1):13-8.

Dai, J,. Xie, W,. Brady, TL,. Gao, J,. & Voytas, DF. (2007). Phosphorylation regulates integration of the yeast Ty5 retrotransposon into heterochromatin. *Mol Cell* 20;27(2):289-99.

Delcuve, GP., Rastegar, M., & Davie, JR. (2009). Epigenetic control. *J Cell Physiol* 219(2):243–50.

Dietert, RR., Dietert, JM. (2008).Potential for early-life immune insult including developmental immunotoxicity in autism and autism spectrum disorders: focus on critical windows of immune vulnerability. *J Toxicol Environ Health B Crit Rev* 11(8):660–80.

Dillon, N. (2006). Gene regulation and large-scale chromatin organization in the nucleus. *Chromosome Res* 14(1):117–26.

Durand, CM., Kappeler, C., Betancur, C., Delorme, R., Quach, H., Goubran-Botros, H., Melke, J., Nygren, G., Chabane, N., Bellivier, F., Szoke, A., Schurhoff, F., Rastam, M., Anckarsäter, H., Gillberg, C., Leboyer, M., & Bourgeron, T. (2006). Expression and genetic variability of PCDH11Y, a gene specific to Homo sapiens and candidate for susceptibility to psychiatric disorders. *Am J Med Genet B (Neuropsychiatr Genet)* 5;141(1):67-70.

Emad, Y., Ragab, Y., Zeinhom, F., El-Khouly, G., Abou-Zeid, A., & Rasker, JJ. (2008). Hippocampus dysfunction may explain symptoms of fibromyalgia syndrome. A study with single-voxel magnetic resonance spectroscopy. *J Rheumatol* 35(7):1371-7.

Fayed, N., Garcia-Campayo, J., Magallón, R., Andrés-Bergareche, H., Luciano, JV., Andres, E., & Beltrán, J. (2010). Localized 1H-NMR spectroscopy in patients with fibromyalgia: a controlled study of changes in cerebral glutamate/glutamine, inositol, choline, and N-acetylaspartate. *Arthritis Res Ther* 12(4):R134.

Fraga MF, Ballestar E, Paz MF, Ropero S, Setien F, Ballestar ML, Heine-Suñer,D., Cigudosa JC, Urioste M, Benitez J, Boix-Chornet M, Sanchez-Aguilera A, Ling C, Carlsson E, Poulsen P, Vaag A, Stephan Z, Spector TD, Wu YZ, Plass C, & Esteller M.(2005). Epigenetic differences arise during the lifetime of monozygotic twins. *Proc Natl Acad Sci* U S A. Jul 26;102(30):10604-9.

Funke, F., Gerich, FJ., & Müller M.(2011). Dynamic, semi-quantitative imaging of intracellular ROS levels and redox status in rat hippocampal neurons. *Neuroimage* 54(4):2590-602.

García-Campayo, J; Fayed, N; Serrano-Blanco, I; & Roca, Miquel. (2009). Brain dysfunction behind functional symptoms: neuroimaging and somatoform, conversive, and dissociative disorders. *Current Opinion in Psychiatry* 22: 224-231

Garofalo, G., Ragusa, RM., Argiolas, A., Scavuzzo, C., Spina, E., & Barletta, C. (1993) Evidence of chromosomal fragile sites in schizophrenic patients. *Ann Genet.*36(2):132-5.

Gericke, GS., Simonic, I., Cloete, E., Buckle, C., & Becker, PJ. (1995). Increased chromosomal breakage in Tourette Syndrome predicts the possibility of variable multiple gene involvement in spectrum phenotypes: Preliminary findings and hypotheses. *American Journal of Medical Genetics (Neuropsychiat Genet)* 60:444-447.

Gericke, GS. (1998). Chromosomal fragility may be indicative of altered higher-order DNA organization as the underlying genetic diathesis in complex neurobehavioral disorders. *Med Hypotheses* 50(4):319-26.

Gericke, GS. (2006). Reactive oxygen species and related haem pathway components as possible epigenetic modifiers in neurobehavioural pathology. *Med Hypotheses* 66(1):92-9.

Gericke, GS. (2006). Chromosomal fragility, structural rearrangements and mobile element activity may reflect dynamic epigenetic mechanisms of importance in neurobehavioural genetics..*Med Hypotheses* 66(2):276-85.

Gericke, GS. (2010). Common chromosomal fragile sites (CFS) may be involved in normal and traumatic cognitive stress memory consolidation and altered nervous system immunity. *Med Hypotheses* 74(5):911-8.

Gibson, KR. (2002). Evolution of human intelligence: the roles of brain size and mental construction. *Brain Behav Evol* 59(1-2):10-20

Gilmore, EC., Nowakowski, RS., Caviness Jr, VS., & Herrup, K.. (2000). Cell birth, cell death, cell diversity and DNA breaks: how do they all fit together? *Trends Neurosci* 23(3):100–5.

Glover, TW., Arlt, MF., Casper, AM., & Durkin, SG. (2005). Mechanisms of common fragile site instability. *Hum Mol Genet* 14 Spec No. 2:R197-205.

Goldschmidt, R. (1982). *The Material Basis of Evolution.* Yale University Press, ISBN:9780300028232, New Haven.

González, E., Elorza, J., & Failde, I. (2010). Fibromyalgia and psychiatric comorbidity: their effect on the quality of life patients. *Actas Esp Psiquiatr* 38(5):295-300.

Gow, JW., Hagan, S., Herzyk, P., Cannon, C., Behan, PO., & Chaudhuri, A. (2009). A gene signature for post-infectious chronic fatigue syndrome. *BMC Med Genomics* 25;2:38.

Grandbastien, MA. (2004). Stress activation and genomic impact of plant retrotransposons. *J Soc Biol* 198(4):425-32.

Gupta, S., Kim, SY., Artis, S., Molfese, DL., Schumacher, A., Sweatt, JD., Paylor, RE., & Lubin, FD. (2010). Histone methylation regulates memory formation. *J Neurosci* 30(10):3589-99.

Guterman, A., Richter-Levin, G. (2006). Neuromodulators of LTP and NCAMs in the amygdala and hippocampus in response to stress. *EXS* 98:137–48.

Hawkins, RD., Hon, GC., & Ren, B. (2010). Next generation genomics: an integrative approach. *Nature Reviews Genetics* 11, 476-486

Hayashi, MT., Masukata, H. (2011). Regulation of DNA replication by chromatin structures: accessibility and recruitment. *Chromosoma*. Feb;120(1):39-46.

Hilschman, N., Barnikol, HU., Barnikol-Watanabe, S., Götz, H., Kratzin, H., & Thinnes, FP. (2001). The immunoglobulin-like genetic predetermination of the brain: the protocadherins, blueprint of the neuronal network. *Naturwissenschaften* 88(1):2-12.

Hinsch, H., Hannenhalli, S. (2006). Recurring genomic breaks in independent lineages support genomic fragility. *BMC Evol Biol* 6:90.

Hirayama, T., Yagi, T. (2006). The role and expression of the protocadherin-alpha clusters in the CNS. *Curr Opin Neurobiol* 16(3):336-42.

Holliday, KL., Nicholl, BI., Macfarlane, GJ., Thomson, W., Davies, KA., & McBeth, J. (2010). Genetic variation in the hypothalamic-pituitary-adrenal stress axis influences susceptibility to musculoskeletal pain: results from the EPIFUND study. *Ann Rheum Dis* 69(3):556-60.

Hsu, E, Pulham, N, Rumfelt, LL, & Flajnik, MF. (2006). The plasticity of immunoglobulin gene systems in evolution. *Immunol Rev* 210:8-26.

Ishiwata, K. (2009). Strategy for development of imaging biomarkers. *Nihon Shinkei Seishin Yakurigaku Zasshi* 29(2):67-71.

Jablonka, E, Raz, G. (2009). Transgenerational epigenetic inheritance:Prevalence, Mechanisms and Implications for the Study of Heredity and Evolution. *The Quarterly Review of Biology* 84: 131–176.

Jackson, JA, Trevino, AV, Herzig, MC, Herman, TS, & Woynarowski, JM.. (2003). Matrix attachment region (MAR) properties and abnormal expansion of AT island minisatellites in FRA16B fragile sites in leukemic CEM cells. *Nucleic Acids Res* 31(21):6354–64.

Jorgensen, RA. (2004). Restructuring the Genome in Response to Adaptive Challenge: McClintock's Bold Conjecture Revisited. *Cold Spring Harb Symp Quant Biol* 69: 349-354

Kaushal, D., Contos, JJ., Treuner, K., Yang, AH., Kingsbury, MA., Rehen, SK., McConnell, MJ., Okabe, M., Barlow, C., & Chun, J. (2003). Alteration of gene expression by chromosome loss in the postnatal mouse brain. *J Neurosci* 23(13):5599-606.

Karayiorgou, M., Simon, TJ., & Gogos, JA. (2010). 22q11.2 microdeletions: linking DNA structural variation to brain dysfunction and schizophrenia. *Nat Rev Neurosci* 11(6):402-16.

Kingsbury, MA., Friedman, B., McConnell, MJ., Rehen, SK., Yang, AH., Kaushal, D.,& Chun, J. (2005). Aneuploid neurons are functionally active and integrated into brain circuitry. *Proc Natl Acad Sci* 102(17):6143-7.

Lee, JA., Lupsk,i JR. (2006). Genomic rearrangements and gene copy-number alterations as a cause of nervous system disorders. *Neuron* 52(1):103–21.

Levenson, JM., Sweatt, JD. (2006). Epigenetic mechanisms: a common theme in vertebrate and invertebrate memory formation. *Cell Mol Life Sci* 63(9):1009–16.

Liebich, I., Bode, J., Reuter, I., & Wingender E. (2002). Evaluation of sequence motifs found in scaffold/matrix-attached regions (S/MARs). *Nucleic Acids Res* 30(15):3433-42.Litman, GW., Cannon, JP., & Dishaw LJ. (2005). Reconstructing immune phylogeny: new perspectives. *Nat Rev Immunol* 11:866-79.

Lubin, FD., Sweatt, JD. (2007). The IkappaB kinase regulates chromatin structure during reconsolidation of conditioned fear memories. *Neuron* 55(6):942-57.

Lutz, J., Jäger, L., de Quervain, D., Krauseneck, T., Padberg, F., Wichnalek, M., Beyer, A., Stahl, R., Zirngibl, B., Morhard, D., Reiser, M., & Schelling, G. (2008). White and gray matter abnormalities in the brain of patients with fibromyalgia: a diffusion-tensor and volumetric imaging study. *Arthritis Rheum* 58(12):3960-9.

Madlung ,A., Comai L. (2004) The effect of stress on genome regulation and structure. *Ann Bot (Lond)* 94(4): 48 1–95.

McCauley, LA., Joos, SK., Barkhuizen, A., Shuell, T., Tyree, WA., & Bourdette, DN. (2002). Chronic fatigue in a population-based study of Gulf War veterans. *Arch Environ Health* 57:340-8.

McClintock, B. (1987). *The Discovery and Characterization of Transposable Elements: the Collected Papers of Barbara McClintock.* Garland, New York

McFarlane, RJ., Whitehall, SK. (2009). tRNA genes in eukaryotic genome organization and reorganization. *Cell Cycle* 8(19):3102-6.

Meaney, MJ. (2001). Maternal care gene expression and the transmission of individual differences in stress reactivity across generations, *Ann. Rev. Neurosci* 24:161–192.

Meaney, MJ., Syzf, M. (2005). Environmental programming of stress responses through DNA methylation: life at the interface between a dynamic environment and a fixed genome. *Dialogues Clin. Neurosci* 7:103–123.

Miki, R., Hattori, K., Taguchi, Y., Tada, MN., Isosaka, T., Hidaka, Y., Hirabayashi, T., Hashimoto,R., Fukuzako, H., & Yagi, T. (2005). Identification and characterization of coding single-nucleotide polymorphisms within human protocadherin-alpha and -beta gene clusters. *Gene* 349:1-14.

Miyata, S., Hatton, GI. (2002). Activity-related, dynamic neuron-glial interactions in the hypothalamo-neurohypophysial system. *Microsc Res Tech* 56(2):143-57.

Morange, M. (2009), What history tells us XVII. Conrad Waddington and the nature of life. *J Biosci* 34(2):195-8.

Murr, R. (2010). Interplay between different epigenetic modifications and mechanisms. *Adv Genet* 70:101-41.

Natelson, BH. (2010). Chronic fatigue syndrome and fibromyalgia: a status report in 2010. *MD Advis* 3(3):18-25.

Nakayama, T., Yamashita, M. (2008). Initiation and maintenance of Th2 cell identity. *Curr Opin Immunol* 20(3):265-71.

Nelson, W., Luo, M., Ma, J., Estep, M., Estill, J., He, R., Talag, J., Sisneros, N., Kudrna, D.,Kim, H., Ammiraju, JS., Collura, K., Bharti, AK., Messing, J., Wing, RA., SanMiguel, P., Bennetzen, JL., & Soderlund, C. (2008). Methylation-sensitive linking libraries enhance gene-enriched sequencing of complex genomes and map DNA methylation domains. *BMC Genomics* 9:621.

Nelson, ED., Monteggia, LM. (2011). Epigenetics in the mature mammalian brain: Effects on behavior and synaptic transmission. *Neurobiol Learn Mem* Mar 30. [Epub ahead of print]

Niederberger, E., Geisslinger, G. (2008). The IKK-NF-kappaB pathway: a source for novel molecular drug targets in pain therapy? *FASEB J* 22(10):3432-42.

Orozco, LD, Cokus, SJ, Ghazalpour, A, Ingram-Drake, L, Wang, S, van Nas, A, Che, N, Araujo, JA, Pellegrini, M., & Lusis, AJ. (2009). Copy number variation influences gene expression and metabolic traits in mice. *Hum Mol Genet* 18(21):4118-29.

Pancer, Z., Cooper, MD. (2006). The evolution of adaptive immunity. *Annu Rev Immunol* 24:497-518.

Pedrosa, E., Stefanescu, R., Margolis, B., Petruolo, O., Lo, Y., Nolan, K., Novak, T., Stopkova, P., & Lachman, HM. (2008). Analysis of protocadherin alpha gene enhancer polymorphism in bipolar disorder and schizophrenia. *Schizophr Res* 102(1-3):210-9.

Potkin, SG., Macciardi, F., Guffanti, G., Fallon, JH., Wang,Q., Turner,JA., Lakatos,A., Miles,MF.,Lander, A., Vawter,MP., & Xie,X. (2010). Identifying gene regulatory networks in schizophrenia. *Neuroimage* 53(3):839-847.

Puliti, A., Rizzato, C., Conti, V., Bedini, A., Gimelli, G., Barale, R., & Sbrana, I. (2010). Low-copy repeats on chromosome 22q11.2 show replication timing switches, DNA flexibility peaks and stress inducible asynchrony, sharing instability features with fragile sites. *Mutat Res* 1;686:74- 83.

Raghavan, SC., Kirsch, IR., & Lieber, MR. (2001). Analysis of the V(D)J recombination efficiency at lymphoid chromosomal translocation breakpoints. *J Biol Chem* 276(31):29126–33.

Rajendran, RS., Zupanc, MM., Lösche, A., Westra, J., Chun, J., & Zupanc, GK. (2007). Numerical chromosome variation and mitotic segregation defects in the adult brain of teleost fish. *Dev Neurobiol* 67(10):1334-47.

Re, A., Cora, D., Puliti, AM., Caselle, M., & Sbrana I. (2006). Correlated fragile site expression allows the identification of candidate fragile genes involved in immunity and associated with carcinogenesis. *BMC Bioinformatics* 7:413.

Rehen, SK., Yung, YC., McCreight, MP., Kaushal, D., Yang, AH., Almeida, BS., Kingsbury, MA.,Cabral, KM., McConnell, MJ., Anliker, B., Fontanoz ,M., & Chun, J. (2005). Constitutional aneuploidy in the normal human brain. *J Neurosci* 25(9):2176-80.

Rooney, S., Chaudhuri, J., & Alt, FW. (2004). The role of the non-homologous end-joining pathway in lymphocyte development. *Immunol Rev* 200:115-31.

Roth, DB., Roth, SY. (2000). Unequal access: regulating V(D)J recombination through chromatin remodeling. *Cell* 103(5):699-702.

Savelyeva, L., Sagulenko, E., Schmitt, JG., & Schwab, M. (2006). Low-frequency common fragile sites: link to neuropsychiatric disorders? *Cancer Lett* 232(1):58-69.

Sbrana, I., Zavattari ,P., Barale, R., & Musio, A. (1998). Common fragile sites on human chromosomes represent transcriptionally active regions: evidence from camptothecin. *Hum Genet* 102(4):409-14.

Schatz, DG. (2004). Antigen receptor genes and the evolution of a recombinase. *Semin Immunol* 16(4):245-56.

Seckl, JR., Holmes, MC. (2007). Mechanisms of disease: glucocorticoids, their placental metabolism and fetal 'programming' of adult pathophysiology. *Nat Clin Pract Endocrinol Metab* (6):479-88.

Shaklai, S., Amariglio, N., Rechavi, G., & Simon, AJ. (2007). Gene silencing at the nuclear periphery. *FEBS J* 274(6):1383–92.

Simonic, I., Gericke, GS. (1996). The enigma of common fragile sites. *Hum Genet* 97:524-31.

Simonic, I., Ott, J. (1996). Novel etiological hypotheses imply new analysis methods for schizophrenia genetics. *Schizophr Res* 20(1-2):235-7.

Singh, SM., McDonald, P., Murphy, B., & O'Reilly, R. (2004). Incidental neurodevelopmental episodes in the etiology of schizophrenia: an expanded model involving epigenetics and development. *Clin Genet* 65(6):435-40.

Sjakste, NI., Sjakste, TG. (2007). Possible involvement of DNA breaks in epigenetic regulation of cell differentiation. *Genetika* 43(5):581–600.

Skinner, MK. (2011). Role of epigenetics in developmental biology and transgenerational inheritance. *Birth Defects Res C Embryo Today* 93(1):51-5.

Stribinskis, V., Ramos, KS. (2006). Activation of human long interspersed nuclear element 1 retrotransposition by benzo(a)pyrene, an ubiquitous environmental carcinogen. *Cancer Res* 66(5):2616-20.

Striedter, GF. (1998). Progress in the study of brain evolution: from speculative theories to testable hypotheses. *Anat Rec* 253(4):105–12.

Sun, JG., Han, S., Ji, H., Zheng, Y., & Ling, SC. (2007). Expression of RAG-1 in brain during mouse development. *Zhejiang Da Xue Xue Bao Yi Xue Ban* 36(2):161-6.

Trapman, J., Dubbink, HJ. (2007). The role of cofactors in sex steroid action. *Best Pract Res Clin Endocrinol Metab* 21(3):403–14.

Turner, JD., Pelascini, LP., Macedo, JA., & Muller, CP. (2008). Highly individual methylation patterns of alternative glucocorticoid receptor promoters suggest individualized epigenetic regulatory mechanisms. *Nucleic Acids Res* 36(22):7207-18.

Turner, AI., Tilbrook, AJ. (2006). Stress, cortisol and reproduction in female pigs. *Soc Reprod Fertil Suppl.* 62:191-203.

Urnovitz, HB., Tuite, JJ., Higashida, JM., & Murphy, WH. (1999). RNAs in the sera of Persian Gulf War veterans have segments homologous to chromosome 22q11.2. *Clin Diagn Lab Immunol* 6(3):330-5.

Valdés, M., Collado, A., Bargalló, N., Vázquez, M., Rami, L., Gómez, E., & Salamero, M. (2010). Increased glutamate/glutamine compounds in the brains of patients with fibromyalgia: a magnetic resonance spectroscopy study. *Arthritis Rheum* 62(6):1829-36.

Wallace, DC. (2010). The epigenome and the mitochondrion: bioenergetics and the environment. *Genes Dev* 24(15):1571-3.

Varmuza, S. (2003). Epigenetics and the renaissance of heresy. *Genome* 46: 963-957

Waerzeggers, Y., Monfared, P., Viel,T., Winkeler,A., & Jacobs, AH. (2010). Mouse models in neurological disorders:applications of non-invasive imaging. *Biochim Biophys Acta* 1802: 819-839.

Wang, T., Zeng, J., Lowe, CB., Sellers, RG., Salama, SR., Yang, M., Burgess, SM., Brachmann, RK., & Haussler, D. (2007). Species-specific endogenous retroviruses shape the transcriptional network of the human tumor suppressor protein p53. *Proc Natl Acad Sci U S A* 104(47):18613-8.

Wang, YH. (2006). Chromatin structure of human chromosomal fragile sites. *Cancer Lett* 232(1):70-8.

Weaver, IC., Meaney, MJ., & Szyf, M. (2006). Maternal care effects on the hippocampal transcriptome and anxiety-mediated behaviors in the offspring that are reversible in adulthood, *Proc. Natl. Acad. Sci. USA* 103:3480–3485.

Williams, SK., Truong, D., & Tyler, JK. (2008). Acetylation in the globular core of histone H3 on lysine- 56 promotes chromatin disassembly during transcriptional activation. *Proc Natl Acad Sci U S A* 105(26):9000-5.

Wilson, AS., Power, BE., & Molloy, PL. (2007). DNA hypomethylation and human diseases. *Biochim Biophys Acta* 1775(1):138-62.

Wise, SS., Thompson, WD., Aboueissa, AM., Mason, MD., & Wise, JP. (2007). Particulate depleted uranium is cytotoxic and clastogenic to human lung cells. *Chem Res Toxicol* 20(5):815-820.

Wood, PB., Ledbetter, CR., Glabus, MF., Broadwell, LK., & Patterson, JC. (2009). Hippocampal metabolite abnormalities in fibromyalgia: correlation with clinical features. *J Pain* 10(1):47-52.

Woynarowski, JM. (2004). AT islands - their nature and potential for anticancer strategies. *Curr Cancer Drug Targets* 4(2):219-34.

Wu, Q. (2005). Comparative genomics and diversifying selection of the clustered vertebrate protocadherin genes. *Genetics* 169(4):2179-88.

Yagi, T. (2003). Diversity of the cadherin-related neuronal receptor/protocadherin family and possible DNA rearrangement in the brain. *Genes Cells* 8(1):1-8.

Yang, AH., Kaushal, D., Rehen, SK., Kriedt, K., Kingsbury, MA., McConnell, MJ., & Chun, J. (2003). Chromosome segregation defects contribute to aneuploidy in normal neural progenitor cells. *J Neurosci* 23(32):10454- 62.

Yurov, YB., Iourov, IY., Vorsanova., SG, Liehr., T, Kolotii, AD., Kutsev, SI., Pellestor, F., Beresheva, AK., Demidova, IA., Kravets, VS., Monakhov, VV., & Soloviev, IV. (2007). Aneuploidy and confined chromosomal mosaicism in the developing human brain. *PLoS One* 2(6):e558.

Zukin, RS., Richter, JD., & Bagni, C. (2009). Signals, synapses, and synthesis: how new proteins control plasticity. *Front Neural Circuits* 3:14.

# 18

# Abnormal Brain Density in Victims of Rape with PTSD in Mainland China: A Voxel-Based Analysis of Magnetic Resonance Imaging Study

Shuang Ge Sui[1], Ling Jiang Li[1], Yan Zhang[1], Ming Xiang Wu[2] and Mark E. King[3]
[1]*Mental Health Institute, Second Xiangya Hospital, Central-South University*
[2]*ShenZhen People's Hospital*
[3]*Faculty of Education, The University of Hong Kong, HHSAR*
*P. R. China*

## 1. Introduction

Posttraumatic stress disorder (PTSD) is a relatively common and predictable psychological syndrome (Miller, 1999). PTSD occurs in a proportion of individuals exposed to severe psychological trauma (Kasai et al., 2006) and in which the individual responds with fear, helplessness, or horror (Danckwerts & Leathem, 2003). Individuals with PTSD suffer from intrusive memories about the traumatic event, persistent avoidance of stimuli associated with the trauma, and persistent symptoms of increased arousal. These symptoms become uncontrollable and disabling (Bremner & Charney, 1994) that serious threaten human health and social function. Due to its debilitating nature, PTSD has emerged as an important public health problem in the general population (Sareen et al., 2007).

In recent years, a great deal of research has been directed towards understanding the etiology, phenomenology, neurobiology, clinical characteristics and treatment of PTSD (Nemeroff et al., 2006). However, a number of core psychological processes underlying PTSD have yet to be elucidated (Shin et al., 2006; Liberzon & Sripada, 2008). Over the past decade, findings from neuroimaging studies have allowed for tremendous advances in our understanding of the experience of emotions in healthy individuals and the dysregulation of these processes associated with PTSD. These studies have been useful in both generating hypotheses on the neurobiology of normative human responses to trauma and complementing our understanding of the wide-ranging alterations in trauma survivors who develop PTSD.

Structural neuroimaging studies have focused primarily on hippocampal volumetry (Geuze et al., 2005) as well as the prefrontal cortex (Geuze et al., 2008a) and other brain structures. Hippocampal morphology has been correlated with severity of PTSD symptomatology (Gilbertson et al., 2002; Villarreal & King, 2004). However, the results have been inconsistent, with studies reporting significant reductions or increases, as well as unchanged volumes. For example, studies have shown that patients with PTSD are associated with bilateral lower hippocampal volume (Bossini & Castrogiovanni, 2007; Bremner et al., 2003; Emdad et al., 2006; Lindauer et al., 2004a; Vythilingam et al., 2005; Li et al., 2006), which are considered to be either due to atrophy of the hippocampus as a consequence of suffering from PTSD due to excessive stress (Bremner et al., 1995; Gurvits et al., 1996) or that hippocampal volume to be a risk factor for developing PTSD (Gilbertson et al., 2002). Other studies report unchanged hippocampal volumes in female patients with chronic PTSD traumatized by intimate partner violence (Fennema-Notestine et al., 2002), those traumatized by witnessing a plane crash at the same air show (Jatzko et al., 2006a), elderly PTSD patients (Golier et al., 2006), and adult burn patients (Winter & Irle, 2004). Opposite trends in abused juveniles were found in other studies. (Tupler & De Bellis, 2006). A recent meta-analysis, however, confirmed the presence of significantly smaller hippocampal and left amygdala volumes in patients with PTSD compared to controls with and without trauma exposure (Karl et al., 2006). The findings of previous studies suggest that abnormal hippocampal volume was not a necessary and sufficient condition of PTSD.

Several studies have shown that the medial prefrontal cortex, which includes the anterior cingulate cortex and medial frontal cortex, are involved in the process of extinction of fear conditioning and the retention of extinction (Milad et al., 2006). Research on abnormalities in the prefrontal cortex in PTSD patients suggested decreased volume (Fennema-Notestine et al., 2002; Carrion et al., 2001; Richert et al., 2006; Hakamata et al., 2007), while some findings suggested increased volume of the middle-inferior and ventral regions of the prefrontal cortex (Richert et al., 2006).

The cerebellum has been considered only as a classical subcortical center for motor control (Botez, 1993). Botez et al. found that the patients with bilateral cerebellar damage showed deficits in the non-motor and behavioural functions including execution, attention, learning, and cognition (Botez, 1993; Ciesielski & Knight, 1994; Gao et al., 1996). Gao et al. found that the lateral cerebellar output (dentate) nucleus is not activated by the control of movement per se, but is strongly engaged during passive and active sensory tasks (Gao et al., 1996). Recent research of the cerebellum's contribution to cognitive processing and emotional processing have increased enormously, showing that the cerebellum is responsible for sensory perception, learning, memory, attention, linguistic, emotional control and conflict resolution processing (Mandolesi et al., 2001; Bischoff-Grethe et al., 2002; Vokaer et al., 2002; Claeys et al., 2003; Guenther et al., 2005; Allen et al., 2005; Konarski et al., 2005; Schmahmann & Caplan, 2006; Gianaros et al., 2007; Schweizer et al., 2007).

Anatomical studies revealed that via the thalamus, the cerebellum interacts with multiple areas of the prefrontal cortex and subcortex limbic lobe (Middleton & Strick, 2001; Zhu et al., 2006). The cerebellum influences several areas of the prefrontal cortex via the thalamus (Middleton & Strick, 2001). Gold and Buckner found a region in the right lateral cerebellum which exhibited a pattern similar to the left inferior frontal gyrus during semantic decisions on words and phonological decisions on pseudowords (Gold & Buckner, 2002). Patients with degenerative cerebellar diseases show high rates of cognitive impairment or psychiatric symptoms (Leroi et al., 2002; Liszewski et al., 2004), and neuroimaging studies have found that mood disorders were activated in the cerebellum (Liotti et al., 2000; Phan et al., 2002). The study by Gianaros et al. found that healthy individuals show heightened stressor-induced neural activation in the cingulate cortex, bilateral prefrontal cortex, and cerebellum while performing a standardized Stroop color-word interference task (Gianaros et al., 2007); however, studies of the cerebellum in PTSD patients have been very limited. In two positron emission tomography (PET) studies, abnormal activities in the cerebellum of PTSD subjects were found, including higher regional cerebral blood flow (Bonne et al., 2003) and augmented glucose absorption activity (Molina et al., 2010). Bellis et al. found that the left, right, and total cerebellum were smaller in maltreated children and adolescents with PTSD. They also found that cerebellar volume was positively correlated with the age of onset of the trauma that led to PTSD and negatively correlated with the duration of the trauma (Bellis & Kuchibhatla, 2006). Even with these findings, no precise results were found in cerebellum sub-areas.

In addition to findings related to the hippocampus and medial prefrontal cortex, many current functional neuroimaging studies have identified that other brain areas such as the prefrontal cortex, temporal lobe, parietal lobe, limbic lobe and cerebellum may also be implicated in PTSD (Bonne et al., 2003; Lanius et al., 2005; Molina et al., 2010; Bremner, 2006, Bremner et al., 2008; Geuze et al., 2008b). Brain functional imaging studies from patients with PTSD showing increased amygdala function and decreased medial prefrontal/anterior cingulate function during fear acquisition are hypothesized to represent a neural correlate of the failure of extinction seen in PTSD (Bremner , 2006, Bremner et al., 2008). A functional magnetic resonance imaging study comparing veterans with and without PTSD reveals that those with PTSD had overactivation of the temporal gyrus during the encoding phase, and underactivation of the bilateral middle temporal gyrus in the retrieval phase (Geuze et al., 2008b). Another functional magnetic resonance imaging study comparing PTSD patients and control subjects' connectivity maps in the left ventrolateral thalamus reveals that PTSD subjects had higher covariations between activations in he left ventrolateral thalamus and in the right insula, left parietal lobe, right middle frontal gyrus, and superior temporal gyrus (Lanius et al., 2005). Fluorodeoxyglucose positron emission tomography (FDG-PET) researches also indicate relatively diminished activity in the limbic, frontal and prefrontal cortex; relatively augmented activity in the fusiform cortex and in the cerebellum in patients with PTSD (Bonne et al., 2003; Molina et al., 2010). The findings of functional neuroimaging studies suggest that there are more brain areas that may be affected in PTSD, but only a few studies have found corresponding structural abnormalities in these brain areas. In contrast to the considerable research on subcortical structure volumetry, few studies to date have been directed to gray matter reductions in the cortex. It is evident that structural neuroimaging studies will allow for the testing of hypotheses of an association between PTSD and abnormal gray matter. Although volumetry findings reveal changes in the volume of specific brain regions, most of these studies defined particular regions-of-interests (ROIs) and measured their size and hemispheric asymmetry using traditional morphometric techniques with high-resolution magnetic resonance images (MRI). The disadvantage of this method is that some important brain areas may be neglected, and the process of drawing ROIs may introduce additional errors. Furthermore, the measurement of volume may not accurately reflect changes in the internal structure of the brain. In recent years, a fully automated voxel-based morphometry (VBM) technique has allowed for the examination of cerebral asymmetries across the entire brain directly (Corbo et al., 2005; Kasai et al., 2008; Luders et al., 2004), which can compensate for the subjectivity of ROI approaches. The VBM technique has been used for assessing regional gray matter density (GMD) (per unit volume in native space) in PTSD patients and revealed abnormal GMD in the hippocampus, anterior cingulate cortex, and insula (Emdad et al., 2006; Jatzko et al., 2006a; Richert et al., 2006; Kasai et al., 2008; Luders et al., 2004).

Most previous PTSD studies in the West focused on the disorder caused by various traumatic events, such as war (Vythilingam et al., 2005; Bremner et al., 1995; Pavic et al., 2007), disaster (Jatzko et al., 2006a, b; Abe et al., 2006; Li et al., 2006; Yamasue et al., 2003), and sexual abuse (Bremner et al., 2003; Tupler&De Bellis, 2006). Although considerable research has focused on rape-related PTSD, limited studies have been carried out in the context of Mainland China. In this study, rape was defined as an event that occurred without the victim's consent that involved the use or threat of force to penetrate the victim's vagina or anus by penis, tongue, fingers, or object, or the victim's mouth by penis (Tjaden & Thoennes, 2000). Interestingly, evidence indicates that the incidence rate of PTSD induced by rape is the highest among all kinds of trauma (Rothbaum et al., 1992).

In the current study, we employed VBM to explore differences in GMD between victims of rape (VoR) with and without PTSD, as well as in healthy comparison (HC) subjects. Based on findings from previous neuroimaging studies (Milad et al., 2006; Carrion et al., 2001; Richert et al., 2006; Hakamata et al., 2007; Bonne et al., 2003; Lanius et al., 2005; Molina et al., 2010; Bremner et al., 2006, 2008; Geuze et al., 2008b), we hypothesized that VoR with PTSD would show structural changes in extensive brain areas, including the prefrontal, temporal, parietal and limbic regions, compared to VOR without PTSD and to HC.

## 2. Material and methods

### 2.1 Subjects

We conducted a cross-sectional study on VoR and HC in Guangdong Province, People's Republic of China. Subjects living and working in Guangdong who met the criteria of being female, at least 18 years old, right-handed, with an educational attainment above secondary school level were included. Exclusion criteria for VoR and HC were a history of neurological or brain trauma and alcohol or drug use/abuse. Additional exclusion criteria for VoR included a previous or current psychiatric diagnosis other than PTSD, and for HC included any previous or current DSM-IV psychiatric disorder. The Ethics Committee of the Second Xiangya Hospital, Central South University, the People's Republic of China approved the study protocol. Written informed consent was obtained from all subjects in the study. The sample size for this study was projected based on previous research (Lindauer et al., 2004a; Fennema-Notestine et al., 2002; Jatzko et al., 2006a; Abe et al., 2006) where sample sizes ranging from eight to twenty were reported.

VoR subjects: VoR subjects were recruited in two stages. In the first stage, 53 potential subjects were recruited from (a) four public psychological consulting clinics; (b) referred to the clinics by a non-government organization (NGO) specializing in assisting victims of sexual assault; and (c) through advertisements in local newspapers requesting VoR for brain imaging studies. As an incentive for participation, six months free psychological counseling and medical therapy were offered. In the second stage, psychiatrists in the four consulting clinics explained the study to the 53 potential subjects and requested consent to participate in this study. As a result, 23 VoR met the inclusion/exclusion criteria and gave written informed consent.

Healthy Comparison (HC) Subjects: The HC subjects for this study were also recruited through a two-stage process. First, after obtaining the major demographic characteristics (i.e. gender, race, age, height, weight, and educational years) of VoR, we published notices across the province to recruit female health workers with similar demographic characteristics. A total of 65 volunteers agreed to participate and were screened according to inclusion/exclusion criteria. The health status of the HC was determined based on health check reports, as well as an illness history interview conducted by a doctor and a psychiatrist. In the second stage, the exact number of HC was recruited to best match the major demographic characteristics of each case of VoR with PTSD.

In this study, all subjects were measured with the Trauma History Questionnaire (THQ) (Green et al., 1996) and the Posttraumatic Stress Disorder Checklist Civilian Version (PCL-C)

(Ruggiero et al., 2003). In addition, two independent, clinically experienced psychiatrists interviewed VoR subjects using the Clinician-Administered PTSD Scale (CAPS) (Blake et al., 1995). The PCL-C was used to predict PTSD diagnoses, and the CAPS was used to differentiate PTSD and non-PTSD VoR subgroups. A senior psychiatrist confirmed the final diagnosis of PTSD.

### 2.2 MRI data acquisition

Images were obtained from using a research-dedicated Siemens Avanto 1.5 Tesla MRI scanner. The T1-weighted anatomical images were acquired using a three-dimensional gradient-echo sequence, with TR=11 msec, TE=4.94 msec, number of averages=1, matrix=256×224 pixels, field of view=256mm×224mm, with a flip angle of 15°. 176 sagittal slices with a 1 mm slice thickness were acquired with no interslice gap. There was a voxel resolution of 1×1×1mm 3. The total acquisition time was 5 minutes and 34 seconds.

### 2.3 MRI data analysis

Voxel-based morphometry was implemented by using the Statistical Parametric Mapping software (SPM2) (Wellcome Department of Imaging Neuroscience, London, England; www.fil.ion.ucl.ac.uk) (Friston et al., 1995). First, images were spatially normalized to the Montreal Neurological Institute (MNI) space with the standard $T_1$-MRI template (Mazziotta et al., 1995) implemented in the SPM2 program, and re-sliced into a final voxel size of $1 \times 1 \times 1 mm^3$ using tri-linear interpolation. The spatially normalized images were then segmented into three compartments: gray matter, white matter and cerebrospinal fluid. Furthermore, a Jacobian determinant was not introduced to modulate the resulting gray matter images so the voxel's values indicate the absolute density of the local gray matter. Finally, the segmented gray matter images from VoR with PTSD, VoR without PTSD, and HC were smoothed with a 12-mm full-width at half-maximum isotropic Gaussian kernel (Ashburner & Friston, 2000). The result of between-groups comparisons of gray matter images were performed in the general linear model.

Because we are particularly interested in exploring increases/decreases in GMD in VoR with PTSD compared to VoR without PTSD and HC, two-sample t-tests were performed in the VBM analysis in a voxel-by-voxel manner. Consistent with previous studies (Liberzon et al., 2007; Hou et al., 2007), the significance threshold was set to $p < 0.005$ corrected for multiple comparisons with a minimal cluster size of >50 voxels. The significant regions were superimposed onto SPM2's standard $T_1$-weighted brain images. Based on previous research (Milad et al., 2006; Carrion et al., 2001; Richert et al., 2006; Hakamata et al., 2007; Bonne et al., 2003; Lanius et al., 2005; Molina et al., 2010; Bremner et al., 2006, 2008; Geuze et al., 2008b), we hypothesized that compared with HC, VoR with PTSD would show gray matter abnormalities in the prefrontal, temporal, parietal and limbic regions. We used the small volume correction (SVC) tool in the SPM2 package with the specific purpose of restricting comparisons to specific voxels located in these regions. This approach permits the implementation of hypothesis-driven analyses with corrections for the pre-specified ROIs rather than corrections for the whole brain.

## 3. Results

Following the initial interview, among the 23 VoR subjects, 13 met the DSM-IV diagnostic criteria for current PTSD and 10 VoR did not meet the criteria for PTSD. Based on the study protocol, 13 HC were recruited to match VoR with PTSD. All subjects were scanned with an MRI, however, due to too many head movements during MRI scanning, a total of five subjects (2 PTSD, 2 non-PTSD, and 1 HC) were removed. As a result, the final sample consisted of 11 VoR with PTSD (ages 18-31), 8 VoR without PTSD (ages 23-33), and 12 HC (ages 22-33).

The three groups did not differ significantly on major demographics (i.e., age, height, weight, and educational years). In addition, the average interval between rape trauma and data acquisition did not differ significantly between VoR with and VoR without PTSD. Even so, VoR with PTSD scored significantly higher on PTSD symptomatology ($P<0.001$) compared to VoR without PTSD and HC. None of the participants in this study received medication prior to neuroimaging acquisition. The results are summarized in Table 1.

| | VoR (n=19) | | Healthy Comparison (n=12) | F | *t* | *p* |
|---|---|---|---|---|---|---|
| | PTSD(n=11) | Non-PTSD(n=8) | | | | |
| | | **Age (years)** | | | | |
| Mean | 25.55 | 27.50 | 26.42 | .614 | - | .55 |
| SD | 4.01 | 4.00 | 3.45 | | | |
| | | **Education (years)** | | | | |
| Mean | 14.73 | 15.63 | 14.83 | .91 | - | .41 |
| SD | 1.62 | 1.92 | 1.12 | | | |
| | | **Hight (CM)** | | | | |
| Mean | 157.82 | 159.25 | 160.67 | .83 | - | .45 |
| SD | 5.44 | 5.81 | 4.77 | | | |
| | | **Weight (KG)** | | | | |
| Mean | 49.00 | 51.13 | 50.88 | 0.41 | - | .67 |
| SD | 4.13 | 6.19 | 6.81 | | | |
| **Trauma event** | raped | raped | none | - | - | - |
| | | **Interval (months)** | | | | |
| Mean | 45.45 | 53.50 | - | - | -.31 | . 76 |
| SD | 55.68 | 55.54 | - | | | |
| | | **PCL-C score** | | | | |
| Mean | 60.36 | 34.63 | 22.58 | 60.32 | - | .000 |
| SD | 8.39 | 8.96 | 7.89 | | | |
| | | **CAPS score** | | | | |
| Mean | 74.45 | 15.88 | - | - | 14.70 | .000 |
| SD | 8.30 | 8.95 | - | | | |

VoR, Victims of Rape; PTSD, post-traumatic stress disorder; SD, standard deviation; CM, centimeter; KG, kilogram; Interval, time between raped trauma occurrence and scan; PCL-C, Post-traumatic Stress Disorder Checklist Civilian Version; CAPS, Clinician-Administered PTSD Scale.

Table 1. Demographic and clinical characteristics of VoR with and without PTSD and Healthy Comparison

### 3.1 Differences in GMD between VoR with PTSD and HC

The areas found to have abnormal GMD in VoR with PTSD compared to HC are shown in Figure 1. The cortical areas with decreased GMD in VoR with PTSD compared to HC are listed in Part A of Figure 1. These areas include the left medial frontal cortex (A-1), right medial frontal cortex (A-2), the left middle frontal cortex (A-3), the left middle temporal gyrus (A-4), and the left fusiform cortex (A-5). The areas with increased GMD are listed in Part B of Figure 1, and include the right posterior cingulate cortex (B-1), the left pre-central cortex (B-2), right pre-central cortex (B-3), the left inferior parietal lobule (B-4), right inferior parietal lobule (B-5), and the right post-central cortex (B-6). The MNI coordinates, voxel t values, k values (cluster size > 50), and corresponding Brodmann Areas (BA) are detailed in Table 2. Regions displayed are for $p < .005$.

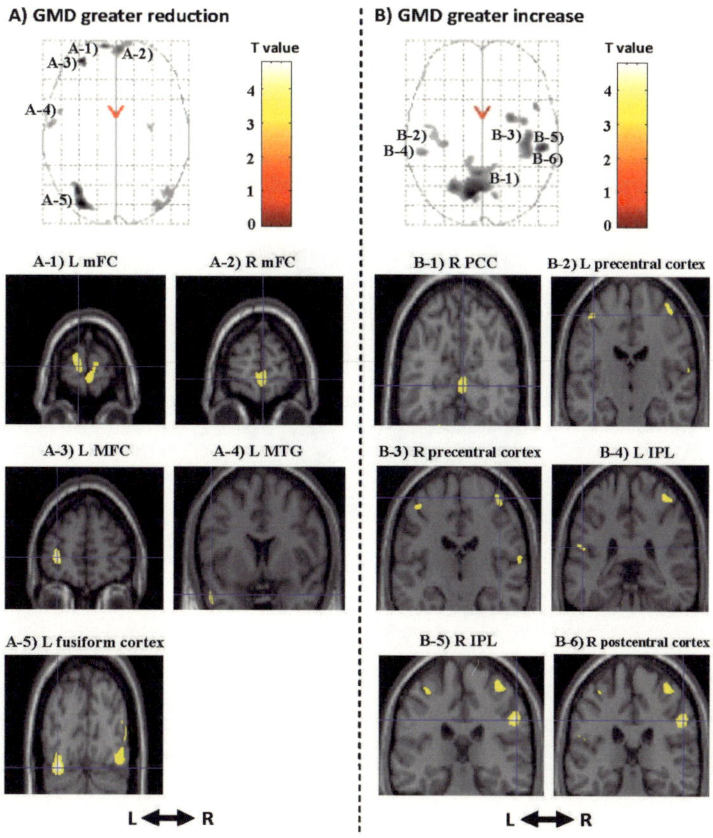


Fig. 1. Brain regions showing abnormalities in GMD in VoR with PTSD versus Healthy Comparison

Part A shows the cortical areas with decreased gray-matter density (GMD) in Victims of Rape with post-traumatic stress disorder compared to Healthy Comparison. Part B shows the areas with increased GMD.

L: left; R: right; mFC: medial prefrontal cortex; MFC: middle frontal cortex; MTG: middle temporal gyrus; PCC: posterior cingulate cortex; IPL: inferior parietal lobule.

| k | Voxel t value | MNI coordinates (x, y, z) | Region | Brodmann Area | *p* |
|---|---|---|---|---|---|
| | | | Greater reduction | | |
| 143 | 3. 85 | -968 11 | Left medial frontal cortex | 10 | 0.001 |
| 318 | 3.73 | 4 64 -4 | Right medial frontal cortex | 10 | 0.001 |
| 398 | 4.67 | -31 54 2 | Left middle frontal cortex | 10 | 0.000 |
| 51 | 3.11 | -51 7 -26 | Left middle temporal gyrus | 21 | 0.003 |
| 718 | 4.75 | -31 -82 -18 | Left fusiform cortex | 19,20 | 0.000 |
| | | | Greater increase | | |
| 449 | 3.57 | 4 -64 7 | Right posterior cingulate | 30,23 | 0.001 |
| 240 | 3.02 | -41 -16 55 | Left pre-central cortex | 4 | 0.003 |
| 343 | 3.77 | 42 -18 62 | Right pre-central cortex | 4,6 | 0.001 |
| 64 | 3.34 | -53 -34 21 | Left inferior parietal lobule | 40 | 0.002 |
| 211 | 3.77 | 57 -27 33 | Right inferior parietal lobule | 40 | 0.001 |
| 412 | 4.17 | 55 -28 35 | Right post-central cortex | 2,3 | 0.000 |

PTSD, Post-traumatic Stress Disorder; k, cluster size; Regions displayed are for p < .005, k >50.

Table 2. Gray-matter density in Victims of Rape with PTSD versus Healthy Comparison

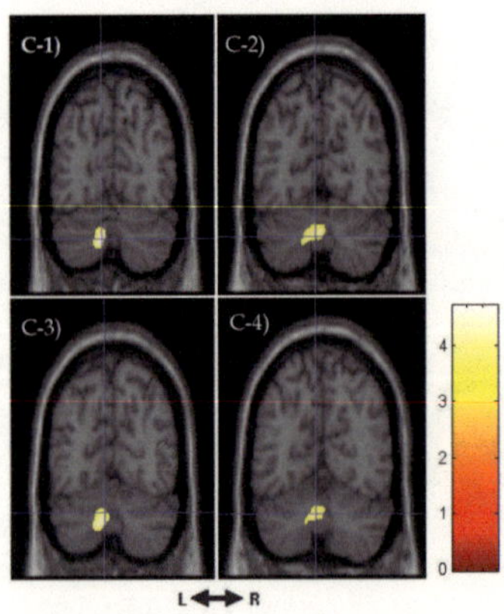


L: left; R: right; (C-1) Pyramis (x = -9, y = -72, z = -36; k = 519, t = 4.70); (C-2) uvula (x = -4, y = -66, z = -35; k = 256, t = 4.02); (C-3) declive (x = -6, y = -69, z = -30; k = 213, t = 3.84); and (C-4) nodule (x = -4, y = -63, z = -31; k = 147, t = 3.93); Coordinates presented are in Montreal Neurological Institute space.

Fig. 2. Significantly increased cerebellum density in VoR with PTSD versus Healthy Comparison

The PTSD Group showed increased cerebellum density compared with controls in the left side, specifically in the pyramis, uvula, declive, and nodule (see Figure 2).

### 3.2 Differences in GMD between VoR with and without PTSD

The areas found to have abnormal GMD in VoR with PTSD compared to the VoR without PTSD are shown in Figure 3. The cortical areas with decreased GMD are listed in Part C of Figure 3. These areas include the right uncus (D-1), the left middle temporal gyrus (D-2), and the left fusiform cortex (D-3). The areas with increased GMD are listed in Part D of

| k | Voxel t value | MNI coordinates (x, y, z) | Region | Brodmann Area | p |
|---|---|---|---|---|---|
| | | | Greater reduction | | |
| 173 | 4.23 | 27 -10 -35 | Right uncus | 20,28 | 0.000 |
| 314 | 5.56 | -55 -1 -26 | Left middle temporal gyrus | 21 | 0.000 |
| 53 | 5.23 | -54 -1 -27 | Left fusiform cortex | 20 | 0.000 |
| | | | Greater increase | | |
| 993 | 5.31 | -48 -8 39 | Left pre-central cortex | 6,4 | 0.000 |
| 607 | 6.03 | -55 -29 21 | Left inferior parietal lobule | 40 | 0.001 |
| 270 | 3.79 | 54 -23 33 | Right post-central cortex | 2 | 0.000 |

Table 3. Gray-matter density in VoR with PTSD versus VoR without PTSDVoR, Victims of Rape; PTSD, post-traumatic stress disorder; *k*, cluster size; Regions displayed are for $p <$ .005, *k>50.*

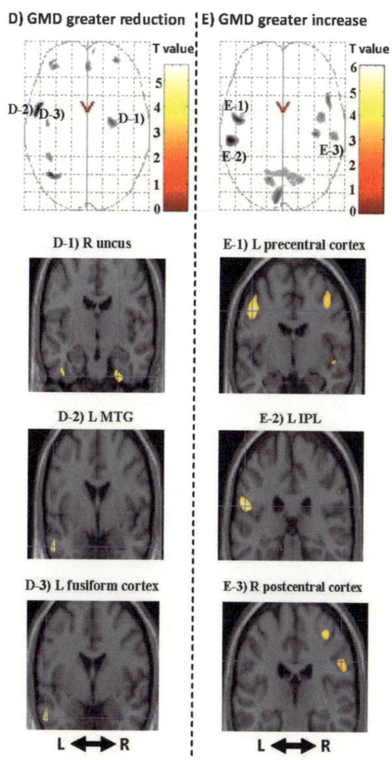


Part C shows the cortical areas with decreased gray-matter density (GMD) in Victims of Rape (VoR) with post-traumatic stress disorder (PTSD) compared to VoR without PTSD. Part D shows the areas with increased GMD.
L: left; R: right; MTG: middle temporal gyrus; IPL: inferior parietal lobule.

Fig. 3. Brain regions showing abnormalities in GMD in VoR with PTSD versus VoR without PTSD

Figure 2, and include the left pre-central cortex (E-1), the left inferior parietal lobule (E-2), and the right post-central cortex (E-3). The MNI coordinates, voxel t values, k values (cluster size > 50), and corresponding BA are detailed in Table 3. Regions displayed are for $p < .005$.

## 4. Discussion

This cross-sectional study employed VBM to examine brain density abnormalities among VoR with PTSD compared to VoR without PTSD and HC in mainland China. The findings of this study support the hypothesis that changes in brain density are associated with the pathophysiology of rape-induced PTSD.

### 4.1 The frontal cortex

The structural abnormalities in the medial and middle frontal cortex found in VoR with PTSD are supported by previous studies (Shin et al., 2006; Fennema-Notestine et al., 2002; Richert et al., 2006; Hakamata et al., 2007). In addition to such structural findings, functional neuroimaging studies have also shown dysfunction in these cortical areas (Bremner et al., 1999a, 2003; Lanius et al., 2004, 2006; Lindauer et al., 2004b, 2008; Morey et al., 2008). It is therefore possible that altered GMD in the medial and middle frontal cortex may contribute to their hypofunction. However, in the current study, VoR with PTSD had GMD reductions in the left middle frontal cortex and the bilateral medial frontal cortex relative to the HC, but no significant differences relative to VoR without PTSD. This result suggests that severe psychological trauma may change brain gray matter of the medial and middle frontal cortex, but that such plastic changes to these cortical brain structures may not underlie the pathophysiology of PTSD.

Compared to VoR without PTSD and HC, VoR with PTSD had significant bilateral increases in GMD of the pre-central gyrus, which mainly consists of the premotor cortex and the supplementary motor area. Studies indicate the importance of the supplementary motor area in motor tasks that demand retrieval of motor memory (Tanji, 1994). The premotor cortex, located in the pre-central cortex (BA6), seems to play a major role in language (Duffau et al., 2003). Functional neuroimaging studies on PTSD suggest abnormal functional activities in this cortical area. Empirical studies have shown that PTSD groups are characterized by relatively more activation in the pre-central cortex than non-PTSD and healthy comparisons (Bonne et al., 2003; Bremner et al., 1999a; Lanius et al., 2006; Shaw et al., 2002; Jatzko et al., 2006b). These findings suggest that increases in GMD of the pre-central cortex may be involved in the neural basis of motor and linguistic PTSD symptomatology.

### 4.2 The parietal lobule

The parietal lobule, including the superior and inferior parietal lobule (BA7, BA40) is implicated in memory, recognition, and deductive reasoning (Xie et al., 2004; Knauff et al., 2002). In this study, compared to VoR without PTSD and HC, VoR with PTSD had significant increases in GMD of the inferior parietal lobule. This indicates that the inferior parietal lobule might play an important role in the pathophysiology of PTSD. Additionally, one PET study showed that chronic PTSD patients presented relatively diminished activity in the post-central regions (Molina et al., 2010), which mainly consist of the primary somatic sensory cortex and secondary somatic sensory cortex (Geng et al., 2006). Increases in GMD in the post-central cortex may be associated with the dysfunction related with PTSD.

### 4.3 The temporal gyrus

Our study showed significant GMD decreases in the left middle temporal gyrus in VoR with PTSD compared to HC. Studies comparing veterans with and without PTSD reveals that those with PTSD had overactivation of the temporal gyrus during the resting state (Molina et al., 2010) and the encoding phase (Geuze et al., 2008b), and underactivation of the bilateral middle temporal gyrus in the retrieval phase (Geuze et al., 2008b). Functional neuroimaging studies reveals significant activation in left middle temporal gyrus in response to empathy judgments in post-therapy PTSD (Farrow et al., 2005) and higher levels of activation in the middle temporal gyrus in dissociative PTSD (Lanius et al., 2006). Empirical evidence suggests that the fusiform cortex is specialized for face processing (Rossion et al., 2000; Rhodes et al., 2004). Research also indicates relatively augmented activity in the fusiform cortex in patients with PTSD (Bonne et al., 2003; Molina et al., 2010). The reduced GMD of the middle temporal gyrus and fusiform cortex found in this study implicates these regions in the dysfunction of memory and dissociative symptoms in PTSD.

### 4.4 The limbic lobe

In the present study, VoR with PTSD had significant increases in GMD in the right posterior cingulate cortex compared to HC. Meta-analyses have revealed that the prominent themes in the posterior cingulate cortex are episodic memory retrieval and pain (Nielsen et al., 2005), visuospatial processing and assessment of threat (Nemeroff et al., 2006), as well as fear conditioning (Doronbekov et al., 2005). Comparison of connectivity maps by functional connectivity analyses (Lanius et al., 2004) reveals that subjects with PTSD showed greater correlations in interregional brain activity than subjects without PTSD in the right posterior cingulate cortex (BA 29). Functional neuroimaging studies have found increased activation in the posterior cingulate cortex in victims with PTSD compared to victims without PTSD and to healthy controls (Bremner et al., 1999a, b, 2003; Doronbekov et al., 2005; Sachinvala et al., 2000). These indicate that dysfunction in the posterior cingulate cortex may underlie pathological symptoms provoked by traumatic reminders of sexual assault among VoR with PTSD.

### 4.5 The cerebellum

We found that the density of cerebellum, which plays an important role in motor and cognition (Mandolesi et al., 2001; Bischoff-Grethe et al., 2002; Vokaer et al., 2002; Claeys et al., 2003; Guenther et al., 2005; Allen et al., 2005; Konarski et al., 2005; Schmahmann & Caplan, 2006; Gianaros et al., 2007; Schweizer et al., 2007), was increased in patients with PTSD. Combination of early studies about structural abnormal (Leroi et al., 2002; Liszewski et al., 2004; Bellis & Kuchibhatla, 2006) and functional abnormal (Bonne et al., 2003; Molina et al., 2010; Gianaros et al., 2007; Liotti et al., 2000; Phan et al., 2002) in the cerebellum in PTSD patients, the finding is consistent with our hypothesis that the cerebellum was involved in the neuropathology of cognitive processing and emotional processing in PTSD patients. Furthermore, the density increased in the cerebellum while decreased in the prefrontal cortex. According to the anatomical studies that the cerebellum interacts with the prefrontal cortex via the thalamus (Middleton & Strick, 2001; Zhu et al., 2006), and the functional studies that the cerebellum influences several areas of the prefrontal cortex via the thalamus (Middleton & Strick, 2001) and exhibits a pattern similar to the frontal cortex during semantic decisions (Gold & Buckner, 2002), the findings suggest that the cerebellum may be involved in the functional compensation for the pathological changes in the neuro-circuitry of PTSD.

Earlier studies in the cerebellum of PTSD patients found correlations with abnormal blood flow and glucose absorption (Bonne et al., 2003; Molina et al., 2010) and abnormal volume (Bellis & Kuchibhatla, 2006) in the cerebellum also. This study extends the literature on cerebellum structure involvement in PTSD. This finding, if replicated in larger patient samples, may serve as a marker of brain dysfunction in PTSD, and thus allows for the study of cerebellum pathophysiology before and throughout the course and treatment of PTSD. It should be noted that whilst the sample size (11 VoR with PTSD) of this study meets the threshold of research reported in the literature （Jatzko et al., 2006a; Hou et al., 2007）, it was nevertheless limited in terms of its statistical power. A further limitation is the potential for selection bias in both the VoR Group and HC. Given the social stigma attached to VoR in the Chinese cultural context that often results in sexual shame, fear and anxiety over disclosure of the rape, guilt over derogating family honor, self-scrutiny and self-blame after the fact, and even blame of the victim, contribute to the potential selection bias in the VoR Group. Regarding the selection bias in HC, it was not our intention for this group (12 HC) to be representative of the general population, nor were the 65-pooled controls. This group was particularly designed to match the VoR with PTSD regarding the major demographic characteristics. However, given the fact that HC were recruited from healthy workers, selection bias from the healthy-worker effect should be borne in mind.

The use of a cross-sectional design is another significant limitation of this study. The shared variance estimated between variables in a cross-sectional design does not allow for a critical examination of causal relationships among them. Consequently, we cannot state categorically whether changes in brain density were the cause or the effect of trauma exposure/PTSD.

## 5. Conclusion

The abnormal density of cerebral regions in VoR with PTSD supports the hypothesis that PTSD is associated with structural plastic changes to brain. The results suggest that the medial frontal cortex, pre-central cortex, posterior cingulate cortex, post-central cortex, inferior parietal lobule, and cerebellum are likely to contribute to the neural mechanisms underlying PTSD. These findings suggest that the pre-central cortex of PTSD may be involved in the neural basis of motor and linguistic PTSD symptomatology; the middle temporal gyrus and fusiform cortex may be implicated in the dysfunction of memory and dissociative symptoms in PTSD; the posterior cingulate cortex may underlie pathological symptoms provoked by traumatic reminders of PTSD; the inferior parietal lobule of PTSD might play an important role in the dysfunction of memory, recognition, and deductive reasoning; and the cerebellum may contribute to the functional compensation for the pathological changes in the neuro-circuitry of PTSD. These findings may lead to a better understanding of the basis of brain structure for clinical symptoms with VoR of PTSD. Also, they can be benefit to the researches of PTSD treatment.

Future studies call for exploring experiences of rape and associated PTSD symptomatology by using case-control or longitudinal designs, investigating the effect of the specific social and cultural meanings of rape, examining the impact on individuals' posttraumatic response and coping ability, and looking into the relation between brain GMD and PTSD symptoms. In addition, the findings of this study need to be confirmed in the future and in different subgroups of PTSD patients.

## 6. Acknowledgments

We acknowledge support from grant from the National Natural Science Foundation of China (30830046 to Lingjiang Li and Shuangge Sui), the National Science and Technology Program of China (2007BAI17B02 to Lingjiang Li), and the National 973 Program of China (2009CB918303, 2006CB5000800 to Lingjiang Li).

## 7. References

Abe, O., Yamasue, H., Kasai, K., Yamada, H., Aoki, S., Iwanami, A., Ohtani, T., Masutani, Y., Kato, N., & Ohtomo, K. (2006). Voxel-based diffusion tensor analysis reveals aberrant anterior cingulum integrity in posttraumatic stress disorder due to terrorism. *Psychiatry Research-Neuroimaging*, Vol. 146, No. 3, pp. 231-242

Allen, G., McColl, R., Barnard, H., Ringe, WK., Fleckenstein, J., & Cullum, CM. (2005). Magnetic resonance imaging of cerebellar-prefrontal and erebellar-parietal functional connectivity. *Neuroimage*, Vol. 28, No. 1, pp. 39-48

Ashburner, J. & Friston, KJ. (2000). Voxel-based morphometry - The methods. *Neuroimage*, Vol. 11, pp. 805-821

Bellis, MD. & Kuchibhatla, M. (2006). Cerebellar volumes in pediatric maltreatment-related posttraumatic stress disorder. *Biological Psychiatry*, Vol. 60, No. 7, pp. 697-703

Bischoff-Grethe, A., Ivry, RB., & Grafton, ST. (2002). Cerebellar involvement in response reassignment rather than attention. *The Journal of Neuroscience.*, 22, No. 2, pp. 546-553

Blake, DD., Weathers, FW., Nagy, LM., Kaloupek, DG., Gusman, FD., Charney, DS., & Keane, TM. (1995). The Development of a Clinician-Administered PTSD Scale. *Journal of Traumatic Stress*, Vol. 8, No. 1, pp. 75-90

Bonne, O., Gilboa, A., Louzoun, Y., Brandes, D., Yona, I., Lester, H., Barkai, G., Freedman, N., Chisin, R., & Shalev, AY. (2003). Resting regional cerebral perfusion in recent posttraumatic stress disorder. *Biological Psychiatry*, Vol. 54, No. 10, pp. 1077-1086

Bossini, L. & Castrogiovanni, P. (2007). Pre- and posttreatment neuroimaging of PTSD: Focus on hippocampal volume. *Journal of Psychosomatic Research*, No. 63, pp. 310-310

Botez, MI. (1993). Cerebellum and non-motor behaviour. *Romanian journal of neurology and psychiatry*, Vol. 31, No. 3-4, pp. 189-193

Bremner, JD. & Charney, DS. (1994). Neurobiology of Posttraumatic Stress Disorder - Implications for Treatment. In: *Current Therapeutic Approaches to Panic and Other Anxiety Disorders*, Darcourt, G., Mendlewjcz, J., Racagni, G., Brunello, N. (Eds.), Vol. 8, pp. 171-186

Bremner, JD., Randall, P., Scott, TM., Bronen, RA., Seibyl, JP., Southwick, SM., Delaney, RC., Mccarthy, G., Charney, DS., & Innis, RB. (1995). MRI-Based Measurement of Hippocampal Volume in Patients with Combat-Related Posttraumatic-Stress-Disorder. *The American Journal of Psychiatry*, Vol. 152, pp. 973-981

Bremner, JD., Staib, LH., Kaloupek, D., Southwick, SM., Soufer, R., & Charney, DS. (1999a). Neural correlates of exposure to traumatic pictures and sound in Vietnam combat veterans with and without posttraumatic stress disorder: A positron emission tomography study. *Biological Psychiatry*, Vol. 45, pp. 806-816

Bremner, JD., Narayan, M., Staib, LH., Southwick, SM., McGlashan, T., & Charney, DS. (1999b). Neural correlates of memories of childhood sexual abuse in women with and without posttraumatic stress disorder. *The American Journal of Psychiatry*, Vol. 156, pp. 1787-1795

Bremner, JD., Vythilingam, M., Vermetten, E., Southwick, SM., McGlashan, T., Staib, LH., Soufer, R., & Charney, DS. (2003). Neural correlates of declarative memory for emotionally valenced words in women with posttraumatic stress disorder related to early childhood sexual abuse. *Biological Psychiatry*, Vol. 53, No. 10, pp. 879-889

Bremner, JD. (2006). Traumatic stress: effects on the brain. *Dialogues Clinical Neuroscience*, Vol. 8, No. 4, pp. 445-461

Bremner, JD., Elzinga, B., Schmahl, C., & Vermetten, E. (2008). Structural and functional plasticity of the human brain in posttraumatic stress disorder. In: *Progress in Brain Research*, de Kloet, ER., Oitzl, MS. & Vermetten E. (Eds.), Vol. 167, pp. 171-186

Carrion, VG., Weems, CF., Eliez, S., Patwardhan, A., Brown, W., Ray, RD., & Reiss, AL. (2001). Attenuation of frontal asymmetry in pediatric posttraumatic stress disorder. *Biological Psychiatry*, Vol. 50, No. 12, pp. 943-951

Ciesielski, KT. & Knight, JE. (1994). Cerebellar abnormality in autism: a nonspecific effect of early brain damage? *Acta Neurobiologiae Experimentalis*, Vol. 54, No. 2, pp. 151-154

Claeys, KG., Orban, GA., Dupont, P., Sunaert, S., Hecke, PV., & Schutter, ED. (2003). Involvement of multiple functionally distinct cerebellar regions in visual discrimination: a human functional imaging study. *Neuroimage*, Vol. 20, No. 2, pp. 840-854

Corbo, V., Clement, MH., Armony, JL., Pruessner, JC., & Brunet, A. (2005). Size versus shape differences: Contrasting voxel-based and volumetric analyses of the anterior cingulate cortex in individuals with acute posttraumatic stress disorder. *Biological Psychiatry*, Vol. 58, No. 2, pp. 119-124

Danckwerts, A. & Leathem, J. (2003).Questioning the Link Between PTSD and Cognitive Dysfunction. *Neuropsychology Review*, Vol. 13, pp. 221-235

Doronbekov, TK., Tokunaga, H., Ikejiri, Y., Kazui, H., Hatta, N., Masaki, Y., Ogino, A., Miyoshi, N., Oku, N., Nishikawa, T., & Takeda, M. (2005). Neural basis of fear conditioning induced by video clip: Positron emission tomography study. *Psychiatry and Clinical Neurosciences*, Vol. 59, No. 2, pp. 155-162

Duffau, H., Capelle, L., Denvil, D., Gatignol, P., Sichez, N., Lopes, M., Sichez, JP., & Van Effenterre, R. (2003). The role of dominant premotor cortex in language: a study using intraoperative functional mapping in awake patients. *Neuroimage*, Vol. 20, No. 4, pp. 1903-1914

Emdad, R., Bonekamp, D., Sondergaard, HP., Bjorklund, TB., Agartz, I., Ingvar, M., & Theorell, TR. (2006). Morphometric and psychometric comparisons between non-substance- abusing patients with posttraumatic stress disorder and normal controls. *Psychotherapy and Psychosomatics*, Vol. 75, pp. 122-132

Farrow, TFD., Hunter, MD., Wilkinson, ID., Gouneea, C., Fawbert, D., Smith, R., Lee, KH., Mason, S., Spence, SA., & Woodruff, PWR. (2005). Quantifiable change in functional brain response to empathic and forgivability judgments with resolution of posttraumatic stress disorder. *Psychiatry Research-Neuroimaging,* Vol. 140, No. 1, pp. 45-53

Fennema-Notestine, C., Stein, MB., Kennedy, CM., Archibald, SL., & Jernigan, TL. (2002). Brain morphometry in female victims of intimate partner violence with and without posttraumatic stress disorder. *Biological Psychiatry,* Vol. 52, No. 11, pp. 1089-1101

Friston, KJ., Holmes, AP., Worsley, KJ., Poline, JB., Frith, CD., & Frackowiak, RSJ. (1995). Statistical parametric maps in functional imaging: A general linear approach. *Human Brain Mapping,* Vol. 2, pp. 189-210

Gao, JH., Parsons, LM., Bower, JM., Xiong, JH., & Fox, PT. (1996). Cerebellum implicated in sensory acquisition and discrimination rather than motor control. *Science,* Vol. 272, No. 5261, pp. 545-547

Geng, JJ., Eger, E., Ruff, CC., Kristjansson, A., Rotshtein, P., & Driver, J. (2006). On-line attentional selection from competing stimuli in opposite visual fields: Effects on human visual cortex and control processes. *Journal of Neurophysiology,* Vol. 96, No. 5, pp. 2601-2612

Geuze, E., Vermetten, E., & Bremner, JD. (2005). MR-based in vivo hippocampal volumetrics: 2. Findings in neuropsychiatric disorders. *Molecular Psychiatry,* Vol. 10, pp. 160-184

Geuze, E., Vermetten, E., Goebel, R., & Westenberg, H. (2008a). Thinner prefrontal cortex in veterans with posttraumatic stress disorder. *Biological Psychiatry,* Vol. 41, No. 3, pp. 675-681

Geuze, E., Vermetten, E., Ruf, M., de Kloet, CS., & Westenberg, HGM. (2008b). Neural correlates of associative learning and memory in veterans with posttraumatic stress disorder. *Journal of Psychiatric Research,* Vol. 42, No. 8, pp. 659-669

Gianaros, PJ., Jennings, JR., Sheu, LK., Derbyshire, SW., & Matthews KA. (2007). Heightened Functional Neural Activation to Psychological Stress Covaries With Exaggerated Blood Pressure Reactivity. *Hypertension,* Vol. 49, pp. 134-140

Gilbertson, M., Shenton, M., Ciszewski, A., Kasai, K., Lasko, N., Orr, S., & Pitman, R. (2002). Smaller hippocampal volume predicts pathologic vulnerability to psychological trauma. *Nature Neuroscience,* Vol. 5, No. 11, pp. 1242-1247

Gold, BT. & Buckner, RL. (2002). Common prefrontal regions coactivate with dissociable posterior regions during controlled semantic and phonological tasks. *Neuron.,* Vol. 35, No. 4, pp. 803-812

Golier, JA., Harvey, PD., Legge, J., & Yehuda, R. (2006). Memory performance in older trauma survivors - Implications for the longitudinal course of PTSD. *Psychobiology of Posttraumatic Stress Disorder: A Decade of Progress,* Vol. 1071, pp. 54-66

Green, BL. (1996).Trauma History Questionnaire. In: *Measurement of stress, trauma, and adaptation,* Stamm, BH, (Ed.), pp. 366-369, Sidran Press, Lutherville, MD

Guenther, FH., Ghosh, SS., & Tourville, JA. (2005). Neural modeling and imaging of the cortical interactions underlying syllable production. *Brain and Language*, Vol. 96, No. 3, pp. 280-301

Gurvits, TV., Shenton, ME., Hokama, H., Ohta, H., Lasko, NB., Gilbertson, MW., Orr, SP., Kikinis, R., Jolesz, FA., McCarley, RW., & Pitman, RK. (1996). Magnetic resonance imaging study of hippocampal volume in chronic, combat-related posttraumatic stress disorder. *Biological Psychiatry*, Vol. 40, No. 11, pp. 1091-1099

Hakamata, Y., Matsuoka, Y., Inagaki, M., Nagamine, M., Hara, E., Imoto, S., Murakami, K., Kim, Y., & Uchitomi, Y. (2007). Structure of orbitofrontal cortex and its longitudinal course in cancer-related post-traumatic stress disorder. *Neuroscience Research*, Vol. 59, No. 4, pp. 383-38

Hou, CL., Liu, J., Wang, K., Li, LJ., Liang, M., He, Z., Liu, Y., Zhang, Y., Li, WH., & Jiang, TZ. (2007). Brain responses to symptom provocation and trauma-related short-term memory recall in coal mining accident survivors with acute severe PTSD. *Brain Research*, Vol. 1144, pp. 165-174

Jatzko, A., Rothenhofer, S., Schmitt, A., Gaser, C., Demirakca, T., Weber-Fahr, W., Wessa, M., Magnotta, V., & Braus, DF. (2006a). Hippocampal volume in chronic posttraumatic stress disorder (PTSD): MRI study using two different evaluation methods. *Journal of Affective Disorders*, Vol. 94, No. 1-3, pp. 121-126

Jatzko, A., Schmitt, A., Demirakca, T., Weimer, E., & Braus, D. (2006b). Disturbance in the neural circuitry underlying positive emotional processing in post-traumatic stress disorder (PTSD) - An fMRI study. *European Archives of Psychiatry and Clinical Neuroscience*, Vol. 256, No. 2, pp. 112-114

Karl, A., Schaefer, M., Malta, LS., Dorfel, D., Rohleder, N., & Werner, A. (2006). A meta-analysis of structural brain abnormalities in PTSD. *Neuroscience and Biobehavioral Reviews*, Vol. 30, No. 7, pp. 1004-1031

Kasai, K., Yamasue, H., Araki, T., Sakamoto, H., & Kato, N. (2006). Structural and Functional Neuroimaging in Posttraumatic Stress Disorder. In: *PTSD: Brain Mechanisms and Clinical Implications*. Kato, N., Kawata, M., & Pitman, RK. (Eds.), pp. 203-209, Springer, Tokyo, Japan.

Kasai, K., Yamasue, H., Gilbertson, MW., Shenton, ME., Rauch, SL., & Pitman, RK. (2008). Evidence for Acquired Pregenual Anterior Cingulate Gray Matter Loss from a Twin Study of Combat-Related Posttraumatic Stress Disorder. *Biological Psychiatry*, Vol. 63, No. 6, pp. 550-556

Knauff, M., Mulack, T., Kassubek, J., Salih, HR., & Greenlee, MW. (2002). Spatial imagery in deductive reasoning: a functional MRI study. *Cognitive Brain Research*, Vol. 13, No. 2, pp. 203-212

Konarski, JZ., McIntyre, RS., Grupp, LA., & Kennedy, SH. (2005). Is the cerebellum relevant in the circuitry of neuropsychiatric disorders? *Journal of Psychiatry & Neuroscience*, Vol. 30, No. 3, pp. 178-186

Lanius, RA., Williamson, PC., Densmore, M., Boksman, K., Neufeld, RW., Gati, JS., & Menon, RS. (2004). The nature of traumatic memories: A 4-T fMRI functional connectivity analysis. *The American Journal of Psychiatry*, Vol. 161, pp. 36-44

Lanius, RA., Williamson, PC., Bluhm, RL., Densmore, M., Boksman, K., Neufeld, RWJ., Gati, JS., & Menon, RS. (2005). Functional connectivity of dissociative responses in posttraumatic stress disorder: A functional magnetic resonance imaging investigation. *Biological Psychiatry*, Vol. 57, No. 8, pp. 873-884

Lanius, RA., Bluhm, R., Lanius, U., & Pain, C. (2006). A review of neuroimaging studies in PTSD: Heterogeneity of response to symptom provocation. *Journal of Psychiatric Research*, Vol. 40, No. 8, pp. 709-729

Leroi, I., O'Hearn, E., Marsh, L., Lyketsos, CG., Rosenblatt, A., Ross, CA., Brandt, J., & Margolis, RL. (2002). Psychopathology in patients with degenerative cerebellar diseases: a comparison to Huntington's disease. *The American Journal of Psychiatry*, Vol. 159, pp. 1306-1314

Li, L., Chen, S., Liu, J. Zhang, J., He, Z., & Lin, X. (2006). Magnetic resonance imaging and magnetic resonance spectroscopy study of deficits in hippocampal structure in fire victims with recent-onset posttraumatic stress disorder. *The Canadian Journal of Psychiatry*, Vol. 51, No. 7, pp. 431-437

Liberzon, I., King, AP., Britton, JC., Phan, KL., Abelson, JL., & Taylor, SF. (2007). Paralimbic and medial prefrontal cortical involvement in neuroendocrine responses to traumatic stimuli. *The American Journal of Psychiatry*, Vol. 164, pp. 1250-1258

Liberzon, I. & Sripada, CS. (2008). The functional neuroanatomy of PTSD: A critical review. *Stress Hormones and Post Traumatic Stress Disorder: Basic Studies and Clinical Perspectives, Progress in Brain Research*, Vol. 167, pp. 151-169, ISSN 0079-6123

Lindauer, RJL., Vlieger, EJ., Jalink, M., Olff, M., Carlier, IVE., Majoie, CBLM., den Heeten, GJ., & Gersons, BPR. (2004a). Smaller hippocampal volume in dutch police officers with posttraumatic stress disorder. *Biological Psychiatry*, Vol. 56, No. 5, pp. 356-363

Lindauer, RJL., Booij, J., Habraken, JBA., Uylings, HBM., Olff, M., Carlier, IVE., den Heeten, GJ., van Eck-Smit, BLF., & Gersons, BPR. (2004b). Cerebral blood flow changes during script-driven imagery in police officers with posttraumatic stress disorder. *Biological Psychiatry*, Vol. 56, No. 11, pp. 853-861

Lindauer, RJL., Booij, J., Habraken, JBA., van Meijel EPM., Uylings, HBM., Olff, M., Carlier, IVE., den Heeten, GJ., van Eck-Smit, BLF., & Gersons, BPR. (2008). Effects of psychotherapy on regional cerebral blood flow during trauma imagery in patients with post-traumatic stress disorder: a randomized clinical trial. *Psychological Medicine*, Vol. 38, No. 4, pp. 543-554

Liotti, M., Mayberg, HS., Brannan, SK., McGinnis, S., Jerabek, P., & Fox, PT. (2000). Differential limbic-cortical correlates of sadness and anxiety in healthy subjects: implication for affective disorders. *Biological Psychiatry*, Vol. 48, No. 1, pp. 30-42

Liszewski, CM., O'Hearn, E., Leroi, I., Gourley, L., Ross, CA., & Margolis, RL. (2004). Cognitive Impairment and Psychiatric Symptoms in 133 Patients With Diseases Associated With Cerebellar Degeneration. *The Journal of Neuropsychiatry and Clinical Neurosciences*, Vol. 16, No. 1, pp. 109-112

Luders, E., Gaser, C., Jancke, L., & Schlaug, G. (2004). A voxel-based approach to gray matter asymmetries. *Neuroimage*, Vol. 22, No. 2, pp. 656-664

Mandolesi, L., Leggio, MG., Graziano, A., Neri, P. & Petrosini, L. (2001). Cerebellar contribution to spatial event processing: involvement in procedural and working memory components. *European Journal of Neuroscience*, Vol. 4, No. 12, pp. 2011-2022

Mazziotta, JC., Toga, AW., Evans, A., Fox, P., & Lancaster, J. (1995). A probabilistic atlas of the human brain: theory and rationale for its development. The International Consortium for Brain Mapping (ICBM). *NeuroImage*, Vol. 2, No. 2, pp. 89–101

Middleton, FA. & Strick, PL. (2001). Cerebellar projections to the prefrontal cortex of the primate.*The Journal of Neuroscience*, Vol. 21, No. 2, pp. 700-712

Milad, MR., Rauch, SL., Pitman, RK., & Quirk, GJ. (2006) Fear extinction in rats: Implications for human brain imaging and anxiety disorders. *Biological Psychology*, Vol. 73, No. 1, pp. 61-71

Miller, L. (1999). Atypical psychological responses to traumatic brain injury: PTSD and beyond. *Neurorehabilitation*, Vol. 13, No. 2, pp. 79-90

Molina, ME., Isoardi, R., Prado, MN., & Bentolila, S. (2010). Basal cerebral glucose distribution in long-term post-traumatic stress disorder. *World Journal of Biological Psychiatry*, Vol. 11, No. 2, pp. 493-501

Morey, RA., Petty, CM., Cooper, DA., Labar, KS., & McCarthy, G. (2008). Neural systems for executive and emotional processing are modulated by symptoms of posttraumatic stress disorder in Iraq War veterans. *Psychiatry Research-Neuroimaging*, Vol. 162, No. 1, pp. 59-72

Nemeroff, CB., Bremner, JD., Foa, EB., Mayberg, HS., North, CS., & Stein, MB. (2006). Posttraumatic stress disorder: A state-of-the-science review. *Journal of Psychiatric Research*, Vol. 40, No. 1, pp. 1-21

Nielsen, FA., Balslev, D., & Hansen, LK. (2005). Mining the posterior cingulate: Segregation between memory and pain components. *Neuroimage*, Vol. 27, No. 3, pp. 520-532

Pavic, L., Gregurek, R., Rados, M., Brkljacic, B., Brajkovic, L., Simetin-Pavic, I., Ivanac, G., Pavlisa, G., & Kalousek, V. (2007). Smaller right hippocampus in war veterans with posttraumatic stress disorder. *Psychiatry Research-Neuroimaging*, 154, No. 2, pp. Vol. 191-198

Phan, KL., Wager, T., Taylor, SF., & Liberzon, I. (2002). Functional neuroanatomy of emotion: a meta-analysis of emotion activation studies in PET and fMRI. *Neuroimage*, Vol. 16, No. 2, pp. 331-348

Rhodes, G., Byatt, G., Michie, PT., & Puce, A. (2004). Is the fusiform face area specialized for faces, individuation, or expert individuation? *Journal of Cognitive Neuroscience*, Vol. 16, No. 2, pp. 189-203

Richert, KA., Carrion, VG., Karchemskiy, A., & Reiss, AL. (2006). Regional differences of the prefrontal cortex in pediatric PTSD: an MRI study. *Depression and Anxiety*, Vol. 23, No. 1, pp. 17-25

Rossion, B., Dricot, L., Devolder, A., Bodart, JM., Crommelinck, M., de Gelder, B., & Zoontjes, R. (2000). Hemispheric asymmetries for whole-based and part-based face processing in the human fusiform gyrus. *Journal of Cognitive Neuroscience*, Vol. 12, No. 5, pp. 793-802

Rothbaum, BO., Foa, EB., Riggs, D.S, Murdock, T., & Walsh, W. (1992). A Prospective Examination of Posttraumatic-Stress-Disorder in Rape Victims. *Journal of Traumatic Stress*, Vol. 5, No. 3, pp. 455-475

Ruggiero, K.J, Ben, KD., Scotti, JR., & Rabalais, AE. (2003). Psychometric Properties of the PTSD Checklist—Civilian Version. *Journal of Traumatic Stress*, Vol. 16, No. 5, pp. 495-502

Sachinvala, N., Kling, A., Suffin, S., Lake, R., & Cohen, M. (2000). Increased regional cerebral perfusion by 99mTc hexamethyl propylene amine oxime single photon emission computed tomography in post-traumatic stress disorder. *Military Medicine*, Vol. 165, No. 6, pp. 473-479

Sareen, J., Cox, BJ., Stein, MB., Afifi, TO., Fleet, C., & Asmundson, GJG. (2007). Physical and mental comorbidity, disability, and suicidal behavior associated with posttraumatic stress disorder in a large community sample. *Psychosomatic Medicine*, Vol. 69, No. 3, pp. 242-248

Schmahmann, JD. & Caplan, D. (2006). Cognition, emotion and the cerebellum. *Brain*, 129, No. 2, pp. 290-292

Schweizer, TA., Oriet, C., Meiran, N., Alexander, MP., Cusimano, M., & Stuss, DT. (2007). The Cerebellum Mediates Conflict Resolution. *Journal of Cognitive Neuroscience*, Vol. 19, No. 12, pp.1974-1982

Shaw, ME., Strother, SC., McFarlane, AC., Morris, P., Anderson, J., Clark, CR., & Egan, GF. (2002). Abnormal functional connectivity in posttraumatic stress disorder. *NeuroImage*, Vol. 15, No. 3, pp.661-674

Shin, LM., Rauch, SL., & Pitman, RK. (2006). Amygdala, Medial Prefrontal Cortex, and Hippocampal Function in PTSD. *Annals of the New York Academy of Sciences*, Vol. 1071, pp. 67-79

Tanji, J. (1994). The Supplementary Motor Area in the Cerebral-Cortex. *Neuroscience Research*, Vol. 19, No. 3, pp. 251-268

Tjaden, P. & Thoennes, N. (2000). Full Report of the Prevalence, Incidence, and Consequences of Violence Against Women: Findings From the National Violence Against Women Survey, In: *National Criminal Justice Reference Service*, 11/2000, Available from http://www.ncjrs.gov/app/Publications/abstract.aspx?ID=183781

Tupler, LA. & De Bellis, MD. (2006). Segmented hippocampal volume in children and adolescents with posttraumatic stress disorder. *Biological Psychiatry*, Vol. 59, No. 6, pp.523-529

Villarreal, G. & King, CY. (2004). Neuroimaging studies reveal brain change in posttraumatic stress disorder. *Psychiatric Annals*, Vol. 34, No. 11, pp.845-856

Vokaer, M., Bier, JC., & Elincx, S., Claes, T., Paquier, P., Goldman, S., Bartholome, EJ., & Pandolfo, M. (2002). The cerebellum may be directly involved in cognitive functions. *Neurology*, Vol. 58, No. 6, pp. 967-970

Vythilingam, M., Luckenbaugh, DA., Lam, T., Morgan, CA., Lipschitz, D., Charney, DS., Bremner, JD., & Southwick, SM. (2005). Smaller head of the hippocampus in Gulf War-related posttraumatic stress disorder. *Psychiatry Research-Neuroimaging*, Vol. 139, pp. 89-99

Winter, H. & Irle, E. (2004). Hippocampal volume in adult burn patients with and without posttraumatic stress disorder. *The American Journal of Psychiatry*, Vol. 161, No. 12, pp.2194-2200

Xie, S., Xiao J., Bai J., & Jiang, X. (2004). Memory tasks in normal aged volunteers: an fMRI study. *China Journal of Medical Imaging Technology*, Vol. 20, pp. 571-574

Yamasue, H., Kasai, K., Iwanami, A., Ohtani, T., Yamada, H., Abe, O., Kuroki, N., Fukuda, R., Tochigi, M., Furukawa, S., Sadamatsu, M., Sasaki, T., Aoki, S., Ohtomo, K., Asukai, N., & Kato, N. (2003). Voxel-based analysis of MRI reveals anterior cingulate gray-matter volume reduction in posttraumatic stress disorder due to terrorism. *Proceedings of the National Academy of Sciences of the United States of America*, Vol. 100, No. 15, pp. 9039-9043

Zhu, J., Yung, W., Chow, BK., Chan, Y., & Wang, J. (2006). The cerebellar-hypothalamic circuits: Potential pathways underlying cerebellar involvement in somatic-visceral integration. *Brain Research Reviews*, Vol. 52, No. 1, pp. 93-106

19

# PTSD, Neuroimaging and Psychotherapy: A Fruitful Encounter

Julio F.P. Peres, PsyD, PhD.
*Radiology Clinic – Universidade Federal de São Paulo, SP,*
*Psychotraumatology Clinic - Hospital Perola Byington, SP,*
*Brazil*

## 1. Introduction

Most of us have dealt with a traumatic event of some kind such as loss, accident, or illness, or will be dealing with one at some point in our lives. Psychological trauma is closely related to the development of posttraumatic stress disorder (PTSD), involving three sets of symptoms: (i) reliving trauma (traumatic memories, nightmares, intrusive thoughts); (ii) emotional avoidance/numbness (affective distance, emotional anaesthesia); and (iii) increased arousal (irritability, insomnia and hypervigilance) (American Psychiatric Association, 1994). Lifetime prevalence of PTSD-triggering traumatic events may be as much as 50-90%, and actual prevalence in the general population is about 8% (Kessler et al., 1995; Vieweg et al., 2006), while partial PTSD (pPTSD) in an at-risk groups have been estimated at approximately 30% (Weiss et al., 1992). After noting that individuals who do not meet the full set of diagnostic criteria for PTSD may suffer from clinically significant symptoms of PTSD (Weiss et al., 1992), the concept of pPTSD or subthreshold PTSD was introduced to describe subsyndromal forms of PTSD (Blanchard et al., 1995; Stein et al. 1997). Thus, exposure to traumatic stressors and psychological trauma is widespread, with a wide range of cognitive and behavioral responses/outcomes among trauma survivors (Peres et al., 2009; 2011).

One of the main psychological sequelae of traumatic experiences is conditioning of specific fears. In addition to PTSD, traumatic events can significantly influence major depression, somatoform disorders, panic and anxiety disorders, obsessive-compulsive disorders, phobic disorders, and substance abuse (Peres et al., 2009). Although traumatic events are associated with PTSD in the literature, traumatized people do not meet DSM-IV (Diagnostic and Statistical Manual of Mental Disorders, 4th Edition) criteria for PTSD in many cases and often present a range of psychoform or somatoform symptoms. Considerable overlap in symptoms and disease comorbidity has been noted for medically unexplained symptoms in the primary care setting, such as chronic fatigue syndrome, low back pain, irritable bowel syndrome, primary headaches, fibromyalgia, temporomandibular joint disorder, major depression, panic attacks, and PTSD (Peres et al., 2009). Epidemiologic surveys increasingly point to a relation between exposure to traumatic events and more health care utilization, adverse health outcomes, onset of specific diseases, and premature death (Corrigan et al., 2005; Keane et al., 2006). Certain characteristics of traumas, particularly peritraumatic cognitive response and related cognitions, appear to heighten the risk for PTSD (Peres et al.,

2009). How people process stressors may be critical in determining whether or not trauma will be experienced, as well as the different constellation of symptoms if traumatization is characterized.

A single traumatic event can be processed in very different ways by individuals who experienced the same traumatic episode (Peres et al., 2005; 2011). The psychopathological signs of trauma are not static over time, nor is the form of the expression of traumatic memories. This fluidity is a consequence of the sensitization that is driven by reminders of the traumatic event and the vulnerability of memory to being modified with repeated recall (Peres et al., 2008; 2011). The sensitization of neural pathways involved in this reactivity is central to understanding the neurobiology of PTSD. The purpose of this chapter is to attempt to integrate both neuroimaging and psychotherapeutic findings in relation to PTSD, so that integration might bring greater efficacy to the treatment of psychologically traumatized patients.

## 2. A single disorder with many different facets

In life-threatening situations, mammals tend to react in two ways: "fight or flight" or "freezing". In light of adaptive evolutionary theory, both types of responses lead to adaptive gains for survivors. The defensive cascade animal model shows that several animals flee from or confront other predators, whereas others "pretend" to be dead when captured (Broman-Fulks et al., 2006). More than 100 studies have pointed to a distinction between simple and complex PTSD; therefore, some researchers have sought to include the dissociative subtype in the DSM-V (van der Kolk, 2006). Although based on recent literature, "freeze, flight, fight, fright, faint" provides a more comprehensive description of the human acute stress response sequence than current descriptions (Bracha et al., 2004). Two main behavioral systems are involved in PTSD: (1) hyperstimulation of sympathetic reactivity with expressive activity of the adrenergic system typically involved in fight or flight responses, and (2) dissociation with parasympathetic reactivity involved in freeze responses (Bremner et al., 2003). Supporting these two PTSD subtypes is a model of risk factors for PTSD developed after a study with a group of acutely burned people. Two pathways to PTSD were discerned: 1) from the size of the burn and level of pain following the acute anxiety, and then to PTSD; and 2) from the size of the burn to the level of acute dissociation following the burn, and then to PTSD. Together these pathways accounted for almost 60% of variance in PTSD symptoms and constituted a model with excellent fit indices. These findings support a model of complex etiology for childhood PTSD in which two independent pathways may be mediated by different biobehavioral systems (Saxe et al., 2005). Similar results were found in a different sample of sexually abused children. Independent pathways—anxiety/arousal and dissociation—through which sexually abused children are likely to develop later PTSD symptoms, accounted for about 57% of variance in PTSD symptoms (Kaplow et al., 2005). The finding that high levels of dissociative symptoms may be related to suppression of autonomic physiological responses to stress supports Bremner's conceptualization of dissociative symptoms as comprising one of two subtypes of the acute stress response, differing physiologically as well as subjectively from a predominantly hyperarousal or intrusive symptom response (Creamer et al., 2005). The dissociative subtype may be seen in adults with a history of sexual abuse during childhood who present a consistent picture of dissociative amnesia, which occurs more often in victims of interpersonal violence during childhood than in combat soldiers and accident victims (who do not present hyperarousal symptoms).

### 2.1 Subtype I

In a situation of unknown risk, heart and visceral alterations point to autonomous nervous system hyperactivity, whereas a subjective state of arousal potentiates an immediate search for syntheses and parameters for generating behavior. Peripheral and metabolic alterations (eg, tachycardia, mydriasis) reflect hyperactivity of the sympathetic nervous system and the hypothalamus-hypophysis-adrenal (HPA) axis leading to an immediate self-preservation response (Peres et al., 2007). Neurofunctional studies with hyperarousal PTSD patients using symptom provocation paradigms (in most cases, the retrieval of traumatic memories) suggest that the difficulty of synthesizing, classifying, and integrating a traumatic memory in narrative form may be related to the decreased activity of the prefrontal cortex involved in reducing negative feedback from the activity of the amygdala (Shin et al., 2004). Studies have implicated the HPA and the sympathetic-adrenal-medullar stress axes as key components of this pathogenic process (Boscarino et al., 2006). The relationship between anxiety level and performance is no longer advantageous after a certain point. Self-generated information flooding into sensory pathways affects the perceptual processing of data from surroundings, thus hampering the ability to formulate new hypotheses and syntheses.

Trauma-related studies involving epinephrine (E), norepinephrine (NE), and serotonin (5-HT) suggested that alterations in NE, E, and 5-HT may have relevance for symptoms commonly seen in survivors with PTSD, including hypervigilance, exaggerated startle, irritability, impulsivity, aggression, and intrusive memories (Southwick et al., 1999). Studies related to the role of NE in arousal, orienting to novel stimuli, selective attention, and vigilance demonstrated heightened noradrenergic neuronal reactivity, increased □-2 receptor sensitivity and exaggerated arousal in organisms that have been exposed to chronic uncontrollable stress. The way an individual cognitively processes a traumatic event may trigger an anxious/arousal or a dissociative reaction.

### 2.2 Subtype II

Tonic immobility (TI) is a possible component of the fear response characterized by freezing or immobility in situations involving extreme fear coupled with physical restraint, and is observed in 30% to 40% of rape victims (Kaplow et al., 2005). A study of TI in victims of childhood sexual abuse (CSA)—female undergraduates ($n$ = 39) and female psychiatric inpatients ($n$ = 41)—showed that more than 52% of all participants reported TI in response to CSA. TI reports were associated with greater current psychological impairment (Heidt et al., 2005) and may be typical not only of rape and sexual abuse victims, but other kinds of directly experienced traumas as well (Bados et al., 2008).

Emotional factors play a role in many reflex TI manifestations referred to as *feigning death*. Whether orienting and defense responses provide a valid model in humans has yet to be proven, but the dissociative response in certain trauma cases resembles animal TI. Bovin and colleagues (2008) asked whether TI mediates relations between perceived inescapability, peritraumatic fear, and PTSD symptom severity among sexual assault survivors. Their findings indicated that TI fully mediated relations between perceived inescapability and overall PTSD symptom severity, as well as re-experiencing and avoidance/numbing symptom clusters. Beyond the hyperarousal PTSD model, TI may be a pathway through which trauma survivors develop severe PTSD symptoms. Supporting this hypothesis, psychophysiological changes associated with peritraumatic dissociation in female recent-rape victims were studied, as well as the relation between these changes and PTSD symptoms. Individuals in the high peritraumatic dissociation group showed a significantly different pattern of physiological responses from those in the low dissociation group. There was suppression of autonomic physiological responses in the former group, which also showed a discrepancy between self-reports of distress and objective physiological indicators in the laboratory setting (low heart rate and skin conductance), whereas high measures of subjective suffering were observed while volunteers talked about rape. On the other hand, the low dissociation group showed increased sympathetic system response (heart rate and skin conductance) during the same task. These findings support the hypothesis that in addition to the anxiety/arousal subtype, there is a dissociative subtype of persons with PTSD symptoms who exhibit diminished physiological reactivity (Griffing et al., 2006). Another study found that female rape victims with acute PTSD who scored high on the Peritraumatic Dissociative Experiences Questionnaire exhibited suppression of physiological responses during exposure to trauma-related stimuli (Kaufman et al., 2002).

Routes to traumatic amnesia from dissociative detachment (loss of emotional content leading to loss of factual content) and from dissociative compartmentalization (failure in integration) are frequent in PTSD subtype II patients. Women with high disability pain were more likely to have experienced child abuse, adult sexual assault, more severe spousal abuse, lifetime abuse-related injuries, and PTSD symptoms.

Neuroimaging studies found distinct neural reciprocities for the two types of responses. The first pattern of sympathetic excitability involved attenuation of medial-prefrontal cortex activity and heightened amygdala activity leading to continuous autonomic arousal and state of alert. The second pattern (dissociative) showed heightened activity of the medial-prefrontal cortex resulting in inhibition of amygdala activity, blunting the sympathetic response and leading to emotional numbing (Peres et al., 2011).

## 3. Neuroimaging studies of sufferers of traumatic memories

Single photon emission computed tomography (SPECT), positron emission tomography (PET), and functional magnetic resonance imaging (fMRI) neuroimaging techniques have provided information about the dynamics of brain activity in sufferers of traumatic memories. The neural substrates underlying traumatic memories have been induced with personalised narrative trauma scripts, images, sounds and virtual reality equipment. The diversity of findings and the heterogeneity of symptomatology amongst people suffering psychological traumas suggest it may not be possible to identify one specific neural circuit underlying PTSD. Nevertheless, neuroimaging studies of symptom provocation have identified some consistent patterns, including reduced left hemisphere activity, and hypo perfusion in the anterior cingulate (AC), dorsolateral prefrontal cortex, hippocampus, and Broca's area. Other areas have shown consistently increased activation, including the parahippocampal gyrus, posterior cingulate, and amygdale. Less consistent findings include bilateral reduction in activation of the thalamus and fusiform gyrus, and increase in activation of the right insula and cerebellum (Peres et al., 2005).

Rauch and colleagues (1996) were the first to use PET and personalised script-driven imagery to temporarily provoke symptoms in individuals with PTSD. The study revealed increased perfusion in limbic and paralimbic structures of the right hemisphere, including the orbit frontal cortex, insular cortex, anterior temporal pole, and middle temporal cortex. Broca's area in the left inferior frontal cortex showed significantly decreased blood flow during provocation of traumatic memories, though not all studies have replicated this finding (McFarlane et al., 1997; Peres et al., 2007).

There is consensus that limbic and paralimbic regions are involved in the expression of emotional memories (Grillon et al., 1996; Shalev et al., 2000; Shalev, 2002; Moscovitch et al., 2005). More specifically, activation of the amygdala and anterior paralimbic structures is implicated in the processing of negative emotions such as fear. Studies of war veterans with PTSD, during visualisation of combat images showed increased activation of the anterior ventral cingulate gyrus and right amygdala, and reduced activity in Broca's area (Shin et al., 1999; Pissiota et al., 2002) A SPECT study by Liberzon and colleagues (1999) using combat veterans with and without PTSD and healthy controls, found left amygdala activation in response to combat sounds in PTSD patients only, but no amygdala activity in response to neutral sounds. Similarly, Rauch and colleagues (2000) found that people with PTSD showed greater activation of the right amygdala when shown frightening faces, compared to the controls.

PET has been used to study veterans to measure patterns of neural activity associated with traumatic images and sounds. Decrease in activity of the left prefrontal cortex (PFC) and anterior cingulate cortex of those individuals has also been demonstrated (Bremner et al., 1999). In another study with war veterans, fMRI was used to measure changes in activation of the left anterior cingulate cortex in response to a cognitive activation model - counting stroop for combat-related, negative, and neutral words (Shin et al., 2001). Individuals with PTSD showed decreased activity in the left PFC and AC when compared to the control group. In contrast, other SPECT studies of war veterans, did not find differential activity in these regions in response to trauma-related stimuli in PTSD, but found increased activity in the middle prefrontal cortex that was not correlated with symptoms (Shin et al., 1999; Zubieta et al., 1999). Two PET studies of women victims of childhood sexual abuse utilized directed scripts of neutral images and events related to the trauma (Bremner et al., 2002; Bremner et al., 1999). The scripts evoked memories of abuse experiences in all women, and resulted in increased bilateral activation of the posterior cingulate and motor cortex, but there was no differential activity in the middle prefrontal cortex or AC in women with PTSD relative to controls. Liberzon and colleagues (1999) and Zubieta and colleagues (1999) conducted a SPECT using similar methodology, involving war veterans with PTSD, publishing findings on PFC activity, which appeared to modulate the response to fear. In contrast to the typical findings, a regional increase in blood flow (not decrease) was found in PFC in individuals with PTSD. This discrepancy may that relate to the selection of this region in a region-of-interest analysis, which was derived from a separate control group or a confounding variable of a dissociative subtype of PTSD. Lanius and colleagues (2004), using a script-driven symptom provocation paradigm, have observed greater activity in the right posterior cingulate, right parietal lobe, and right occipital lobe, in PTSD and less activity in the left hemisphere. These findings support the suggestion of the inherently nonverbal nature of traumatic memory recall in PTSD subjects, compared to a more verbal pattern of traumatic memory recall in subjects without PTSD.

Despite some inconsistencies, there are reproducible neuroimaging findings in studies of traumatic memories. Functional neuroimaging has revealed greater activation of the right amygdala and anterior paralimbic regions, structures which are known to be involved in processing negative emotions, deactivation of the Broca's area and other non-limbic cortical regions, and decreased activity of the left PFC and cingulate cortex in response to trauma-related stimuli in individuals with PTSD (Hull et al., 2002; Pitman et al., 2001; Peres et al., 2007).

However, there is also evidence to suggest that the failure of the medial prefrontal cortex/anterior cingulate network to regulate amygdala activity may extend beyond the situations of threat reminders associated with traumatic memory (Bremner et al., 1999), as these circuits are also implicated in the processing of facial expression and affect (Phillips et al., 1997), and have been found to be abnormal in PTSD (Rauch et al., 2000; Felmingham et al., 2003). The exact nature of the disruption of the networks in PTSD is unclear, but such findings suggest that there is an abnormality in the networks involved in these processing affective states. The finding of Felmingham and colleagues (2003) was of particular interest, and demonstrated less ability to differentiate between fearful and resting facial expression in PTSD, possibly reflective of the emotional numbing symptom in PTSD, which has disruptive socially implications.

Williams and colleagues (2005) explored the time course of activations associated with processing of fearful faces in PTSD and found that while traumatic emotions had a primary impact on the medial prefrontal systems, there was also a breakdown of the laterality of AC responses, which intensified with repeated exposure. The lack of coupling of the amygdala and AC in the PTSD subjects may account for the disruption of spatio-temporal activity observed in this disorder.

Another body of research has examined the processing of non-trauma-related stimuli in PTSD (Semple et al., 1993; Weber et al., 2005). This line of research is of particular interest for two reasons. It explores the question as to whether there are differences between PTSD subjects and controls in their ability to manage their day-to-day environment (Clark et al., 2003). PTSD patients demonstrated reduced activity in the left dorsolateral and inferior parietal cortex, indicative of decreased recruitment of these key areas involved in verbal working memory updating. Event-related potential (ERP) data from these same subjects (Weber et al., 2005) showed an abnormal pattern of cortical source activity during this updating process in PTSD, with a strong reduction in left fronto-parietal activity, systems involved in attention, working memory and interactions with medial temporal areas during episodic memory. The abnormalities that have been identified raise the question as to whether the difficulties that individuals with PTSD have dealing with traumatic reminders may, in part, reflect a more pervasive abnormality of information processing (McFarlane et al., 1997). There is extensive work demonstrating ERP abnormalities in PTSD (Karl et al., 2006).

One of the challenges in interpreting these data is understanding the extent to which such changes are indicative of primary pathology in the processing of traumatic memories or whether they are part of compensatory changes which would represent partial resilience - the ability to overcome difficulties and build a satisfactory quality of life - to trauma exposure. Britton and colleagues (2005) found decreased activation to the amygdala to the neutral memories in PTSD and increased activation to the traumatic reminders in both PTSD and trauma exposed individuals who did not develop PTSD. In general, the pattern of activation for PTSD patients was midway between those for combat-exposed and non-traumatized controls, indicating they may have partial or less effective regulation of amygdala activation than combat-exposed controls. PTSD patients also showed a failure of activation in the AC and diminished medial prefrontal cortex activity in response to traumatic memories. These findings emphasise that the interaction between neural circuits, rather than activity of specific neuroanatomical regions is central to understanding the neurobiology of PTSD. The AC is of importance in the monitoring of emotional experience (Bush et al., 2000) and the greater intensity of negative emotions in PTSD may represent a failure of this region to exert appropriate top down inhibition (Britton et al., 2005).

One interesting study (investigated the temporal dynamics of amygdala activity in PTSD, and found increased early amygdala responses, which in the left hemisphere correlated with symptom severity (Protopopescu et al., 2005). PTSD patients also failed to show the normal pattern of habituation to threat-related words (unrelated to trauma), and instead showed a pattern suggestive of sensitization. In summary, this pattern of reactivity and increasing responsiveness to threat stimuli in PTSD provides valuable neurobiological insights into the difficulty that patients have in modulating their reactivity. Chung and colleagues (2006) in a SPECT study in a resting condition, found increased blood flow in limbic regions and decreased perfusion in the superior frontal gyrus and parietal and temporal regions in PTSD, further suggesting general dysregulation of regions involved in memory and emotion in PTSD.

An fMRI study explored the processing of social cognitions associated with empathy judgments in PTSD (Farrow et al., 2005). Participants were scanned pre- and post- modified cognitive behavioural therapy, with healthy people showing increased activation in the left middle temporal gyrus associated with empathy judgments and posterior cingulate gyrus activation associated with forgivability judgments. In patients, activity of regions activated by empathy and forgivability judgments increased as PTSD symptoms resolved, suggesting networks that might underpin the symptoms of social withdrawal and emotional numbing.

Intense or overwhelming experiences may trigger different responses, and studies have shown interindividual variability in the processing of life events and basic emotions (Eugene et al., 2003). Rather than simply passively registering reality, acquisition of information is conceived as an intrinsically active dynamic process of deconstruction and reconstruction of the external world on the basis of patterns of stimulations exciting the sensory receptors (Palmer et al., 2004). Sensory data from the outside world are deconstructed and used to build percepts, or perceptual representations. In order to cope with enormous amounts of sensory information being processed simultaneously - to generate adaptive behavior on the basis of this information - the nervous system has to collect them in a single percept. This process of building a representation (known as the "binding problem") gives rise to a perceptual unit, or synthesis, which depends on neural activity manifesting a state of spatial-temporal coherence to define the percept produced, even though it may be spread across several cortical circuits. A sensory stimulation pattern may generate one synthesis in a certain neutral situation but another very different one in situations in which these stimuli are accompanied by emotionally valenced events. The forming of atypical perceptual syntheses associated with events of highly emotional content may be related to several of the perceptual disorders involved in PTSD. For instance, dissociated PTSD subjects have distorted body perceptions (Griffin et al., 1997). The traumatized individuals' perceptive "binding" may occur in a dysfunctional manner: the nervous system may not succeed in grouping - or synthesizing - sensory information gathered from the environment in a coherent and functional manner. Strategies for altering maladapted syntheses/bindings formed by traumatic events may provide an important tool for exposure and cognitive restructuring therapy. For instance, a traumatized individual may use new associations (new "pathways" - or neural circuitry) based on their own experiences of solving problems to constitute perceptual "bindings".

Whether an event is traumatic or not will depend on an individual's perceptual neural-circuitry processing and underlying resilience - significantly influenced by subjectivity (Creamer et al., 2005) - which is the ability to cope effectively and adapt in the face of loss, hardship or adversity (Bonanno et al., 2004.; Block et al.., 1996). Resilient individuals reported fewer posttraumatic symptoms after combat and showed greater ability to optimize emotional functioning through the use of alternative cognitive strategies (Bonanno et al., 2004; Florian et al., 1995). Neuroscientists have yet to comprehensively research this field (Peres et al., 2011). Examining neural mechanisms underlying psychological trauma or resilience is difficult given the heterogeneous symptoms and peculiarities of traumatic memories (key symptoms of PTSD). There are several methodological challenges and complex factors to control such as: (i) traumatized individuals typically present various comorbidities (e.g. major depression, substance abuse, etc.), (ii) traumatic events of different kinds (violence, accidents, loss, etc.) involve distinct sensory levels and modalities of memories (visual, tactile, olfactory, auditory, affective), (iii) different PTSD symptoms and emotions may accompany specific neural interactions during retrieval of traumatic memories (e.g. dissociative experiences are psychoneurophysiologically different from hyperarousal experiences, thus it is now clear that the division of PTSD into more specific subtypes is necessary in future diagnostic manuals to better categorise patterns of symptomatology and the respective neural substrates involved), (iv) the heterogeneous nature of trauma may pose difficulties when inducing reproducible responses in patients, or comparable activations in healthy control subjects, (v) the recency of the memories being studied is often different (memory expression may be modified over time, causing changes in the neural substrates involved). In the last ten years, however, neuroimaging research has yielded important information on heightened amygdala responsivity in PTSD patients during symptomatic states, and has found that medial prefrontal cortex (mPFC) responsivity is inversely associated with PTSD-symptom severity (Shin et al., 2006). Nevertheless, the directionality of the PFC to amygdala-activity correlation has been inconsistent: negative in PTSD cases but positive in controls, suggesting coupling only in psychopathology (Shin et al., 2005; Peres et al., 2008; 2011).

### 3.1 Comprehending neuroimaging findings

As advances are made in interpreting the meaning of neuroimaging findings, this work may lead to important refinements of therapeutic interventions for the treatment of traumatized patients (Peres et al., 2008). Clinical studies suggest that abnormalities in interpretation, synthesis, and integration of emotionally salient episodes play a crucial role in experiences being received as traumatic (Van Der Kolk, 1997).

Decreased hippocampal volume, often associated with PTSD, may have etiological significance for dissociation and errors in interpretation of information related to threats (Gilbertson et al., 2002). Moreover, reduction or blockage of hippocampal integrative function can fragment the various aspects of the memory of the traumatic experience into body sensations, smells, and sounds that seem strange and separate from other life experiences (Van Der Kolk, 1997). It has been proposed previously that impaired hippocampal functional may contribute to the fragmentation of experience in patients with PTSD (Lamprecht et al., 2002).

People exposed to personalised narratives of their trauma who have PTSD demonstrate a different pattern of activation, highlighting networks that are more associated with affective processing and less associated with linguistic representation. It appears that disruption of activity in the left frontal region is of particular importance in PTSD (Pissiota et al., 2002; Van Der Kolk, 1997) and the propensity to engage right hemisphere networks. It has been suggested that the left hemisphere sequentially organizes information and is responsible for problem solving and categorization operations (Hull et al., 2002; Van Der Kolk, 1997), which may explain why traumatic memories are experienced as 'belonging to the present', as brain regions necessary for sequencing and categorizing experiences are not adequately activated (Peres et al., 2007; 2011).

Individuals with PTSD were examined with SPECT before and after treatment with Eye Movement Desensitization and Reprocessing (Levin et al., 1999). Post-treatment, there was increased activity in the AC and left frontal lobe, perhaps influencing neuronal activity in the areas implicated in PTSD, particularly the left hemisphere. The finding of Farrow and colleagues (2005) further indicated that post-treatment there was greater activation of left hemisphere pathways associated with empathetic responses, with concomitant symptomatic improvement in PTSD.

During exposure to traumatic narratives, several studies have also shown a decline in activation in Broca's area of the left inferior frontal gyrus. Shin and colleagues (1999) verified that only individuals with PTSD exhibited a failure of activation in Broca's area and the AC. Other studies have also identified significantly decreased activity in Broca's area, and are perhaps linked with the difficulty PTSD individuals have in assimilating the traumatic event into a narrative structure (Hull et al., 2002; Peres et al., 2007; 2011).

The PFC and AC have been shown to be deactivated during retrieval of traumatic memories in patients with PTSD. These structures may inhibit responses to emotional stimuli (Bryant et al., 2005; Gilboa et al., 2004). In addition, dysfunction of dorsolateral PFC may mediate problems with language, cognition and integration of verbal expression with emotions. Decreased PFC activity may extinguish response to the symptoms of PTSD, attenuating the negative feedback of amygdala activity (Bremner et al., 2002; Nutt et al., 2004; Peres et al., 2007; 2011).

However, studies that have examined the temporal dynamics of these neural networks suggest that one of the key factors in PTSD is a progressive sensitisation and increasing responsivity to non-specific threat stimuli, even in a brief period of time (Protopopescu et al., 2005). The failure to adaptively process threat suggests that in PTSD, there is a propensity for increasing strength of affective responses with time, which disrupts the modulation of affect. Such neuroimaging findings highlight the experience of patients and underscore the disruptions of processing of the external world. Further evidence for a pervasive problem of information processing of non-trauma related stimuli in PTSD (Clark et al., 2003; Karl et al., 2006) suggests that treatment needs to address this aspect of the phenomenology of the disorder. The sense of being confused and aroused by the external world goes beyond specific reminders of the trauma.

Although neuroimaging studies of PTSD are still in an "embryonic" stage, disruption of hippocampal function, deactivation of Broca's area, the left hemisphere, and prefrontal cortex are consistently implicated in the pathophysiology of PTSD, expressed as a difficulty in synthesizing, categorizing, and integrating the traumatic memory (Peres et al., 2008). The subtle impact of the processing of facial expression may impact on the sense of engagement and empathy in the therapeutic setting. These abnormalities occur against the background of a more pervasive disruption of information processing in PTSD of stimuli unrelated to the trauma. These limitations should be considered as an important factor challenging the capacity of these patients to engage in the therapeutic process.

### 3.1.1 Trauma and memory systems

Trauma, in its Greek etymological root, means lesion caused by an external agent. The term psychic trauma was firstly coined by Freud (1895) during his studies on the aetiology of neurosis, in which he stated that psychic traumatism is characterized by excessive excitement related to an individual's tolerance and capacity to integrate and psychically elaborate this stimulus. However, characterization of an event as traumatic does not depend only on the stressor stimulus, and there is no single human response to the same traumatic events or a "universal reaction to trauma" (Jones et al., 2003). The search to understand idiosyncratic responses to trauma has turned to the contribution of personality factors (Bonanno et al., 2004), with the way people process the stressor event appearing to be a critical factor in determining whether an event will be encoded as traumatic or not (Peres et al., 2007).

There are several complex memory systems involved, including declarative memory (Peres et al., 2005). Emotional memories interact with the neural substrates of declarative memory (Erk et al.,1998). Clinical observations clearly demonstrate that unpleasant emotional memories (charged with sadness, disgust, fear, or rage) can lead to maladaptive changes, such as distortions of perception, assessment, and judgment (Fivush et al., 1998). Although such distortions may not characterize a traumatic event, unpleasant emotional memories can remain vivid over time, and serve as references for expression of avoidance behaviours. In contrast, an event of greater emotional impact that is perceived as traumatic can lead to abnormal memory phenomena that are typical of PTSD, including the extreme imprinting of the experience, fragmentation of memories for the event, partial forgetfulness, or even amnesia (Lamprecht et al., 2002; Van Der Kolk, 1997). Studies of adults with a history of sexual abuse during childhood present with a consistent picture of dissociative amnesia, occurring more often in victims of interpersonal violence during childhood than in combat soldiers and accident victims (Williams et al., 1995). Amnesias for emotional and cognitive content appear to be related to the age at which the trauma occurred, as well as the constancy of the stressor event, with younger the age and prolonged duration of the traumatic stressor associated with greater probability of significant amnesia (Loftus et al., 1999). Thus, terrifying experiences can either totally resist integration, or can be etched in an "indelible" manner in a person's memory, and under many circumstances, traumatized individuals report a combination of these two phenomena. For example, in studies of posttraumatic nightmares, some individuals reported they repeatedly experienced the same traumatic scenes without change over a 15-year period. It is curious to note that few patients describe their perceptions as exact representations of sensations experienced at the time of the trauma (Van Der Kolk, 1997; 2006). The permeability of traumatic memories, to cultural influences and changes of their expression over time has been demonstrated (Jones et al., 2003).

Van der Kolk (1997) investigated the differences in recovering memories of traumatic experiences from recovering memories of significant but non-traumatic events. Non-traumatic memory recall was associated with narratives and was without strong sensorial manifestation. In contrast, 78% of individuals questioned about traumatic memories from both childhood and adult traumas, initially reported not having any memory of the event and were unable to give an account of what happened. Regardless of the age at which the trauma occurred, all individuals stated that they initially "remembered" the trauma in the form of sensorial flashbacks, such as visual, olfactory, affective, or auditory impressions, with the awareness and capacity to describe what actually happened developing over time. This study demonstrated the key distinction between the recovery of the traumatic and emotional events was the relative absence of any narrative expression of the traumatic memory.

Functional neuroimaging studies suggest that explicit retrieval is preferentially associated with increased activity in prefrontal and medial temporal regions (Schacter et al., 1998), and the phenomenological awareness that accompanies episodic memories may arise within the hippocampal-frontal memory system. This information has to be bound together to be retrievable as a conscious memory, and the hippocampus is critical to this binding function (Verfaellie et al., 1997). Studies point to an important distinction between hippocampally-dependent and non hippocampally-dependent forms of memory that are affected differently by extreme stress (Brewin et al., 2001; 2003). One form, termed verbally accessible memory (VAM) supports ordinary autobiographical memories that can be modified and interact with other autobiographical knowledge, so that the trauma is represented within a personal context comprising past, present, and future. These traumatic memories are influenced by information that the individual has encoded before, during, and after the traumatic event, and that received sufficient conscious processing to be transferred to long-term memory in a form that can explicitly retrieved and verbally communicated. Another form, termed situationally accessible memory (SAM), contains information that has been obtained from lower-level perceptual processing of the traumatic scene (e.g. visuospatial information that has received little conscious processing) (Hellawell et al., 2002) and from the person's bodily (e.g. autonomic, motor) responses. This form of memory is consistent with the phenomenon of trauma-related 'flashbacks' that are a characteristic of severely traumatized people. Because SAMs do not involve verbal representations, these memories are difficult to communicate and may not therefore interact with other autobiographical knowledge. During periods of intense emotion, reduction of hippocampally-dependent processing of information and formation of SAMs may result in increased probability of amygdala reactivity to trauma reminders and the person experiencing a sense of current threat. A longitudinal study (Peace et al., 2004) of the reliability of memories for trauma and other emotional experiences, demonstrated that traumatic memory imagery tended to persist with no apparent decrement, whereas emotional memories were subject to considerable distortion over time. The findings converge on the non-hippocampally dependent nature of traumatic memories, and suggest a tendency of these memories to resist change with the passage of time. Nevertheless, it is clear that that at any time multiple memory systems are activated simultaneously and in parallel and findings suggest that these systems may interact (Poldrack et al., 2003; McDonald et al., 2004). One treatment study, using an exposure and cognitive restructuring process, suggest an interaction between SAM and VAM systems (Peres et al., 2007).

Clinical observation indicates that the narrative organization of mnemonic content, will assist its permeability to change. If an event, once charged with emotions, can be integrated into an individual's autobiographical memory, it tends not to be available anymore as a separate and immutable entity. The memory becomes modified by associated experiences, emotional context and a state of consciousness during the recall process (Peres et al., 2005). Breuer and Freud asserted that bringing early traumatic material to consciousness would allow "abreaction" and quick remission of symptoms, with psychotheraputic approaches favouring the retrieving the mis-stored memory and integrating this memory with narratives. This re-working consisted of building cross-links between the traumatic memory and other memories and thoughts, believed to reintegrate the isolated traumatic memory into "normal" memory systems (Freud, 1895).

### 3.1.2 Implications of neuroimaging findings in psychotherapeutic treatment: The challenge of integration

Questions concerning the neurobiological effects of psychotherapeutic interventions are now given considerable importance within the field of psychiatry and psychology. Neuroimaging studies have provided evidence for changes in cerebral dynamics after pharmacotherapy or psychotherapy (Peres et al., 2008; Rybakowski, 2002). PET, ERP and fMRI studies have provided substantial evidence that cognitive and behavioural changes that occurred within a psychotherapeutic context can cause alterations in the regional cerebral metabolism of patients with obsessive-compulsive disorders (Schawartz et al., 1996), major depression (Brody et al., 2001), as well as in patients with social phobia (Furmark et al., 2002) and specific phobia (Paquette et al., 2003). The findings suggest that the psychotherapeutic interventions have the potential to modify dysfunctional neural circuits associated with the disorders studied (Roffman et al., 2005).

Psychological treatments are presently considered the first-line intervention of choice for sufferers of traumatic memories with PTSD (Foa et al., 2000). According to the Expert Consensus Guideline Series for treatment of PTSD (1999), exposure-based therapy was indicated as a psychological treatment of choice for flashbacks, intrusive thoughts, trauma-related fears, and avoidance. All of the multicomponent treatments that include cognitive interventions have exposure as one of their key elements (Levin et al., 1999; Marks et al., 1998; Peres et al., 2007; 2011). In fact, revisiting traumatic memories can bring therapeutic benefits, as long as a well-structured process of restructuring of the emotional content is employed (Littrell, 1998).

Ehlers and colleagues (2002) evaluated the quality and content of memories of individuals that had been through different traumatic experiences. The authors emphasized the importance of identifying, the moment of greatest emotional salience, so that associations and patterns of arousal established at that moment could be reprocessed. Conscious attention to unfolding events is likely to result in richer VAM representations, and theoretically, sustained attention to flashbacks may promote information transfer between these systems, leading more rapidly to amygdala inhibition (Brewin et al., 2003; 2005). Therefore, it is reasonable to postulate that well designed exposure and cognitive restructuring psychotherapies may enable the critical translation of the fragmented sensory elements of the traumatic memories into a more integrated, narrative representation of the memory (Peres., 2007). In this respect, psychotherapy should facilitate a new framing of the traumatic experience by reviving and strengthening memories of successful coping and self-effectiveness prior to the trauma. These memories, their respective emotional valences and states of consciousness, may be recognized and interconnected with the memory of the trauma during a restructuring session. We found that each time a patient narrated a traumatic episode, the narrative could be structured with new cognitive and emotional elements extracted from reinforced memories of successful coping. Therefore, the reinterpretation and reconstruction of traumatic memories may lead to changes in neural networks involved, and relieve symptoms (Peres et al., 2007).

Increasingly, psychological interventions have focused on exposure-based therapies for cognitive restructuring of past events (Leskin et al., 1998), with the essential component of involving repeated exposure to memories of the traumatic stressor. Is should be noted, however, that confrontation with traumatic memories through debriefing has not been effective in treating individuals with PTSD (Marcks et al., 1998). Thus, confrontation of the memories does not appear to be sufficient to provide a therapeutic effect, but also requires the restructuring and integration of memories. A point worth noting is Breuer and Freud found prepsychoanalytic cathartic treatment alone generally ineffective, and the latter turned to a more narrative type of approach in transference based therapy (Freud et al., 1895). Moreover, we believe it is critical for narrative to involve the search for constructive lessons. Thus, psychotherapy will sensitize the traumatized individual's resilient traits by propitiating access to this repertoire from their pre-trauma life history. Good examples of successful coping by individuals who drew lessons from their traumatic experiences and so developed their resilience may be also provide models for trauma victims when developing new types of cognitive processing.

### 3.1.3 Memory reconstruction

There is consensus that emotionally-charged memories are not static, but rather, are interpretations, new reconstituted versions of the original event (Damasio., et al 2002). Loftus and colleagues (1999) observed the imprecise nature of remembering by examining the phenomenon of false memories. It has also been demonstrated that responses to traumas are guided by emotional beliefs, independently of the precision of the information (Peres et al., 2007; McNally et al., 2003). Thus, neuroscience findings provide crucial insight for psychotherapy, highlighting that emotionally-charged memories are peculiar representations of an event, distant from the original episode, but salient in their significance for the individual.

We postulate that the re-interpretation and reconstruction of traumatic memories can be used with exposure and cognitive restructuring psychotherapies, to alleviate some of the distressing symptoms of PTSD, by changing the nature of the representations of the traumatic event. It is therefore, crucial to consider that the most important modulators of the acquisition, formation, and evocation of traumatic memories are the emotions involved and the individuals' conscious access to the memories (Baddelev et al., 2000; Dolan et al., 2002). The retrieval of traumatic memories, whether spontaneous or provoked, occurs in an altered state of consciousness. Vermetten and Bremner (Vermetten et al., 2004) reviewed remarkable similarities in neuroimaging studies of traumatic recall and hypnotic processes. The same brain structures - thalamus, hippocampus, amygdala, medial prefrontal cortex, and anterior cingulate cortex - were involved in both research lines. We propose that therapeutic interventions focussing on emotions and the conscious processing of these events will modulate the memory for these events, effectively changing the interactions between underlying neural networks. It is argued that this shift of consciousness, will results in changes in the perception of the same event (Dietrich et al., 2003). Retrieval and interpretation of the original altered states of consciousness also permit the transformation of "early" traumatic memory into "later" explicit memory (Brenneis et al., 1996). In accordance, Breuer suggested hypnosis might be useful to access and modulate that altered state of consciousness and remobilize memory systems for the purpose of cross linking them with narrative memory functions (Freud et al., 1895). Other work supports the idea that the use of altered states of consciousness can be an effective tool in the formation of new patterns of perception involving thought, feelings, and behaviour (Horowitz et al., 1972; Kasorow et al., 1999). By re-experiencing the trauma in different states of consciousness and, consequently, acquiring different perceptions of the same traumatic event, the individual may efficiently transfer information from the non-hippocampally-dependent memory store to the hippocampally-based memory system (Peres et al., 2007; Peres et al., 2005). In many cases, the trauma per se must be accessed before mourning can proceed. In this respect, Pierre Janet's hypnotherapy and its approach based on a dissociation model has been used satisfactorily for cases in which traumatic grief occurs when psychological trauma obstructs mourning (van der Hart et al., 1990).

Psychotherapy can be informed by the neuroimaging literature in relation to the difficulties PTSD patients have with processing both trauma-related and trauma-neutral information. The challenge is to be able to grasp the experience of an individual whose registration of the environment is fundamentally different from normal perception, and explore the attribution of meaning. Neuroimaging research highlights that a large component of a patient's cognitive and affective experience, has changed their capacity to create meaning and manage their perceptions of those experiences, particularly with regard to interpretations of their current environment. The challenge of the psychotherapy is to draw the patient out of this world by facilitating changes in perception and meaning.

When a traumatic memory can be reconstructed and reintegrated in this way, it loses intensity and evolves from a traumatic memory into an emotional one. Psychotherapy can facilitate the search for a narrative and integrated translation of the traumatic event, so the experience can be understood and conveyed in communicable language. We argue that psychotherapeutic interventions involving exposure and cognitive restructuring, and accommodating the altered states of consciousness during traumatic memory retrieval, will make an important contribution to the treatment of PTSD. Moreover, other psychotherapeutic strategies related to mirror neurons can offer a satisfactory outcome of traumatized people submitted to psychotherapy, as follows.

## 4. Mirror neurons

The mirror property of certain neurons was discovered at the University of Parma when science was once again helped by chance when Fogassi was in a laboratory, within the field of vision of a monkey subjected to a neurophysiological study, when he reached for a grape using a random gesture similar to one the monkey used to perform certain tasks. Fellow researchers observed that the same neurons in the monkey showed activation although it had not performed the motor task (Rizzolatti et al. 1996). After this surprising observation, neurophysiological research conducted by Rizzolatti and colleagues (2000; 2001) showed a class of visual-motor neurons in the monkey's premotor cortex, which were named mirror neurons. These neurons were activated when a particular action was performed or when the monkey observed a similar action being performed by another individual. Comparison between observing and performing an action involves not only the premotor cortex, but also pathways extending to the posterior parietal lobe. The process of sensory-motor integration is supported by the frontal-parietal network, which provides an internal copy of actions observed as a means of explicitly generating the same actions. Based on these 1996 findings, European and American neuroscientists, by using different techniques in different laboratories, observed the presence of mirror properties in human neurons distributed in several other areas, such as Broca's region, which is related to verbal expression (Rizzolatti and Arbib, 1998; Rizzolatti and Craighero, 2004). Mirror neurons have been studied while subjects observe other individuals performing an action and while they themselves perform the same action, along with a number of other useful strategies. Iacoboni and colleagues (2005) conducted fMRI studies of 23 healthy individuals observing three types of visual stimuli: grasping actions without context; context itself (scenes containing objects); and grasping in two different contexts. In the last situation, the context suggested an intention associated with the action of holding or gripping something (drinking tea or cleaning a table). The actions inserted in context, compared with the two other tasks, produced a significant increase in activity in the posterior area of the lower frontal gyrus and the ventral premotor cortex. Discussion of the findings from neurofunctional studies, besides locating circuits associated with imitation and intention, has included theories of social cognition - how we interpret the world around us and therefore how we relate to events in our lives.

### 4.1 Mirroring and empathy

The mirror property was also observed in neurons involved in the task of simulating "mind reading". The theory of mind studies the ability to understand what is going on in other people's minds and is partly related to empathy (from the Greek empatheia, meaning 'to feel as if inside'). These neural substrata seem to facilitate certain aspects of the ability to represent other people's mental states through a conceptual system (Gallese and Goldman, 1998). Mirror neurons have been observed during cognitive processes such as social intersubjectivity, imitation, learning, empathy, and contagious behavior such as yawning or laughing (Hurley and Chater, 2005). Mirroring properties may well have been important filters or a selective mechanism for survival in our ancestral past when responding to conflict or fleeing from eminent threat. One school of thought in the neurosciences argues that mirror neurons probably influenced social skills, use of tools and language. We know that autistic individuals experience difficulty in grasping social plasticity, and this fact, together with the absence of substantive findings on the physiopathology of this disorder, plus recent findings relating to mirroring properties of certain neurons, has prompted specific research on autistic children such as Dapretto and colleagues (2006). It was found that normally developing children activated mirror neurons in the limbic system via the insula when the emotional significance of imitation was experienced and understood, but the same neural circuit was not activated in autistic children. Following these findings, further studies have suggested that autism is associated with altered neural activity patterns during imitation, which includes circuits integrating areas serving visual, proprioceptive, and emotional functions. Researchers have suggested that this deficient integration may impair social-cognitive functions in these individuals (Williams et al., 2006).

Many neuroscientists believe that mirror neurons dissolve the barrier between I and the other (Oberman et al., 2005). Singer and colleagues (2004) showed an interesting similarity in relation to the involvement of the insula, cingulate, thalamus, and cerebellum in the phenomenon of empathy. These areas were activated when an individual observes another person feeling a painful stimulus. However, only structures involved in affective responses - rather than sensory circuits - were activated. The mirror properties of this circuit involve consciousness of the person's experiences and an emotional understanding of them, but not a precise sensory replica, since the observer does not experience the pain itself. Gallese (2006) reviewed that there was activation in the same circuits while experiencing comprehension of other people's emotions. In another fMRI study, the insula was activated when a subject experienced not only a basic emotion, such as the aversion caused by inhaling an odor, but also when the same subject visualized the face of another person feeling this aversion (Wicker et al, 2003). The wide range of neurofunctional research in humans (Peres and Nasello, 2008) means that neuroscience can now describe the activity of mirror neurons as a mechanism through which we experience empathy and recognize other individuals' intentions by observing their behavior, and mirroring this model when generating similar behavior.

### 4.2 Posttraumatic stress disorder, mirroring and psychotherapy

Our hypothesis is that psychotherapists may use mirror properties with PTSD patients by showing them behavioral paradigms based on individuals who successfully coped with similar traumas. On this basis, a new experimental design has been used in a recent fMRI study of traumatized individuals (Farrow et al., 2005). Thirteen patients were examined while performing three tasks that involved: (1) speculation as to another person's intention; (2) empathy; (3) decision to forgive other people; and each task was compared with the baseline involving social judgments. These PTSD individuals were subjected to a program based on behavioral therapy. Activation occurred in the same areas of the brain as those indicated in previous studies of healthy subjects, including activation in the left middle temporal as a response to empathy, and posterior cingulate in response to forgiveness decisions in post-therapy examinations. These areas were correlated with reduced PTSD symptoms. The authors suggest that time and therapy were probably the factors causing neural "normalization" in relation to these cognitive social tasks, for which PTSD individuals usually show limitations. Being able to understand other people's intentions while paying attention to their actions is a fundamental factor in social behavior. In fact, emotional numbing and social isolation are among the main PTSD symptoms (American Psychiatric Association, 1994).

Several studies have suggested that group therapy (or debriefing) is not appropriate for PTSD patients since they show no improvement, and symptoms get worse in some cases (Lewis, 2003). In the light of what we know of mirroring properties today, it is understandable that sharing painful experiences without positive models of successful coping may simply reflect and emphasize suffering instead of relieving it. On the other hand, groups such as Alcoholic Anonymous or Narcotics Anonymous bring together people seeking to end their dependency; they offer a new perspective by using repeated examples of other people coping successfully, and they have contributed to the recovery of these individuals (Vederhus and Kristensen, 2006).

Certain personality traits work to "protect" the individual during exposure to stressful events (Bonanno, 2004). One of them is self-confidence, which comprises three characteristic attitudes: the search for meaning or significance in everyday life; the notion that it is possible to affect the outcome of events; the belief that learning and development are a consequence of both positive and negative experiences. The decisive factor in developing resilience is related to the way in which an individual perceives and processes experiences (Peres et al., 2005; 2007; 2011). Therefore sensitizing the reinforcement of resilient traits is an important aspect for psychotherapy of trauma victims, and mirror neurons may be involved in this process. Observation and simulation of coping behavior may provide individuals with models not previously apprehended by those who continue to show symptoms of the disorder, thus sensitizing their own experience of coping successfully. Although PTSD patients present a constellation of symptoms and frequently verbalize their inability to act differently, "observing" successful examples of dealing with trauma may sensitize their actions, since new behavioral paradigms may be "copied." An important element here is that psychotherapy for trauma victims should render the perception of new opportunities for generating adaptive behavior easier. In our experience, we noted that "visualizing a path in advance is a fundamental step toward taking it." However, the question is raised: is it really that simple?

The complexity of human processing obviously goes beyond simple conditioning. An important part of this process includes patients accessing their own repertories of resilient attitudes, which may reinforce strategies used in the past to overcome other difficulties experienced prior (as a child, teenager or adult) to the traumatic event (Peres et al., 2005; Peres et al., 2007). Some theories suggest that understanding others people's minds, especially their judgments and intentions, is a prerequisite for imitation and learning (Tomasello et al, 1993). Opposing this view, there is now a growing consensus among philosophers, psychologists, and neuroscientists in relation to the belief that imitation and learning are connected to perception of the other "like me" (Meltzoff, 2005). Meltzoff developed the idea that imitation and learning occur when three circumstances coincide: (1) the observer produces similar behavior to the model; (2) the perception of an action causes the observer's response; (3) equivalence between the actions of "I" and "other" plays a role in generating the response. In this respect, imitation is based on the repertoire of an observer, who identifies himself or herself with a model. Therefore, observation of examples of people who learned from their traumatic experiences and grew on that basis may occur once individuals have recognized their values, talents, and ability to recover but are still lacking a model to cope with the current trauma. In the same way that watching the behavior of professional tennis or soccer players, or any other sport, will not lead to an exact copy of their movements, but the basics may be incorporated in the observer's non-professional repertoire, examples of successfully coping will be superimposed on the treated individual's own models for coping. Internal representations of the body states associated with actions, emotions, and sensations are evoked within the observer, as if he/she would be doing a similar action or experiencing a similar emotion or sensation. Mirror neuron systems are likely to be the neural correlate of this mechanism. By means of a shared neural state realized in two different bodies, the "objectual other" becomes "another self" (Gallese, 2006). The search for therapeutic meaning through the construction of resilient narratives was correlated with higher prefrontal cortex activity and reduced PTSD symptoms (Peres et al., 2007). Therefore, it is crucial for patients to be aware that their capabilities, having been reinforced in advance, can be the basis for assimilating new specific examples of coping with trauma. In the context of exposure and cognitive restructuring therapy, films and overcoming reports may provide an opportunity to revise traumatic memories by incorporating other percepts based on healthy examples. Such cognitive faculty of reinterpretation and reconstruction of emotionally charged memories may be used to good effect in exposure and cognitive restructuring therapy (Peres et al., 2007; 2011). Retrieving examples of individuals themselves being successful at other points in their lives, or highlighting other victims of psychological trauma who have managed to regain a satisfactory quality of life may ease therapeutic restructuring. Although the University of Parma monkey clearly identified with the Italian researcher's gesture, we are far from recognizing all the nuances of gestures and expressions humans derive from others and what they communicate. It is also important to remember that just as we observe and mirror the behavior of others, the same happens in relation those observing us. Our own examples of successful coping may increase awareness in our children, friends, patients, and colleagues. In this respect, Galileo Galilei left us a good example as inspiration for our "mirroring", when he said: "You cannot teach a man anything; you can only help him find it within himself." We would add that it is not a question of psychotherapists telling patients "how to do it" on an intellectual level, but rather stimulating their awareness in their ability to choose paths predictive of a better quality of life (Peres et al., 2005). We now illustrate a practical example of neuroimaging and psychotherapy integration for the benefit of traumatized patients.

## 5. Police officers under attack: Resilience implication of an fMRI study

For the first time, in 2011, it was possible to examine the neurofunctional reciprocities of a homogeneous set of traumatized individuals through control of complex variables (free of comorbidities and medications, no need for washout, same age of traumatic memory, same traumatic event also experienced by resilient individuals) in relation to coping (Group 1), continuity (Group 2) and spontaneous resilience to trauma (Group 3) (Peres et al., 2011). After psychotherapy, Group 1 was comparable to Group 3 resilient policemen in terms of symptom scores and neural expressions related to traumatic memory retrieval. The findings underline the importance of psychotherapy for shortening the period of suffering and/or avoiding symptoms becoming chronic – since Group 2 pPTSD policemen (not subjected to psychotherapy) continued to present the same symptoms with signs of worsening, whereas all those subjected to psychotherapy presented a reduction of at least 37% in total CAPS scores.

Evidence from neuroimaging research indicates that the PFC underlies many cognitive skills (Wood et al., 2003). Current and previous findings related to mPFC deactivation report that pPTSD and PTSD patients experience difficulty in activating this area, which is related to cognitive categorization and labeling of internal states (Peres et al., 2007; Shin et al., 2006). Higher brain regions such as the mPFC fail to diminish exaggerated arousal and distress symptoms mediated via the amygdala, and this may be related to the pathological responses found in psychologically traumatized victims (Peres et al., 2008). The hypothesis that primary pathology in PTSD may be amygdala hyper-responsivity rather than deficient mPFC suggests 'bottom-up' activation of the amygdala on the mPFC (Gilboa et al., 2004). Most neuroimaging studies of PTSD show reduced mPFC activity (Peres et al., 2007; Lanius et al., 2001), and some find increased amygdala activity during threat processing (Peres et al., 2008; Shin et al., 2006).

Integrating sensory traces of memories into structured therapeutic narratives is one of the main challenges for psychotherapies applied to trauma victims (Peres et al., 2008; Shin et al.,

2006), and pPTSD individuals require the same level of care (Carlier et al., 1995). Neural correlations with post-psychotherapy improvement were quite marked: as CAPS and narrative Traumatic Memory Inventory (TMI) scores improved, mPFC activation increased and amygdala activation decreased. Group 1's increased mPFC activation correlated with post-psychotherapy symptom improvement, which suggests that more active cognitive mPFC processing affected the resilience of pPTSD subjects. Because the PFC plays a major role in integrating cortical functioning and mediating perception and storage of memories in the cortical system, this region may be particularly important for processing traumatic memories and the subsequent development of PTSD symptoms (McFarlane et al., 2002).

Research has pointed to the nonverbal nature of traumatic memory recall in PTSD subjects, compared to a more verbal pattern of traumatic memory recall in healthy subjects (Lanius et al., 2004). Psychotherapy may help to build narratives and resilient integrated translations of fragmented traumatic memories via mPFC, and thus weaken their sensory content while strengthening them cognitively. We found that all three groups activated the mPFC while retrieving pleasant and neutral memories in the first and second scans, which suggests preservation of the declarative memory system in pPTSD subjects for non-traumatic events (Lanius et al., 2004; Peres et al., 2008). On the basis of our results for Group 1 and 2, we would postulate that diminished mPFC activity when processing stressor information during periods of intense emotional arousal heightens the probability of the amygdala being activated. It was interesting to note that increased mPFC activity was concomitant with less amygdala activity for a traumatic memory in both the "resilient" and "pPTSD after psychotherapy" groups.

The TMI scores showed that retrieval of memory of traumatic events was emotionally and sensorially less intense for Group 1 after psychotherapy. They were able to communicate their memories in a more structured narrative, like Group 3, which showed a well-defined narrative structure and low scores for sensory modalities of traumatic memory on both TMI measures. Unlike the psychotherapy group, in the second set of symptom measurements, Group 2 did not show significantly better scores in terms of psychological improvement and the sensory modalities of traumatic memory remained similar.

Previous research on correlations between CAPS and BOLD signals show that improvements in patients' symptoms were related to higher levels of PFC activity and less amygdala activity (Peres et al., 2008; Shin et al., 2006). The higher TMI narrative scores for the traumatic memory after psychotherapy were also correlated with higher levels of mPFC activity, strengthening the evidence for involvement of this region in the psychotherapy applied. The therapeutic effects may be largely due to extinction learning (Charney et al., 2004; Phelps et al., 2004), which builds a new response hierarchy and gradually replaces the previous association with fear. The similarities between Group 1 post-psychotherapy and Group 3 in relation to neural expression and symptom scores show that resilience can be developed and psychotherapy can affect this learning process.

Emotional flexibility is a critical mechanism underlying the ability of resilient people to successfully adapt to ever-changing environments (Bonanno, 2004; Block et al., 1996 Charney et al., 2004). Resilient police officers scored high on religiosity and two indicators of resilient coping were observed: seeking spiritual support and collaborative religious coping. This cognitive reserve related to supportive feelings may have influenced their resilient processing. Fear extinction is also mediated by inhibitory control of the mPFC over amygdala-based fear processes (Phelps et al., 2004) and exposure-based treatment of PTSD is thought to facilitate extinction learning (Shin et al., 2006; Charney et al., 2004) and therefore successful coping with trauma.

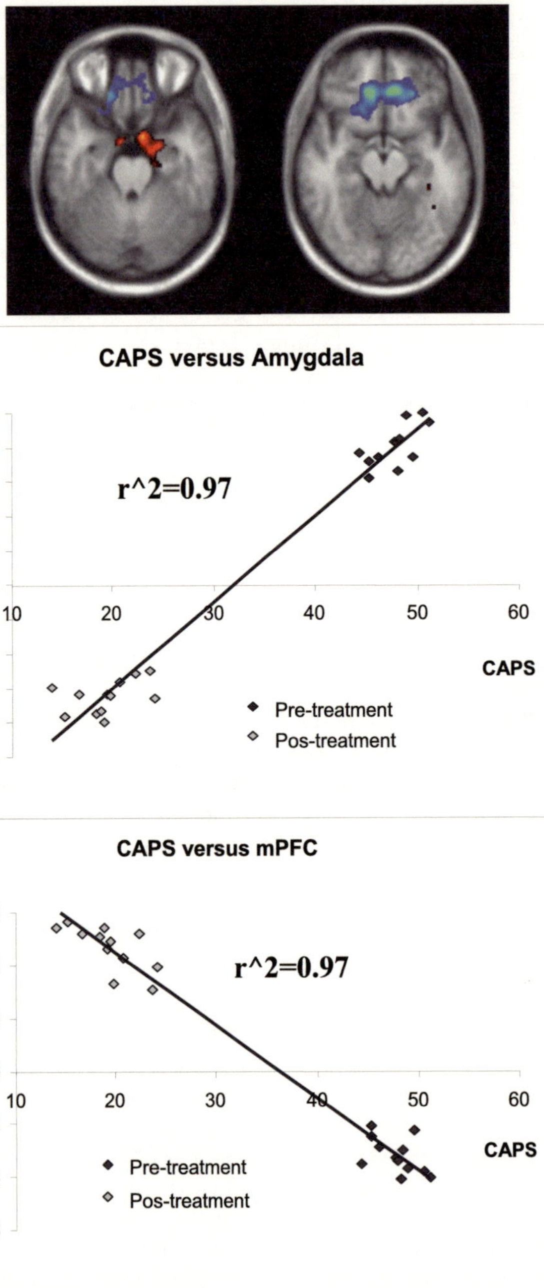


Fig.1. Correlation between changes in BOLD and changes in total severity of posttraumatic stress disorder (Clinician-Administered PTSD Scale, or CAPS) following ECRT. The functional maps display the areas where changes in BOLD activity in medial prefrontal cortex (mPFC) and amygdala correlated with changes in total CAPS score. The scatter plots display the direction of these correlations (increase in total CAPS on the horizontal axis, extent of BOLD activity on the vertical axis).

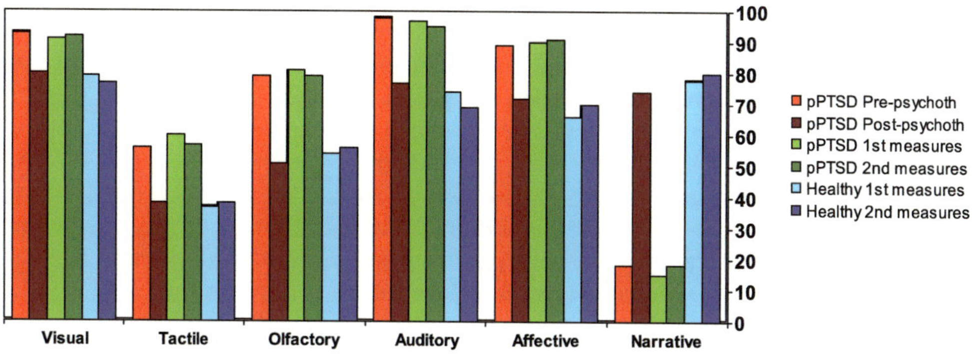


Fig.2. Memory modality and intensity scores of traumatic memory obtained after both fMRI scans for Group 1 (red), 2 (green) and 3 (blue). Traumatic memory was affectively and sensorially less intense, and narrative scores were higher for Group 1 after psychotherapy. The sensory, affective and narrative modalities of traumatic memory remained similar for Group 2 on first and second measures. Group 3 showed a well-defined narrative structure and low scores for sensory modalities of traumatic memory on both measures.

Several studies show greater suppression of cortisol release in PTSD individuals than in non-PTSDs (Yehuda et al., 1995 ; 1998; Grossman et al. 2003; Newport et al., 2004), supporting the hypothesis that PTSD is associated with enhanced negative feedback regulation of the hypothalamic-pituitary-adrenal (HPA) axis. Indeed, lower cortisol levels may also be a risk factor that affects peritraumatic reactivity and increases the likelihood of developing more pronounced PTSD symptoms (Yehuda et al., 1998; Delahanty et al., 2000). However, most studies have examined HPA axis alterations by comparing a sample of chronic, highly symptomatic PTSD patients with healthy controls (Yehuda et al., 1998; Grossman et al. 2003; Newport et al., 2004). Contrary to our hypothesis, the present study found that cortisol release was normal and as expected for the age group for both pPTSD and healthy police officers, which shows that non-chronic pPTSD police officers may not present an enhanced negative feedback regulation of the HPA axis, so a PTSD-risk factor may not be characterized if psychological assistance is provided promptly.

## 6. Conclusions

Psychotherapy appears efficacious in enabling sufferers of psychological trauma to better cope with the memories of their traumatic experience, with the reconstruction of the traumatic memories (Peres et al., 2007). Emotionally-charged memories are subjective representations of an event, often distorted and distant from the original episode, but salient in their significance to the individual (Creamer et al., 2005). Although there is a marked degree of inter individual variability in the processing of memory of life-events and basic emotions, we postulate that the re-interpretation and reconstruction of traumatic memories will be efficacious in relieving PTSD symptomatology. This process will influence the neural networks sub serving these experiences, leading to the formation of new memories that are less fragmented and available for narrative expression, an idea that is consistent with neuroimaging and clinical observations. Understanding the neural processes associated with successful response to psychotherapy may point to specific mechanisms that can be modified to enhance treatment response. In accordance with previous studies (Felmingham et al., 2007; Bryant et al., 2008; Peres et al., 2007; 2011) mPFC has a key involvement in this learning process, and psychotherapy may influence the development of a more narrative pattern of trauma. Thus, the modulation of neural circuitry, involving PFC and the amygdalar complex, is a crucial aspect in the development of a psychotherapeutic approach which favours the search for narrative and integrative translations of the sensory fragmented traumatic memory. Words are the vehicles for the therapeutic process, which is related to the attribution of meanings to past events. Our data showed that the predictors of resilience were self-efficacy, empathy and optimism in addition to supportive feeling as traits that can boost resilient processing, therefore future research should address these cognitive strategies that contribute to better responses to psychotherapy (Peres et al., 2007; 2011). Further research is required for better understanding of mechanisms for processing traumatic experiences aligned with recovery in chronic PTSD samples and the same type of neuroimaging design looks promising. The work of building bridges between psychotherapy and neuroimaging must continue. Future multicentre studies addressing specific types of traumatic memories, and the age at which they were formed should be encouraged. The growing understanding of the neurobiology of emotionally-charged memories and their modulation may inform treatment of the victims of psychological trauma. Construction of coherent bridges between psychotherapy and neuroimaging must continue, in order that the two complementary and interdependent bodies of work can bring greater efficacy to the treatment of psychologically traumatized patients.

## 7. References

American Psychiatric Association. Diagnostic and statistical manual of mental disorders. 4th ed. Washington (DC): American Psychiatric Association; 1994.

Bados A, Toribio L, Garcia-Grau E: Traumatic events and tonic immobility. Span J Psychol, 11:516–521, 2008.

Blanchard EB, Hickling EJ, Vollmer AJ, Loos WR, Buckley TC, Jaccard JJ. Short-term follow-up of post-traumatic stress symptoms in motor vehicle accident victims. Behaviour Research and Therapy, 33:369-377, 1995.

Block J, Kremen AM. IQ and ego-resiliency: conceptual and empirical connections and separateness. Journal of Personality and Social Psychology, 70(2):349-61, 1996.

Bonanno GA. Loss, trauma, and human resilience: have we underestimated the human capacity to thrive after extremely aversive events? American Psychology, 59(1):20-8, 2004.

Boscarino JA: A prospective study of PTSD and early-age heart disease mortality among Vietnam veterans: implications for surveillance and prevention. Psychosom Med, 70:668–676, 2008.

Bovin MJ, Jager-Hyman S, Gold SD. Tonic immobility mediates the influence of peritraumatic fear and perceived inescapability on posttraumatic stress symptom severity among sexual assault survivors. J Trauma Stress, 21:402–409, 2008.

Bracha HS: Can premorbid episodes of diminished vagal tone be detected via histological markers in patients with PTSD? Int J Psychophysiol, 51:127–133, 2004.

Bremner JD, Vythilingam M, Vermetten E, et al.: Cortisol response to a cognitive stress challenge in posttraumatic stress disorder (PTSD) related to childhood abuse. Psychoneuroendocrinology, 28:733–750, 2003.

Bremner JD. Functional Neuroanatomical Correlates of Traumatic Stress Revisited 7 Years Later, This Time with Data. Psychopharmacology Bulletin, 37:6-27, 2003.

Bremner, J. D., Staib, L. H., Kaloupek, D. G., Southwick, S. M., Soufer, R., & Charney, D. S. Neural correlates of exposure to traumatic pictures and sounds in Vietnam combat veterans with and without posttraumatic stress disorder: A positron emission tomography study. Biological Psychiatry, 45(7): 806-816, 1999.

Bremner, J.D. Neuroimaging studies in posttraumatic stress disorder. Current Psychiatry Reports, Aug; 4(4):254-263, 2002.

Brenneis, C..B. Memory systems and the psychoanalytic retrieval of memories of trauma. Journal of American Psychoanalysis Association. 44(4):1165-1187, 1996.

Brewin CR: Risk factor effect sizes in PTSD: what this means for intervention. J Trauma Dissociation, 6:123–130, 2005.

Brewin, C.R.A cognitive neuroscience account of posttraumatic stress disorder and its treatment. Behaviour Research and Therapy, 39(4):373-393, 2001.

Brewin, C.R., Holmes, E.A. Psychological theories of posttraumatic stress disorder. Clinical Psychology Review, 23(3):339-376, 2003.

Britton J, Luan Phan K, Taylor S, Fig L, Liberzon I Corticolimbic Blood Flow in Posttraumatic Stress Disorder During Script-Driven Imagery. Biological Psychiatry, 57:832– 884, 2005.

Brody, A.L., Saxena, S., Schwartz, J..M., Stoessel, P.W., Maidment, K, Phelps, M.E., Baxter, L.R. Jr. Regional brain metabolic changes in patients with major depression treated with either paroxetine or interpersonal therapy. Archives of General Psychiatry, 58(7): 631-640, 2001.

Broman-Fulks JJ, Ruggiero KJ, Green BA, et al.: Taxometric investigation of PTSD: data from two nationally representative samples. Behav Ther, 37:364–380, 2006.

Bryant RA, Felmingham K, Kemp A, Das P, Hughes G, Peduto A, Williams L. Amygdala and ventral anterior cingulate activation predicts treatment response to cognitive behaviour therapy for post-traumatic stress disorder. Psychological Medicine; 38(4):555-561, 2008.

Bryant, R.A., Felmingham, K.L., Kemp, A.H., Barton, M., Peduto, A.S., Rennie, C., Gordon, E. and Williams, L.M. Neural Networks of Information Processing in Posttraumatic Stress Disorder: A Functional Magnetic Resonance Imaging Study. Biol Psychiatry, 58:111–118, 2005.

Bush, G., Lu, P., Posner, M.I. Cognitive and emotional influences in the anterior cingulate cortex. Trends Cognitive Science, 4:215-222, 2000.

Carlier IV, Gersons BP. Partial Posttraumatic Stress Disorder (PTSD): The Issue of Psychological Scars and the Ocurrence of PTSD Symptoms. The Journal of Nervous and Mental Disease, 183(2):107-109, 1995.

Charney DS. Psychobiological mechanisms of resilience and vulnerability: implications for successful adaptation to extreme stress. American Journal of Psychiatr, 161(2):195-216, 2004.

Chung YA, Kim SH, Chung SK, Chae JH, Yang DW, Sohn HS, Jeong J. Alterations in cerebral perfusion in posttraumatic stress disorder patients without re-exposure to accident-related stimuli. Clin Neurophysiol, 117(3):637-644, 2006.

Clark, C.R., McFarlane, A.C., Morris, P., Weber, D.L., Sonkilla, C., Shaw, M., Marcina,.J., Tochon-Danguy, and Egan, G.F. Cerebral Function in Posttraumatic Stress Disorder during Verbal Working Memory Updating: A Positron Emission Tomography Study. Biological Psychiatry, 53:474-481, 2003.

Corrigan, P.W., Watson, A.C. Findings from the National Comorbidity Survey on the frequency of violent behavior in individuals with psychiatric disorders. Psychiatry Res, 136(2-3):153-162, 2005.

Creamer, M., McFarlane, A. C. & Burgess, P. Psychopathology following trauma: the role of subjective experience. Journal of Affective Disorders, 86, 175-182, 2005.

Damasio, A.R. Remembering when. Scientific American, 287(3):66-73, 2002.

Dapretto M, Davies MS, Pfeifer JH, Scott AA, Sigman M, Bookheimer SY, Iacoboni M. Understanding emotions in others: mirror neuron dysfunction in children with autism spectrum disorders. Nat Neurosci, 9(1):28-30, 2006.

Delahanty DL, Raimonde AJ, Spoonster E. Initial posttraumatic urinary cortisol levels predict subsequent PTSD symptoms in motor vehicle accident victims. Biological Psychiatry, 48(9):940-7, 2000.

Dietrich, A. Functional neuroanatomy of altered states of consciousness: The transient hypofrontality hypothesis. Consciousness and Cognition, 12: 231–256, 2003.

Dolan, R.J. Emotion, cognition, and behavior. Science, 8;298(5596):1191-1194, 2002.

Ehlers, A., Hackmann, A., Steil, R., Clohessy, S., Wenninger, K., Winter, H. The nature of intrusive memories after trauma: the warning signal hypothesis. Behaviour Research and Therapy, 40(9):995-1002, 2002.

Erk, S., Kiefer, M., Grothe, J., Wunderlich, A.P., Spitzer, M., Walter, H. Emotional context modulates subsequent memory effect. Neuroimage 18(2):439-47, 2003.

Eugene, F., Levesque, J., Mensour, B., Leroux, J.M., Beaudoin, G., Bourgouin, P., Beauregard, M.The impact of individual differences on the neural circuitry underlying sadness. Neuroimage, 19(2 Pt 1):354-64, 2003.

Farrow TF, Zheng Y, Wilkinson ID, Spence SA, Deakin JF, Tarrier N, Griffiths PD, Woodruff PW.Quantifiable change in functional brain response to empathic and forgivability judgements with resolution of posttraumatic stress disorder. Psychiatry Research: Neuroimaging, 140; 45– 53, 2005.

Felmingham K, Kemp A, Williams L, Das P, Hughes G, Peduto A, Bryant R. Changes in anterior cingulate and amygdala after cognitive behavior therapy of posttraumatic stress disorder. Psychological Science, ;18(2):127-9, 2007.

Felmingham, K.L., Bryant, R.A., Gordon, E. Processing angry and neutral faces in post-traumatic stress disorder: an event-related potentials study. Neuroreport, 15:14(5):777-780, 2003.

Fivush, R. Children's recollections of traumatic and nontraumatic events. Development and Psychopathology, 10(4): 699-716, 1998.

Florian V, Mikulincer M, Taubman O. Does hardiness contribute to mental health during a stressful real-life situation? The roles of appraisal and coping. Journal of Personality and Social Psychology, 68(4):687-95, 1995.

Foa, E. B., Keane, T. M., Friedman, M. J. Effective treatments for PTSD: Practice guidelines from the International Society for Traumatic Stress Studies. New York, Guilford Press, 2000.

Freud, S. Studies on Hysteria [with Breuer, J]. In The Standard Edition of the Complete Works of Sigmund Freud, Vol. 2 J. Strachy, Ed. and Trans.: Hogarth. London, P189-221, 1895.

Furmark, T., Tillfors, M., Marteinsdottir, I., Fischer, H., Pissiota, A., Langstrom, B., Fredrikson, M. Common changes in cerebral blood flow in patients with social phobia treated with citalopram or cognitive-behavioral therapy. Archives of General Psychiatry, 59(5):425-433, 2002.

Gallese V, Goldman A. Mirror neurons and the simulation theory of mind-reading. Trends Cogn Sci 12:493–501, 1998.

Gallese V. Intentional attunement: a neurophysiological perspective on social cognition and its disruption in autism. Brain Res, 24;1079(1):15-24, 2006.

Gilbertson, M.W., Shenton, M.E., Ciszewski, A., Kasai, K., Lasko, N.B, Orr, S.P., Pitman, R.K. Smaller hippocampal volume predicts pathologic vulnerability to psychological trauma. Nature Neuroscience, 5(11):1242-1247, 2002.

Gilboa A, Shalev AY, Laor L, Lester H, Louzoun Y, Chisin R, Bonne O. Functional Connectivity Of The Prefrontal Cortex And The Amygdala In Posttraumatic Stress Disorder. Biological Psychiatry, 55:263–272, 2004.

Griffin MG, Resick PA, Mechanic MB. Objective assessment of peritraumatic dissociation: psychophysiological indicators. Am J Psychiatry, 154(8):1081-8, 1997.

Griffing S, Lewis CS, Chu M, et al.: Exposure to interpersonal violence as a predictor of PTSD symptomatology in domestic violence survivors. J Interpers Violence, 21:936–954, 2006.

Grillon, C., Southwick, S.M., Charney, D.S. The psychobiological basis of posttraumatic stress disorder. Molecular Psychiatry, 1:278-297, 1996.

Grossman R, Yehuda R, New A, Schmeidler J, Silverman J, Mitropoulou V, Sta Maria N, Golier J, Siever L. Dexamethasone suppression test findings in subjects with personality disorders: associations with posttraumatic stress disorder and major depression. American Journal of Psychiatry, 160(7):1291-8, 2003.

Heidt JM, Marx BP, Forsyth JP: Tonic immobility and childhood sexual abuse: a preliminary report evaluating the sequela of rape-induced paralysis. Behav Res Ther, 43:1157–1171, 2005.

Hellawell, S.J., Brewin, C.R. A comparison of flashbacks and ordinary autobiographical memories of trauma: cognitive resources and behavioural observations. Behaviour Research and Therapy, 40(10):1143-1156, 2002.

Horowitz M, Wilner N, Alvarez W: Impact of Event Scale: a measure of subjective stress. Psychosom Med, 41: 209–218, 1979.

Horowitz, M.J. Image formation: clinical observations and a cognitive model. In: Sheehan P, editor. The function and nature of imagery .New York: Academic Press. p281-309, 1972.

Hull, A.M. Neuroimaging findings in post-traumatic stress disorder. Systematic review. British Journal of Psychiatry, 181:102-10, 2002.

Hurley, S. & Chater, N. Perspectives on Imitation: From Neuroscience to Social Science, Volume 2: Imitation, Human Development, and Culture. Cambridge, MA: The MIT Press, 2005.

Iacoboni M, Molnar-Szakacs I, Gallese V, Buccino G, Mazziotta JC. Grasping the Intentions of Others with One's Own Mirror Neuron System. PLoS Biol 3(3): e79, 2005.

Jones, E., Vermaas, R.H., McCartney, H., Beech, C., Palmer, I., Hyams, K., Wessely, S. Flashbacks and post-traumatic stress disorder: the genesis of a 20th-century diagnosis. British Journal of Psychiatry, 182:158-163, 2003.

Kaplow JB, Dodge KA, Amaya-Jackson L, Saxe GN: Pathways to PTSD, part II: sexually abused children. Am J Psychiatry, 162:1305–1310, 2005.

Karl, A., Malta, L., Maercker, L. Meta-analytic review of event related potential studies in post-traumatic stress disorder. Biological Psychology, 71: 123-147, 2006.

Kaufman ML, Kimble MO, Kaloupek DG, et al.: Peritraumatic dissociation and physiological response to trauma-relevant stimuli in Vietnam combat veterans with posttraumatic stress disorder. J Nerv Ment Dis, 190:167–174, 2002.

Keane TM, Marshall AD, Taft CT: Posttraumatic stress disorder: etiology, epidemiology, and treatment outcome. Annu Rev Clin Psychol, 2:161–197, 2006.

Kessler RC, Sonnega A, Bromet E, Hughes M, Nelson CB. Posttraumatic stress disorder in the National Comorbidity Survey. Archives of General Psychiatry, 52:1048–60, 1995.

Lamprecht, F., Sack, M. Posttraumatic stress disorder revisited. Psychosomatic Medicine, 64(2):222-237, 2002.

Lanius RA, Bluhm R, Lanius U, Pain C. A review of neuroimaging studies in PTSD: heterogeneity of response to symptom provocation. J Psychiatr Res, 40(8):709-29, 2006.

Lanius RA, Williamson PC, Boksman K, Densmore M, Gupta M, Neufeld RW, Gati JS, Menon RS. Brain activation during script-driven imagery induced dissociative responses in PTSD: a functional magnetic resonance imaging investigation. Biol Psychiatry, 15;52(4):305-11, 2002.

Lanius RA, Williamson PC, Densmore M, Boksman K, Gupta MA, Neufeld RW, Gati JS, Menon RS. Neural correlates of traumatic memories in posttraumatic stress disorder: a functional MRI investigation. American Journal of Psychiatry, 158(11):1920-2, 2001.

Lanius RA, Williamson PC, Densmore M, Boksman K, Neufeld RW, Gati JS, Menon RS.The nature of traumatic memories: a 4-T FMRI functional connectivity analysis. American Journal of Psychiatry, 161(1):36-44, 2004.

Lanius, R.A., Hopper, J.W. & Menon, R.S. Individual differences in a husband and wife who developed PTSD after a motor vehicle accident: a functional MRI case study. American Journal of Psychiatry, 160 (4): 667-669, 2003.

Leskin GA, Woodward SH, Young HE, Sheikh JI: Effects of comorbid diagnoses on sleep disturbance in PTSD. J Psychiatr Res, 36:449–452, 2002.

Leskin, G.A., Kaloupek, D.G., Keane, T.M. Treatment for traumatic memories: review and recommendations. Clinical Psychology Review, 18(8):983-1001, 1998.

Levin, P., Lazrove, S., van der Kolk, B. What psychological testing and neuroimaging tells us about the treatment of Posttraumatic Stress Disorder by Eye Movement Desensitization and Reprocessing. Journal of Anxiety Disorder, 13 (1-2): 159-172, 1999.

Lewis, S. J. Do one-shot preventive interventions for PTSD work? A systematic research synthesis of psychological debriefings. Aggression and Violent Behavior, 8:329–343, 2003.

Liberzon, I., Taylor, S.F., Amdur, T.D., Chamberlain, K.R., Minoshima, S., Koeppe, R.A., Fig, L.M. Brain activation in PTSD in response to trauma-related stimuli. Biological Psychiatry, 45 (7): 817-826, 1999.

Littrell, J. Is the reexperience of painful emotion therapeutic? Clinical Psychology Review, 8(1):71-102, 1998.

Loftus, E.F., Polage, D.C. Repressed memories. When are they real? How are they false? Psychiatric Clinics of North America, 22(1):61-70, 1999.

Marks I, Lovell K, Noshirvani H, Livanou M, Thrasher S. Treatment of posttraumatic stress disorder by exposure and/or cognitive restructuring: A controlled study, Archives of General Psychiatry, 55:317-325, 1998.

McDonald, R.J., Devan, B.D., Hong, N.S. Multiple memory systems: the power of interactions. Neurobiology Learning and Memory, 82(3):333-346, 2004.

McFarlane AC, Yehuda R, Clark CR. Biologic models of traumatic memories and post-traumatic stress disorder. The role of neural networks. Psychiatric clinics of North America, 25(2):253-70, 2002.

McFarlane, A. C. & Yehuda, R. Resilience, vulnerability and the course of posttraumatic reactions. In Van der Kolk, B. A., McFarlane, A. C., & Weisaeth, L., (ed.) Traumatic Stress: The Effects of Overwhelming Experience on Mind, Body and Society. New York: Guilford, 1996.

McFarlane, A.C. The prevalence and longitudinal course of PTSD: Implications for the Neurobiological Models of PTSD. In R. Yehuda & A. C. McFarlane (Eds.), Psychobiology of posttraumatic stress disorder. New York: Annals of the New York Academy of Sciences, 821:10-23, 1997.

McNally, R.J. Progress and controversy in the study of posttraumatic stress disorder. Annual Review of Psychology, 54(1):229-252, 2003.

Meltzoff, A. N. Imitation and other minds: The "Like Me" hypothesis. In S. Hurley and N. Chater (Eds.), Perspectives on Imitation: From Neuroscience to Social Science (Vol. 2 pp. 55-77) Cambridge, MA: MIT Press, 2005.

Moscovitch, M., Rosenbaum, S., Gilboa, A., Addis, D.R., Westmacott, R., Grady, C., McAndrews, M.P., Levine, B., Black, S., Winocur, G. and Nadel, L. Functional neuroanatomy of remote episodic, semantic and spatial memory: a unified account based on multiple trace theory. J Anat, 207(1): 35–66, 2005.

Newport DJ, Heim C, Bonsall R, Miller AH, Nemeroff CB. Pituitary-adrenal responses to standard and low-dose dexamethasone suppression tests in adult survivors of child abuse. Biological Psychiatry, 55(1):10-20, 2004.

Nutt, J.D., Malizia, A.L. Structural and functional brain changes in posttraumatic stress disorder. Journal of Clinical Psychiatry, 65 Suppl 1. 11-17, 2004.

Oberman LM, Hubbard EM, McCleery JP, Altschuler EL, Ramachandran VS, Pineda JA. EEG evidence for mirror neuron dysfunction in autism spectrum disorders. Brain Res Cogn Brain Res, 24(2):190-8, 2005.

Palmer I: No pain, no gain. Part II. A personal conceptualisation of PTSD and post traumatic psychological difficulties. J R Army Med Corps, 150:67–71, 2004.

Paquette, V., Levesque, J., Mensour, B., Leroux, J.M., Beaudoin, G., Bourgouin, P., Beauregard, M. "Change the mind and you change the brain": effects of cognitive-behavioral therapy on the neural correlates of spider phobia. Neuroimage, 18(2):401-409, 2003.

Peace, K., Porter, S. A longitudinal investigation of the reliability of memories for trauma and other emotional experiences. Applied Cognitive Psychology, 54(1):211-219, 2004.

Peres J, Mercante J, Nasello AG: Psychological dynamics affecting traumatic memories: implications in psychotherapy. Psychol Psychother, 78(4):431–447, 2005.

Peres JF, McFarlane A, Nasello AG, Moores KA. Traumatic memories: bridging the gap between functional neuroimaging and psychotherapy. Australian New Zealand Journal of Psychiatry, 42(6):478-88, 2008.

Peres JF, Newberg AB, Mercante JP, Simão M, Albuquerque VE, Peres MJ, Nasello AG. Cerebral blood flow changes during retrieval of traumatic memories before and after psychotherapy: a SPECT study. Psychological Medicine, 37(10):1481-91, 2007.

Peres JFP, Foester B, Santana LG, Fereira MD, Nasello AG, Savoia M, Moreira-Almeida A, Lederman H. Police officers under attack: Resilience implications of an fMRI study. J Psychiatr Res, 45(6):727-34, 2011.

Peres, J. F. P.; Nasello, A. G. Psychotherapy and neuroscience: toward closer integration. International Journal of Psychology, 43(6):943-957, 2008.

Peres, J.F.P. and Nasello, A.G. Posttraumatic stress disorder neuroimaging findings and their clinical implications. Rev Psiquiatr Clin, 32, (4): 189-201, 2005.

Peres, J.F.P.; Gonçalves, A.L.; Peres, M.F. Psychological trauma in chronic pain: implications of PTSD for fibromyalgia and headache disorders. Curr Pain Headache Rep, 13(5):350-357, 2009.

Peres, JFP, Moreira-Almeida, A, Nasello, AG, Koenig, HG. Spirituality and Resilience in Trauma Victims. Journal of Religion and Health, 46:343-50, 2007.

Phelps EA, Delgado MR, Nearing KI, LeDoux JE. Extinction learning in humans: role of the amygdala and vmPFC. Neuron, 43(6):897-905, 2004.

Phillips, M.L., Young, A.W., Senior, C., Brammer, M., Andrew, C., Calder, A.J., Bullmore, E.T., Perrett, D.I., Rowland, D., Williams, S.C., Gray, J.A., David, A.S. A specific neural substrate for perceiving facial expressions of disgust. Nature, 2:389 (6650):495-498, 1997.

Pissiota, A., Frans, O., Fernandez, M., von Knorring, L., Fischer, H., Fredickson, M. Neurofunctional correlates of posttraumatic stress disorder: a PET symptom provocation study. European Archives Psychiatry Clinical Neuroscience, 252 (2): 68-75, 2002.

Pitman, R.K., Shin, L.M., Rauch, S.L. Investigating the pathogenesis of posttraumatic stress disorder with neuroimaging. Journal of Clinical Psychiatry, 62 Suppl 17:47-54, 2001.

Poldrack, R.A., Packard, M.G. Competition among multiple memory systems: converging evidence from animal and human brain studies. Neuropsychologia, 41(3):245-251, 2003.

Protopopescu, X., Pan, H., Tuescher, O., Cloitre, M., Goldstein, M., Engelien, W., Epstein, J., Yang, Y., Gorman, J., LeDoux, J., Silbersweig, D., Stern, E. Differential time courses and specificity of amygdala activity in posttraumatic stress disorder subjects and normal control subjects. Biol Psychiatry, 1:57(5):464-473, 2005.

Rauch, S.L. Symptom provocation study of Post-traumatic Stress Disorder using Positron Emission Tomography and Script-driven imagery. Archives of General Psychiatry, 53(5):380-387, 1996.

Rauch, S.L., Whalen, P.J., Shin, L.M., McInerney ,S.C., Macklin, M.L., Lasko, N.B., Orr, S.P., Pitman, R.K. Exaggerated amygdala response to masked facial stimuli in posttraumatic stress disorder: a functional MRI study. Biological Psychiatry, 47 (9): 796-776, 2000.

Rizzolatti G, Craighero L. The mirror-neuron system. Annu Rev Neurosci, 27:169-92, 2004.

Rizzolatti G, Fadiga L, Gallese V, Fogassi L. Premotor cortex and the recognition of motor actions. Brain Res Cogn Brain Res, 3(2):131-41, 1996.

Rizzolatti G, Fogassi L, Gallese V. Cortical mechanisms subserving object grasping and action recognition: A new view on the cortical motor functions. In: Gazzaniga MS, editor. The new cognitive neurosciences, 2nd edition, p. 539–52. Cambridge, MA: MIT Press, 2000.

Rizzolatti G, Fogassi L, Gallese V. Neurophysiological mechanisms underlying the understanding and imitation of action. Nat Rev Neurosci, 2:661–70, 2001.

Roffman, J.L., Marci, C.D., Glick, D.M., Dougherty, D.D., Rauch, S.L. Neuroimaging and the functional neuroanatomy of psychotherapy. Psychological Medicine, 35(10):1385-1398, 2005.

Rybakowski, J. Neurobiological aspects of psychotherapy theory and practice Psychiatria Polska, 36(1):5-15, 2002.

Saxe GN, Stoddard F, Hall E, et al.: Pathways to PTSD, part I: children with burns. Am J Psychiatry, 162:1299–1304, 2005.

Schacter, D.L., Buckner, R.L. On the relations among priming, conscious recollection, and intentional retrieval: evidence from neuroimaging research. Neurobiology Learning and Memory, 70(1-2):284-303, 1998.

Schwartz, J.M., Stoessel, P.W., Baxter, L.R. Jr., Martin, K..M., Phelps, M.E. Systematic changes in cerebral glucose metabolic rate after successful behavior modification treatment of obsessive-compulsive disorder. Archives of General Psychiatry, 53(2):109-113, 1996.

Semple, W.E., Goyer, P., McCormick, R., Morris, E., Compton, B., Muswick, G. Preliminary report: brain blood flow using PET in patients with posttraumatic stress disorder and substance-abuse histories. Biol Psychiatry, 34(1-2):115-118, 1993.

Shalev AY. Acute stress reactions in adults. Biol Psychiatry, 1;51(7):532-543, 2002.

Shalev, A.Y., Peri, T., Brandes, D., Freedman, S., Orr, S.P., Pitman, R.K. Auditory startle response in trauma survivors with posttraumatic stress disorder: a prospective study. Am J Psychiatry, 157(2):255-261, 2000.

Shin LM, Orr SP, Carson MA, et al.: Regional cerebral blood flow in the amygdala and medial prefrontal cortex during traumatic imagery in male and female Vietnam veterans with PTSD. Arch Gen Psychiatry, 61:168–176, 2004.

Shin LM, Rauch SL, Pitman RK. Amygdala, medial prefrontal cortex, and hippocampal function in PTSD. Annals of the New York Academy of Sciences, 1071:67-79, 2006.

Shin LM, Wright CI, Cannistraro PA, Wedig MM, McMullin K, Martis B. A Functional Magnetic Resonance Imaging Study Of Amygdala And Medial Prefrontal Cortex Responsesto Overtly Presented Fearful Faces In Posttraumatic Stressdisorder. Archives of General Psychiatry, 62:273–281, 2005.

Shin, L.M., McNally, R.J., Kosslyn, S.M., Thompson, W.L., Rauch, S.L., Alpert, N.M., Metzger, L.J., Lasko, N.B., Orr, S.P., Pitman, R.K. Regional cerebral blood flow during script-driven imagery in childhood sexual abuse-related PTSD: A PET investigation. American Journal of Psychiatry, 156(4):575-584, 1999.

Shin, L.M., Whalen, P.J., Pitman, R.K., Bush, G., Macklin, M.L., Lasko, N.B., Orr, S.P., McInerney, S.C., Rauch, S.L. An fMRI study of anterior cingulate function in posttraumatic stress disorder. Biological Psychiatry, 50 (12):932-942, 2001.

Simeon D, Yehuda R, Knutelska M, Schmeidler J. Dissociation versus posttraumatic stress: cortisol and physiological correlates in adults highly exposed to the World Trade Center attack on 9/11. Psychiatry Res, 15;161(3):325-9, 2008.

Singer T, Seymour B, O'Doherty J, Kaube H, Dolan RJ, Frith CD. Empathy for pain involves the affective but not sensory components of pain. Science, 303:1157–62, 2004.

Southwick SM, Paige S, Morgan CA 3rd, et al.: Neurotransmitter alterations in PTSD: catecholamines and serotonin. Semin Clin Neuropsychiatry, 4:242–248, 1999.

Stein MB, Walker JR, Hazen AL, Forde DR. Full and partial posttraumatic stress disorder: findings from a community survey. Am J Psychiatry, 154(8):1114-9, 1997.

The expert consensus guideline series. Treatment of posttraumatic stress disorder. The Expert Consensus Panels for PTSD. J Clin Psychiatry, 60(Suppl 16):3–76, 1999.

Tomasello M, Savage-Rumbaugh S, Kruger AC. Imitative learning of actions on objects by children, chimpanzees, and enculturated chimpanzees. Child Dev, 64(6):1688-705, 1993.

van der Hart O, Brown P, Turco RN: Hypnotherapy for traumatic grief: janetian and modern approaches integrated. Am J Clin Hypn, 32:263–271, 1990.

van der Kolk BA: Clinical implications of neuroscience research in PTSD. Ann N Y Acad Sci, 1071:277–293, 2006.

van Der Kolk, B.A. The Psychobiology of Traumatic Memory: Clinical Implications of Neuroimaging Studies. Annals of the New York Academy of Sciences, 821: 98-113, 1997.

Vederhus, J.K., Kristensen, O. High effectiveness of self-help programs after drug addiction therapy. BMC Psychiatry, 23;6:35, 2006.

Verfaellie, M., Keane, M..M. The neural basis of aware and unaware forms of memory. Seminars in Neurology, 17(2):153-161, 1997.

Vermetten, E., Bremner, J.D. Functional brain imaging and the induction of traumatic recall: a cross-correlational review between neuroimaging and hypnosis. International Journal of Clinical and Experimental Hypnosis, 52(3):280-312, 2004.

Vieweg WV, Julius DA, Fernandez A, Beatty-Brooks M, Hettema JM, Pandurangi AK. Posttraumatic stress disorder: clinical features, pathophysiology, and treatment. American Journal of Medicine, 119(5):383-90, 2006.

Weber, D.L., Clark, C.R., McFarlane, A.C., Moores, K.A., Morris, P., Egan, G.F. Abnormal frontal and parietal activity during working memory updating in post-traumatic stress disorder. Psychiatry Research: Neuroimaging, 140: 27-44, 2005.

Weiss DS, Marmar CR, Schlenger WE, Fairbank JA, Jordan BK, Hough RL, Kulka RA. The prevalence of lifetime and partial stress disorder in Vietnam Theater veterans. Journal of Traumatic Stress, 5(3):365-376, 1992.

Wicker B, Keysers C, Plailly J, Royet JP, Gallese V, Rizzolatti G. Both of us disgusted in My insula: the common neural basis of seeing and feeling disgust. Neuron, 30;40(3):655-64, 2003.

Williams JH, Waiter GD, Gilchrist A, Perrett DI, Murray AD, Whiten A. Neural mechanisms of imitation and 'mirror neuron' functioning in autistic spectrum disorder. Neuropsychologia, 44(4):610-21, 2006.

Williams, L.M. Recovered memories of abuse in women with documented child sexual victimization histories. Journal of Traumatic Stress, 8: 649-676, 1995.

Williams, L.M., Kemp, A.H., Felmingham, K., Barton, M., Olivieri, G., Peduto, A., Gordon, E., Bryant, R. Trauma modulates amygdala and medial prefrontal response to consciously attended fear. NeuroImage, 29: 347-357, 2005.

Wood JN, Grafman J. Human prefrontal cortex: processing and representational perspectives. Nature Review Neuroscience, 4(2):139-47, 2003.

Yehuda R, Boisoneau D, Lowy MT, Giller EL Jr. Dose-response changes in plasma cortisol and lymphocyte glucocorticoid receptors following dexamethasone administration in combat veterans with and without posttraumatic stress disorder. Archives of General Psychiatry, 52(7):583-93, 1995.

Yehuda R, McFarlane AC, Shalev AY. Predicting the development of posttraumatic stress disorder from the acute response to a traumatic event. Biol Psychiatry, 44(12):1305-13, 1998.

Zubieta, J.K., Chinitz, J.A., Lombardi, U., Fig, L.M., Cameron, O.G., Liberzon, I. Medial frontal cortex involvement in PTSD symptoms: a SPECT study. Journal of Psychiatry Research, 33(3):259-264, 1999.